PROCEDURES

KINN'S

THE ADMINISTRATIVE MEDICAL ASSISTANT

AN APPLIED LEARNING APPROACH

KINN'S
THE ADMINISTRATIVE
MEDICAL ASSISTANT

AN APPLIED LEARNING APPROACH

13TH EDITION

Deborah Proctor, EdD, RN
Adjunct Faculty Member
Butler County Community College
Butler, Pennsylvania

Brigitte Niedzwiecki RN, MSN, RMA
Medical Assistant Program Director & Instructor
Chippewa Valley Technical College
Eau Claire, WI

Julie Pepper, BS, CMA (AAMA)
Medical Assistant Instructor
Chippewa Valley Technical College
Eau Claire, Wisconsin

Payel Bhattacharya Madero, MBA, RHIT
Adjunct Faculty
Cal State Fullerton University
Fullerton, California

ELSEVIER

ELSEVIER

3251 Riverport Lane
St. Louis, Missouri 63043

Notices

International Standard Book Number: 978-0-323-39672-1

Executive Content Strategist: Jennifer Janson
Content Development Manager: Ellen Wurm-Cutter
Senior Content Development Specialist: Becky Leenhouts
Publishing Services Manager: Julie Eddy
Senior Project Manager: Richard Barber
Design Direction: Paula Catalano

Printed in Canada

Last digit is the print number: 9 8 7 6 5 4 3 2

Working together
to grow libraries in
developing countries

www.elsevier.com • www.bookaid.org

PREFACE

Medical assisting as a profession has changed dramatically since *The Office Assistant in Medical and Dental Practice,* by Portia Frederick and Carol Towner, was first published in 1956. Each subsequent edition of this textbook has reflected the age in which it was published. Now, *Kinn's The Medical Assistant: An Applied Learning Approach,* thirteenth edition, in its 60th year of publication, continues to represent a long-standing commitment to high-quality medical assisting education with its engaging, straightforward writing style and demonstrated positive outcomes. Hundreds of instructors in classrooms across the country have used this text to teach thousands of students over the years. Many of these students have gone on to teach students of their own with this very same trusted resource. To continue the use and growth of this text and its features, the thirteenth edition continues to offer the most comprehensive, up-to-date, and innovative approach to teaching this subject today.

This textbook has endured throughout the years because it has been able to keep pace with an ever-changing profession while producing students who are well trained and qualified to enter medical practices across the country. This dependability is the reason the market continues to rely on this text, edition after edition. Underlying this dependability is a foundation of pedagogic features that has stood the test of time and that has been expanded and improved upon yet again in this latest edition. Such features include the following:

- An easy-to-read, highly interactive writing style that engages students through practical applications of medical assistant competencies.
- An emphasis on skill development, with procedural steps outlining each skill, supported by rationales that provide meaning to each step.
- A pedagogic framework based on the use of learning objectives, vocabulary terms, and supportive student supplements.
- A package of supportive materials to accommodate a wide variety of student learning types and instructor teaching styles.

NEW TO THIS EDITION

- **Updated Art Program.** The artwork throughout has been updated and modernized, providing a more attractive textbook for student use. Many new photographs and line drawings throughout support the revised content more effectively and are more relevant to the actual healthcare setting. New images show up-to-date equipment, provide more disease examples, and better illustrate key procedural steps.

- **New chapter on Competency-Based Education for Medical Assisting.** The emphasis of competency mastery is high to meet accreditation standards. This chapter helps set the stage for medical assisting students to understand their programming and how the road to mastery will affect their ability to attain a job.
- **New Chapter on The Health Record.** The manner in which the medical record is maintained in a medical office has changed dramatically with the move to the EHR. This chapter reviews how the medical assistant maintains and interacts with the medical record.
- **Learning Objectives are listed in the same order as the flow of content.** The learning objectives are tied to curriculum competencies. This feature makes it easy to see where the learning objectives are covered to aid in review of the material and measurement of competency coverage.
- **Procedures are integrated into the TOC.** Provides a quick reference to where the procedures will be covered and in what order.
- **Professional Behaviors boxes.** The medical assistant must develop the ability to interact professionally with patients, families, co-workers, and other members of the healthcare team. These boxes provide tips on professional behavior that are specific to each chapter's content.

EVOLVE

The Evolve site features a variety of student resources, including Chapter Review Quizzes, new Procedure Videos, Medical Terminology Audio Glossary, practice CMA and RMA exams, and much more! The instructors' Evolve Resources site consists of TEACH Instructor Resources, including Lesson Plans, PowerPoint Presentations, Answer Keys for Chapter Review Quizzes, and a retooled Test Bank with more than 2000 questions.

STUDY GUIDE AND PROCEDURE CHECKLIST MANUAL

The Study Guide provides students with the opportunity to review and build on information they have learned in the text through vocabulary reviews, case studies, workplace applications, and more. The updated Procedure Checklists include CAAHEP and ABHES competencies that can be traced to the online correlation grid.

FEATURES

A Scenario is presented at the beginning of each chapter so the student can envision a real-world situation when reading the chapter content.

Scenario questions provide a way for students to apply the concepts they are learning and think about decisions they would make in real situations.

Learning Objectives emphasize the cognitive and performance objectives presented in the chapter.

Each chapter contains a vocabulary list with definitions so students can first familiarize themselves with the important terms associated with each chapter.

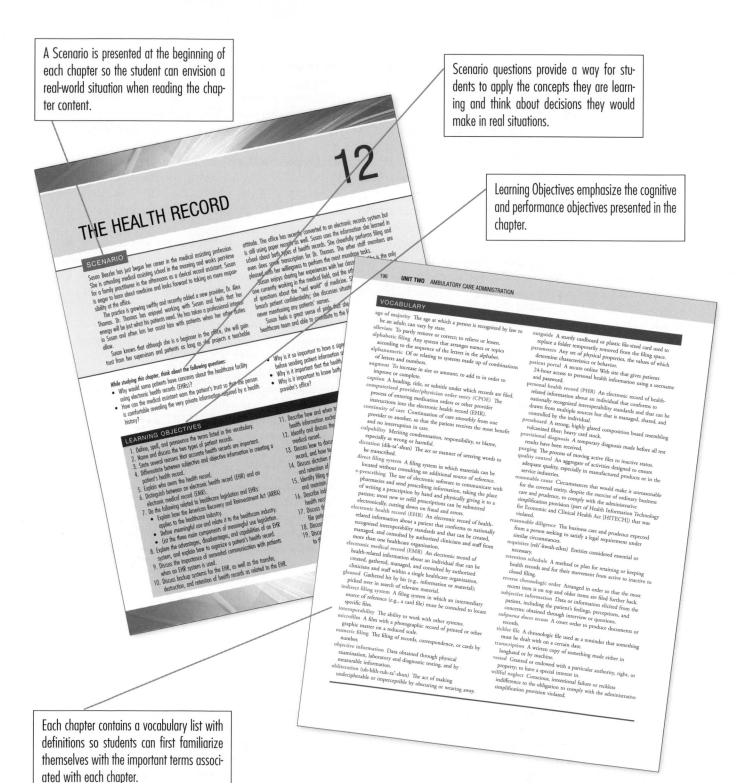

386 **UNIT FIVE** FUNDAMENTALS OF CLINICAL MEDICAL ASSISTING

Pathogens Standard. Healthcare facilities must establish specific policies and procedures for the management of an exposure incident (e.g., accidental needlestick) and the exposed employee.

Compliance Guidelines

Because the Bloodborne Pathogens Standard is written to cover employees working in all health fields, only some of the regulations apply to the ambulatory care setting. Safety and infection control fundamentals go beyond hand washing and knowledge of the disease cycle. The information is presented here as it applies to the medical assisting profession.

Barrier Protection

Medical assistants routinely should use appropriate barrier precautions when contact with blood or other body fluids is expected. Barrier protection, or PPE, includes specialized clothing or equipment that prevents the healthcare worker from coming in contact with blood or other potentially infectious material, thereby preventing or minimizing the entry of infectious material into the body. Barrier devices include disposable gloves, face masks, face shields, protective glasses, shoe covers, laboratory coats, barrier gowns, mouthpieces, and resuscitation bags (Figure 20-5).

Since the implementation of Standard Precautions, the use of disposable examination gloves is required in healthcare facilities. Because of the frequent allergic reactions associated with latex products, facilities now use nonlatex gloves. If the facility where you work still uses latex gloves, signs of an allergic reaction include localized **urticaria**, dermatitis, conjunctivitis, and **rhinitis**. Hypersensitive reactions can be systemic, producing asthma symptoms or **anaphylaxis**. If a healthcare worker or a patient shows signs of sensitivity to latex, the healthcare provider is required to provide products made of nonallergenic materials. Gloves must be worn if the medical assistant is at all likely to be involved in any of the following activities (Procedure 20-1):

- Touching a patient's blood, body fluids, mucous membranes, or skin that is not intact.

- Handling items and surfaces contaminated with blood and body fluids.
- Performing venipuncture, finger sticks, injections, and other vascular procedures.
- Assisting with any surgical procedure. If a glove is torn during the procedure, the glove should be removed, the hands washed carefully, and a new glove put on as soon as possible.
- Handling, processing, and disposing of all specimens of blood and body fluids.
- Cleaning and decontaminating spills of blood or other body fluids.

The same pair of gloves cannot be worn for the care of more than one patient; new disposable gloves must be used for each individual patient.

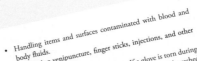

Safety Alert

Protective equipment contaminated with body fluids of any kind must be removed and placed in a designated area or biohazard container. The hands or any other exposed areas must be washed or flushed as soon as possible. Face shields that cover the mouth, nose, and eyes must be worn whenever splashes, sprays, or droplets are possible. Utility gloves may be reused if they are intact (i.e., have no cracks, tears, or punctures). All PPE must be removed before the medical assistant leaves the medical facility (Figure 20-6).

CRITICAL THINKING APPLICATION 20-5

Rosa is caring for an injured 3-year-old child with an open wound on his right knee. She puts on disposable gloves to clean the wound, and the mother demands to know why. How can she explain her actions?

Environmental Protection

Environmental protection refers to minimizing the risk of occupational injury by isolating or removing any physical or mechanical health hazard in the medical workplace. Every medical assistant must adhere to these safety rules.

- Read warning labels on biohazard containers and equipment.
- Minimize splashing or spraying of potentially infectious materials. Blood that splatters onto open areas of the skin or mucous membranes is a proven mode of HBV transmission.
- Bandage any breaks or lesions on your hands before gloving.
- If any body surface is exposed to potentially infectious material, scrub the area with antimicrobial soap and warm, running water as soon as possible after the exposure.
- If your eyes come in contact with body fluids, continuously flush them with water as soon as possible for a minimum of 15 minutes using an eye wash unit. A stationary unit connected to warm, running water is the best method for properly flushing potentially infectious material out of the eyes (Figure 20-7 and Procedure 20-2).
- Contaminated needles and other sharps should never be recapped, bent, broken, or resheathed; needle units must have protective safety devices to cover the contaminated needle after injection.

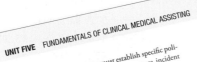

FIGURE 20-5 Personal protective equipment.

Critical Thinking Application boxes prompt students to apply what they have learned as they read and study the chapter.

Safety Alert boxes alert students to important safety information and reinforce the importance of safety in the profession.

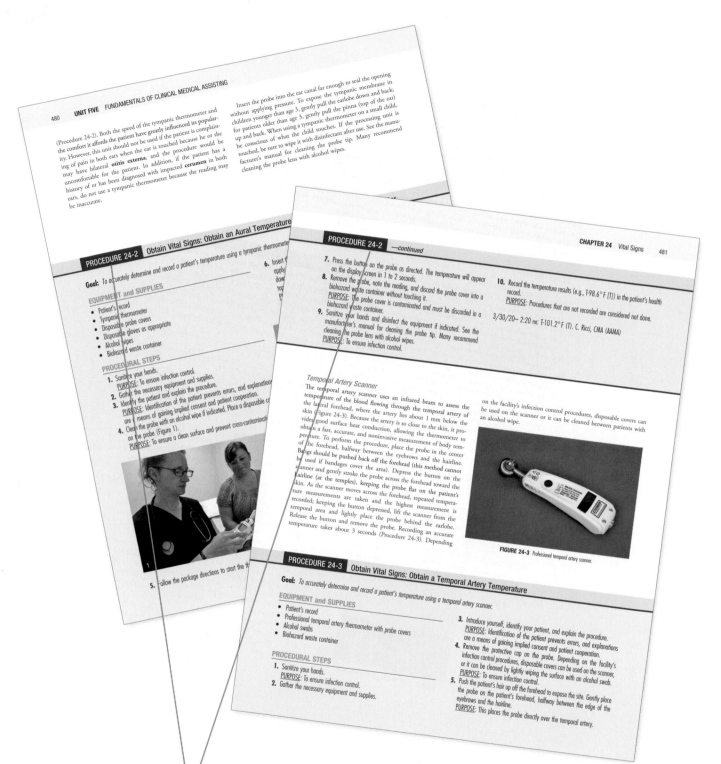

480   **UNIT FIVE**   FUNDAMENTALS OF CLINICAL MEDICAL ASSISTING

(Procedure 24-2). Both the speed of the tympanic thermometer and the comfort it affords the patient have greatly influenced its popularity. However, this unit should not be used if the patient is complaining of pain in both ears when the ear is touched because he or she may have bilateral **otitis externa**, and the procedure would be uncomfortable for the patient. In addition, if the patient has a history of or has been diagnosed with impacted **cerumen** in both ears, do not use a tympanic thermometer because the reading may be inaccurate.

Insert the probe into the ear canal far enough to seal the opening, without applying pressure. To expose the tympanic membrane in children younger than age 3, gently pull the earlobe down and back; for patients older than age 3, gently pull the pinna (top of the ear) up and back. When using a tympanic thermometer on a small child, be conscious of what the child touches. If the processing unit is touched, be sure to wipe it with disinfectant after use. See the manufacturer's manual for cleaning the probe tip. Many recommend cleaning the probe lens with alcohol wipes.

PROCEDURE 24-2   Obtain Vital Signs: Obtain an Aural Temperature

Goal: To accurately determine and record a patient's temperature using a tympanic thermometer.

EQUIPMENT and SUPPLIES

- Patient's record
- Tympanic thermometer
- Disposable probe covers
- Disposable gloves as appropriate
- Alcohol wipes
- Biohazard waste container

PROCEDURAL STEPS

1. Sanitize your hands.
   PURPOSE: To ensure infection control.
2. Gather the necessary equipment and supplies.
3. Identify the patient and explain the procedure.
   PURPOSE: Identification of the patient prevents errors, and explanations are a means of gaining implied consent and patient cooperation. Place a disposable cover
4. Clean the probe with an alcohol wipe if indicated. Place a disposable cover on the probe (Figure 1).
   PURPOSE: To ensure a clean surface and prevent cross-contamination.

6. Insert the apply down top P

5. Follow the package directions to start the th

PROCEDURE 24-2   —continued

7. Press the button on the probe as directed. The temperature will appear on the display screen in 1 to 2 seconds.
8. Remove the probe, note the reading, and discard the probe cover into a biohazard waste container without touching it.
   PURPOSE: The probe cover is contaminated and must be discarded in a biohazard waste container.
9. Sanitize your hands and disinfect the equipment if indicated. See the manufacturer's manual for cleaning the probe tip. Many recommend cleaning the probe lens with alcohol wipes.
   PURPOSE: To ensure infection control.

CHAPTER 24   Vital Signs   481

10. Record the temperature results (e.g., T-98.6° F [T]) in the patient's health record.
    PURPOSE: Procedures that are not recorded are considered not done.

3/30/20— 2:20 PM: T-101.2° F (T). C. Ricci, CMA (AAMA)

Temporal Artery Scanner

The temporal artery scanner uses an infrared beam to assess the temperature of the blood flowing through the temporal artery of the lateral forehead, where the artery lies about 1 mm below the skin (Figure 24-3). Because the artery is so close to the skin, it provides good surface heat conduction, allowing the thermometer to obtain a fast, accurate, and noninvasive measurement of body temperature. To perform the procedure, place the probe in the center of the forehead, halfway between the eyebrows and the hairline. Bangs should be pushed back off the forehead (this method cannot be used if bandages cover the area). Depress the button on the scanner and gently stroke the probe across the forehead toward the hairline (at the temples), keeping the probe flat on the patient's skin. As the scanner moves across the forehead, repeated temperature measurements are taken and the highest measurement is recorded; keeping the button depressed, lift the scanner from the temporal area and lightly place the probe behind the earlobe. Release the button and remove the probe. Recording an accurate temperature takes about 3 seconds (Procedure 24-3). Depending on the facility's infection control procedures, disposable covers can be used on the scanner or it can be cleaned between patients with an alcohol wipe.

FIGURE 24-3 Professional temporal artery scanner.

PROCEDURE 24-3   Obtain Vital Signs: Obtain a Temporal Artery Temperature

Goal: To accurately determine and record a patient's temperature using a temporal artery scanner.

EQUIPMENT and SUPPLIES

- Patient's record
- Professional temporal artery thermometer with probe covers
- Alcohol swabs
- Biohazard waste container

PROCEDURAL STEPS

1. Sanitize your hands.
   PURPOSE: To ensure infection control.
2. Gather the necessary equipment and supplies.

3. Introduce yourself, identify your patient, and explain the procedure.
   PURPOSE: Identification of the patient prevents errors, and explanations are a means of gaining implied consent and patient cooperation.
4. Remove the protective cap on the probe. Depending on the facility's infection control procedures, disposable covers can be used on the scanner, or it can be cleaned by lightly wiping the surface with an alcohol swab.
   PURPOSE: To ensure infection control.
5. Push the patient's hair up off the forehead to expose the site. Gently place the probe on the patient's forehead, halfway between the edge of the eyebrows and the hairline.
   PURPOSE: This places the probe directly over the temporal artery.

Step-by-step Procedure boxes demonstrate how to perform and document procedures encountered in the healthcare setting.

- Write out the entire word and refrain from using abbreviations and emoticons.
- Use proper capitalization, grammar, sentence structure, and punctuation. Check the spelling of the e-mail before sending it. Most e-mail software has a spell-checker.
- Be concise, accurate, and clear in your message.
- Always end your e-mail with "Thank you" or "Sincerely" and your complete name. For business e-mails, include contact information after your name, including the agency's address, phone number, and fax number.
- Leave white space (i.e., one blank line) between the salutation, paragraphs, and your complete name.
- Zip large attachments before sending the files. **Zip** is a computer program that compresses a file or folder, making it smaller and easier to send. The receiver uses an unzip program to extract the contents.
- Many e-mail programs have features such as (!) urgent or a response box that sends an e-mail back to the sender when the e-mail is opened by the recipient. Use the urgent feature only for crucial e-mails.

8-14

CRITICAL THINKING APPLICATION

Christiana receives an e-mail from a patient that is in all capital letters. How might she perceive the situation with the patient? How could she verify her perceptions? How should she handle this situation?

Some healthcare facilities may also include language in e-mails related to confidentiality and whom to contact if the e-mail was sent to the wrong address. Medical assistants must adhere to the facility's confidentiality rules when communicating with or about patients. Copies of e-mail communications should be uploaded to the patient's EHR for a permanent record of the electronic communication.

EHR software frequently contains clinical messaging or clinical e-mail features. This feature is an e-mail within the EHR. The clinical messaging feature provides secure communication for healthcare employees to converse about the patient. For instance, the message may be sent from the receptionist to the medical assistant regarding a patient who called requesting a refill. The medical assistant can then follow up with the provider regarding the refill.

Faxed Communication

Fax (short for facsimile) machines send and receive documents using the phone lines. In the healthcare facility, the fax machine

may be part of a copy machine, or the computers may have software that allows faxes to be sent and received. As communications technology has advanced, the use of fax machines has decreased, but they are still an important piece of equipment in the ambulatory care center.

When sending a fax, you must adhere to HIPAA and HITECH rules. Healthcare facilities usually have a required face sheet (the first sheet) that includes confidentiality language, which instructs the recipient, if he or she is not the intended party, to destroy the fax and contact the medical facility. Besides the confidentiality statement, the face sheet should include the contact information for sender and recipient, the date, and the total number of pages.

CLOSING COMMENTS

Patient Education

If the medical assistant is responsible for preparing patient education materials using the computer's word processing program, it is important that these materials contain correct grammar, spelling, punctuation, and sentence structure. The appearance of brochures and documents created by the ambulatory care center staff reflects on the medical practice. The medical assistant should proofread all documents carefully before printing them.

Legal and Ethical Issues

The medical assistant should keep a copy of all documents produced using word processing. A copy of any document sent to a patient must also be uploaded into the patient's EHR. All patient-related documents are confidential, and the medical assistant must ensure the security and privacy of the information.

Professional Behaviors

Written communication in any form requires the medical assistant to be respectful, polite, and professional. It is important to proofread all written communication before it is sent to the recipient. Spell-checker tools can help identify misspelled words and sometimes incorrect usage of grammar and punctuation. However, these tools cannot always identify a word used incorrectly; only proofreading can capture those errors. Proofreading also allows the reader to reassess the tone of the communication, making sure it is appropriate. Finally, the medical assistant should recheck the spelling of the person's name and address for accuracy. A well-composed message gives the reader a reassuring sense of the accuracy and professionalism of the healthcare facility's staff.

NEW! Professional Behaviors boxes provide tips on professional behavior that are specific to each chapter's content.

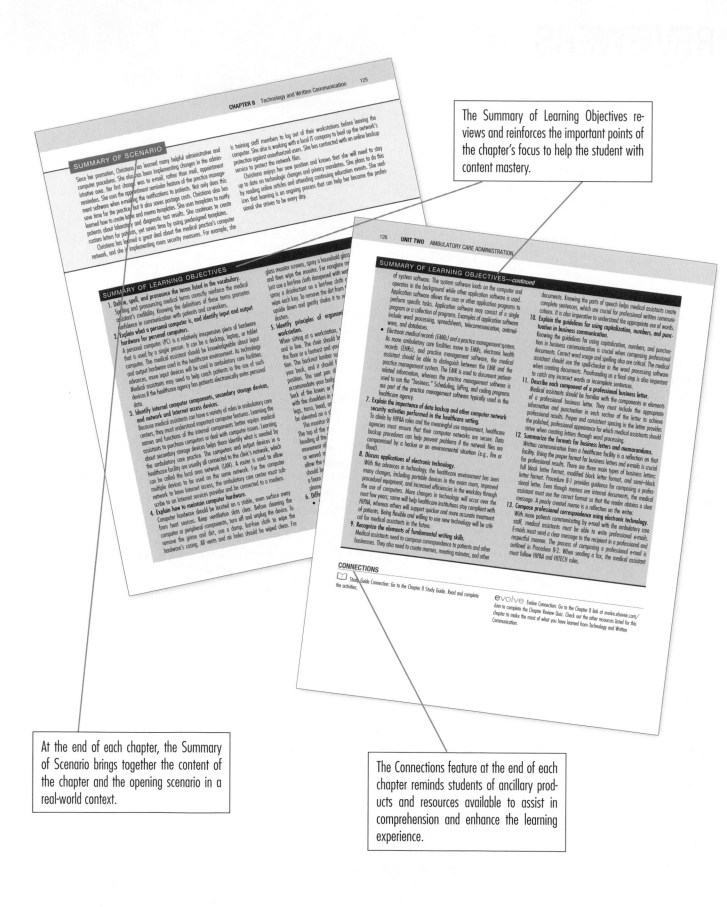

The Summary of Learning Objectives reviews and reinforces the important points of the chapter's focus to help the student with content mastery.

At the end of each chapter, the Summary of Scenario brings together the content of the chapter and the opening scenario in a real-world context.

The Connections feature at the end of each chapter reminds students of ancillary products and resources available to assist in comprehension and enhance the learning experience.

REVIEWERS

Brenda G. Abplanalp, RN, BSN, MSEd
Director
Pennsylvania College of Technology
Williamsport, Pennsylvania

Pam Alt, RN, MSN, RMA
Medical Assistant Program Director
Mid-State Technical College
Marshfield, Wisconsin

Deborah A. Balentine, MEd, RHIA, CCS, CCS-P, CHTS-TR
Adjunct Instructor—Adult Education
City Colleges of Chicago
Chicago, Illinois

Janet K. Baumann, BS, CMA (AAMA), EMT-B
Medical Assistant Program Director
Northcentral Technical College
Wausau, Wisconsin

Cynthia A. Bloss, AA, RMA, BMO
Instructor, Clinical Liaison
Southeastern College
Clearwater, Florida

Marquitta Breeding, CMA (AAMA)
Wallace State Community College
Hanceville, Alabama

Leon Deutsch, RMA, BS, MEd
Dean of Teaching & Learning
Grayson College
Denison, Texas

Jennifer Dietz, BS, CMA (AAMA), PBT (ASCP)^{CM}
Assistant Professor
Cuyahoga Community College—Metropolitan Campus
Cleveland, Ohio

Tracie Fuqua, BS, CMA (AAMA)
Medical Assistant Program Director
Wallace State Community College
Hanceville, Alabama

Deborah S. Gilbert, RHIA, MBA, CMA
Assistant Professor of School of Allied Health
Dalton State College
Dalton, Georgia

Kimberly Annette Head, DC, BS, BA
Director of CE Healthcare Programs
Collin College
Plano, Texas

Judith K. Kline, RMA, NCMA, CCMA, CMAA, AHI, NCET, NCICS, NCPT
Professor
Miami Lakes Educational Center & Technical College
Miami Lakes, Florida

Jennifer K. Lester, BA, NHA, AMT
Medical Administrative Instructor
Charleston Job Corps Center & Bridge Valley Community & Technical College Workforce Program
Charleston, West Virginia

Michelle C. Maus, MBA, BS, PhD, ABD
Department Chair/Assistant Professor
Tiffin University
Tiffin, Ohio

Tammy McClish, MEd, CMA (AAMA), RTARRT
Allied Health Instructor
The University of Akron
Akron, Ohio

Brigitte Niedzwiecki, RN, MSN, RMA
Medical Assistant Program Director & Instructor
Chippewa Valley Technical College
Eau Claire, Wisconsin

Cynthia B. Orlando, CAHI, OBT, NRCMA
Instructor
Eastern College of Health Vocations
New Orleans, Louisiana

Julie Pepper, BS, CMA (AAMA)
Medical Assistant Instructor
Chippewa Valley Technical College
Eau Claire, Wisconsin

Melanie Shearer, MS, MT (ASCP) PBT^{CM}, CMA (AAMA)
Medical Assisting Associate Professor
Cuyahoga Community College
Cleveland, Ohio

CONTENTS

UNIT TWO

Ambulatory Care Administration

Brigitte Niedzwiecki and Julie Pepper

UNIT SIX

Career Development

Brigitte Niedzwiecki and Julie Pepper

COMPETENCY-BASED EDUCATION AND THE MEDICAL ASSISTANT STUDENT

1

Shawna Long is a newly admitted student in a medical assistant (MA) program at your school. Shawna is anxious about starting classes and very concerned that she may not be a successful student. She had trouble with some of her classes in high school and must continue to work part time while taking medical assistant classes. Based on what you discover about the learning process in this chapter, see whether you can help Shawna take steps toward success.

While studying this chapter, think about the following questions:

- What is competency-based education and how can it help Shawna learn and achieve skills?
- Why is it important for Shawna to understand how she learns best?
- Time management is a crucial part of being a successful student and a successful medical assistant. What are some methods Shawna can implement to help her manage her time as effectively as possible?

- Shawna will face many problems and challenges while working through the MA program. How can she develop workable strategies for dealing with these issues?
- What is the role of assertiveness in effective professional communications?
- Studying may be a challenge for Shawna. What skills can she use to help her learn new material and prepare for examinations?

LEARNING OBJECTIVES

1. Define, spell, and pronounce the terms listed in the vocabulary.
2. Discuss competency-based education and adult learners.
3. Summarize the importance of student portfolios in proving academic success and skill competency.
4. Examine your learning preferences and interpret how your learning style affects your success as a student.
5. Differentiate between adaptive and nonadaptive coping mechanisms.
6. Apply time management strategies to make the most of your learning opportunities.
7. Integrate effective study skills into your daily activities.
8. Design test-taking strategies that help you take charge of your success.
9. Incorporate critical thinking and reflection to help you make mental connections as you learn material.
10. Analyze healthcare results as reported in graphs and tables.
11. Apply problem-solving techniques to manage conflict and overcome barriers to your success.
12. Relate assertiveness, aggressiveness, and passive behaviors to professional communication and discuss the role of assertiveness in effective communication.

VOCABULARY

competencies Mastery of the knowledge, skills, and behaviors that are expected of the entry-level medical assistant.

critical thinking The constant practice of considering all aspects of a situation when deciding what to believe or what to do.

empathy (em′-puh-the) Sensitivity to the individual needs and reactions of patients.

learning style The way an individual perceives and processes information to learn new material.

mnemonic A learning device (e.g., an image, a rhyme, or a figure of speech) that a person uses to help him or her remember information.

perceiving (pur-sev′-ing) How an individual looks at information and sees it as real.

processing (pro′-ses-ing) How an individual internalizes new information and makes it his or her own.

reflection (re-flek′-shun) The process of thinking about new information so as to create new ways of learning.

stressor An event, activity, condition, or other stimulus that causes stress.

For many years the curriculum for medical assistant programs has been based on student achievement of specific **competencies**. According to the Medical Assisting Education Review Board (MAERB):

> Medical assistants graduating from programs accredited by the Commission on Accreditation of Allied Health Education Programs (CAAHEP) will demonstrate critical thinking based on knowledge of academic subject matter required for competence in the profession. They will incorporate the cognitive knowledge in performance of the psychomotor and affective domains in their practice as medical assistants in providing patient care.

The Accrediting Bureau of Health Education Schools (ABHES) also bases its recommended curriculum on student achievement of identified competencies:

> The depth and breadth of the program's curriculum enables graduates to acquire the knowledge and competencies necessary to become an entry-level professional in the medical assisting field. Competencies required for successful completion of the program are delineated, and the curriculum ensures achievement of these entry-level competencies through mastery of coursework and skill achievement. Focus is placed on credentialing requirements and opportunities to obtain employment and to increase employability.

National curriculum standards for the education of medical assistants are based on recognized competencies that employers expect entry-level medical assistants to have. The 2015 Core Curriculum for Medical Assistants established by the MAERB must be followed for programs accredited by CAAHEP. Those completing a CAAHEP-accredited program must demonstrate core entry-level competencies in knowledge of subject matter, be able to perform the psychomotor skills needed in an ambulatory care center, and have appropriate behavioral competencies to respond professionally and with **empathy** toward patients and their families. The 12 academic subjects in a CAAHEP-approved curriculum are as follows:

I. Anatomy and Physiology
II. Applied Mathematics
III. Infection Control
IV. Nutrition
V. Concepts of Effective Communication
VI. Administrative Functions
VII. Basic Practice Finances
VIII. Third Party Reimbursement
IX. Procedural and Diagnostic Coding
X. Legal Implications
XI. Ethical Considerations
XII. Protective Practices

ABHES also offers accreditation for medical assisting programs. The organization focuses its curriculum requirements on student competency achievement with 11 required areas of study:

1. General Orientation [to the field of medical assisting]
2. Anatomy and Physiology
3. Medical Terminology
4. Medical Law and Ethics
5. Psychology of Human Relations
6. Pharmacology
7. Records Management
8. Administrative Procedures
9. Clinical Procedures
10. Medical Laboratory Procedures
11. Career Development

What does this mean for you, the medical assistant student? To meet national standards, your MA program must comply with competency-based learning in multiple areas. The most important characteristic of competency-based education is that it measures learning and skill achievement over time. Students progress through the program by demonstrating their competence, which means they prove they have mastered the knowledge, skills, and professional behaviors required to achieve competency in a particular task. For example, one of the basic skills you must achieve as a medical assistant student is taking an accurate blood pressure. Some students will have more difficulty consistently achieving this goal than others, but each student must be able to take a blood pressure accurately before he or she can move on in the curriculum.

ADULT LEARNERS AND COMPETENCY-BASED EDUCATION

Competency-based learning is ideal for adult learners who are attempting to understand new information and achieve new skills. Educators recognize that adult learners come to the classroom with different work-related experiences and educational backgrounds. Therefore, adult students have a wide range of understanding about the knowledge and skills that must be achieved in the program. Adult students also learn material at different rates. Competency-based education recognizes these qualities of adult learners and takes advantage of them. Let's go back to the blood pressure example. Perhaps you took a healthcare lab in high school, in which you learned to take blood pressures; another student may have worked in a long-term care facility, where he was responsible for monitoring vital signs throughout the day. You both may need just a review of the anatomy and physiology aspects of a patient's blood pressure. However, other students in the class will not know anything about this skill. With competency-based education, your instructor can design laboratory activities that meet all students' needs, including your own.

CRITICAL THINKING APPLICATION   **1-1**

Can you think of any examples of how competency-based education might help you succeed as a medical assistant student? Come up with two possibilities and share them with your classmates.

PORTFOLIOS

Have you taken a class in the past that required you to develop a portfolio? Portfolios are frequently used in an Art or English class to demonstrate student skills and learning achievements. Generally, a portfolio is a collection of student materials that demonstrates learning. An advantage of developing a portfolio for a medical assistant program is that you can decide which pieces of your work best demonstrate your learning and skill achievement over time. Why would this be beneficial to you?

In a competency-based program, you must achieve a series of skills, not only to complete the program, but also to prove to future employers that you are competent in all the identified skills an entry-level medical assistant should have. Once you complete the program and are looking for your first medical assistant position, how can you prove to potential employers that you are competent in all required skills? What can you bring to an interview that summarizes your abilities? A comprehensive portfolio that you develop throughout the courses you take in your MA program contains materials that you can use to demonstrate the knowledge and skills you have accumulated throughout your course of study. A comprehensive portfolio includes examples of work completed in each course and proof of the skills achieved.

A comprehensive portfolio can be used to create an interview portfolio that is tailored to prove your competency in the skills outlined in a specific job description. (Interview portfolios are discussed in more detail in the chapter, Career Development and Life Skills.) For example, as a new graduate, you see an ad for a medical assistant position in a local pediatrician's office that is looking for an individual who is competent in electronic health records (EHRs), knowledgeable about immunizations, and who knows how to perform basic coding skills. If you have retained copies of all of your achievements in those designated areas in a comprehensive portfolio, you can pull out those specific copies to create a job interview portfolio that demonstrates your knowledge base and skill level. Items that you can feature in a comprehensive portfolio include:

- Samples of projects completed throughout your courses of study, to demonstrate your learning in a variety of subjects. For example, perhaps in one of your courses, you developed a list of community resources that could help patients with a variety of needs. Including this project demonstrates your knowledge of local agencies that might prove useful to the patient population of a healthcare facility where you are seeking employment. Another project may require you to investigate a specific disease process, including expected signs and symptoms, diagnostics, and treatment details. This project would demonstrate your knowledge of a disease process, management of patients, diagnostic studies, and medications. Other assignments may require you to demonstrate your administrative knowledge and skills, such as EHR skills, basic practice finances, and coding capabilities.
- Samples of key procedural checklists that show evidence of your achievement of skills in measuring and recording vital signs and performing hands-on skills, such as electrocardiography (ECG), phlebotomy, medical laboratory procedures, infection control, administration of medication, therapeutic communication, third-party reimbursement, medical law and ethics applications, and emergency preparedness and practices. Collecting copies of competency achievement documentation in all these areas will help you demonstrate entry-level job readiness during an interview.
- Copies of awards (e.g., scholarships, dean's list), to demonstrate your academic achievements.
- Copies of any certifications you have achieved (e.g., cardiopulmonary resuscitation [CPR] and First Aid and Safety), to demonstrate your readiness for employment in a healthcare facility.
- Letters of recommendation from current employers, faculty members, and others, to highlight your personal and work-related qualities.

Collecting material for a comprehensive portfolio should start with the very first course in the MA program in which you are enrolled. Choose examples of work that demonstrate your completion of core requirements, in addition to competency achievement across the curriculum. You then will have all the materials needed to create a specific interview portfolio for each job interview you earn.

WHO YOU ARE AS A LEARNER: HOW DO YOU LEARN BEST?

You have taken the first step toward becoming a successful student by choosing your profession and field of study. The medical assistant profession is both challenging and rewarding. Becoming a medical assistant opens the doors to a wide variety of opportunities in both administrative and clinical practice at ambulatory or institutional healthcare facilities. To become a successful medical assistant, you first must become a successful student. This chapter helps you discover the way you learn best and provides multiple strategies to assist you in your journey toward success.

CRITICAL THINKING APPLICATION   **1-2**

Consider your history as a student. What do you think helped you succeed? What do you think needs improvement? Create a plan for improvement that includes two or three ways you can become a more successful student. Be prepared to share this plan with your classmates.

Think about what you do when you are faced with something new to learn. How do you go about understanding and learning the new material? Over time you have developed a method for **perceiving** and **processing** information. This pattern of behavior is called your **learning style**. Learning styles can be examined in many different ways, but most professionals agree that a student's success depends more on whether the person can "make sense" of the information than on whether the individual is "smart." Determining your individual learning style and understanding how it applies to your ability to learn new material are the first steps toward becoming a successful student (Figure 1-1).

Learning Style Inventory

For you to learn new material, two things must happen. First, you must perceive the information. This is the method you have developed over time that helps you examine new information and recognize it as real. Once you have developed a method for learning about the new material, you must *process* the information. Processing the information is how you internalize it and make it your own. Researchers believe that each of us has a preferred method for learning new material. By investigating your learning style, you can figure out how to combine different approaches to perceiving and processing information that will lead to greater success as a student.

The first step in learning new material is determining how you perceive it, or as some experts explain, what methods you use to learn the new material. Some learners opt to watch, observe, and use **reflection** to think about and learn the new material. These students are *abstract perceivers,* who learn by analyzing new material, building

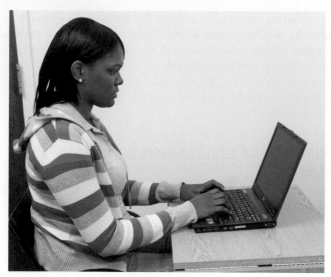

FIGURE 1-1 Student learning.

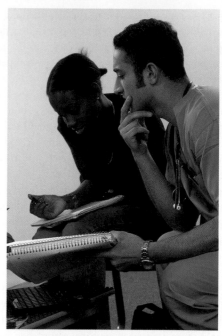

FIGURE 1-2 Learning in a small group.

theories about it, and using a step-by-step approach to learning. Other students need to perform some activity, such as rewriting notes from class, making flash cards, and outlining chapters, to learn new information. Students who learn by "doing" are called *concrete perceivers.* Concrete learners prefer to learn things that have a personal meaning or that they believe are relevant to their lives. So, which type of perceiver do you think you are? Before you actually learn new material, do you need time to think about it, or do you prefer to "do" something to help you learn the material?

The second step in learning new material is information processing, which is the way learners internalize the new information and make it their own. New material can be processed by two methods. *Active processors* prefer to jump in and start doing things immediately. They make sense of the new material by using it *now.* They look for practical ways to apply the new material and learn best with practice and hands-on activities. *Reflective processors* have to think about the information before they can internalize it. They prefer to observe and consider what is going on. The only way they can make sense of new material is to spend time thinking and learning a great deal about it before acting. Which type of information processor do you think you are? Do you prefer to jump in and start doing things to help you learn, or do you need to analyze and consider the material before you can actually learn it?

Using Your Learning Profile to Be a Successful Student: Where Do I Go From Here?

No one falls completely into one or the other of the categories just discussed. However, by being aware of how we generally prefer first to perceive information and then to process it, we can be more sensitive to our learning style and can approach new learning situations with a plan for learning the material in a way that best suits our learning preferences.

Your preferred perceiving and processing learning profile will fall into one of the following four stages of the Learning Style Inventory, which was created by David Kolb of Case Western Reserve University.

- *Stage 1* learners have a *concrete reflective* style. These students want to know the purpose of the information and have a personal connection to the content. They like to consider a situation from many points of view, observe others, and plan before taking action. They feel most comfortable watching rather than doing, and their strengths include sensitivity toward others, brainstorming, and recognizing and creatively solving problems. If you fall into this stage, you enjoy small-group activities and learn well in study groups.

- *Stage 2* learners have an *abstract reflective* style. These students are eager to learn just for the sheer pleasure of learning, rather than because the material relates to their personal lives. They like to learn lots of facts and arrange new material in a clear, logical manner. Stage 2 learners plan studying and like to create ways of thinking about the material, but they do not always make the connection with its practical application. If you are a stage 2 learner, you prefer organized, logical presentations of material and therefore enjoy lectures and readings and generally dislike group work. You also need time to process and think about new material before applying it.

- *Stage 3* learners have an *abstract active* style. Learners with this combination learning style want to experiment and test the information they are learning. If you are a stage 3 learner, you want to know how techniques or ideas work, and you also want to practice what you are learning. Your strengths are in problem solving and decision making, but you may lack focus and may be hasty in making decisions. You learn best with hands-on practice by doing experiments, projects, and laboratory activities. You enjoy working alone or in small groups (Figure 1-2).

- *Stage 4* learners are *concrete active* learners. These students are concerned about how they can use what they learn to make a difference in their lives. If you fall into this stage, you like to relate new material to other areas of your life. You have leadership capabilities, can create on your feet, and usually are vocal in a group, but you may have difficulty completing your work on time. Stage 4 learners enjoy teaching others and working in groups and learn best when they can apply new information to real-world problems.

CRITICAL THINKING APPLICATION   **1-3**

- Consider the two ways to perceive new material. Are you a concrete perceiver, who ties the information to a personal experience, or are you an abstract perceiver, who likes to analyze or reflect on the meaning of the material? Choose the type you think most accurately describes your method of learning.
- Now, think about the way you process learning. Are you an active processor, who always looks for the practical applications of what you learn, or are you a reflective processor, who has to think about new material before internalizing it?
- After completing this activity, write down the combination of your perceiving and processing learning styles and share it with your instructor.

To get the most out of knowing your learning profile, you need to apply this knowledge to how you approach learning. Each of the learning stages has pluses and minuses. When faced with a learning situation that does not match your learning preference, see how you can adapt your individual learning profile to make the best of the information. For example, if you are bored by lectures, look for an opportunity to apply the information being presented to a real problem you are facing in the classroom or at home. If you are an abstract perceiver, take time outside of class to think about new information so that you are ready to process it into your learning system. If you benefit from learning in a group, make the effort to organize review sessions and study groups. If you learn best by teaching others, offer to assist your peers with their learning. By taking the time now to investigate your preferred method of learning, you will perceive and process information more effectively throughout your school career.

CRITICAL THINKING APPLICATION   **1-4**

Take a few minutes to reflect on a time when you really enjoyed learning about something new. How was the material presented, and what did you do to "make it your own"? What do you need to do to become a more effective learner?

COPING MECHANISMS

Have you ever thought about how you deal or cope with stressful situations? We each have our own ways of managing stress or conflict. We've developed these methods over time, and whether they are effective depends on the individual's personality and life experiences; the environment or situational specifics that surround the

issue; and the type of stress involved. For example, perhaps you have other demands on your time besides those related to school. Perhaps you are worried about money, house work, children, jobs, and so on. All these things can contribute to individual stress levels. Coping strategies are the methods we consciously use to solve problems and attempt to minimize the stress associated with them.

CRITICAL THINKING APPLICATION   **1-5**

Make a list of five things that cause stress in your life. Next to each item, write down how you typically would cope with that stressor.

Myths About Stress

The following are some commonly held beliefs about stress that, in fact, are not true. See how many of these myths are part of your beliefs about stress.

Myth 1: Stress is always negative. If not managed in a positive way, stress can be very damaging. However, stress can also motivate us to work harder and achieve more, so it can be quite beneficial in our lives. Can you think of an example of stress as a positive influence in your life?

Myth 2: We all respond to stress in the same way. The perception of a stressful situation is individualized, and each person responds to stress in his or her own way. For example, students typically are stressed about exams, but each individual student perceives that stress and responds to it differently.

Myth 3: If no symptoms are evident, then stress does not exist. Stress is always present. If you have developed adaptive coping mechanisms, you may not display the symptoms of stress, such as worry, anxiety, or difficulty sleeping. Nonetheless, stress is present in all our lives.

Myth 4: We should ignore the symptoms of stress unless they drastically affect our lives. Manageable symptoms of stress include headache, backache and upset stomach. However, these minor problems are warnings that worse health issues can develop if we continue to mismanage stress levels.

From the Explorables. Available at https://explorable.com/myths-about-stress?gid=1600. Accessed June 5, 2015.

Strategies used to reduce stress are called *adaptive,* or *constructive, coping mechanisms.* For example, if finding time to study for an exam is stressful, an adaptive response to this stress is to use time management strategies, such as planning study hours in advance to avoid the stress of last-minute preparation. However, some coping strategies may actually increase stress levels. These are identified as *nonadaptive coping mechanisms.* Therefore, if you have a big project due and you procrastinate to the last minute to start working on it, your anxiety over the project may result in even more stress.

Adaptive coping mechanisms can help a person gain control over a stressful situation. Negative, or nonadaptive, strategies may be effective short term but often lead to long-term stress. The good news is that coping mechanisms are learned behaviors. It is possible to replace coping mechanisms that do not work with ones that are more successful.

One of the keys to managing stress in your life is to maintain your health. If you are eating properly, exercising regularly, and consistently getting enough sleep, you are much more capable of managing stress. Mentally managing your stress levels is also really important. Learning relaxation techniques, using positive self-talk, implementing time management strategies, expressing how you feel, and honestly communicating with others are all factors that can help you manage your stress levels more effectively.

Adaptive and Nonadaptive Coping Mechanisms

Adaptive Coping Mechanisms:
- Using humor to cope with a painful situation
- Gathering information about the cause of a problem
- Learning new skills to manage a problem
- Trying to derive meaning from a stressful situation
- Accepting the responsibility or blame
- Using distraction to manage negative feelings
- Practicing relaxation methods
- Using positive self-talk
- Seeking social support for the issue
- Anticipating a stressful situation and planning a coping strategy
- Getting adequate nutrition, exercise, and sleep

Nonadaptive Coping Mechanisms
- Compartmentalizing thoughts and emotions
- Anticipating or rehearsing stressful events
- Avoiding anxiety by relying on something (e.g., alcohol or drugs) or someone to cope with stress
- Doing everything you can to avoid stressful situations
- Running away, either physically or mentally, to escape a stressful situation

---

CRITICAL THINKING APPLICATION   1-6
Look back on the list of **stressors** in your life and how you typically responded to each. Is there anything you have learned from your reading that might help you better cope with stress? Next to each stressor, add an adaptive coping mechanism that could help.

TIME MANAGEMENT: PUTTING TIME ON YOUR SIDE

One of the most complicated tasks for a professional medical assistant is to manage time effectively. No other workplace can compete with the distractions and demands of a busy healthcare facility. Do you think you practice effective time management skills? Do you believe that you are in control of your time, or do you think that other people or situations control it? How frequently do you say that you just do not have enough time to do what you are supposed to do, let alone those things you would like to do? Time management gives you the opportunity to spend time in the way you choose. Effective time management is also crucial to your success as a student and as a future healthcare professional (Figure 1-3).

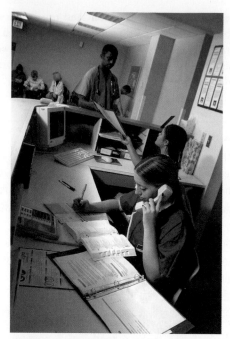

FIGURE 1-3 Time management in a busy medical practice.

How to Put Time on Your Side

The following time management skills are designed to help you deal effectively with the demands on your time. Highlight the ones you think will be most useful in helping you deal with your situation.

1. **Determine your purpose.** What do you want to accomplish this semester, in this course, or in this unit of study? What do you want to achieve as a student? What is one thing you can do to help achieve your goals?
2. **Identify your main concern.** Besides school, what other demands do you have on your time? Based on the learning goals you have established, what do you need to do to accomplish your goals?
   - *Plan time:* Schedule projects in advance, and make notes to yourself on deadlines.
   - *Guard time:* Avoid distractions (e.g., television, music, cell phones, social media) that interfere with your concentration. Notice how others abuse your time. Learn to say no to outside demands on your time.
   - *Discover time:* Think about what you do with your time all day long. Are there instances where you could "steal" time from something to "create" more time in your schedule? For example, maybe you spend time carpooling kids to activities or waiting for a class to start. Can you keep your books with you and use that downtime to highlight part of a chapter or create flash cards for an upcoming test?
   - *Assign time:* Ask for help when you need it from friends and family.
3. **Be organized.** What materials (e.g., books, research, supplies) do you need to have an effective study session? What preparation is needed to make the most of your time?
   - *Record time:* Use a day planner or calendar, either paper or electronic, to note the due dates for assignments and tests. If a paper or project is due on a specific date, put a reminder in your day planner to start the project on a specific date so that you are sure to have it done when it is due.

- *Optimal time:* Take advantage of the time of day when you study and learn the best. Schedule study time during your peak performance time. If you are an early riser, make time for homework first thing in the day; if you are a night owl, do your homework at night. Plan on dedicating at least some of your optimal time to your school work.

4. **Stop procrastinating.** If you avoid working on your goals, you may not achieve them. Examine the following suggestions as ways to break the procrastination cycle.

  - *Make the work meaningful: What is important about the work you are putting off and what are the benefits of getting it done?* Reflect on your long-range goals. Is it important to do a good job on the work so you can earn an acceptable grade, do well in the course, complete the medical assisting program, and ultimately find employment?
  - *Plan work deadlines:* Break assignments into achievable sections that can be completed in the time slots available. Schedule those work sections in your day planner so that you do not forget deadlines for assignments.
  - *Ask for help:* Let your support system know you have work to get done. Ask them for encouragement to stay on track. If you have school-age children, you can set an excellent example by planning "family" homework sessions. You can get some of your work done while acting as a role model for learning behaviors for your children. Let your partner know when due dates are looming or tests are scheduled. Ask for help in meeting day-to-day demands so that you can study or prepare for school.
  - *Prioritize:* If you keep avoiding a certain task, re-evaluate its priority. If it is really worth worrying about, get started now, not later. Don't waste time worrying about how you are going to get things done. Spend that time actually working on the projects that worry you the most.
  - *Reward yourself:* Create a reward that is meaningful and something for which you will work. If you want to spend time with your family or friends on the weekend, develop a plan and stick to it so that you can share that special time as a reward.

5. **Remember you.** It is very easy to become overwhelmed with responsibilities both in school and at home. Part of successful time management includes setting aside time to do things you enjoy. You have chosen a profession that can be very demanding. Now is the time to remember that you have to take care of yourself in addition to meeting your professional and personal responsibilities.

CRITICAL THINKING APPLICATION   1-7

How do you spend your time? For 3 days this week, write down the amount of time you spend on each activity. How much television do you watch? How much time do you spend talking or texting on the phone and checking social media? How about driving time, visiting time, work time, time for family and friends, and so on? At the end of the 3-day period, add up the amount of time you spent on your daily activities. Do you recognize any time you might be wasting? Can you implement any of the suggested time management strategies to make more time available?

STUDY SKILLS: TRICKS FOR BECOMING A SUCCESSFUL STUDENT

So far in this chapter, we have looked at the influence of individual learning styles and time management on learning success. Now we will investigate some ideas that are useful for learning new material. These study skills include memory techniques, active learning, brain tricks, reading methods, and note-taking strategies.

Several techniques can help you store and remember information. The first of these involves organizing information into recognizable groups so that the brain can find it easily. You can organize information by getting the big picture first before trying to learn the details. One way to implement this strategy is to skim a reading assignment before actually reading and taking notes on the material, thus getting a general impression of what you need to learn before tackling the details. Depending on your learning style, it may also help to find a way of making the new information meaningful. Think about your educational goals and how the new material will help you achieve those goals.

Another way of remembering material is to create an association with something you already know. If new material is grouped with already stored material, the brain remembers it much more easily. For example, maybe you took a biology class in high school and learned the basics about human anatomy and physiology. Try to create a link between what you previously learned and the detail of the new information you are expected to learn now. Or maybe you have a family member who suffers from a particular disease. Think about that individual's signs and symptoms while learning more details about the disease so that you can apply your learning to his or her situation.

A useful study skill for some learners is to be physically active while learning. Some students learn best if they walk or talk out loud while studying. Besides encouraging learning, moving and talking while studying relieves boredom and keeps you awake. Another way to be actively involved in learning is to use pictures or diagrams to represent the material you are studying. Some people are visual learners, and creating pictures of the material is the easiest method for them to retain the information. Other students find that rewriting notes, making lists of information, creating flash cards, color-coding notes, or highlighting important material in a textbook helps them retain the material. Writing also helps students who need to "do" something to learn.

Studying goes much more smoothly if you work with your brain rather than against it. If you tend to get anxious and worried while studying, you may be acting as your own worst enemy. One way of dealing with a topic you are anxious about is to overlearn it. If material is overlearned, you are much less likely to experience test anxiety. Another method for remembering material is to review it quickly after class. This mini-review helps the new information become part of your long-term memory system.

Many students find creating songs, dances, or word associations an effective way to learn and remember new material. Putting details into a familiar song and moving to it can help trick the brain into remembering the information. This is especially helpful when trying to learn anatomy and physiology. For example, think about one of your favorite songs and "dance" your way through the blood flow through the heart. Or, if you are finding the organization of the body especially tricky to remember, such as the movement of food through the gastrointestinal (GI) system, create a **mnemonic** that helps you remember the information. The most common one suggested for the parts of the intestines is: **D**ow **J**ones **I**ndustrial **C**limbing **A**verage **C**losing **S**tock **R**eport. The first letter of each word stands for an anatomic part of the intestines—*d*uodenum, *j*ejunum, *i*leum, *c*ecum, *a*ppendix, *c*olon, *s*igmoid, and *r*ectum. You can make up your own mnemonics or memory tricks to help you learn complicated material.

Another excellent way of learning information is to actually teach it to someone else. Teaching requires you to have a good understanding of the material and the ability to describe it for others. It can be an effective reinforcement of complicated material.

A great deal of the learning process is expected to take place from assigned readings. You can use several methods to make reading assignments more meaningful. If you find a reading assignment challenging or difficult to understand, the first step is to take the time to read it again. Sometimes the first time through the material is not enough to gain understanding. As you read, highlight important words or thoughts and stop periodically to summarize the material. Some students find outlining new material helpful. This is another way to use active learning to help you make the information "your own."

If you get bored while reading, use your body; walk or talk your way through the assignment. Take the time to look up words or terms you do not understand or ask your instructor or tutor for help. The best way to determine whether you have learned anything from your reading is to try to explain the material to someone else. For example, you can meet with other students and explain to them what you learned. If you can do that effectively, you know you have acquired the knowledge needed from the reading assignment.

Many students find effective note taking a challenge. The big question is, "How much of what the instructor says do I actually need to write down?" The first step in effective note taking is to come to class prepared. The more familiar you are with the material, the easier it will be to determine the important parts of the instructor's lecture. Pay attention to the instructor and look for clues to what he or she thinks is important. Ask questions about the material if you do not understand it, rather than writing down information that makes no sense to you. Think critically about what you hear before you write it down so you can start to build relationships among the things you want or need to know.

If your instructor uses PowerPoint presentations to teach a lesson, request copies of the slides before the lecture so you have an opportunity to review them as you are doing your reading. Many courses have an online website where PowerPoints or other lecture materials are available for review. Take advantage of these added materials to be prepared for each class so that you can ask questions about anything you don't understand. In addition, this textbook has an extensive online site (i.e., Evolve) that you can access for learning resources. Investigate the site and see whether something there can help you reach your learning goals.

When it comes to actual note taking, some strategies can make the process of recording notes an active learning tool. Organize the information as much as possible while you are writing or typing, either in an outline or a paragraph format. If you take notes on a laptop or tablet, make sure your typing skills are good enough for you to keep up with the flow of information and that you review

your notes shortly after class to fill in any missing details. If you take notes on paper, use only one side of the page (for easier reading) and leave blank spaces where needed to fill in details later. Use key words to help you remember the material, and create pictures or diagrams to help visualize it. If permitted, use tape recorders and make sure you have copies of any handouts or notes distributed by your instructor that cover material written on the board or provided in a PowerPoint presentation. If your instructor refers the class to a YouTube video or other website, transcribe the site address correctly to refer to it at a later time. Another helpful tool is to develop your own system of abbreviations to help simplify the note-taking process.

The most effective way to use your notes is to review them shortly after class. This is the time to add details, clarify information, or make notes about asking the instructor for explanations during the next class. You could even exchange notes with students you trust to compare information (Figure 1-4). Some students find it beneficial to create a computerized copy of their notes (if they wrote them out on paper) or to rewrite them. This gives you an opportunity to learn the material as you transcribe it. As you are reviewing your notes, you also can draw mind maps of the information or diagram outlines to help you better understand and remember the material.

Creating mind maps is a way of representing the main idea of a topic and supporting important details with a figure or picture. Healthcare textbooks present complicated concepts with multiple main ideas, each with its own important details. Mind maps are a way of combining complex details and organizing them into a format that is easier to remember. The spider map (Figure 1-5)

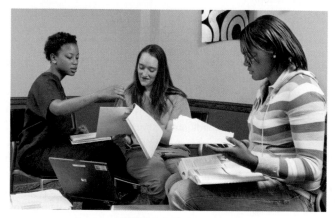

FIGURE 1-4 Sharing notes.

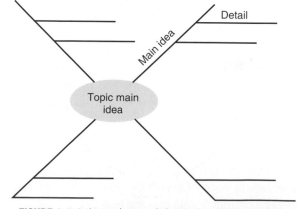

FIGURE 1-5 Spider map showing multiple main ideas with supporting details.

presents a method for including several main ideas with details in one study guide. The fishbone map (Figure 1-6) can be used to learn complicated causes of disease. The chain-of-events map (Figure 1-7) displays the cause and effect of events, such as infection control or the history of medicine. The cycle map (Figure 1-8) shows the connection between factors, such as in the chain of infection. Creating your own mind maps is a way of making the information more meaningful and easier for you to understand and remember.

Although many techniques can help you study, perhaps the most important one is your attitude toward learning. Some students fall into the "I can't possibly learn this material" trap. That type of attitude only leads to self-defeat. The way to overcome barriers is first

to recognize that they exist. Once you know your weak spots, use the suggested study skills to improve in those areas. Do not be afraid to ask questions or to ask for help if you do not understand the material. Use as many different strategies as necessary to become a successful student.

> ### CRITICAL THINKING APPLICATION 1-8
> Write down at least two barriers to learning that you face. Review the study skills suggestions and choose four to try out. Use them over the next week to help you learn new material. Reflect on whether the chosen study skills helped you learn the material better.

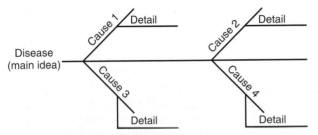

FIGURE 1-6 Fishbone map used to describe causes of disease.

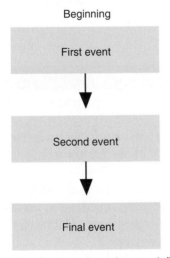

FIGURE 1-7 Chain-of-events map showing the cause and effect of events.

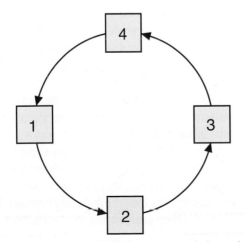

FIGURE 1-8 Cycle map illustrating the way one action leads to another.

TEST-TAKING STRATEGIES: TAKING CHARGE OF YOUR SUCCESS

What happens when you do not know the answer to the first question on a test? What if you do not know the next one? Are you able to go on without panicking? Many people find taking tests the most challenging part of being a successful student. Multiple approaches are available that you can use to take charge of your success and improve your ability to take tests. These include such strategies as adequate preparation, controlling negative thoughts during test time, and understanding ways to manage various types of questions.

The first step is to go into a test adequately prepared. Use the time management skills already outlined in this chapter to prepare for the big day. Recognize and use your preferred learning style to overlearn the material and increase your confidence. Use memory tools (e.g., flash cards, checklists, and mind maps) to help you visualize the material. Form a study group if you are the type of learner who benefits from studying in groups. Schedule and plan study time, and reward yourself for your hard work. It also is important to go into the test rested and relaxed; therefore, you should eat, exercise to relieve stress, and sleep before the test so that you are as alert as possible.

Before you start the test, make sure you read the directions carefully. If possible, begin with the easiest or shortest questions to build your confidence. Be aware of the amount of time allotted for the examination, and pace yourself accordingly. As you go through the test, look for clues to answers in other questions. During test time, remember to use positive self-talk at the first indication of panic. Repeatedly remind yourself that you are well prepared; relax and think about the material before you get worried. You need to stop negative thoughts as soon as they arise and instead visualize yourself being successful. Use slow, deep breathing to relax and, if helpful, close your eyes for a minute and visualize a relaxing place before you go on with the test.

Certain strategies are useful for answering different types of questions. With multiple choice questions, try to identify key words or clues in each question. Read the question carefully and answer it in your head before you review the provided answers. If you are not absolutely sure of the answer, make an educated guess or follow your instincts in choosing an answer. If there are answers that you know are not correct, that can eliminate the "all of the above" answer choice. By eliminating the answers that you know are incorrect, you can focus on the other answer choices.

"True or false" questions give you a 50/50 chance of being correct. Remember that if any part of the question is not true, then the statement is false. Again, check the statements for key words that help indicate the direction of the answer. Look for qualifying terms (e.g., *always, never, sometimes*) that are the key to understanding the meaning of the true or false statement.

CRITICAL THINKING APPLICATION   **1-9**

Think about a time you experienced test anxiety. Write down the details of the situation and how you felt. Choose four test-taking strategies you think would be beneficial in handling similar situations in the future.

BECOMING A CRITICAL THINKER: MAKING MENTAL CONNECTIONS

The ability to process information and arrive at reasonable conclusions is crucial to all healthcare workers. The process of **critical thinking** involves (1) sorting out conflicting information, (2) weighing your knowledge about that information, (3) ignoring or letting go of personal biases, and (4) deciding on a reasonable belief or action. Critical thinking is actually an active search for the truth.

Critical thinking could be described as thorough thinking, because it requires learners to keep an open mind to all possibilities. Successful students are thorough thinkers because they must determine the facts about a topic and come to logical conclusions about the material. Critical thinkers also are inquisitive learners; they constantly analyze and sort out conflicting information to reach conclusions.

A crucial step in critical thinking is evaluating the results of your learning. Reflection is the key to critical thinking. "How did I learn what I learned?" and "What does it mean in my life?" are questions that must be asked consistently to continue to learn. Becoming a successful student, and ultimately a successful member of the allied health team, requires critical thinking skills.

Tables and Graphs

Tables and graphs can be helpful tools in many aspects of healthcare, but you must take the time to analyze the information they include so that you process it accurately. For example, the body mass index (BMI) table you will learn about in the chapter, Nutrition and Health Promotion, and the growth chart graphs you will learn to use in the chapter, Assisting in Pediatrics, provide significant information about the health status of individual patients. In addition, tables throughout this textbook outline and summarize details about coding, health insurance, disease processes, medications, and treatments. To maximize your learning throughout the medical assistant program, you should use the information in tables and graphs to help prepare yourself to work as an entry-level medical assistant.

A graph is a diagram or picture that represents information and its relationships. Analyzing graphs is useful for determining a general

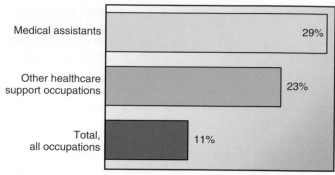

FIGURE 1-9 Projected percentage change in employment of medical assistants (2012 to 2022).

trend; for example, Figure 1-9 shows the projected increase in employment opportunities for medical assistants from 2012 to 2022. The bar graph clearly demonstrates the projected percentage of changes in employment opportunities for medical assistants. Figure 1-10 shows the projected change in total employment of select healthcare occupations. Can you see how graphs can help you understand a concept much easier than if the data were written out in paragraph form? More than one type of graph can be used to represent a single set of information.

How to Analyze a Graph

1. *Read the title and the axes of a graph to determine the information included.*

   The *x*-axis is the line on a graph that runs horizontally (left to right), and the *y*-axis is the line that runs vertically (up and down). For example, in Figure 1-10, different healthcare occupations are listed along the *y*-axis, and projected job opportunities (in hundreds of thousands) are listed on the *x*-axis. Based on your interpretation of this information, how many positions did the Bureau of Labor Statistics project for medical assistants?

2. *Determine the general trend of the graph.*

   For example, if you review the growth chart graph of a 2-year-old girl, you would be able to see whether her height and weight have consistently increased over time or whether she has had a sudden increase (maybe a growth spurt) or a decrease that might reflect a recent illness.

3. *Graphs can also be useful in visualizing information that doesn't seem to fit.*

   For example, if you are responsible for measuring the length and weight of a 4-month-old infant and the measurements that you took are markedly different (either larger or smaller) than the measurements recorded at the last well-child examination, perhaps your measurements are incorrect. If you check them again and come up with the same numbers, document your results but inform the provider of the differences so the provider can investigate the changes with the baby's caregiver. Can you see how being able to use graphs can help you gain insight into patient healthcare results?

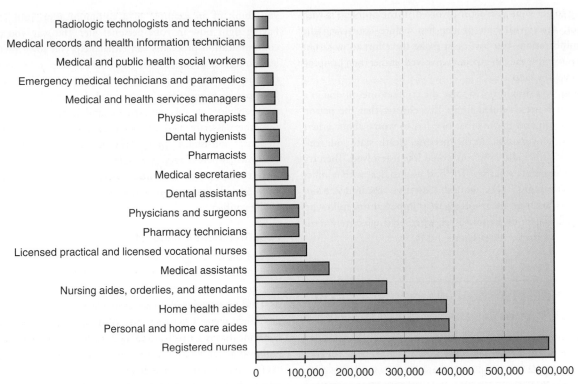

FIGURE 1-10 Projected change in total employment of select health care occupations, 2006-2016. Bureau of Labor Statistics, http://www.bls.gov/spotlight/2009/health_care/home.htm. Accessed August 31, 2015.

PROBLEM SOLVING AND CONFLICT MANAGEMENT

As a future member of the healthcare team, you frequently will face problems and conflict. Although we usually look at these situations as negative factors in our lives, problem solving and conflict management actually give us the opportunity to affect a potentially negative situation in a positive way. Learning how to manage problems can be very useful for your practice as a medical assistant and for your success as a student.

The first step in reaching an equitable solution to a problem or conflict is to identify the central issue. How many times have you known that you were upset about something but were not really sure why you felt that way? You cannot solve a problem or resolve a negative situation unless you are sure of what is at the root of your feelings. You need to understand the problem and gather as much information about the situation as possible before you decide to act. One way to do this is to ask yourself these questions:

- When does the situation occur and under what circumstances?
- How does it make me feel?
- Is someone else involved? Who? Is it the same person every time?
- What interferes with making a decision or resolving the conflict?

Once you understand the situation and how you feel about it, you need to decide whether it is worth the effort to resolve it. Prioritize your involvement. Sometimes situations and problems may arise that you are unable to resolve or that you may decide are not important enough to act on. For example, one of the students in your class occasionally checks her phone during lectures. You find her behavior distracting at times, but does it bother you enough to

do something about it? If it does, then you need to try to resolve the conflict. However, if it is a minor problem, then maybe it isn't worth the effort to talk to her about it. After you have gathered the details about the problem or conflict and you have decided it is important enough to act on, it is time to determine possible solutions. One way to do this is to ask for advice or brainstorm ideas with individuals you respect. Sometimes another person can give you special insight into the problem that you were unable to see on your own. After brainstorming for possible solutions, you should get feedback on the workability of the suggested solutions. An alternative to brainstorming possible solutions to the problem is to list the pros and cons of possible solutions on a piece of paper. Simply looking at a list of the positive and negative aspects of the solution may clarify how you could solve the problem. Before deciding on a particular solution, make sure you critically analyze the consequences of each proposed solution: Which one best meets your needs and has the potential for providing an outcome you can live with?

Finally, you are ready to implement the chosen solution. However, your work is not over yet. You need to evaluate the outcome of your decision and see whether it truly did meet your needs. If not, it may be time to review other possible solutions and try another approach.

Conflict management requires some additional consideration. If you are in conflict with a peer, an instructor, or a co-worker, it is important to follow certain guidelines. First of all, regardless of the situation, you should follow the chain of command to reach a reasonable resolution to the conflict. If you are in conflict with another student, then you should attempt to work it out with that person before trying to get your instructor involved. If the problem is with an instructor, meet with him or her first before contacting the school's administration. You first must make the effort to work out the issue directly with the other person involved, rather than jumping to another level for help.

In addition, you should try to solve the conflict one-on-one in a private place at a prescheduled time. This ensures that the person will meet with you and that neither one has to worry about others overhearing the conversation. At the meeting, clearly state your feelings about the conflict and how you would like it resolved. Then try to come to an agreeable solution. The best way to deal with conflict situations is through open, honest, assertive communication. However, just as with problem solving, it is important to follow up on the decided course of action to see whether it effectively dealt with the source of the conflict (Figure 1-11).

CRITICAL THINKING APPLICATION   **1-10**

Think about a serious problem you are currently facing. Use the brainstorming and/or pros and cons method for creating solutions to the problem. Implement your chosen solution, and follow up on its effectiveness. Did the problem-solving process help you manage the situation more effectively?

ASSERTIVE, AGGRESSIVE, AND PASSIVE COMMUNICATION

Effective communication is crucial in the healthcare environment. As a medical assistant, you are expected to communicate clearly and empathetically with patients, families, peers, and other healthcare professionals. Your ability to display professional communication behaviors will determine your success in this new profession. Can

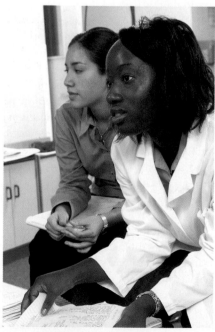

FIGURE 1-11 Dealing with conflict.

you think of an example of a communication problem you are having right now in your personal life? The way you respond to communication problems can either help you solve them fairly or lead to serious problems. We learn how to respond to conflict from the time we are young children. This learned behavior can range from passive to aggressive to assertive behaviors. Passive communication behaviors are on one extreme, and aggressive responses are on the other; assertive styles balance responses in the middle. Passive responses consistently protect the interests of another person over your own, whereas aggressive behaviors demand that your needs be met at the expense of another. Assertive communication strategies attempt to defend both your rights and those of the other individual in the conflict.

Assertive Communication

One of the challenges faced by workers in a healthcare environment is acting assertively when necessary. Assertive communication allows you to express your thoughts and feelings honestly and enables you to stand up for yourself in a reasonable, rational manner without an emotional scene. However, most of us are not born assertive; it is a behavior that must be learned, and many of us must practice it over and over again before it becomes a natural response.

Passive, or nonassertive, individuals often feel hurt when they are taken advantage of or are anxious about dealing with conflict. Just because they comply with what they are told to do or do not argue when they are treated unfairly does not mean that they are not upset about the situation. Often these individuals internalize their hurt and anxiety and eventually have an angry outburst because of built-up stress. Aggressive individuals, on the other hand, take advantage of others, appear self-righteous, and act in a superior way to get what they want. People who act aggressively may humiliate or hurt others to achieve their goals or to have their own needs satisfied.

Passive and Aggressive Behaviors and Language

An individual with passive or nonassertive body language displays the following behaviors when attempting to deal with conflict:
- Keeps the eyes downcast
- Shifts his or her weight when talking
- Has a slumped posture or wrings the hands
- Whines or uses a hesitant tone of voice
- May use the following phrases:
  - "Maybe" or "I guess"
  - "I wonder if you could…"
  - "Would you mind very much if…"
  - "It's not really important."

An aggressive person displays the following behaviors:
- Leans forward and points a finger when talking
- Raises the voice or sounds arrogant
- May use the following phrases:
  - "You'd better…"
  - "If you don't watch out…"
  - "Do it or else!"
  - "You should do it this way!"

Learning how to respond assertively in a potentially challenging situation enables us to be honest and direct with others while at the same time being emotionally honest with ourselves. The goal of assertive behavior is to treat others with respect while acknowledging our own feelings about the problem.

The first step in becoming assertive is to describe the situation and how it makes you feel. Perhaps you have a co-worker who is taking advantage of you; coming to work late, taking long breaks, not answering the phones, and so on. How does that make you feel? Are you angry, hurt, or disappointed? Decide which word best describes your feelings and, using an "I" sentence, clearly state how you feel about the situation. Be specific about the problem. If your statement is too general (e.g., "I am very hurt when you act like that"), the person you are confronting can either misunderstand or ignore you because he or she does not know specifically what is wrong. A statement such as, "I am very hurt that you take advantage of me by consistently being late for work, taking long breaks, and not helping with answering the phones," makes the problem very clear and expresses your feelings when the behavior occurs.

Acting assertively takes practice, practice, practice. In addition, just because you deliver a clear, concise, assertive message does not mean that the problem will be solved that quickly. Your assertive words must be combined with assertive body language to deliver a clear message about how serious you consider the situation. Remember, 80% to 90% of a message is nonverbal. Therefore, your "I" message must be accompanied by assertive behavior, including establishing eye contact and slightly raising your voice to get the individual's attention. And just because you deliver the perfect message does not mean you will always get what you want. The message may have to be repeated; do you really think someone who is habitually late for work is going to start showing up on time because of one assertive message? However, regardless of the outcome, you will feel better because you have honestly communicated how you feel about the situation, and you are actively working on a resolution of the problem.

CRITICAL THINKING APPLICATION   **1-11**

Do you consider yourself passive (nonassertive), assertive, or aggressive? Think about a recent conflict situation. How did you respond? Could assertive behaviors help you solve the problem while making you feel better about yourself?

Professional Behaviors Box

Perhaps the most difficult thing for you to learn is the art of assertiveness; that is, honestly informing others how you feel about a conflict situation, why you feel that way, and what changes you would like to see. The professional medical assistant faces many challenging situations. Communicating assertively helps you therapeutically resolve those conflicts. In addition, as a professional medical assistant, you are expected to act as the patient's advocate. To perform this crucial duty adequately, you must learn to communicate assertively with other individuals and organizations to meet the needs of your patients.

SUMMARY OF SCENARIO

One of the things Shawna can do to improve her learning is to determine her individual learning style. By understanding how she typically perceives and processes new information, she can plan the best methods for learning new material. In addition to understanding who she is as a learner, Shawna needs to practice successful coping mechanisms and time management skills to keep up with school and work responsibilities. Assertive communication, effective problem solving, and developing study skills that work for her are also keys to her success as a student.

SUMMARY OF LEARNING OBJECTIVES

1. **Define, spell, and pronounce the terms listed in the vocabulary.**
   Spelling and pronouncing medical terms correctly reinforce the medical assistant's credibility. Knowing the definitions of these terms promotes confidence in communication with patients and co-workers.

2. **Discuss competency-based education and adult learners.**
   The most important characteristic of competency-based education is that it measures learning and skill achievement over time. Students progress by demonstrating their competence, which means they prove that they have mastered the knowledge, skills, and professional behaviors required to achieve competency in a particular task.

3. **Summarize the importance of student portfolios in proving academic success and skill competency.**
   A portfolio is a collection of student materials that demonstrates learning. A comprehensive portfolio is developed throughout the courses in a medical assistant program and contains materials that demonstrate the knowledge and skills achieved by the student throughout the course of

study. A comprehensive portfolio includes examples of work completed in each course and proof of the skills achieved. It can be used to create individual interview portfolios that demonstrate knowledge and skill achievement.

4. **Examine your learning preferences and interpret how your learning style affects your success as a student.**
   Learning preferences are the ways you like to learn and that have proven successful in the past. Your learning style is determined by your individual method of perceiving or examining new material and the way you process it or make it your own. People are either concrete or abstract perceivers and either active or reflective processors.

5. **Differentiate between adaptive and nonadaptive coping mechanisms.**
   Adaptive coping mechanisms help a person gain control over a stressful situation; negative or nonadaptive strategies may be effective short term but often lead to long-term stress.

Continued

SUMMARY OF LEARNING OBJECTIVES—*continued*

6. **Apply time management strategies to make the most of your learning opportunities.**

   Using effective time management strategies, such as setting goals, prioritizing, getting organized, and avoiding procrastination, results in a more successful student and an effective medical assistant.

7. **Integrate effective study skills into your daily activities.**

   Study skills, such as memory techniques, active learning, brain tricks, effective reading methods, note-taking strategies, and mind maps, all help students to be more successful.

8. **Design test-taking strategies that help you take charge of your success.**

   Test-taking strategies include preparing adequately for the examination, controlling negative thoughts during the examination, and understanding how to deal with different types of questions.

9. **Incorporate critical thinking and reflection to help you make mental connections as you learn material.**

   Critical thinking can be defined as *thorough thinking* because it considers all sides of the information without bias. Reflection is the process of thinking about or reviewing information before acting.

10. **Analyze healthcare results as reported in graphs and tables.**

    Tables and graphs can be helpful tools in many aspects of healthcare, but you must take the time to analyze the information they present so that you process it accurately. Tables are used to outline and summarize significant healthcare information, and graphs diagram or create a picture that represents information and its relationships. To maximize your learning throughout the medical assistant program, you should use the information in tables and graphs to help prepare you to perform as an entry-level medical assistant.

11. **Apply problem-solving techniques to manage conflict and overcome barriers to your success.**

    Problem-solving and conflict management techniques are crucial to your success. First, identify the central issue and how you feel about it; then, consider possible solutions and their potential results, implement the chosen solution, and analyze the results.

12. **Relate assertiveness, aggressiveness, and passive behaviors to professional communication and discuss the role of assertiveness in effective communication.**

    Passive responses consistently protect the interests of another person over your own, whereas aggressive behaviors demand that your needs be met at the expense of another. Assertive communication strategies attempt to defend both your rights and those of the other individual in the conflict.

    Assertive communication allows you to express your thoughts and feelings honestly and enables you to stand up for yourself in a reasonable, rational manner without an emotional scene. Learning how to respond assertively in a potentially challenging situation enables us to be honest and direct with others while at the same time being emotionally honest with ourselves. The goal of assertive behavior is to treat others with respect while acknowledging our own feelings about the problem.

CONNECTIONS

Study Guide Connection: Go to the Chapter 1 Study Guide. Read and complete the activities.

evolve Evolve Connection: Go to the Chapter 1 link at *evolve.elsevier.com/kinn* to complete the Chapter Review Quiz. Check out the other resources listed for this chapter to make the most of what you have learned from Competency-Based Education and the Medical Assistant Student.

THE MEDICAL ASSISTANT AND THE HEALTHCARE TEAM

2

SCENARIO

Carmen Angelos is a new student in a medical assisting program accredited by the Commission on Accreditation of Allied Health Education Programs (CAAHEP) at Butler County Community College. Carmen is returning to school after working at a local pharmacy for 5 years, where she became very interested in pursuing a career in medical assisting. She has been out of high school for a few years but is very excited about her new career choice.

While studying this chapter, think about the following questions:

- Why is it important to learn about professional medical assisting organizations?
- What is a typical job description for an entry-level medical assistant?
- What allied health professionals might you work with as a medical assistant?
- Why is it important for medical assisting students to learn about the various healthcare facilities and medical specialties?
- How will scope of practice and standards of care determine your role as a medical assistant?

LEARNING OBJECTIVES

1. Define, spell, and pronounce the terms listed in the vocabulary.
2. Summarize the history of medicine and its significance to the medical assisting profession.
3. Identify national departments and agencies that focus on health.
4. List professional medical assisting organizations.
5. Discuss the typical job description of a medical assistant and describe the role of the medical assistant as a patient navigator.
6. Identify a variety of allied health professionals who are part of the healthcare team.
7. Summarize the various types of medical specialties and healthcare facilities.
8. Define a patient-centered medical home (PCMH) and discuss its five core functions and attributes.
9. Differentiate between scope of practice and standards of care for medical assistants, and compare and contrast provider and medical assistant roles in terms of standard of care.

VOCABULARY

accreditation (uh-kre-duh-ta′-shun) The process by which an organization is recognized for adherence to a group of standards that meet or exceed the expectations of the accrediting agency.

allopathic (al-o-path′-ik) A system of medical practice that treats disease by the use of remedies, such as medications and surgery, to produce effects different from those caused by the disease under treatment; medical doctors (MDs) and osteopaths (DOs) practice allopathic medicine; also called *conventional medicine*.

complementary and alternative medicine (CAM) A group of diverse medical and healthcare systems, practices, and products that are not generally considered part of conventional medicine. Complementary medicine is used in combination with conventional medicine (allopathic or osteopathic); alternative medicine is used instead of conventional medicine.

contamination (kun-ta-mu-na′-shun) The process by which something becomes harmful or unusable through contact with something unclean.

holistic (ho-lis′-tik) A form of healing that considers the whole person (i.e., body, mind, spirit, and emotions) in individual treatment plans.

hospice (hos′-pus) A concept of care that involves health professionals and volunteers who provide medical, psychological, and spiritual support to terminally ill patients and their loved ones.

indicator An important point or group of statistical values that, when evaluated, indicates the quality of care provided in a healthcare facility.

negligence Conduct that falls below the standards of behavior established by law; a *negligent act* is one that does not meet the standards of what is expected of a reasonably prudent person acting under similar circumstances.

subluxations (sub-luk-sa′-shuns) Slight misalignments of the vertebrae or a partial dislocation.

triage The process of sorting patients to determine medical need and the priority of care.

Medical assistants are multiskilled healthcare workers who function under the direction of a licensed provider and are primarily employed in outpatient or ambulatory care facilities, such as medical offices and clinics. According to the U.S. Bureau of Labor Statistics, medical assisting is one of the nation's fastest growing careers, and employment opportunities are projected to grow 29% through 2022.

This growth in job opportunities for medical assistants is due to multiple factors, including a steady increase in the aging population as baby-boomers spur demand for preventive health services from physician offices and ambulatory care centers. Since medical assistants are trained in both administrative and clinical skills they are perfect employees to meet the needs of this increasing population. In addition, the Affordable Care Act has given millions of uninsured Americans the opportunity to have health insurance, which means physician practices and clinics will be caring for an ever-increasing number of patients. The switch to electronic health records (EHRs) in ambulatory care centers will also open up employment opportunities for medical assistants who are trained in EHR computer software.

THE HISTORY OF MEDICINE

Although religious and mythologic beliefs were the basis for care for the sick in ancient times, evidence suggests that drugs, surgery, and other treatments based on theories about the body were used as early as 5,000 BC. Moses presented rules of health to the Hebrews in approximately 1205 BC. He was the first advocate of preventive medicine and is considered the first public health officer. Moses knew that some animal diseases could be passed to humans and that **contamination** existed; therefore, a religious law was developed forbidding humans to eat or drink from dirty dishes. The people of that era believed that doing so would defile their bodies, and they would lose their souls.

Hippocrates, known as the Father of Medicine, is the most famous of the ancient Greek physicians. He was born in 450 BC on the island of Cos in Greece. He is best remembered for the Hippocratic Oath, which has been administered to physicians for more than 2,000 years. To this day, most graduating medical school students swear to some form of the oath (Figure 2-1). Hippocrates is credited with taking mysticism out of medicine and giving it a scientific basis. During this period of history, most believed that illness was caused by demonic possession; to cure the illness, the demon had to be removed from the body. Hippocrates' clinical descriptions of diseases and his volumes on epidemics, fevers, epilepsy, fractures, and instruments were studied for centuries. He believed that the body had the capacity to heal itself and that the physician's role was to help nature. He described four "humors": blood, phlegm, yellow bile, and black bile, which he believed must be in balance for the body to maintain a healthy state.

Medical knowledge developed slowly, and distribution of such knowledge was poor. In the seventeenth century, European academies or societies were established, consisting of small groups of men who met to discuss subjects of mutual interest. One of the earliest academies was the Royal Society of London, formed in 1662. In the United States, medical education was greatly influenced by the Johns Hopkins University School of Medicine in Baltimore, Maryland, established in the early 1890s. The school admitted only college graduates with at least one year's training in the natural sciences. The clinical education at Johns Hopkins was superior because the school partnered with Johns Hopkins Hospital, which had been created expressly for teaching and research by members of the medical faculty. Table 2-1 presents selected medical pioneers and their achievements.

I swear to fulfill, to the best of my ability and judgment, this covenant:

I will respect the hard-won scientific gains of those physicians in whose steps I walk, and gladly share such knowledge as is mine with those who are to follow.

I will apply, for the benefit of the sick, all measures [that] are required, avoiding those twin traps of overtreatment and therapeutic nihilism.

I will remember that there is art to medicine as well as science, and that warmth, sympathy, and understanding may outweigh the surgeon's knife or the chemist's drug.

I will not be ashamed to say "I know not," nor will I fail to call in my colleagues when the skills of another are needed for a patient's recovery.

I will respect the privacy of my patients, for their problems are not disclosed to me that the world may know. Most especially must I tread with care in matters of life and death. If it is given me to save a life, all thanks. But it may also be within my power to take a life; this awesome responsibility must be faced with great humbleness and awareness of my own frailty. Above all, I must not play at God.

I will remember that I do not treat a fever chart, a cancerous growth, but a sick human being, whose illness may affect the person's family and economic stability. My responsibility includes these related problems, if I am to care adequately for the sick.

I will prevent disease whenever I can, for prevention is preferable to cure.

I will remember that I remain a member of society, with special obligations to all my fellow human beings, those sound of mind and body as well as the infirm.

If I do not violate this oath, may I enjoy life and art, respected while I live and remembered with affection thereafter. May I always act so as to preserve the finest traditions of my calling and may I long experience the joy of healing those who seek my help.

Written in 1964 by Louis Lasagna, Academic Dean of the School of Medicine at Tufts University, and used in many medical schools today.

FIGURE 2-1 Modern version of the Hippocratic Oath.

TABLE 2-1   Medical Pioneers and Their Achievements

NAME	ACHIEVEMENT	NAME	ACHIEVEMENT
Andreas Vesalius (1514-1564)	Father of modern anatomy; wrote first anatomy book	Robert Koch (1843-1910)	Developed Koch's postulates, a theory of causative agents for disease; discovered the cause of cholera
William Harvey (1578-1657)	Discovered the circulatory system	William Roentgen (1845-1923)	Discovered the x-ray
Anton van Leeuwenhoek (1632-1723)	First to observe microbes through a lens; developed the first microscope	Walter Reed (1851-1902)	Proved that yellow fever was transmitted by mosquito bites while in the U.S. Army serving in Cuba
John Hunter (1728-1793)	Founder of scientific surgery	Paul Ehrlich (1854-1915)	Injected chemicals for the first time to treat disease (syphilis)
Edward Jenner (1749-1823)	Developed smallpox vaccine	Marie Curie (1867-1934)	Discovered radium and polonium
Ignaz Semmelweis (1818-1865)	First physician to recommend hand washing to prevent puerperal fever; believed there was a connection between performing autopsies and then delivering babies that caused puerperal fever in new mothers	Alexander Fleming (1881-1955)	Discovered penicillin
		Albert Sabin (1906-1993)	Developed the oral live-virus vaccine for polio 10 years after Salk developed the first injected vaccine
Florence Nightingale (1820-1910)	Founder of nursing	Virginia Apgar (1909-1974)	Founded neonatology; developed the Apgar score, which assesses the status of newborns
Clara Barton (1821-1912)	Established the American Red Cross	Jonas Salk (1914-1955)	Developed the first safe and effective injectable vaccine for polio
Elizabeth Blackwell (1821-1910)	First woman in the United States to earn a Doctor of Medicine degree	Christiaan Barnard (1922-2001)	Performed the first human heart transplant
Louis Pasteur (1822-1895)	Father of bacteriology and preventive medicine; developed pasteurization and established the connection between germs and disease	Edwin Carl Wood (1929-2011)	Pioneered the technique of in vitro fertilization (IVF)
Joseph Lister (1827-1912)	Father of sterile surgery; developed antiseptic methods for surgery	David Ho (1952-)	Research pioneer in acquired immunodeficiency syndrome (AIDS)

The History of Medical Assisting

As the practice of medicine became more organized and more complicated, some physicians hired nurses to help in their office practices. Gradually, the administrative part of running a practice became increasingly complicated and time-consuming, and physicians realized that they needed an assistant with both administrative and clinical training. Nurses were likely to have training only in clinical skills; therefore, many physicians began training individuals—medical assistants—to assist with all the office duties.

The first medical assistants started working in individual physicians' offices with on-the-job training to help out when an extra pair of hands was needed. Today medical assisting is one of the most respected allied health fields in the industry, and training is readily available through community colleges, junior colleges, and private educational institutions throughout the United States.

CRITICAL THINKING APPLICATION   **2-1**
- In Table 2-1, review the list of individuals who have made significant contributions to medicine. Which one do you believe had the greatest impact on modern healthcare?
- Consider how the medical assisting profession began. How do you think advances in medicine throughout history have affected the current practice of medical assisting?

NATIONAL DEPARTMENTS AND AGENCIES THAT FOCUS ON HEALTH

In the United States, the following agencies focus primarily on health and on safety in the workplace.

- *Department of Health and Human Services (HHS):* The principal U.S. department for providing essential human services and protecting the health of all Americans, especially those unable to help themselves. The HHS is made up of more than 300 programs covering research; child services, including immunizations; financial assistance for low-income families; programs for the elderly; and oversight of Medicare and Medicaid programs.
- *Centers for Disease Control and Prevention (CDC):* The principal U.S. federal agency concerned with health. It conducts research on health-related issues and serves as a clearinghouse for information and statistics associated with healthcare. The divisions of the CDC focus on specific health-related issues; some of these divisions are the National Center for HIV, STD, and TB Prevention; the Public Health Practice Program Office; the National Center on Birth Defects and Developmental Disabilities; and the National Center for Health Statistics. The CDC establishes regulations that affect all healthcare facilities.
- *National Institutes of Health (NIH):* The NIH is part of the HHS and seeks to improve the health of the American people. It supports and conducts biomedical research into the causes and prevention of diseases and uses a modern communications system to furnish biomedical information to the healthcare professions. It consists of 27 different institutes and centers, in addition to the National Library of Medicine. Thousands of research projects are under way in NIH laboratories and clinics at any given time. The NIH also provides funding for research projects conducted at universities, medical schools, and hospitals.
- *Occupational Safety and Health Administration (OSHA):* An agency of the Department of Labor responsible for establishing and enforcing regulations to protect individuals in the workplace. OSHA's influence in the healthcare setting is far-reaching, especially in the areas of infection control and the development of the Bloodborne Pathogens Standard to protect healthcare workers and patients from contracting infectious diseases in a healthcare setting.

PROFESSIONAL MEDICAL ASSISTING ORGANIZATIONS

In 1955 the Kansas Medical Assistants Society initiated a meeting to consider the creation of a national organization. This resulted in the formation of the American Association of Medical Assistants (AAMA) in 1956, which remains the only association devoted exclusively to the medical assisting profession. Maxine Williams, CMA-A, was elected the first AAMA president in 1957. In 1959 a Certification Committee was appointed to develop the AAMA Certification Program, and the first certification examinations were administered in 1963.

In 1974 the U.S. Office of Education recognized AMA/AAMA as an official accrediting agency for medical assisting programs in public and private institutions. In 1993 the **accreditation** process was restructured and became the responsibility of the Commission on Accreditation of Allied Health Education Programs (CAAHEP). Only graduates of CAAHEP-accredited programs or of programs accredited by the Accrediting Bureau of Health Education Schools (ABHES) can sit for the National Certification Examination to become Certified Medical Assistants (CMA [AAMA]). The AAMA has continued to grow; in 2014, it reported that the number of certified medical assistants (CMA [AAMA]) with current credentials exceeded 75,000. More information about the AAMA is available on the organization's website: *www.aama-ntl.org/*.

The American Medical Technologists (AMT) was founded in 1939 as a nationally recognized certification agency for multiple allied health professionals, including Medical Laboratory Technician (MLT), Phlebotomy Technician (RPT), Medical Assistant (RMA), Medical Administrative Specialist (CMAS), and Dental Assistant (RDA). The AMT certification examinations are developed, administered, and analyzed by a committee of subject matter experts. Once certification has been granted, applicants automatically become members of the AMT and earn the credential RMA. AMT is accredited by the National Commission for Certifying Agencies (NCCA). Additional information on the AMT is available on the organization's website: *www.americanmedtech.org/*.

The National Healthcareer Association (NHA) was established in 1990 to offer certification examinations in a number of allied health programs; for example, certification is granted for pharmacy, phlebotomy, and electrocardiography (ECG) technicians. The NHA also offers two different medical assisting certifications: Certified Clinical Medical Assistant (CCMA) and Certified Medical Administrative Assistant (CMAA). The NHA is not involved in program curriculum standards or program accreditation. It simply offers certification if the applicant can successfully pass the NHA examination developed for each particular medical discipline. You can find out more about the certifications offered through the NHA at the company's website: *www.nhanow.com/*.

MEDICAL ASSISTANT JOB DESCRIPTION

Medical assistants are the only allied health professionals specifically trained to work in ambulatory care settings, such as physicians' offices, clinics, and group practices. That training includes both clinical and administrative skills, covering a multitude of medical practice needs. The skills performed by an entry-level medical assistant depend on his or her place of employment, but all graduates of accredited programs are taught a similar skill set.

Clinical skills include:

- Assisting during physical examinations
- Performing patient screening procedures
- Assisting with minor surgical procedures, including sterilization procedures
- Performing electrocardiograms (ECGs)
- Obtaining and recording vital signs and medical histories
- Performing phlebotomy
- Performing tests permitted by the Clinical Laboratory Improvement Amendments (i.e., CLIA-waived tests)
- Collecting and managing laboratory specimens
- Following OSHA regulations on infection control
- Administering vaccinations and medications as ordered by the practitioner

- Performing patient education and coaching initiatives within the scope of practice
- Documenting accurately in a paper record or an EHR
- Performing first aid procedures as needed
- Performing infection control procedures
- Applying therapeutic communication techniques
- Adapting to the special needs of a patient based on his or her developmental life stage, cultural diversity, and individual communication barriers
- Acting as a patient advocate or navigator, including referring patients to community resources
- Acting within legal and ethical boundaries

Administrative skills include:
- Answering telephones
- Managing patient scheduling
- Creating and maintaining patient health records
- Documenting accurately in a paper record and an EHR
- Performing routine maintenance of facility equipment
- Performing basic practice finance procedures
- Coordinating third-party reimbursement
- Performing procedural and diagnostic coding
- Communicating professionally with patients, family members, practitioners, peers, and the public
- Managing facility correspondence
- Performing patient education and coaching initiatives within the scope of practice
- Following legal and ethical principles
- Complying with facility safety practices

These lengthy lists of capabilities that make up the basic skill set are not all that is expected of entry-level medical assistants; they also play a significant role as the patient's advocate (Figure 2-2). Current research describes this role as being a "patient navigator." If you have ever had a loved one who was very ill and required medical attention from a number of different practitioners and allied health specialty groups, you understand what a complex and overwhelming task it can be to make decisions and coordinate a loved one's care. Dr. Harold P. Freeman, a surgical oncologist at Harlem Hospital, pioneered the concept of patient navigation in 1990. His goal was to eliminate the barriers to timely cancer screening, diagnosis, treatment, and supportive care so often experienced by medically underserved or minority communities. These individuals consistently faced financial, cultural, healthcare system, and communication barriers. In 2005 policymakers in Congress passed the Patient Navigator Outreach and Chronic Disease Prevention Act, which authorized the Secretary of Health and Human Services to make grants through 2010 for the development of patient navigator programs. A total of $25 million was awarded over 5 years to develop community-based navigation programs, and the Center to Reduce Cancer Health Disparities was created at the NIH.

Data from navigator programs show that they can improve the diagnosis of cancer and treatment outcomes. Studies of the original navigation program at Harlem Hospital showed that patient 5-year survival rates for breast cancer improved from 39% before development of the program to 70%.

Since its origin at Harlem Hospital, the program designed to help cancer patients has expanded and spread to other medical disciplines. The Affordable Care Act (ACA) requires that "insurance navigators" be available to help consumers research and enroll in health insurance through the law's health insurance marketplace.

CRITICAL THINKING APPLICATION   2-2

Medical assistants have long been encouraged to act as patient advocates in the ambulatory care setting. Given their multilevel training, medical assistants can help patients navigate through a wide variety of confusing issues. Let's think about how you could help a patient and family navigate the following scenario:

Mrs. Kate Glasgow is an 82-year-old patient in the primary care practice where you work. Mrs. Glasgow recently suffered a mild cerebrovascular accident (CVA), and her son is trying to help coordinate her care. Mrs. Glasgow does not understand when or how to take her new medications; she is concerned about whether her health insurance will cover the cost of frequent clinic appointments and assistive devices; she doesn't understand how to prepare for an MRI the provider ordered; and she dislikes having to have blood drawn every week. Based on what you have learned about the job description of a medical assistant, how can you help navigate Mrs. Glasgow and her family through this complex and challenging medical regimen? What specific actions could help Mrs. Glasgow and her son mange her care?

ALLIED HEALTH PROFESSIONALS

The definition of an allied health professional can vary, but it loosely refers to those who can act only under the authority of a licensed medical practitioner (e.g., MD, DO, optometrist, dentist, pharmacist, podiatrist, or chiropractor). Allied health professionals include respiratory therapists, radiation therapists, occupational therapists, physical therapists, technologists of various types, dental hygienists, medical assistants, phlebotomists, pharmacy technicians, and other professionals who do not independently diagnose and prescribe treatment, but perform diagnostic procedures, therapeutic services, and provide care.

The allied health professions fall into two broad categories: technicians (assistants) and therapists. Technicians are trained to perform procedures, and their education lasts 2 years or less. They are required to work under the supervision of medical providers or licensed therapists. This part of the allied health field includes, among others,

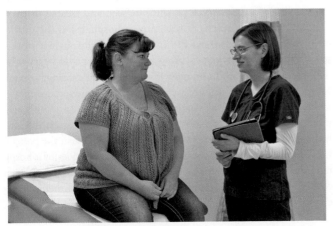

FIGURE 2-2 Medical assistant counseling a patient.

physical therapy assistants, medical laboratory technicians, radiology technicians, occupational therapy assistants, recreational therapy assistants, respiratory therapy technicians, and medical assistants (Table 2-2).

The educational process for nurses and therapists is more intensive. These professions require a state-issued license and an advanced degree, showing that the individual is trained to evaluate patients, diagnose conditions, develop treatment plans, and understand the rationale behind various treatments (Table 2-3).

Allied health professionals typically work as part of a healthcare team, which is what you will do as a professional medical assistant.

As a new medical assistant, you will enter the ranks of an ever-growing group of allied health professionals that provide services for patients in a variety of settings in today's healthcare system. Allied health professionals comprise nearly 60% of the healthcare workforce. The term "allied health" is used to identify a cluster of health professions, encompassing as many as 200 careers. In the United States, about 5 million allied health professionals work in more than 80 different professions; they represent approximately 60% of all healthcare providers.

MEDICAL PROFESSIONALS

Physicians and providers (e.g., nurse practitioners and physician assistants) are portals of entry or first contacts for patients seeking medical care. After the initial assessment or with the diagnosis of a more complex health issue, patients may be referred to a medical specialist for further examination and treatment. Primary care providers (PCPs) are often referred to as "gatekeepers," because most insurance policies require that patients first must be assessed and, if possible, treated by the PCP before they are referred to a specialist for more advanced assessment and care.

Doctors of Medicine

Medical doctors (Doctor of Medicine [MD]) are considered **allopathic** physicians. They are the most widely recognized type of physician. They diagnose illness and disease and prescribe treatment for their patients. MDs have a wide variety of rights, including writing prescriptions, performing surgery, offering wellness advice, and performing preventive medicine procedures. Becoming an MD requires 4 years of undergraduate university training (premed) and 4 years of medical school. Regardless of where premed students attend college, a national standard of course work is required to apply to medical school. They must take entry and advanced levels of biology, physics, organic and inorganic chemistry, mathematics, English, humanities, and social sciences. The United States has approximately 125 allopathic medical schools. After medical school, the student faces 3 to 8 years of residency programs, depending on the medical specialty he or she pursues. After completion of a residency program, a physician can obtain board certification in one or more of 37 different specialty areas recognized by the American Board of Medical Specialties (Table 2-4). An MD must have a state license to practice, and continuing education is required to maintain the license. Graduates of foreign medical schools usually can obtain a license in the United States after passing an examination and completing a residency program in this country.

Doctors of Osteopathy

Osteopathic physicians (Doctor of Osteopathy [DO]) complete requirements similar to those of MDs to graduate and practice medicine. Osteopaths use medicine and surgery, in addition to osteopathic manipulative therapy (OMT), in treating their patients. Andrew Taylor Still is considered the father of osteopathic medicine, which he established in 1874. He believed in a more **holistic** approach to medicine, and although he was an MD, he founded the American School of Osteopathy in Kirksville, Missouri. The school originally was chartered to offer an MD degree but later focused more on the osteopathic approach. DOs stress preventive medicine and holistic patient care, in addition to a special focus on the musculoskeletal system and OMT. Premed students moving toward osteopathic medicine complete the same undergraduate course work as allopathic candidates and 4 years of medical studies at a school for osteopathic medicine. Over the years there have become fewer differences between allopathic and osteopathic programs, with many DO physicians earning residency programs in the same institutions as MDs.

Doctors of Chiropractic

Chiropractors (Doctor of Chiropractic [DC]) typically are thought of as "bone doctors," but they actually focus on the nervous system to help patients live healthier lives. The nervous system is the master system of the body, controlling and coordinating all the other systems. Information from the environment, both internal and external, moves through the spinal cord to get to the brain, and in the same manner, information from the brain moves through the spinal cord to reach the body in a two-way flow of communication. The intention of the chiropractic adjustment is to remove any disruptions or distortions of this energy flow that may be caused by slight misalignments, which chiropractors call **subluxations**. Chiropractic colleges require undergraduate studies in biology, organic and inorganic chemistry, physics, English, and the humanities and then 3 to 4 years studying chiropractic services. Chiropractic care is one of the most common fields of **complementary and alternative medicine (CAM)**.

Hospitalists

Hospitalists are physicians whose primary professional focus is the general medical care of hospitalized patients. Most hospitalists are employed by the healthcare facility instead of having individual freestanding offices in which patients are seen and treated. Perhaps the most attractive benefit of becoming a hospitalist is the quality of life for the physician and his or her family. Hospitalists work a specific, set number of hours each week and receive a set salary from their employers. In addition, most institutions that employ hospitalists cover these physicians with blanket malpractice insurance, saving the practitioner the expense of costly premiums. Although the hospitalist is in charge of the patient while the person is in the hospital, if the patient has a PCP, he or she may still visit the patient. Of course, the patient is not required to use the services of a hospitalist and may be cared for by the attending physician of his or her choice. The hospitalist would still refer the patient to medical specialists as needed for more advanced care.

Text continued on p. 25

TABLE 2-2   Allied Health Occupations Recognized by the American Medical Association

TITLE	CREDENTIAL	JOB DESCRIPTION
Anesthesiology assistant	AA	Functions as a specialty physician assistant under the direction of a licensed and qualified anesthesiologist; assists in developing and implementing the anesthesia care plan.
Art therapist	ATR	Uses drawings and other art and media forms to assess, treat, and rehabilitate patients with mental, emotional, physical, and/or developmental disorders.
Athletic trainer	ATC	Provides a variety of services, including injury prevention, assessment, immediate care, treatment, and rehabilitation after physical injury or trauma.
Audiologist	CCC-A	Identifies individuals with symptoms of hearing loss and other auditory, balance, and related neural problems; assesses the nature of those problems and helps individuals manage them.
Blood bank technology specialist	SBB	Performs routine and specialized tests in blood center and transfusion services, using methods that conform to the accepted standards in the blood bank industry.
Diagnostic cardiovascular sonographer/technologist	RDCS, RVT	Using invasive or noninvasive techniques (or both), performs diagnostic examinations and therapeutic interventions for the heart and blood vessels at the request of a physician.
Clinical laboratory science/medical technologist	MT, MLT	In conjunction with pathologists, performs tests to diagnose the causes and nature of disease; also develops data on blood, tissues, and fluids of the human body using a variety of methodologies.
Counseling-related professional	LPC, LMHC	Deals with human development through support, therapeutic approaches, consultation, evaluation, teaching, and research; practices the art of helping people to grow.
Cytotechnologist	CT	Works with pathologists to evaluate cellular material from all body sites, primarily through use of the microscope; examines specimens for normal and abnormal cytologic changes, including malignancies.
Dance therapist	DTR, ADTR	Uses the psychotherapeutic properties of movement as a process that furthers the emotional, cognitive, social, and physical integration of the patient as a tool for healing.
Dental assistant, dental hygienist, dental laboratory technician	CDA, RDH, CDT	Performs a wide range of tasks, from assisting the dentist to teaching patients how to prevent oral disease and maintain oral health.
Diagnostic medical sonographer	RDMS	Uses medical ultrasound to gather sonographic data, which can aid the diagnosis of a variety of conditions and diseases; also monitors fetal development.
Dietitian, dietetic technician	DTR	Integrates and applies the principles of food science, nutrition, biochemistry, physiology, food management, and behavior to achieve and maintain good health.
Electroneurodiagnostic technologist	REEG-T	Records and studies the electrical activity of the brain and nervous system; obtains interpretable recordings of patients' nervous system function.
Genetics counselor	IGC	Provides genetic services to individuals and families seeking information about the occurrence or risk of a genetic condition or birth defect.
Health information management professional	RHIA, RHIT	Provides expert assistance in the systems and processes for health information management, including planning, engineering, administration, application, and policy making.
Kinesiotherapist	RKT	Provides rehabilitation exercise and education designed to reverse or minimize debilitation and enhance the functional capacity of medically stable patients.

Continued

TABLE 2-2   Allied Health Occupations Recognized by the American Medical Association—*continued*

TITLE	CREDENTIAL	JOB DESCRIPTION
Massage therapist	MT	Applies manual techniques, and may apply adjunctive techniques, with the intention of positively affecting the health and well-being of a patient or client.
Medical assistant	CMA, RMA, CCMA, CMAA	Functions as a member of the healthcare delivery team and performs both administrative and clinical procedures and duties; a multiskilled health professional.
Medical illustrator	MI	Specializes in the visual display and communication of scientific information; creates visuals and designs communication tools for teaching both medical professionals and the public.
Music therapist	MT-BC	Uses music in a therapeutic relationship to address the physical, emotional, cognitive, and social needs of individuals of all ages; assesses the strengths and needs of clients and patients.
Nuclear medicine technologist	RT	Uses the nuclear properties of radioactive and stable nuclides to make diagnostic evaluations of anatomic or physiologic conditions of the body; also provides therapy with unsealed radioactive sources.
Ophthalmic laboratory technician, medical technician/technologist	COT, COMT	Collects data and performs clinical evaluations; performs tests and protocols required by ophthalmologists; assists in the treatment of patients.
Orthoptist	CO	Performs a series of diagnostic tests and measurements on patients with visual disorders; helps design a treatment plan to correct disorders of vision, eye movements, and alignment.
Orthotist/prosthetist	RTO, RTP, RTPO	Designs and fits devices (orthoses) to patients who have disabling conditions of the limbs and spine and/or partial or total absence of a limb.
Perfusionist	CCP	Operates extracorporeal circulation and autotransfusion equipment during any medical situation in which the patient's respiratory or circulatory function must be supported or temporarily replaced.
Pharmacy technician	CPhT	Assists pharmacists with duties that do not require the expertise or judgment of a licensed pharmacist.
Radiation therapist, radiographer	RRTD	Delivers prescribed dosages of radiation to patients for therapeutic purposes; provides appropriate patient care and maintains accurate records of the treatment provided.
Rehabilitation counselor	CRC	Determines and coordinates services to assist people with disabilities in moving from psychological and economic dependence to independence.
Respiratory therapist, respiratory therapy technician	RRT, CRT, RPFT, CPFT	Evaluates, treats, and manages patients of all ages with respiratory illnesses and other cardiopulmonary disorders. Advanced respiratory therapists exercise considerable independent judgment.
Surgical assistant	CSA	Assists in exposure, hemostasis, closure, and other intraoperative technical functions that help surgeons carry out a safe operation with optimal results for the patient.
Surgical technologist	ST, CST	Helps prepare patients for surgery and maintain the sterile field in the surgical suite, making sure all members of the surgical team follow sterile technique.
Therapeutic recreation specialist	CTRS	Uses treatment, education, and recreation services to help people with illnesses, disabilities, and other conditions develop and use their leisure in ways that enhance their health.

TABLE 2-3   Licensed Healthcare Professions

TITLE	CREDENTIAL	JOB DESCRIPTION
Certified nurse midwife	CNM	RN with additional training and certification; performs physical exams; prescribes medications, including contraceptive methods; orders laboratory tests as needed; provides prenatal care, gynecologic care, labor and birth care, and health education and counseling to women of all ages.
Diagnostic cardiac sonographer or vascular technologist	DCS or DVT	Assists in the diagnosis and treatment of cardiac and vascular diseases and disorders; performs noninvasive tests, including echocardiographs and electrocardiographs.
Emergency medical technician	EMT	Progresses through several levels of training, each providing more advanced skills. EMT's medical education encompasses managing respiratory, cardiac, and trauma cases and often emergency childbirth. Some states also recognize specialties in the EMT field, such as EMT-Cardiac, which includes training in cardiac arrhythmias, and EMT-Shock Trauma, which includes starting intravenous fluids and administering specific medications.
Licensed practical or vocational nurse	LPN or LVN	Provides bedside care, assisting with the day-to-day personal care of inpatients; assesses patients, documents their progress, and administers medications and intravenous fluids when allowed by law; often works in hospitals or skilled nursing facilities and in physicians' offices.
Medical technologist	MT	Performs diagnostic testing on blood, body fluids, and other types of specimens to assist the provider in arriving at a diagnosis.
Nurse anesthetist	NA	RN who administers anesthetics to patients during care provided by surgeons, physicians, dentists, or other qualified health professionals.
Nurse practitioner	NP	Provides basic patient care services, including diagnosing and prescribing medications for common illnesses; must have advanced academic training, beyond the registered nurse (RN) degree, and also must have extensive clinical experience.
Occupational therapist	OT	Assists in helping patients compensate for loss of function.
Paramedic	Paramedic	Specially trained in advanced emergency skills to aid patients in life-threatening situations.
Physical therapist	PT	Assists patients in regaining their mobility and improving their strength and range of motion. They devise treatment plans in conjunction with the patient's physician.
Physician assistant	PA	Provides direct patient care services under the supervision of a licensed physician; trained to diagnose and treat patients as directed by the physician, and in most states are allowed to write prescriptions; take patient histories, order and interpret tests, perform physical examinations, and make diagnostic decisions.
Radiology technician	RT	Uses various machines to help the provider diagnose and treat certain diseases; machines may include x-ray equipment, ultrasonographic machines, and magnetic resonance imaging (MRI) scanners.
Registered dietitian	RD	Thoroughly trained in nutrition and the different types of diets patients require to improve or maintain their condition. They design healthy diets for patients during hospital stays and can help plan menus for home use. They also teach patients about their recommended diet.
Registered nurse	RN	Provides direct patient care, assesses patients, and determines care plans; they have many career options.
Respiratory therapist	RT	Commonly uses oxygen therapy to assist with breathing; also performs diagnostic tests that measure lung capacity. Most RTs work in hospitals. All types of patients receive respiratory care, including newborns and geriatric patients.

TABLE 2-4   Examples of Medical Specialties

SPECIALTY	PRACTITIONER'S TITLE	DESCRIPTION
Allergy and immunology	Allergist/immunologist	Allergists/immunologists are trained to evaluate disorders and diseases of the immune system. This includes conditions such as adverse reactions to drugs and food, anaphylaxis, and problems related to autoimmune diseases, asthma, and insect stings.
Anesthesiology	Anesthesiologist	Anesthesiologists provide pain relief and pain management during surgical procedures and also for patients with long-standing conditions accompanied by pain.
Colon and rectal surgery	Colorectal surgeon	Colorectal surgeons diagnose and treat conditions affecting the intestines, rectum, and anal area, in addition to organs affected by intestinal disease.
Dermatology	Dermatologist	Dermatologists work with adult and pediatric patients in treating disorders and diseases of the skin, hair, nails, and related tissues. Dermatologists are specially trained to manage conditions such as skin cancers, cosmetic disorders of the skin, scars, allergies, and other disorders, both malignant and benign.
Emergency medicine	Emergency physician	Emergency physicians are experts in assessing and treating a patient to prevent death or serious disability. They provide immediate care to stabilize the patient's condition, and then refer the patient to the appropriate professional for further care.
Family medicine	Primary care provider (PCP)	PCPs offer care to the whole family, from newborns to elderly adults. They are familiar with a wide range of disorders and diseases, and preventive care is their primary concern.
General surgery	Surgeon	General surgeons correct deformities and defects and treat diseases or injured parts of the body by means of operative treatment.
Genetics	Medical geneticist	Geneticists are physicians trained to diagnose and treat patients with conditions related to genetically linked diseases. They provide genetic counseling when indicated.
Internal medicine	Internist	Internists are concerned with comprehensive care, often diagnosing and treating those with chronic, long-term conditions. They must have a broad understanding of the body and its ailments.
Neurologic surgery	Neurosurgeon	Neurosurgeons provide surgical care for patients with conditions of the central, autonomic, and peripheral nervous systems.
Neurology/psychiatry	Neurologist/psychiatrist	Neurologists diagnose and treat disorders of the nervous system. Psychiatrists are physicians who specialize in the diagnosis and treatment of people with mental, emotional, or behavioral disorders. A psychiatrist is qualified to conduct psychotherapy and to prescribe medications.
Nuclear medicine	Nuclear medicine specialist	These specialists use radioactive substances to diagnose, treat, and detect disease.
Obstetrics and gynecology	Obstetrician/gynecologist	Obstetricians provide care to women of childbearing age and monitor the progress of the developing child. Gynecologists are concerned with the diagnosis and treatment of the female reproductive system.
Ophthalmology	Ophthalmologist	Ophthalmologists diagnose, treat, and provide comprehensive care for the eye and its supporting structures. These physicians also offer vision services, including corrective lenses.

TABLE 2-4   Examples of Medical Specialties—*continued*

SPECIALTY	PRACTITIONER'S TITLE	DESCRIPTION
Otolaryngology	Otolaryngologist	Otolaryngologists treat diseases and conditions that affect the ear, nose, and throat and structures related to the head and neck. Problems that affect the voice and hearing are also referred to this specialist.
Pathology	Pathologist	Pathologists study the causes of diseases. They study tissues and cells, body fluids, and organs themselves to aid in the process of diagnosis.
Pediatrics	Pediatrician	Pediatricians promote preventive medicine and treat diseases that affect children and adolescents. They monitor the child's growth and development and provide a wide range of health services.
Physical medicine and rehabilitation	Physiatrist	Physiatrists assist patients who have physical disabilities. This may include rehabilitation, patients with musculoskeletal disorders, and patients suffering from pain as a result of injury or trauma.
Plastic surgery	Plastic surgeon	Plastic surgeons work with patients who have a physical defect as a result of some type of injury or condition. They perform reconstructive cosmetic enhancements and elective procedures.
Preventive medicine	Preventive medicine specialist	Preventive medicine specialists are concerned with preventing mental and physical illness and disability. They also analyze current health services and plan for future medical needs.
Radiology	Radiologist	Radiology is a specialty in which x-rays are used to diagnose and treat disease. A diagnostic radiologist specializes in using x-rays, ultrasound, nuclear medicine, computed tomography, and magnetic resonance imaging to detect abnormalities throughout the body.
Thoracic surgery	Thoracic surgeon	Thoracic surgeons are concerned with the operative treatment of the chest and chest wall, lungs, heart, heart valves, and respiratory passages.
Urology	Urologist	Urologists are concerned with the treatment of diseases and disorders of the urinary tract. They diagnose and manage problems with the genitourinary system and practice endoscopic procedures related to these structures.

CRITICAL THINKING APPLICATION   **2-3**

- Investigate the different philosophies of medicine among allopathic, osteopathic, and chiropractic physicians. Discuss with your class the similarities and differences among these three approaches to medicine.
- What experiences have you had with medical doctors (MDs), osteopaths (DOs), or chiropractors (DCs)? How does their training or expertise differ?

Dentists

There is no difference in training between dentists with a "DDS" or a "DMD." The two degrees mean the same thing: the dentist graduated from an accredited dental school. DDS stands for Doctor of Dental Surgery, and DMD stands for Doctor of Medicine in Dentistry or Doctor of Dental Medicine. The university where each dental school is based determines the degree in dentistry that is awarded. The level of education and clinical training required to earn a dental degree are similar to those expected by medical schools. Upon completion of general dentistry training, additional postgraduate training is required to become a dental specialist, such as an orthodontist or periodontist.

Optometrists

The optometrist (OD) is trained and licensed to examine the eyes, to test visual acuity, and to treat vision defects by prescribing correctional lenses and other optical aids. Optometrists study at accredited schools of optometry for 4 years after completing undergraduate studies in the sciences, mathematics, and English. They must be licensed in the state in which they practice. Optometrists should not be confused with ophthalmologists, who are licensed MDs.

Podiatrists

Podiatrists (Doctors of Podiatric Medicine [DPMs]) are educated in the care of the feet, including surgical treatment. Podiatrists are trained to find pressure points and weight-distribution problems. These physicians must complete an undergraduate bachelor's degree in addition to 4 years of training in a podiatric medical school and 3 years of hospital residency training. This training is similar to that of other doctors.

Nurse Practitioners

Nurse practitioners (NPs) provide basic patient care services, including diagnosing and prescribing medications for common illnesses, or they may have additional training and expertise in a specialty area of medicine. These professionals must have advanced academic training beyond the registered nurse (RN) degree and also have vast clinical experience. An NP is licensed by individual states and can practice independently or as a part of a team of healthcare professionals.

Nurse Anesthetists

Nurse anesthetists are registered nurses (RNs) who administer anesthetics to patients during surgical or inpatient diagnostic procedures. They practice in many different healthcare settings, including hospital surgical areas, labor and delivery units, ophthalmology offices, plastic surgery offices, and many others. Certified Registered Nurse Anesthetist (CRNA) must have a Bachelor of Science in Nursing (BSN) or other appropriate baccalaureate degree; a current license as a registered nurse; and at least 1 year's experience in an acute care nursing setting. They also must have graduated from an accredited graduate school of nurse anesthesia program, which can range from 24 to 36 months, and must pass a national certification examination after graduation.

Physician Assistants

A physician assistant (PA) is a certified healthcare professional who provides diagnostic, therapeutic, and preventive healthcare services under the supervision of a medical doctor. Physician assistants must be licensed, which requires completion of a physician assistant program that is typically at the master's degree level. Physician assistants must pass the Physician Assistant National Certifying Examination to practice in any state. They may also complete advanced training to focus on a particular specialty practice.

TYPES OF HEALTHCARE FACILITIES
Hospitals

Hospitals are classified according to the type of care and services they provide to patients and by the type of ownership. There are three different levels of hospitalized care, which are interconnected.

Primary Level of Care
- Smaller city or community hospitals
- Usually serve as the first level of contact between the community members and the hospital setting

Secondary Level of Care
- Both PCPs and specialists provide care
- Larger municipal or district hospitals that provide a wider variety of specialty care and departments

Tertiary Level of Care
- Referral system for primary or secondary care facilities
- Provide care for complicated cases and trauma
- Medical centers, regional and specialty hospitals

Private hospitals are run by a corporation or other organization and usually are designed to produce a profit for the owners or stockholders. *Nonprofit* hospitals exist to serve the community in which they are located and are normally run by a board of directors. The term *nonprofit* sometimes is misleading, because "profit" is different from "making money." A nonprofit hospital or organization may make money in a campaign or fundraiser, but all of the money is returned to the organization. Nonprofit hospitals and organizations must follow strict guidelines in the area of finance and must account to the government for the money brought in and the purposes for which it is used.

A *hospital system* is a group of facilities that are affiliated and work toward a common goal. Hospital systems may include a hospital and a cancer center in a small community or may consist of a group of separate hospitals in a specific geographic region. Many hospital systems are designed as integrated health delivery systems. An integrated delivery system (IDS) is a network of healthcare providers and organizations that provides or arranges to provide a coordinated continuum of services to a defined population and is willing to be held clinically and fiscally accountable for the clinical outcomes and health status of the population served. An IDS may own or could be closely aligned with an insurance product, such as a type of insurance policy. Services provided by an IDS can include a fully equipped community and/or tertiary hospital, home healthcare and **hospice** services, primary and specialty outpatient care and surgery, social services, rehabilitation, preventive care, health education and financing, and community provider offices. An IDS can also be a training location for health professional students, including physicians, nurses, and allied health professionals.

Accreditation is considered the highest form of recognition for the quality of care a facility or organization provides. Not only does it indicate to the public that the facility is concerned with providing high-quality care, it also provides professional liability insurance benefits and plays a role in regulatory agency relicensure and certification efforts. Hospitals and other healthcare facilities are accredited by The Joint Commission, an organization that promotes and evaluates the quality of care in healthcare facilities. Standards or **indicators** have been developed that help determine when patients are receiving high-quality care. The term *quality* refers to much more than whether the patient liked the food served or had to wait to have a procedure or test performed. Categories of compliance include:
- Assessment and care of patients
- Use of medication
- Plant, technology, and safety management
- Orientation, education, and training of staff
- Medical staff qualifications
- Patients' rights

Accreditation by The Joint Commission is required to obtain reimbursement from Medicare, managed care organizations, and insurance companies. Besides accrediting healthcare facilities, The Joint Commission carefully evaluates patient safety. It has established the National Patient Safety Goals, which must be addressed by member facilities. The 2015 safety goals for ambulatory organizations took effect January 1, 2015. They included:

- Identifying patients correctly
- Using medicines safely
- Preventing infection
- Preventing mistakes in safety

All these safety factors are addressed in future chapters.

CRITICAL THINKING APPLICATION   **2-4**

- What types of hospitals are found in your local area, and what services do they provide?
- Are there any patient populations in your area that are underserved? Why might this be the case?

Ambulatory Care

Ambulatory care centers include a wide range of facilities that offer healthcare services to patients who seek outpatient health services. Physicians' offices, group practices, and multispecialty group practices are common types of ambulatory care facilities, and medical assistants can be employed in all of these practices. Group practices may involve a single specialty, such as pediatrics, or may be multispecialty. A multispecialty practice might consist of an internal medicine specialist, an oncologist, a primary care provider, and an endocrinologist.

Usually the providers in the practice refer patients to each other when indicated. This is not only more convenient for the patients, but also more profitable for the members in the practice. A patient seeing a provider for the first time is considered a *new* patient, whereas a patient who has seen the provider on previous occasions is called an *established* patient. Most providers charge new patients more than established patients because the levels of decision making, the extent of the physical examination, and the complexity of the medical history require that more time be directed toward the new patient.

Occupational health centers are concerned with helping patients return to work and productive activity. Often, physical therapy is used in conjunction with rehabilitation services to assist the patient in regaining as much of his or her previous level of ability as possible. Also, freestanding rehabilitation centers can assist patients with a wide range of services. Pain management centers help patients deal with discomfort associated with their condition. Sleep centers diagnose and treat people with sleep problems. Freestanding urgent or emergency care centers provide patients with an alternative to hospital emergency departments (EDs) and are typically open when traditional provider offices are closed.

Surgery has become more convenient because of the number of ambulatory surgical centers that exist today. Many insurance companies now prefer day surgery because it is more cost-effective. A wide variety of outpatient surgical facilities is available, offering procedures in ophthalmology, plastic surgery, and gastrointestinal concerns, including colonoscopies.

Dialysis centers offer services to patients with severe kidney disorders, and many of the larger cities across the country have cancer centers for patients who need treatment by oncologists. Among the many other types of ambulatory care facilities are centers that provide magnetic resonance imaging (MRI), student health clinics, dental clinics, community health centers, and women's health centers.

Other Healthcare Facilities

Several other types of healthcare facilities deserve attention in the broad overview of the healthcare industry. Diagnostic laboratories offer testing services for patients referred by their providers. The enactment of CLIA in 1967 and its amendment in 1988 established that the only laboratory tests that can be performed in a physician's office lab are those designated as *CLIA-waived.* You will learn how to perform many CLIA-waived tests in your medical assistant program. Larger ambulatory care centers may contain an on-site advanced diagnostic laboratory where all studies can be completed. Smaller or independent practices typically have to send non-CLIA-waived tests to an outside diagnostic facility.

Home health agencies or hospital-affiliated home healthcare organizations provide crucial services to patients who require medical follow-up but are not in a hospital setting. Home healthcare includes therapy services, administration of and assistance with medications, wound care, and other services so that the patient can remain at home, yet still obtain consistent medical attention. Hospice care is a type of home health service that provides medical care and support for patients facing end-of-life issues and their families. The goal of hospice is to provide peace, comfort, and dignity while controlling pain and promoting the best possible quality of life for the patient. Some communities have inpatient hospice services available either in a special unit in a hospital or in an independent hospice center.

The Patient-Centered Medical Home

According to the Agency for Healthcare Research and Quality (AHRQ), which is part of the HSS, "The patient-centered medical home is a way of organizing primary care that emphasizes care coordination and communication to transform primary care into what patients want it to be."

The Patient-Centered Medical Home (PCMH) model, sometimes referred to as the *primary care medical home,* is one of the most exciting healthcare delivery reforms occurring today, and it is transforming the organization and delivery of primary care. Research indicates that PCMHs are saving money by reducing hospital and ED visits while at the same time improving patient outcomes. The AHRQ believes that improving our primary care system is the key to achieving high-quality, accessible, efficient healthcare for all Americans. The agency recognizes that health information technology (IT) plays a central role in the successful implementation of the key features of the primary care medical home. According to the AHRQ, the PCMH has five core functions and attributes:

1. *Comprehensive care:* The primary care practice has the potential to provide physical and mental healthcare, prevention and wellness, acute care, and chronic care to all patients in the practice. However, comprehensive care cannot be provided by only the practicing physician. It requires a team of care providers. The healthcare team for a PCMH includes physicians, nurse practitioners, physician assistants, nurses, pharmacists, nutritionists, social workers, educators, and medical assistants. If these specialty individuals are not readily available to smaller physician practices, virtual teams can be created online to link providers and patients to services in their communities.

2. *Patient-centered care:* The PCMH provides primary healthcare that is holistic and relationship-based, always considering the individual patient and all facets of his or her life. However, establishing a partnership with patients and their families requires understanding and respect of each patient's unique needs, culture, values, and preferences. Medical assistants are trained to provide respectful patient care regardless of individual patient factors. The goal of PCMH is to encourage and support patients in learning how to manage and organize their own care. Patients and families are recognized as core members of the care team.

3. *Coordinated care:* The PCMH coordinates care across all parts of the healthcare system, including specialty care, hospitals, home healthcare, and community services. Coordination is especially important when patients are transitioning from one site of care to another, such as from hospital to home. The PCMH works at creating and maintaining open communication among patients and families, the medical home, and members of the broader healthcare team.

4. *Accessible services:* The PCMH is designed to deliver accessible care. This is achieved through establishing policies that create shorter wait times for urgent needs, more office hours, around-the-clock telephone or electronic access to a member of the care team, and alternative methods of communication, such as e-mail and telephone care.

5. *Quality and safety:* The PCMH is committed to delivering quality healthcare by providing evidence-based medicine and shared decision making with patients and families; assessing practice performance and working on improvements; collecting safety data; and measuring and responding to patients' experiences and satisfaction. All of this information is made public to allow an open assessment of the practice and suggestions for possible methods of improvement.

For further information about the PCMH model, refer to the Patient Centered Medical Home Resource Center, Department of Health and Human Services: *http://pcmh.ahrq.gov*

SCOPE OF PRACTICE AND STANDARDS OF CARE FOR MEDICAL ASSISTANTS

Scope of practice is defined as the range of responsibilities and practice guidelines that determine the boundaries within which a healthcare worker practices. What is the scope of practice of a medical assistant? There is no single definition of the scope of practice for medical assistants throughout the United States, but some states have enacted scope of practice laws covering medical assistant practice. These states include Alaska, Arizona, California, Florida, Georgia, Illinois, Maine, Maryland, Montana, Nevada, New Hampshire, New Jersey, New York, Ohio, South Dakota, Virginia, Washington, and West Virginia. Medical assistants working in those states must refer to the identified roles specified in the law. However, for those employed in states without scope of practice laws, medical assistant practice is guided by the norms of that particular location, facility policies and procedures, and individual physician-employers. In some states, medical assistants are overseen by the board of nursing, whereas in others, the board of medicine oversees medical assistants. Make sure you are aware of your state's rules governing medical assistant scope

of practice. Procedure 2-1 outlines how to locate a state's legal scope of practice for medical assistants.

One factor is absolutely true about all practicing medical assistants—they are not independent practitioners. Whether certified or not, regardless of length of training or experience, every medical assistant must practice under the direct supervision of a physician or other licensed provider (e.g., nurse practitioner or physician assistant).

Earlier in this chapter we discussed the typical tasks performed by a medical assistant, so you already know generally what duties medical assistants perform in ambulatory care centers; however, some specific tasks are beyond the scope of practice of medical assistants, including the following:

- Performing telephone or in-person **triage**; medical assistants are not legally authorized to assess or diagnose symptoms
- Prescribing medications or making recommendations about over-the-counter drugs and remedies
- Giving out drug samples without provider permission
- Automatically submitting refill prescription requests without provider orders
- Administering intravenous (IV) medications and starting, flushing, or removing IV lines unless permitted by state law
- Analyzing or interpreting test results
- Operating laser equipment

What is the difference between scope of practice and standards of care? The *scope of practice* for a medical assistant is what has been established by law in some states or by practice norms, institutions, or physician-employers in states without scope of practice laws. *Standards of care,* however, is a legal term that refers to whether the level and quality of patient service provided is the same as what another healthcare worker with similar training and experience in a similar situation would provide. Standards of care set minimum guidelines for job performance. They define what the expected quality of care is and provide specific guidelines on whether the care standard has been met. Medical assistants not meeting the expected standard of care may be charged with professional **negligence** (discussed in greater detail in the chapter, Medicine and Law).

The following are examples of breaks in the standards of care in medical assisting.

- A patient calls reporting a persistent headache for 3 days. You tell the patient to get some rest and take ibuprofen, without referring the call to a provider. What standard of care has been broken?
- A patient asks you to explain his lab report. You do your best to explain what his blood count levels mean. What is the problem here?
- An elderly patient tells you she cannot afford to get her prescriptions filled. The provider is busy, but you know there are samples of the prescribed drug in the medication cupboard, so you give her several packets. Does this follow standard of care?
- A patient tells you her son fell on the playground yesterday, and he is complaining that his arm hurts. You tell the mother it is probably just a strain and suggest she wrap the arm with an elastic bandage. Why is this a problem?
- You overhear a patient calling one of your co-workers "nurse." Should your co-worker correct the patient? Why?

Hopefully you are beginning to see that the practice of medical assisting is limited not only by individual state laws or norms, but also by the standards and scope of practice established by the supervising providers where the medical assistant is employed. Remember, the scope of practice and expected standards of care for licensed medical professionals are quite different from those for medical assisting practice. The medical assistant must refer to the provider for orders and guidance on what behaviors are expected for medical assistants in that facility. The medical assistant can *never* independently diagnose, prescribe, or treat patients. She or he must *always* have the written order of a provider or follow established policies and procedures when performing clinical skills.

PROCEDURE 2-1   Locate a State's Legal Scope of Practice for Medical Assistants

Goal: *To determine the legal scope of practice for medical assistants employed in your home state.*

No single definition of the scope of practice for medical assistants applies throughout the United States. However, some states have enacted scope of practice laws that cover medical assistant practice (i.e., Alaska, Arizona, California, Florida, Georgia, Illinois, Maine, Maryland, Montana, Nevada, New Hampshire, New Jersey, New York, Ohio, South Dakota, Virginia, Washington, and West Virginia). Medical assistants working in those states must refer to the identified roles specified in the law.

In states that do not have scope of practice laws, three main elements guide medical assistant practice: the norms of the particular location; the healthcare facility's policies and procedures; and the instructions of the individual physician employer. In some states medical assistants are overseen by the board of nursing, whereas in others, the board of medicine oversees medical assistants. Make sure you have closely studied and clearly understand your state's rules governing the medical assistant's scope of practice.

EQUIPMENT and SUPPLIES

- Computer with Internet access

PROCEDURAL STEPS

1. Google "medical assistant state scope of practice laws", or refer to the American Association of Medical Assistants website (*www.aama-ntl.org/employers/state-scope-of-practice-laws*).
   PURPOSE: To research scope of practice laws in your home state.
2. Summarize the scope of medical assistant practice in your state, and give details on where you found this information.
   PURPOSE: To learn the legal scope of practice in the state where you are employed.
3. Discuss the scope of practice for medical assistants in your home state with your peers.
   PURPOSE: To reinforce your learning about the legal scope of practice in your home state.

CLOSING COMMENTS

Medical assisting has developed over the years into a profession that makes considerable contributions to quality patient care in ambulatory care centers. Medical assistants are uniquely trained to manage both the administrative and clinical needs of patients in physicians' offices, clinics, and outpatient facilities. One of the crucial roles of medical assistants is to act as the patient's navigator; that is, to help patients understand and comply with complex care issues. The medical assistant joins a wide range of allied health professionals as part of a healthcare team in which all members work together to best meet the needs of patients. Medical assistants can work in a variety of healthcare facilities and alongside medical specialists to care for patients. They also can act as core members of the patient-centered medical home and, along with a variety of community resources, can help provide holistic care to patients in the healthcare system. However, medical assistant practice must align with state and regional scope of practice laws and must meet expected standards of care. Medical assistants must always act under the direction of a physician or provider; they cannot diagnose, prescribe, or treat patients independently.

Patient Education

Some patients have very little knowledge about the healthcare industry and may need instruction and explanations about details important to their healthcare. They often call the healthcare facility with questions; therefore, medical assistants must understand the wide variety of healthcare facilities and medical resources available in the community. Become familiar with community resources to make provider-approved referrals for patients who need help from various sources. If a patient seems to have a need, speak with him or her privately and determine whether any agency or organization might help with the issues at hand. The patient-centered medical home model relies on all healthcare workers to participate in the care of patients.

Legal and Ethical Issues

Medical assistants are responsible for understanding and following the scope of practice in their communities and for always meeting the expected standards of care. Not meeting these responsibilities can result in serious liability for themselves and their employers. Remember, the medical assistant must act under the direct supervision of a physician or licensed provider. You must know the limitations placed on your practice by the state in which you live or by the facility or provider who employs you. There is nothing more important than patient safety, so always act within the guidelines of the law and according to the policies and procedures of the facility where you work. Medical assistants are multiskilled healthcare workers who can have a lasting positive effect on patient outcomes. However, never forget that you do not have the authority or education to diagnose, prescribe, or treat patient clinical problems.

Professional Behaviors

Much of this chapter has focused on an introduction to what it means to be a medical assistant and what you will need to learn so you can perform all the skills expected of an entry-level medical assistant. However, working with patients and providing quality care goes beyond being able to perform administrative and clinical skills. Each patient must be viewed holistically. This means considering the following patient factors:

- What is the patient's physical condition, and how is it affecting his or her life?
- What is the patient's psychological state; is it preventing the person from following treatment regimens?
- Are any communication barriers preventing the patient from understanding the diagnosis or suggested treatment?
- Is the patient's culture, age, or lifestyle preventing him or her from following the provider's orders?
- Are insurance issues or financial problems preventing the patient from following through with treatment plans?

These are just a few of the factors that can affect patient outcomes. Again, because you will be trained in both administrative and clinical duties, you will be in a unique position to understand all the factors that might affect patient care. It is your responsibility to treat all patients with respect and empathy and to do whatever you can to support them throughout the healthcare experience.

SUMMARY OF SCENARIO

Carmen is a bit overwhelmed but very excited about what she has learned about the role of medical assistants in ambulatory care. She finds it hard to believe that she will become competent in all aspects of the typical medical assistant's job description, but she anticipates learning both administrative and clinical skills. She is looking forward to joining the local AAMA chapter so that she can take advantage of professional development opportunities and

networking with other medical assistant professionals and students in her community. Carmen now appreciates the significance of scope of practice and of meeting standards of care, and she is researching the laws affecting medical assistant practice in her state. She can't wait until she is actually able to work with the healthcare team to meet the holistic needs of patients in the practice where she will be employed.

SUMMARY OF LEARNING OBJECTIVES

1. **Define, spell, and pronounce the terms listed in the vocabulary.**
   Spelling and pronouncing medical terms correctly reinforce the medical assistant's credibility. Knowing the definitions of these terms promotes confidence in communication with patients and co-workers.
2. **Summarize the history of medicine and its significance to the medical assisting profession.**
   The history of medicine can be traced to ancient practices as far back as 5,000 BC. In 1205 BC Moses presented rules of health to the Hebrews, thus becoming the first advocate of preventive medicine. Hippocrates, known as the father of medicine, is the most famous of the ancient Greek physicians and is best remembered for the Hippocratic Oath, which has been administered to physicians for more than 2,000 years. The medical assistant profession relies on previous medical discoveries to provide

patients with safe care in today's healthcare environment. Table 2-1 summarizes medical pioneers and their achievements.

3. **Identify national departments and agencies that focus on health.**
   The Department of Health and Human Services (HHS) is the principal U.S. department for providing essential human services and protecting the health of all Americans, especially those unable to help themselves. The Centers for Disease Control and Prevention (CDC) is the federal agency concerned with health; it conducts research on health-related issues and serves as a clearinghouse for information and statistics associated with healthcare. The CDC establishes regulations that affect all healthcare facilities. The National Institutes of Health (NIH) is part of the HHS and seeks to improve the health of the American people; it also supports and conducts biomedical research into the causes and prevention of diseases and uses

SUMMARY OF LEARNING OBJECTIVES—*continued*

a modern communications system to furnish biomedical information to the healthcare professions. The Occupational Safety and Health Administration (OSHA), an agency of the Department of Labor, is responsible for establishing and enforcing regulations to protect individuals in the workplace, including those employed in healthcare.

4. **List professional medical assisting organizations.**

The American Association of Medical Assistants (AAMA) was formed in 1956 and is the only association devoted exclusively to the medical assisting profession. The AAMA is involved in accreditation of medical assisting programs through its association with the Commission on Accreditation of Allied Health Education Programs (CAAHEP), managing the CMA (AAMA) exam, providing professional development opportunities for medical assistants, and supporting and researching issues affecting practicing medical assistants. The American Medical Technologists (AMT) is a nationally recognized certification agency for multiple allied health professionals, including medical assistants (who earn the credential Registered Medical Assistant [RMA]). The National Healthcareer Association (NHA) is a company that offers certification examinations to a number of allied health programs, including two different medical assisting certifications: Certified Clinical Medical Assistant (CCMA) and Certified Medical Administrative Assistant (CMAA). The NHA is not involved in program curriculum standards or program accreditation.

5. **Discuss the typical job description of a medical assistant and describe the role of the medical assistant as a patient navigator.**

Medical assistants are the only allied health professionals specifically trained to work in ambulatory care settings, such as physicians' offices, clinics, and group practices. That training includes both clinical and administrative skills, covering a multitude of medical practice needs. The skills performed by an entry-level medical assistant depend on his or her place of employment, but all graduates of accredited programs are taught a similar skill set.

Medical assistants have long been encouraged to act as patient advocates in the ambulatory care setting. That role is now described as acting as a patient navigator to help patients manage the complexities of their care. Given their multilevel training, medical assistants can help patients navigate through a wide variety of confusing issues.

6. **Identify a variety of allied health professionals who are part of the healthcare team.**

The definition of an allied health professional can vary, but it loosely refers to those who can act only under the authority of a licensed medical practitioner. Allied health professions fall into two broad categories: technicians (assistants) and therapists. Allied health professionals, including professional medical assistants, typically work as part of a healthcare team. Table 2-2 presents a list of allied health occupations, and Table 2-3 shows a list of licensed healthcare professions.

7. **Summarize the various types of medical specialties and healthcare facilities.**

Physicians and other providers (e.g., nurse practitioners and physician assistants) are portals of entry or first contacts for patients seeking medical care. Medical professionals include physicians (MDs, DOs), dentists, chiropractors, optometrists, podiatrists, pharmacists, nurse practitioners, and physician assistants. Table 2-4 presents a list of medical specialties. Healthcare facilities include different levels of hospitals, ambulatory care facilities, and a variety of other institutions that provide specialty care for patients.

8. **Define a patient-centered medical home (PCMH) and discuss its five core functions and attributes.**

The PCMH is also referred to as the *primary care medical home,* a concept that is transforming the organization and delivery of primary care. Improving our primary care system is the key to achieving high-quality, accessible, efficient healthcare for all Americans. The PCMH has five core functions and attributes: (1) comprehensive care, (2) patient-centered care, (3) coordinated care, (4) accessible services, and (5) evidence-based, high-quality, safe care.

9. **Differentiate between scope of practice and standards of care for medical assistants, and compare and contrast provider and medical assistant roles in terms of standards of care.**

Scope of practice is defined as the range of responsibilities and practice guidelines that determine the boundaries within which a healthcare worker practices. The scope of practice for a medical assistant is what has been established by law in some states or by practice norms, institutions, or physician-employers in states without scope of practice laws (see Procedure 2-1). *Standards of care* is a legal term that refers to whether the level and quality of patient service provided is the same as what another healthcare worker with similar training and experience in a similar situation would provide. Standards of care set minimum guidelines for job performance.

The scope of practice and expected standard of care for licensed medical professionals are quite different from those acceptable for a medical assistant. The medical assistant must refer to the provider for orders and guidance on what behaviors are expected for medical assistants in that facility. The medical assistant can never independently diagnose, prescribe, or treat patients. He or she must always have the written order of a provider or follow established policies and procedures when performing clinical skills.

CONNECTIONS

Study Guide Connection: Go to the Chapter 2 Study Guide. Read and complete the activities.

evolve Evolve Connection: Go to the Chapter 2 link at *evolve.elsevier.com/kinn* to complete the Chapter Review Quiz. Check out the other resources listed for this chapter to make the most of what you have learned from The Medical Assistant and the Healthcare Team.

3

PROFESSIONAL BEHAVIOR IN THE WORKPLACE

SCENARIO

Karen Yon has wanted to work in the medical field for most of her adult life. She studied very hard in high school and graduated with honors. She volunteered in a local hospital and then, after working as a server in restaurants for 3 years, she enrolled in medical assisting classes. After her externship, she was offered an entry-level medical assistant position at a primary care practice.

Karen strives to perform all of her duties professionally and compassionately. She maintains a professional image for patients and co-workers. She had found it difficult to learn to be professional at all times and show compassion to patients through just the classroom experience. However, she knew that these were important aspects of her job, and she was able to gain valuable experience in these areas during her externship. Because this is her first job in the medical field, she wants to make a good impression on her employer and contribute to the healthcare team.

While studying this chapter, think about the following questions:

- Why is professionalism an important attribute in the field of medical assisting?
- How can Karen show professional behavior toward all patients in the healthcare setting?
- How can time management strategies help Karen prioritize her responsibilities as a member of the healthcare team?
- Would it benefit Karen to become a member of her local AAMA chapter?

LEARNING OBJECTIVES

1. Define, spell, and pronounce the terms listed in the vocabulary.
2. Explain the reasons professionalism is important in the medical field, and describe work ethics.
3. Discuss the attributes of professional medical assistants, and project a professional image in the ambulatory care setting.
4. Identify obstructions to professional behaviors.
5. Define the principles of self-boundaries.
6. Describe the dynamics of the healthcare team.
7. Apply time management strategies to prioritize the medical assistant's responsibilities as a member of the healthcare team.
8. Summarize the role of professional medical assistant organizations.

VOCABULARY

characteristics Distinguishing traits, qualities, or properties.
demeanor (dih-me′-nur) Behavior toward others; outward manner.
detrimental (deh-truh-men′-til) Obviously harmful or damaging.
disseminate (dih-seh′-muh-na-te) To disburse; to spread around.

reflection A therapeutic communication technique in which a person responds with a feeling term that indicates how the individual feels about a problem. For example, "You sound angry about being scheduled for this diagnostic test."

What is professional behavior? We tend to hold medical personnel to a higher standard of professionalism than those in most other career fields. The medical assistant who works to improve his or her professional approach in the workplace is an asset to the employer and will quickly be promoted to positions of more responsibility in the healthcare industry. Some employers are just as concerned about medical assistants' professional behavior as they are about their ability to perform administrative and clinical skills, because the way the medical assistant approaches and interacts with patients is critical to the success of the practice. Professionalism is useful not only in the workplace; it also is a valuable skill when dealing with other business professionals in everyday life.

THE MEANING OF PROFESSIONALISM

Professionalism is defined as having a courteous, conscientious, and respectful approach to all interactions and situations in the workplace. It is characterized by or conforms to the recognized standard

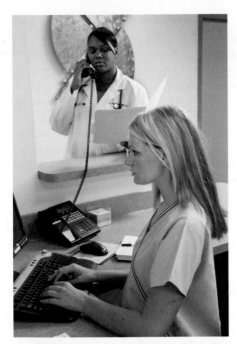

FIGURE 3-1 The professional medical assistant is an asset to the healthcare facility.

ATTRIBUTES OF PROFESSIONAL MEDICAL ASSISTANTS

Patients often see the medical assistant as an extension of the provider and healthcare facility. Therefore, the behavior and attitude of the medical assistant can either positively or negatively affect patients' perception of the quality of care they can expect to receive. As representatives of the healthcare facility, medical assistants must consistently display professionalism through their attitude, appearance, and behavior. Regardless of the situation, the medical assistant must always act professionally.

Many **characteristics** make up the professionalism required of medical assistants. Student medical assistants should begin developing these attributes while in school; these qualities do not appear magically when the student begins working with actual patients. Although we might think that we would always behave appropriately during an externship or in a job setting, the habits developed in school carry over into these experiences. If the behavior is unacceptable, it will be **detrimental** to the medical assistant's professional career. If the medical assistant wishes to advance and receive wage increases, promotions, and the trust of the employer, the attributes discussed in the following sections must be a part of his or her professional behavior.

CRITICAL THINKING APPLICATION   **3-1**
- How can students practice professional behavior while still in the classroom situation?
- When students are practicing administrative and clinical skills, how can they demonstrate proficiency in professional behavior?

---

of care for the profession. Conducting themselves in a professional manner is essential for successful medical assistants. The attitude of those in the medical profession generally is more conservative than that seen in other career fields. Patients expect professional behavior and base much of their trust and confidence in those who show this type of **demeanor** in the healthcare facility (Figure 3-1).

WORK ETHICS

Work ethics are sets of values based on the moral virtues of hard work and diligence. They involve a whole range of activities, from individual acts to the philosophy of the entire facility. The medical assistant should always display initiative and be reliable. A person who has a good work ethic is one who arrives on time, is rarely absent, and always performs to the best of his or her ability. Co-workers become frustrated if another employee consistently arrives late or is absent. This forces the co-workers to take on additional duties and may prevent them from completing their own work. One missing employee can disrupt the entire day; phones may not be answered promptly, and patients may have to wait for appointments because the staff is shorthanded. Also, lunch and other breaks may be shortened because the staff cannot process cases as quickly when an employee does not show up. All employees should know, and follow, the attendance policies of the facility as outlined in the policies and procedures manual.

Most new hires have a probationary period that may last 30 to 90 days. Any absences or tardiness during the probationary period can be grounds to terminate the employee once the probationary period is up or even before that if multiple attendance issues arise. If the medical assistant has an emergency and must be absent or tardy, he or she should make sure to notify the supervisor according to office policy. All employees must be on time and in attendance every day in the healthcare facility. Providers and patients alike expect this reliability.

Courteous and Respectful

Treating patients with courtesy and dignity are crucial to interacting with patients professionally. Courteous behavior is polite, open, and welcoming. Just the simple act of establishing eye contact, greeting patients with a smile, saying "Nice to see you"; "Can you please …"; and "Thank you …" can make a patient feel welcome and respected. Despite patient attitudes or the stressors in your personal and professional life, you must always treat patients with respect. Patients expect to be treated as individuals, not just another health problem. How can the medical assistant achieve the goals of treating others with courteous regard and thoughtful consideration?

- If you are working with an angry or unhappy patient, use therapeutic communication skills to find out about the real issues the patient is concerned about.
- Display positive nonverbal behaviors, including using an even, calm tone of voice; establishing eye contact; and taking the patient into a private area to discuss problems.
- Always use proper grammar, without slang words, to demonstrate your respect for the individual.
- If the patient is from another culture or speaks another language, communicate as best you can, but try either to have a family member present who understands English or to use an interpreter.

- Explain medical treatments and conditions with simple lay language rather than expecting the patient to understand medical terminology.
- Demonstrate interest in patients as individuals.
- Recognize the personal biases that you bring to the field of medical assisting and how they can affect respectful patient care.
- Respect the role of other members of the healthcare team in meeting the needs of patients and families.
- Demonstrate sensitivity to the patient's and the family's needs.
- Maintain patient confidentiality.

Diplomatic and Tactful

A diplomatic and tactful person always attempts to interact honestly without giving offense. The medical assistant must be sensitive to the needs of patients and co-workers, especially if the person you are communicating with is upset. How can you honestly and effectively communicate with someone who is asking you a difficult question or who may become angry about a particular situation? Could your personal belief system and biases affect how you interact with co-workers, patients, and families? What methods can the professional medical assistant use to communicate diplomatically and tactfully with co-workers and patients?

- Respond calmly to problematic situations with **reflection**, making sure the patient knows you recognize how he or she feels about the problem.
- Consistently communicate politely and honestly.
- Gather feedback about the possible causes of the problem.
- Recognize the needs and rights of others and attempt to reach a mutually beneficial resolution to the problem.
- Assess your personal response to the situation and do not allow your personal beliefs and biases prevent you from interacting diplomatically and tactfully with patients, families, and co-workers.
- Provide patient- and family-centered care.
- Show sensitivity to the needs of healthcare team members.

Responsible and Honest

A responsible medical assistant is one who is dependable. The healthcare team must be able to rely on the medical assistant to perform all his or her duties within the accepted standards of care. Practice managers should be confident that once given a task to do, the medical assistant will carry it out accurately and in a timely manner. At the same time, if an error is made or there is a problem performing a particular task, the medical assistant must honestly report these issues to the immediate supervisor. Patient safety is the number one priority, and anytime it is compromised, the medical assistant must report the problem so that the patient can be safeguarded against any further injury. This is true whether the issue is an administrative or a clinical one. Clearly, if you make a mistake when administering a medication, you must immediately report this error. However, an administrative error (e.g., inaccurate coding, making a mistake on an insurance document, or neglecting to make a follow-up appointment for a patient) also can result in significant negative effects on the practice and the patients involved. In addition, your co-workers depend on you to help out as needed and honestly share any problems noted in the workings of the facility. Dependability and honesty are critical components in earning the trust and respect of others.

How can an entry-level medical assistant perform his or her duties with responsibility, integrity, and honesty?

- Interact with patients in a straightforward, honest manner while supplying all the facts, using lay terms so the patient understands and can make educated decisions.
- Be thorough and pay close attention to detail so that the patient is confident you are a responsible professional.
- Never misrepresent yourself or the medical practice.
- Honestly recognize your own limitations and do not hesitate to seek guidance or assistance if you are not sure of a particular administrative or clinical procedure.
- Accept responsibility for your failures or errors and determine how to prevent them from occurring in the future.
- Take on responsibilities that are within your job description willingly and with the intent to perform them to the best of your ability.

Response to Criticism

A reliable way to improve professional behavior is by showing a willingness to respond to constructive criticism. It can be very difficult to receive negative feedback in the workplace. Being told we are doing something wrong can threaten our confidence and self-esteem. However, constructive criticism is a way for us to recognize that there are areas in which we need to improve our skills and develop more professional methods. To grow beyond entry-level skills, the medical assistant must be willing to recognize any weaknesses in practice and use this feedback to go beyond minimal expectations. Becoming defensive or blaming others only causes more problems. Learn to honestly evaluate your own behavior and be willing to use criticism as a means to excel in your profession.

Professional Image

How do you think a professional medical assistant should look? What visually marks an individual as a professional? How you appear affects the way you are treated and what others think of you. Think of the last time you had to go to a doctor's office. What did you like or dislike about the way employees were dressed or their general appearance? Important assumptions are made within seconds of meeting someone, based only on how they look. Let's consider some standard guidelines for the appearance of the professional medical assistant.

Most medical facilities require medical assistants to wear a uniform or scrubs; this gives patients a way to immediately identify employees of the clinic. Besides providing a consistent appearance for everyone who works at the facility, wearing scrubs can be an infection control measure to prevent the passage of "street germs" in the facility. However, scrubs must be clean and pressed and fit properly to establish a professional demeanor. If administrative staff members are permitted to wear street clothes, they must choose professional clothing that is not too tight and projects a professional, businesslike appearance. All staff members should wear the facility's name badge in a clearly visible location so that patients and visitors to the clinic can identify each employee and his or her title.

In addition, hair should be clean and not overly styled. Longer hair must be tied back to prevent it from interfering with patient procedures. Shoes should be clean (most facilities require white athletic shoes), and nails should be cut short and without nail polish (no artificial nails). Longer nails, artificial nails, and polish are an infection control problem because microbes can grow and multiply under the surface of the nails and in the cracks of the polish. Jewelry is another infection control factor, especially rings. Because microorganisms can invade the cracks and crevices of jewelry, facilities typically restrict employees from wearing anything but a plain wedding ring and watch. Tattoos and body piercings are not considered professional, so medical assistants must follow office policy about their appearance. Be careful with makeup; a moderate amount might enhance your appearance, but too much might be offensive to some patients. You also must be careful with the use of colognes or perfumes. Patients might be allergic to strong odors, and many facilities state that employees should not wear any strong scents, to avoid patient discomfort.

OBSTRUCTIONS TO PROFESSIONALISM

At times it is not easy to be a professional. Sometimes patients, co-workers, and supervisors try our patience, and it can be difficult to maintain a professional attitude in these cases. Some of the obstructions to professional behavior are discussed in this section.

Personal Problems and "Baggage"

Everyone has a life outside the workplace, and sometimes we face challenges and difficult times that are hard to put aside. During working hours, our thoughts should be on the job at hand, especially when we are dealing with patients. However, some situations in our lives may be so critical or distracting that we find ourselves thinking of them constantly. This personal baggage can interfere with our ability to perform job duties properly.

When a situation intrudes on our thoughts at work, it often is best to take the time to talk with a supervisor. It is not always necessary to share the intimate details, but a quick explanation that some difficulties are occurring outside of work helps the supervisor understand any changes in habit or attitude. Regardless of whether your supervisor understands your situation, it is always best to be honest about what is happening to you personally so your employer is at least aware of your personal stressors. The professional medical assistant never transfers personal problems or baggage to anyone at the medical facility, especially patients. The workday should be focused on delivering quality patient care; therefore, do not allow personal business to interfere with the time that should be spent assisting patients and the provider. The patient must be the prime concern of all the employees in a medical facility.

CRITICAL THINKING APPLICATION   **3-2**

It often is difficult to keep from thinking about a personal problem while you are working. How can Karen do this if she is concerned about an issue at home?

Rumors and the "Grapevine"

A rumor is talk or widely **disseminated** opinion with no discernible source, or a statement that is not known to be true. The definition alone suggests that spreading rumors should be avoided. Most people enjoy working in an environment in which employees cooperate and get along with each other, but rumors can cause problems with

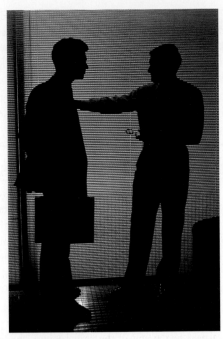

FIGURE 3-2 Gossip and rumors have no place in the medical profession. Avoid employees who participate in this type of activity.

employee morale and often are great exaggerations or manipulations of the truth. By promoting the grapevine, rumors are passed along and become more and more outrageous with each retelling. A medical assistant should refuse to participate in the office rumor mill and should attempt to be cordial and friendly to everyone at work (Figure 3-2). Supervisors regard those who spread or discuss rumors as unprofessional and untrustworthy. In addition, you should always avoid passing along work-related rumors to patients, family, and friends.

Personal Phone Calls and Business

The medical assistant should not take unnecessary phone calls from friends and family at the office. The office phone is a business line and must be used as such, except in emergencies. Using personal cell phones during working hours is not acceptable. Use breaks and lunch hours to take care of business on the phone. Never take a personal call or respond to text messages on a cell phone while working with a patient. If a phone must be carried, place it on the vibrate setting and always step into a hall or break area if a call absolutely must be taken. This should happen only in rare cases. Visitors should not frequent the office, especially the area where the medical assistant is working. If someone must come to the office, always offer the reception area as a waiting room. Visitors should never be allowed to enter patient areas.

Checking personal e-mail also should be avoided in the workplace. Any type of personal business, such as studying, looking up information on the Internet for personal use, Internet shopping, or using social media should be done at home and not in the office. All of these actions distract the medical assistant from the job at hand; the focus should be on serving the patients in the office at all times. Many employees are fired each year for surfing or shopping on the Internet for personal reasons or for checking personal e-mail. Make sure all personal business is handled outside of business hours.

CRITICAL THINKING APPLICATION   3-3

- Karen has a friend who works in a store a few doors down from her office. Her friend has started stopping in daily on her lunch hour to chat with Karen. How can Karen politely discourage this?
- A medical assistant who works with Karen has a sick child at home and wants to check on her periodically throughout the day. How should this situation be handled in a professional way?

ESTABLISHING HEALTHY SELF-BOUNDARIES

Personal or self-boundaries are extremely individual. We all determine our physical, emotional, and mental limits and use them to protect ourselves in both our personal and professional lives. Personal boundaries are developed to protect us from being manipulated or used by others. Each individual's personal boundaries help identify the person as a particular individual with certain thoughts and feelings that separate him or her from others. Self-boundaries help identify each of us as a unique individual. For example, you may not have a problem with a co-worker who refuses to take out the facility garbage at the end of the shift because she is willing to clean the examination rooms, but another co-worker may have a real issue with her refusal to share in all of the facility's jobs.

We must recognize our individual self-boundaries and appreciate their presence in others to develop healthy relationships in both our personal and professional lives. In other words, we expect those we live and work with to recognize and understand our personal limits, but at the same time we must respect the self-boundaries of others. Personal boundaries allow us to preserve our integrity and take responsibility for who we are and how we treat others. Even though we have the right to determine our own self-boundaries, we do not have the right to expect that everyone we interact with will feel the same way we do.

One way of protecting your personal boundaries is to clearly identify and explain them to others. For example, perhaps you enjoy the clinical side of the facility—interacting with patients about their health issues or helping to find community resources for patients in need—more than you enjoy the administrative responsibilities, such as coding and basic practice finances. Share this with your supervisor and co-workers and see whether you can work out a solution. Perhaps you can perform most of the clinical skills needed while another worker who likes to perform administrative skills can do so without interruption. Working out personal differences requires honest communication and compromise so that everyone understands your position and recognizes that you are willing to be a team member. This process starts with you recognizing that your needs and feelings are not more important than those of anyone else, but also that your preferences are just as important and deserve to be recognized. You have a right to personal boundaries, but you must also recognize this right in others.

Awareness of personal boundaries helps us determine the actions and behaviors that we find unacceptable. Healthy self-boundaries make it possible to respect our strengths, abilities, and individuality and those of others. Establishing healthy self-boundaries results in:

- Improved self-confidence
- Better ability to communicate honestly with others
- Relationships based on honesty and respect

THE HEALTHCARE TEAM

To deliver comprehensive quality care, everyone who interacts with patients, from the time they enter the facility to the time they leave, must work as a cooperative member of the healthcare team. If managers were asked to name the most important attributes for medical professionals, teamwork would be high on the list (Figure 3-3). Staff members must work together for the good of the patients. They must be willing to perform duties outside a formal job description if they are needed in other areas of the office. Many supervisors frown on employees who state, "That's not in my job description." A professional medical assistant should perform the duty and later discuss with the supervisor any valid reasons that the task should have been assigned to someone else. However, if the task is illegal, unethical, or places the patient or anyone else in danger, it should not be done. If you are ever concerned about patient safety, you should discuss the situation with your supervisor before performing the task.

Although we all would enjoy working in an office where everyone gets along and likes every other employee, this does not always happen. Personal feelings must be set aside at work, and all employees must cooperate with others to get the job done efficiently. If a medical assistant has an issue with another employee, the first move would be to discuss it privately with the other person. If the situation does not improve, perhaps a supervisor (office or practice manager) should be involved for further discussions. Do not bring the provider into the discussion unless there is no choice because the facility manager is expected to deal with personnel issues (Figure 3-4).

TIME MANAGEMENT

The time management strategies for students discussed in Chapter 1 can also be applied when you begin your work as a professional medical assistant. You often hear the expression to "work smart." This means that we are to use our time efficiently and concentrate on the most important duties first. To do this, we must first prioritize our duties and arrange our schedules to ensure that these duties can be performed. The first way to improve time management is to plan the tasks that need to be done that day. Taking 10 minutes to write down the tasks for the day helps ensure that they are done. Then, stay on schedule throughout the day, unless you are interrupted by

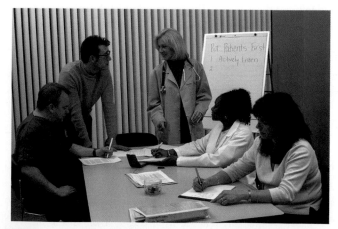

FIGURE 3-3 Teamwork is a vital part of the medical profession. All staff members must work together to care for the patient and perform required duties in the healthcare facility.

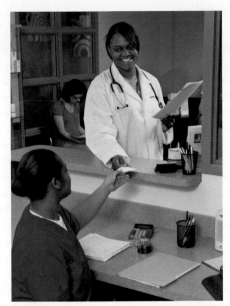

FIGURE 3-4 Knowing which employee to call when help is needed promotes goodwill among employees and often gets a task done more efficiently.

emergencies. Even then, when days are well planned, allowances can be made for emergencies and most tasks can still be completed. The key to managing time is prioritizing.

Prioritizing

Prioritizing is simply deciding which tasks are most important. Many people make a "to do" list for the day's activities, but the secret to success is prioritizing those activities into categories that give order to the tasks.

Most tasks can be prioritized into three general categories: those that must be done that day, those that *should* be done that day, and those that *could* be done if time permits. Once a general list of tasks has been established, review the list and further prioritize it, using a code such as *M* for must, *S* for should, and *C* for could (or this might be further simplified by using the letters *A*, *B*, and *C*). Once the tasks have been divided into these categories, they can be further classified in each section. For instance, if category *A* (must be done that day) has six tasks, they can be numbered in the order they should be performed. The same process is completed with the tasks in categories *B* and *C*. As the tasks are completed, they are checked off for that day. Other categories can be added to customize the list. For example, an *H* category can be used for duties to perform at home, *P* could represent phone calls that need to be made, *E* could represent errands to run, and *EM* might represent e-mails to be sent. Customizing the categories makes the list more user-friendly and helps the user to meet his or her individual needs.

Time Management Strategies

- Organize and review your daily "to do" list. If you honestly believe you can't possibly get everything that is a priority done, ask for help. It is better to admit you can't do it all than to ignore a task that is important.
- Brainstorm with your peers about ways to achieve all the tasks facing everyone each day. Maybe someone can come up with a unique way to solve a problem; but if not, at least all of you will be on the same page.
- Make a master list of important tasks so nothing is forgotten.
- Try to accomplish like tasks in the same block of time. If you have phone calls to return or insurance referrals to complete, do each at the same time to be more efficient.
- Multitask as much as possible to accomplish a variety of responsibilities throughout the day.
- At the end of each day, create a new "to do" list for the next day so that nothing important is forgotten.

CRITICAL THINKING APPLICATION 3-4

How can Karen prioritize her tasks in the administrative medical office? Based on what you know about the typical job description for an administrative medical assistant, what tasks do you think should be a priority?

MEDICAL ASSISTANT ORGANIZATIONS

Participation in a professional medical assistant organization has multiple benefits. According to the American Association of Medical Assistants (AAMA) website (*www.aama-ntl.org/*), becoming a member includes the following benefits:

- AAMA legal counsel represents medical assistants across the United States to fight for the rights of medical assistant practice; in addition, the counsel stays abreast of federal and state laws regarding medical assisting.
- Membership shows a level of seriousness about your chosen profession.
- Members receive a complimentary subscription to *CMA Today*, an informative magazine devoted entirely to the medical assistant profession; each issue (six per year) offers continuing education unit (CEU) articles, medical assisting news, and healthcare information.
- The CMA (AAMA) Exam is one of the credentialing exams offered to medical assistants; members can take the exam at a reduced rate.
  - To be eligible for the CMA (AAMA) Certification/Recertification Examination, the candidate must be a graduate of a medical assisting program accredited by the Commission on Accreditation of Allied Health Education Programs (CAAHEP) or the Accrediting Bureau of Health Education Schools (ABHES).
  - The CMA (AAMA) certification must be renewed every 5 years

Another possible credential for medical assistants is the Registered Medical Assistant (RMA). This credential is awarded by the American Medical Technologists (AMT) organization and is accredited by the National Commission for Certifying Agencies.

Becoming credentialed as a medical assistant has definite benefits. Because credentialed medical assistants have had to pass a national standardized exam, they have the knowledge that allows them to perform well at their jobs and also a credential that is either preferred or required by employers in many facilities. For many new medical assistants, an earned credential improves their chances of getting and keeping a job in today's healthcare environment.

CLOSING COMMENTS

Patients expect and deserve professional behavior from those who work in medical facilities. Display courtesy and respect toward patients, families, and peers. A diplomatic and tactful person always attempts to interact honestly without giving offense. By displaying these attributes, the medical assistant earns the respect of co-workers and becomes indispensable to his or her employer. Behaving in a professional manner in the medical office helps gain the patient's trust. Trust is one of the most important factors in preventing cases of medical liability. Treating patients with care and not subjecting them to negative behaviors keeps the patient-provider relationship strong and conducive to the health and recovery of the patient. Performing as a cooperative team member goes a long way in promoting a positive healthcare environment for the patient. Incorporating time management strategies into each day not only helps you perform tasks more efficiently, but also ensures that no important tasks are left uncompleted. The entry-level medical assistant can promote professional behavior by joining one of the professional medical assistant organizations and seeking national credentialing.

Patient Education

Remember that most patients do not have any medical background and do not understand many of the phrases used by the medical community. Always be patient and courteously explain any aspect of the instructions or details the patient does not understand. Project a professional attitude of diplomacy and respect. If the patient seems concerned about revealing pertinent information, assure the person that medical assistants and the rest of the staff in the facility are bound by rules of patient confidentiality. Before the patient leaves the exam room, make sure to ask, "Do you have any questions?" This gives patients the opportunity to get all their questions answered before they leave the facility. A professional medical assistant does not share personal information with anyone at the medical facility. Refrain from passing along rumors of any type to patients or their families.

Legal and Ethical Issues

The workday should be centered around patient care, so never allow personal business to intrude on time that should be spent assisting patients and the provider. Otherwise, the patient may be left with the impression that the medical assistant, or the entire staff, is unprofessional, and this often leads to trust issues with the individuals employed at the facility. Professional credentialing is becoming more important each year. To safeguard future practice rights, medical assistants should become credentialed as either a CMA (AAMA) or an RMA.

SUMMARY OF SCENARIO

Karen is happy to be employed in a primary care practice in which providing quality patient care is paramount. She is learning to be careful about what she says and to remain focused on the patient instead of any personal difficulties she may be having. Karen knows it is her responsibility to be a team player and to assist the other staff members as much as possible. She maintains a good attitude and gets a strong sense of pride from being a member of the medical profession. She is meticulous about presenting a neat appearance and arrives on time for each workday. She always asks others whether they need help when she has any extra time throughout the day. Karen looks forward to a long relationship with her employer. The rewards she feels as a member of the health team are second to none.

SUMMARY OF LEARNING OBJECTIVES

1. **Define, spell, and pronounce the terms listed in the vocabulary.**
   Spelling and pronouncing medical terms correctly reinforce the medical assistant's credibility. Knowing the definitions of these terms promotes confidence in communication with patients and co-workers.

2. **Explain the reasons professionalism is important in the medical field, and describe work ethics.**
   Professionalism is the characteristic of conforming to the technical or ethical standards of a profession. Professionalism is vital in the medical profession because patients expect and deserve to be treated in a professional way. When the medical assistant acts in a professional way, he or she establishes trust with the patient. Patients notice professional behavior, even when it is not directed at them specifically. They notice how others are treated in the reception room and in other areas of the office. Always act in a professional manner while at work. Work ethics are sets of values based on the moral virtues of hard work and diligence, involving a whole range of activities, from individual acts to the philosophy of the entire facility.

3. **Discuss the attributes of professional medical assistants, and project a professional image in the ambulatory care setting.**
   Professional medical assistants display courteous, respectful behaviors and communicate with tact and diplomacy. They demonstrate responsible and honest behaviors and always act with integrity. Professional medical assistants view constructive criticism as a way of improving their skill level. Important assumptions are made within seconds of meeting someone based only on how they look. Most medical facilities require that medical assistants wear a uniform or scrubs or professional clothing that is not too tight and projects a professional, businesslike appearance. In addition, name badges should be visible; hair should be clean, and longer hair should

SUMMARY OF LEARNING OBJECTIVES—*continued*

be tied back; shoes should be clean; nails should be short and without nail polish (no artificial nails); and no jewelry should be worn.

4. **Identify obstructions to professional behaviors.**

   Everyone has a life outside the workplace, and sometimes we face challenges and difficult times that are hard to put aside. The professional medical assistant never transfers personal problems or baggage to anyone at the medical facility. The medical assistant should refuse to participate in the office rumor mill and should be cordial and friendly to everyone at work. Avoid personal phone calls and visits unless it is an absolute emergency.

5. **Define the principles of self-boundaries.**

   Awareness of personal boundaries helps us determine the actions and behaviors that we find unacceptable. Healthy self-boundaries make it possible to respect our strengths, abilities, and individuality and those of others.

6. **Describe the dynamics of the healthcare team.**

   To deliver comprehensive quality patient care, everyone who interacts with patients, from the time they enter the facility to the time they leave, must work as a cooperative member of the healthcare team.

7. **Apply time management strategies to prioritize the medical assistant's responsibilities as a member of the healthcare team.**

   Medical assistants need to use time efficiently, prioritize duties, and arrange schedules to ensure that duties can be performed in a timely manner. This can be done by planning tasks that need to be done that day. Most tasks can be prioritized into three general categories: those that must be done that day, those that should be done that day, and those that could be done if time permits.

8. **Summarize the role of professional medical assistant organizations.**

   There are definite benefits to becoming credentialed as a medical assistant. Because credentialed medical assistants (i.e., those with a CMA [AAMA] or AMT certificate) have had to pass a national standardized exam, they have proven they have the knowledge to perform well at their jobs. These individuals also have a credential that may be required by healthcare employers.

CONNECTIONS

Study Guide Connection: Go to the Chapter 3 Study Guide. Read and complete the activities.

evolve Evolve Connection: Go to the Chapter 3 link at *evolve.elsevier.com/ kinn* to complete the Chapter Review Quiz. Check out the other resources listed for this chapter to make the most of what you have learned from Professional Behaviors in the Workplace.

4

THERAPEUTIC COMMUNICATION

SCENARIO

Many types of patients seek medical attention and care in an ambulatory care setting. Each patient has different needs and different concerns, even if the diagnoses are similar. Communication and interpersonal skills are vital in meeting those needs and providing optimum care to the patient. However, the patient is not the only individual who must be considered; family members often are crucial to the patient's health and well-being.

Lucille Cloyd is an 83-year-old patient who has been diagnosed with heart disease and is seeing Dr. Neill for treatment. Her daughter, Sarah Smithson,

helps care for her and frequently accompanies her mother to Dr. Neil's office. Mrs. Cloyd is widowed and visits the physician once a month, in addition to receiving home care services. The medical assistant must consider not only the needs of Mrs. Cloyd, but also those of her extended family. Compassion and sensitivity are necessary to care for this patient, in addition to excellent therapeutic communication skills.

While studying this chapter, think about the following questions:

- What communication barriers might exist between patients and healthcare workers?
- How does the medical assistant effectively communicate with a patient's family members?

- How will developing good therapeutic communication skills make the medical assistant more effective?

LEARNING OBJECTIVES

1. Define, spell, and pronounce the terms listed in the vocabulary.
2. Discuss first impressions and patient-centered care.
3. Do the following related to communication paths:
   - Identify styles and types of verbal communication.
   - Identify types of nonverbal communication.
   - Recognize and respond to verbal and nonverbal communication.
4. Recognize communication barriers.
5. Summarize factors that should be considered when communicating with diverse patient populations.
6. Identify techniques for overcoming communication barriers.

7. Do the following related to communication during difficult times:
   - Recognize the elements of oral communication using the sender-receiver process.
   - Apply feedback techniques, including reflection, restatement, and clarification, to obtain information.
   - Discuss open and closed questions or statements
8. Discuss important factors about therapeutic communication across the life span.
9. List and explain the levels of Maslow's hierarchy of needs.

VOCABULARY

congruence Being in agreement, harmony, or correspondence; conforming to the circumstances or requirements of a situation.

stereotype Something conforming to a fixed or general pattern; a standardized mental picture that is held in common by many

and represents an oversimplified opinion, prejudiced attitude, or uncritical judgment.

Therapeutic communication skills developed by the medical assistant help set the tone of care in a healthcare facility. Patients who visit the healthcare facility may not be at their best, and the way the medical assistant reacts to and interacts with them can make an incredible difference in whether they view the facility and those who care for them positively or negatively. These interactions may also affect the patient's treatment and recovery.

FIRST IMPRESSIONS

The opinions formed in the early moments of meeting someone remain in our thoughts long after the first words have been spoken. The first impression involves much more than just physical appearance or dress; it includes attitude, compassion, and therapeutic communication skills that clearly help the patient and family members realize that the medical assistant is interested in who they are and what they need (Figure 4-1).

Delivering quality patient care is the primary objective of the professional medical assistant. Patients are the reason the facility exists. Each patient should be welcomed warmly by name and with a polite greeting. Think for a moment about how it feels to be a new patient entering the unknown territory of a healthcare facility. Staff members of the facility are in familiar surroundings and already have some information about the new patient. However, the patient knows nothing about the staff members. One way to break that barrier is to have all staff members wear name badges, with letters large enough to be read at a distance of 3 feet. Include the staff position if several divisions of responsibility exist (e.g., "medical assistant," "administrative specialist," and "practice manager"). When the patient approaches, make introductions and smile. Smiles should show in the voice and the eyes. Genuinely welcome the patient to the facility. This small effort helps put the patient at ease in the healthcare environment.

To provide high-quality patient care, we must communicate effectively with the patient and provide a warm, caring environment. Positive reactions and interactions with the patient are vital. Because

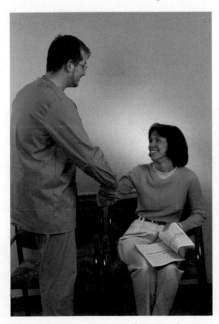

FIGURE 4-1 First impressions are critical in gaining the patient's trust.

medical care by nature is extremely personal, a medical assistant must always remember that each patient is an individual with certain anxieties. These anxieties often cause people to act and react in different ways; therefore, effective verbal and nonverbal communication with each patient is absolutely essential.

Healthcare professionals accept the responsibility of developing helping relationships with their patients. The interpersonal nature of the patient–medical assistant relationship carries with it a certain amount of responsibility to forget one's self-interest and focus on the patient's needs. A medical assistant can elicit either a positive or a negative response to patient care simply by the way he or she treats and interacts with patients. You usually are the first person with whom the patient communicates; therefore, you play a vital role in initiating therapeutic patient interactions.

PATIENT-CENTERED CARE

Healthcare professionals have embraced patient-centered care, an innovative approach to the planning, delivery, and evaluation of healthcare that is grounded in mutually beneficial partnerships among healthcare providers, patients, and families. Patient- and family-centered care applies to patients of all ages and may be practiced in any healthcare setting. Each patient who seeks care has a unique set of needs, including clinical symptoms that require medical attention and issues specific to the individual that can affect his or her care. As patients navigate the healthcare delivery system, providers and their employees must be prepared to identify and address not just the clinical aspects of care, but also the spectrum of each patient's demographic and personal characteristics. Good communication skills are vital to meeting the needs of the patient and his or her support system.

COMMUNICATION PATHS

Verbal Communication

When we communicate verbally with our patients, we use words to deliver the intended message. The two major forms of verbal communication are oral communication and written communication.

Most of us consider talking the only form of verbal communication. However, there are many different styles and methods of sending a patient a voice-related message, including face-to-face discussions, telephone conversations, voicemail, television or radio advertisements, and videos. Verbal communication occurs when we express our thoughts with words. Verbal communication is affected by many factors, including our tone of voice, enunciation of words, use of therapeutic pauses, emphasis on certain terms, and choice of words, including whether we use medical or lay language. Nonverbal behaviors (i.e., the tone of voice we use, facial expressions, and so on) can drastically affect how words are interpreted. All of these factors affect the patient's understanding of our verbal message.

The other form of verbal communication is the written word. When we put our thoughts to paper, such as writing down instructions for a patient, our verbal words are now in written form. A wide variety of written communication is used in the healthcare setting on a routine basis. Examples include patient education handouts, written provider orders (e.g., prescriptions), e-mails describing laboratory results or appointment reminders, letters, faxes, articles, hand-written notes, and text messages. A type of written communication used routinely for all patients is documentation in the health record. Just as with oral communication, we must be careful that written communication is both accurate and comprehensive to prevent patient confusion or medical errors. All written communication carries an added legal burden, so it is crucial that everything that is documented or written down for patient referral is accurate and comprehensive.

Electronic communication, such as e-mails or text messages, is an efficient way of delivering a written message to the patient, but several cautionary notes apply to the use of these methods. First, patient confidentiality must always be secured; for example, messages should be sent only to an e-mail address or cell phone number the patient has approved. Second, there is no way to confirm the patient actually received the message unless he or she is required to respond with a receipt of message or the message is flagged electronically to show that it was received. If the healthcare facility relies on e-mail or text messages to communicate with patients, these systems must be in place to make sure the patient is actually receiving the information. Text messages should be completely written out, without abbreviations or shortcuts; for example, do not use "u" for "you." In addition, it is important to use lay language rather than medical terminology so that the patient can understand the meaning of the message. You also must be careful of the writing style used in an e-mail. Using all capital letters in an e-mail can be interpreted as screaming at the person receiving the e-mail, which can lead to misunderstanding and communication problems.

Nonverbal Communication

Much of what we communicate to our patients is conveyed through the use of conscious or unconscious body language. Our nonverbal actions, such as gestures, facial expressions, and mannerisms, are learned behaviors that are greatly influenced by our family and cultural backgrounds. The body naturally expresses our true feelings; in fact, experts say that more than 90% of communication is nonverbal. This means that, even though the verbal message is an important method of delivering information, the *way* we deliver those words determines how the patient interprets them.

Most of the negative messages communicated through body language are unintentional; therefore, it is important to remember while conducting patient interviews that nonverbal communication can seriously affect the therapeutic process. You can do much to put a patient at ease by the tone of your voice. Your facial expression and the ease and confidence of your movements demonstrate a sincere interest in the patient. Therapeutic use of space and touch also are important ways of sending nonverbal messages to your patients. You should establish eye contact (in most cases), sit in a relaxed but attentive position, and avoid using furniture as a barrier between you and the patient. Give the patient your undivided attention and let your body language inform each patient that you are interested in his or her medical problems (Procedure 4-1).

The key to successful patient interaction is **congruence** between the words used and the body language observed. In other words, if you say to a patient who had an emergency that made him late for his appointment, "I understand you had an unexpected problem that prevented you from getting here on time," but you say it in a doubting or sarcastic tone of voice with your arms crossed and your face disapproving, what message did that patient receive? Effective therapeutic communication means we need to constantly be aware of our body language and work at making sure our nonverbal language matches our words. To be viewed as honest and sensitive to the needs of your patients, you must be aware of your nonverbal behavior patterns. The nonverbal message the patient receives from the medical assistant's listening behavior should be "You are a person of worth, and I am interested in you as a unique individual" (Figure 4-2).

Observing your patient fosters mutual understanding. The purpose of observing nonverbal communication is to become sensitive to or aware of the feelings of others as conveyed by small bits of behavior rather than words. This sensitivity enables you to adapt your behavior to these feelings; to deliberately select your response, either verbal or nonverbal; and thereby to have a favorable effect on others. The favorable effect may consist of providing emotional support, conveying that you care, defusing the patient's fear or anger, or providing an invitation to release pent-up feelings by talking about the situation that aroused the feelings (Figure 4-3). Table 4-1 lists some nonverbal behaviors by patients that may indicate anxiety, frustration, or fear.

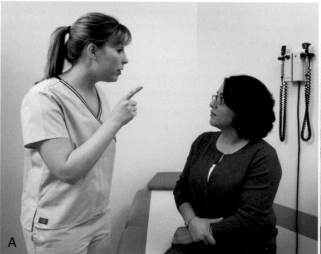
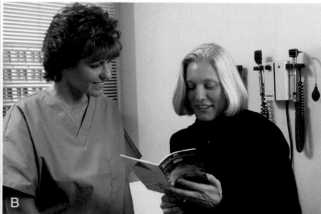

FIGURE 4-2 A, Pointing often is an accusatory gesture and causes discomfort. B, A bright smile helps to put the patient at ease and to relax.

Nonverbal Language Behaviors

Nonverbal behavior—that is, your body language—can have either a positive or negative effect on patient interactions. Positive nonverbal behaviors enhance the patient's experience in the healthcare setting. Communication experts recommend the following:

- When gathering information from a patient, lean toward the patient to show interest.
- Face the patient squarely and at eye level to help make the patient more comfortable and to demonstrate sensitivity and empathy.
- Eye contact is essential for therapeutic communication unless the patient is from a culture that discourages this; many Asian cultures consider eye contact during a conversation very rude.
- A closed posture (crossed arms or legs) may indicate disinterest.
- Be sensitive to the patient's personal space when possible. Maintain a comfortable distance, at least an arm's length away, when interacting with a patient.

- Be careful with body gestures such as hand and arm movements. Gestures, such as nodding your head when the patient talks, can display interest, but too much body movement can be distracting.
- Your tone of voice should reflect your interest in the patient. Speaking too quietly or too loudly can detract from therapeutic communication.
- Continually observe the patient's body language; watch for signs of confusion, boredom, worry, and other emotions so that you can respond appropriately.
- Documenting in an electronic health record can be distracting to both the medical assistant and the patient. Remind yourself to look at the patient frequently, and use encouraging body language to maintain a personal interaction with him or her.

PROCEDURE 4-1   Respond to Nonverbal Communication

Complete this procedure with another student playing the role of the patient. To make the experience more realistic, choose a student about whom you know very little. To maintain the student's privacy, he or she does not have to share any confidential information.

Goal: *To observe the patient and respond appropriately to nonverbal communication.*

Scenario: *Tanya Williams, 36, is a new patient with the CC of intermittent abdominal pain with alternating diarrhea and constipation. Ms. Williams has experienced this discomfort for several months and appears very frustrated. You are working in the administrative side of the practice today and have to gather initial information from Ms. Williams about the history of her complaints, in addition to collecting her insurance information and having her sign several forms. She is sitting with her arms wrapped around her abdomen, tapping her right foot on the floor, and refusing to maintain eye contact. What is her nonverbal behavior telling you, and how can you establish therapeutic communication with this patient?*

EQUIPMENT and SUPPLIES

- Appropriate intake forms for a new patient
- Patient's health record

PROCEDURAL STEPS

1. Greet the patient pleasantly, introduce yourself, and verify her ID and date of birth (DOB). Explain your role.
   PURPOSE: To make the patient feel comfortable and at ease.
2. Ask the patient the purpose of her visit and the onset, duration, and frequency of her symptoms. Pay close attention to her body language to determine whether what she is telling you is congruent with her body language.
   PURPOSE: Nonverbal language naturally expresses the patient's true feelings. Closely observing body language helps you reach more detailed conclusions about patient information.
3. Use restatement, reflection, and clarification to gather as much information as possible about the patient's CC. Make sure all medical terminology is adequately explained.

PURPOSE: Therapeutic communication techniques help the medical assistant gather complete information; using feedback techniques and making sure the patient understands medical terms helps relieve anxiety.

4. Speak in a pleasant, distinct manner, remembering to maintain eye contact with your patient.
   PURPOSE: Positive nonverbal behaviors create a friendly, caring atmosphere. Remain sensitive to the diverse needs of your patient throughout the interview process.
5. Continue to observe the patient's nonverbal behaviors and select the appropriate verbal response to demonstrate your sensitivity to her discomfort, frustration, and anxiety.
   PURPOSE: Displaying sensitivity to and awareness of the patient's nonverbal body language demonstrates your concern for the patient and helps defuse the patient's concerns.

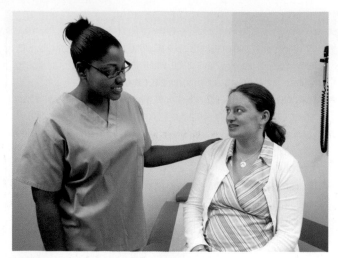

FIGURE 4-3 Touching the patient communicates care and compassion. Careful listening and asking questions helps the patient express thoughts and feelings.

TABLE 4-1 Observation of Nonverbal Communication in Patients

AREA OBSERVED	OBSERVATION	INDICATION
Breathing patterns	Rapid respirations, sighing, shallow thoracic breathing	Anxiety, boredom, pain
Eye patterns	Side-to-side eye movements, looking down at the hands	Anxiety, distrust, embarrassment
Hands	Tapping fingers, cracking knuckles, continuous movement, sweaty palms	Anxiety, worry, fear
Arm placement	Folded across chest, wrapped around abdomen	Anxiety, worry, fear, pain
Leg placement	Tension, crossed and/or tucked under, tapping foot, continuous movement	Frustration, anger

Recognizing and Responding to Verbal and Nonverbal Communications

The medical assistant not only must implement therapeutic communication skills, he or she also must observe the patient to interpret the person's message and level of understanding. In the following critical thinking exercise, the medical assistant uses the therapeutic communication skills discussed in the chapter, including active listening techniques, open and closed questions and statements, positive nonverbal skills, and effective observation of the patient's body language. How would you answer each question?

Communication factors that should be considered in this exercise include the following:

• What nonverbal language is being used by the patient, Mr. Anderson, and how should it be interpreted?
• Mr. Anderson tells the medical assistant he is not following that crazy diet and never will. What therapeutic communication skills can be used to get more information out of Mr. Anderson and to reinforce the physician's recommendations?
• During the discussion Mr. Anderson says he stopped taking the blood pressure medicine because of the side effects. What communication techniques and therapeutic body language can be used to emphasize the need for Mr. Anderson to take his medicine as prescribed?

CRITICAL THINKING APPLICATION   **4-1**

Toby Anderson, a 52-year-old patient, was recently diagnosed with hypertension and prescribed Lotensin bid for treatment. He is being seen today for follow-up measurement of his blood pressure. Mr. Anderson also has issues with his bill, which he wants to discuss with the "woman in charge." He is 45 pounds overweight and was given information about a reduced-calorie, low-sodium diet 1 month ago, but he has not lost any weight. He tells the medical assistant who is trying to help him understand his bill that he is just going to quit coming to the doctor since he isn't getting any better and he can't afford it anyway. He is sitting with his arms across his chest, tapping his foot, and occasionally cracking his knuckles.

COMMUNICATION BARRIERS

Effective therapeutic communication requires the delivery of a clear message to the patient. However, along the way, many communication barriers can cause misunderstanding and misinterpretation of your message. Successful communication relies on knowing what barriers to communication exist and how to navigate around these roadblocks. By understanding what barriers may stand in the way of your attempts at effective communication, you can more successfully sidestep these challenges and engage in patient-centered communication. Communication barriers can arise from both medical assistants and patients. The following sections discuss just some of the communication barriers that the medical assistant might use when interacting with patients.

Providing Unwarranted Assurance

Mrs. Miller says to you, "I know this lump is going to turn out to be cancer." The typical reply is almost automatic: "Don't worry, I'm sure everything will be fine." This type of answer indicates that her anxiety is insignificant and denies her the opportunity to discuss her fears further. A reflective response, such as "You sound really worried about…" acknowledges her feelings and demonstrates empathy and a willingness to listen to her concerns.

Giving Advice

Mrs. Thompson has just finished talking to the physician. She looks at you and says, "Dr. Rowe says I need surgery to get rid of these gallstones. I just don't know. What would you do?" If you tell her how you would handle the situation, you may have shifted the accountability for decision making from her to you, and she has not worked out her own solution. Does this woman really want to know what you would do? Probably not. You could respond to her question with, "Based on what the doctor told you, what do you think you should do?" or "Do you need further information to make your decision?" If the patient continues to question recommendations, the medical assistant should encourage further discussion with the provider.

Using Medical Terminology

You must adjust your vocabulary to fit the patient. The more the patient understands about what is happening and the management of the problem, the better the outcome. Misinterpreted communication is the most common error in patient care. One of the biggest problems for the patient is understanding medical terminology. Closely observe the patient's body language while he or she receives instructions or patient education. If the patient shows signs of not understanding the procedure, ask the patient to repeat back to you the information or instructions. This demonstration–return demonstration form of providing feedback ensures that the patient completely understands what is happening. It also gives the medical assistant the opportunity to clarify any misconceptions.

Leading Questions

While gathering patient information, you ask the patient, "You don't smoke, do you?" By asking questions in this manner, you indicate the preferred answer. Telling you that he or she does smoke would surely meet with your disapproval. Keep your questions positive. A better way of asking would be "Have you ever smoked?" or "Do you use tobacco?"

Talking Too Much

Some medical assistants associate helpfulness with verbal overload. The patient may let you talk at the expense of his or her own need to explain what is wrong. Always remember that when interacting with a patient, you should listen more than you talk. Pay close attention to the patient's body language to make sure you are giving the patient ample opportunity to discuss the health problem or issue.

Stereotyping

Stereotyping is defined as the application of a standardized mental picture that is held in common by members of a group; it represents an oversimplified opinion or a prejudiced attitude. It is unfair to stereotype anyone or categorize the person based on preconceived and often incorrect assumptions. Although sometimes an assumption based on stereotypic categories may have a degree of truth, people should not be judged before you have gotten to know them as individuals. The medical assistant should push preconceived notions aside and look at the individual when forming and building a relationship. In the medical profession, stereotypic categories should not be considered when caring for patients.

Other communication barriers are caused by problems the patient might have. By being sensitive to such problems, the medical assistant can use therapeutic communication techniques to help these patients.

Physical Impairment

Patients may have physical conditions that impair their ability to communicate effectively. This could be a vision or hearing problem or one of many other conditions that make communicating a bit more difficult than usual. The medical assistant should use more descriptive language when speaking with the patient who has a visual disturbance. This helps the patient "see" what is being discussed. A person with diminished hearing may be very sensitive and in denial of the condition. Make sure you have his or her attention and that you are face-to-face with the person while speaking. People who are hearing impaired often are very dependent on lip reading for comprehension. In either case, involve family members or assistive devices to help communicate effectively with the patient.

CRITICAL THINKING APPLICATION   **4-2**
- What must be considered when communicating verbally with an elderly patient?
- How can the medical assistant demonstrate patience with an elderly patient during her appointment when the office is extremely busy?

Language

With non-English-speaking patients, the medical assistant may need to use gestures and more body language to convey messages. In such cases, be alert to the possibility of misunderstanding. Confirm that the message sent is the message the listener received by asking for feedback. Ask the listener to repeat the message, and if family members are present, make sure they, also, have a good understanding of what was communicated. The clinic may employ a bilingual staff member to reduce the chance of miscommunication with those who speak a different language.

SENSITIVITY TO DIVERSITY

Practicing respectful patient care is extremely important when working with a diverse patient population. *Empathy* is the key to creating a caring, therapeutic environment. Empathy goes beyond sympathy. A medical assistant who is empathetic respects the individuality of the patient and attempts to see the person's health problem through his or her eyes, recognizing the effect of all holistic factors on the patient's well-being. Empathetic sensitivity to diversity first requires those interested in healthcare to examine their own values, beliefs, and actions; you cannot treat all patients with care and respect until you first recognize and evaluate your personal biases. We think and act a certain way for many reasons. The first step in understanding the process is to evaluate your individual value system. Why do you have certain attitudes or beliefs about the worth of individuals or things?

CRITICAL THINKING APPLICATION   **4-3**
What do you value most in life? What is important to you? What influences you to act in a certain way? Make a list of five things you value the most and share them with the class. Try to determine why you feel so strongly about those particular things.

Many different factors influence the development of a value system. Value systems begin as learned beliefs and behaviors. Families and cultural influences shape the way we respond to a diverse society. Other factors that influence reactions include socioeconomic and educational backgrounds. To develop therapeutic relationships, you must recognize your own value system to determine whether it could affect your method of interaction. Preconceived ideas about people because of their race, religion, income level, ethnic origin, sexual orientation, or gender can act as barriers to the development of a therapeutic relationship. You will be unable to treat your patients empathetically unless you can connect with them in some way. Personal biases or prejudices are monumental barriers to the development of therapeutic relationships.

CRITICAL THINKING APPLICATION   4-4

Honestly evaluate your personal biases. What do you find unacceptable in people? Do you prejudge an individual based on his or her affiliation with a particular group or because of a certain lifestyle decision? Do these biases create barriers to the development of therapeutic relationships? If so, how can you get beyond these barriers?

Consider the following scenarios and discuss them with your classmates:

- While you are gathering a patient's insurance information, the patient tells you that he has tested positive for the human immunodeficiency virus (HIV). Do you think this will affect your therapeutic relationship?
- A homeless person with very poor hygiene stops in to make an appointment to see the provider. Will this cause a problem with your professional manner?
- You are told by your office manager that an inmate of the county prison is being brought in this afternoon for an examination. Do you think his status will affect your interaction with the patient?
- You are attempting to register a 20-year-old patient who brought her two young children with her to the clinic today. She is a single mother who is pregnant with her third child and receives public assistance. What do you think? Will you have difficulty being empathetic and communicating therapeutically with this young woman?

Sensitivity to Diversity

Regardless of the type of healthcare facility in which you work, you will care for a wide variety of patients. The following are some points to consider when communicating with diverse groups of patients.
- Patients of Asian backgrounds may have been raised in a culture that considers it extremely rude to establish eye contact. Americans view an unwillingness to establish eye contact as a sign of distrust or embarrassment; however, for individuals from Japan or China, lack of eye contact may be a way of demonstrating respect.
- Personal space may be an issue for patients from diverse backgrounds. If a patient appears very uncomfortable with touch or lack of personal space, attempt to accommodate him or her as much as possible.
- Research has shown that older people face unique communication problems in the healthcare environment. When you are caring for an aging individual, it is important to focus patient teaching and information on the patient rather than the family member who may be present.
- Patients may use their religious beliefs and values to understand and cope with their health problems. However, using religion to guide healthcare decisions may result in a conflict with the provider's recommendations. Healthcare workers may need to find a balance between respect for a patient's beliefs and the delivery of high-quality healthcare.

OVERCOMING BARRIERS TO COMMUNICATION

We know that communication barriers exist, but how do we overcome them? Most people who enter the medical field have a natural sense of caring and empathy, but the medical assistant can nurture communication skills by using patience, observation, and sensitivity to patient needs, in addition to therapeutic listening skills. If a patient has a physical impairment, being observant helps with communication issues. Often these patients want to be self-sufficient, so they may not appreciate help with simple tasks. Be patient with them and with those who have a language barrier. Encourage these patients to bring an interpreter so that accurate, quality information can be placed into the health record. Prejudice can be overcome with facts about the source of social bias, and the same is true for stereotyping issues. Even highly abrasive patients can be tolerated when the medical assistant wants to be an effective communicator with all patients. If nothing seems to work, talk to the office manager or provider. In severe cases, the provider may have to speak to the patient, or even suggest that he or she seek a different facility for care.

Communication during Difficult Times

Communication is not an art that comes easily to everyone. It often is difficult to express feelings in an honest, open way. When a crisis occurs, it is much harder to communicate effectively, and we sometimes say things we do not mean. Medical assistants must develop communication skills that can be used in times of trouble. They must be able to understand the reason or reasons a patient or co-worker is unable to communicate.

Patience is important, too, because people are not always at their best when they are concerned about their condition or that of a loved one. Always remain calm when dealing with a person who is experiencing a traumatic event or has any depressive condition. Remember that he or she may be reacting to strong emotions, including fear, anger, doubt, inadequacy, or many others. The key is to listen, to determine the best way to help the patient out of any immediate danger, and to help him or her establish some type of support system (Figure 4-4).

Therapeutic Techniques

The linear communication model describes communication as an interactive process involving the sender of the message, the receiver, and the crucial component of feedback to confirm reception of the message. When two people interact, both usually act as senders and

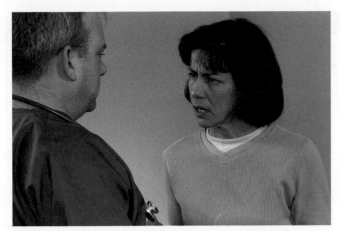

FIGURE 4-4 Remain calm even if a patient becomes verbally aggressive. Attempt to calm the person by listening and expressing empathy whenever possible.

as receivers (or communicators). The *sender* is the person who sends a message through a variety of different channels. *Channels* can be spoken words, written or e-mailed messages, and body language. The sender *encodes* the message, which simply means that he or she chooses a specific means of expression using words and other channels. The receiver *decodes* the message according to his or her understanding of what is being communicated. The message can be sent by a number of different methods or channels, such as face-to-face communication, telephone, e-mail, and letter; however, there is no way to confirm that the message was actually received unless the patient provides *feedback* about what he or she interpreted from the message. Feedback completes the communication cycle by providing a means for us to know exactly what message the patient received and therefore whether it requires clarification.

For example, as a medical assistant, one of your responsibilities will be to provide patient education on how to prepare for diagnostic studies. Let's say you have to explain to an elderly patient how to prepare for a colonoscopy. Even though you provide a detailed explanation of the preparation procedure, in addition to a handout explaining the step-by-step process, how do you really know whether the patient understands (has received the message you sent)? You ask the patient to provide feedback by explaining the process back to you. As a member of the healthcare team, you must become an effective communicator. You will play a vital role in collecting and documenting patient information. If your methods of collection or recording are faulty, the quality of patient care may be seriously impaired.

In summary, the verbal messages you send are only part of the communication process. You have a specific context in mind when you send your words, but the receiver puts his or her own interpretations on them. The receiver attaches meaning determined by his or her past experiences, culture, self-concept, and current physical and emotional states. Sometimes these messages and interpretations do not coincide. Feedback from the patient is crucial in determining whether the patient understood the message. Successful communication requires mutual understanding by both the interviewer and the person being interviewed.

Active Listening Techniques

Listening is just as important to good communication as the spoken word. *Hearing* is the process, function, or power of perceiving sound, whereas *listening* is defined as paying attention to sound or hearing something with thoughtful attention. Patients need to know that the medical assistant is listening. Sometimes it is hard to listen. We may not be able to listen effectively because we are distracted by our own thoughts. Perhaps the situations occurring in our own lives make the conversation we are hearing seem meaningless and unimportant. Or so many messages may be attacking at once that we are unable to focus on any specific one to listen to what is being communicated. At other times, we may simply be too tired to listen, or we may have prejudged the speaker and decided that we do not need to listen. However, while working with patients, the medical assistant must be diligent not only in hearing the words being spoken, but also in listening to them and to what the patient is attempting to communicate.

Active listeners go beyond hearing the patient's message to concentrating, understanding, and listening to the main points in the discussion. Active listening techniques encourage patients to expand on and clarify the content and meaning of their messages. They are very useful communication tools to implement when a patient is agitated or upset because these methods help the medical assistant clarify the important details of the patient's chief complaint.

Three processes are involved in active listening: restatement, reflection, and clarification.

- *Restatement* is simply paraphrasing or repeating the patient's statements with phrases such as "You are saying…" or "You are telling me the problem is…"

- *Reflection* involves repeating the main idea of the conversation while also identifying the sender's feelings. For example, if the mother of a young patient is expressing frustration about her child's behavior, a reflective statement identifies that feeling with the response "You sound frustrated about…" Or, if a patient expresses concern about being able to pay surgical bills, an appropriate reflective statement recognizes the patient's feelings: "You appear anxious about…" Reflective statements clearly demonstrate to patients that you are not only listening to their words; you also are concerned and are attending to their feelings.

- *Clarification* seeks to summarize or simplify the sender's thoughts and feelings and to resolve any confusion in the message. Questions or statements that begin with "Give me an example of…" or "Explain to me about…" or "So what you're saying is…" help patients focus on their chief concern and give you the opportunity to clear up any misconceptions before documenting patient information.

Listening is not a passive role in the communication process; it is active and demanding. You cannot be preoccupied with your own needs, or you will miss something important. For the duration of a patient interaction, no one is more important than this particular patient. Listen to the way things are said, the tone of the patient's voice, and even to what the patient may not be saying out loud but is saying very clearly with body language (Procedure 4-2).

Helpful Listening Guidelines

- Listen to the main points of the discussion.
- Attend to both verbal and nonverbal messages.
- Be patient and nonjudgmental.
- Do not interrupt.

- Never intimidate your patient.
- Use active listening techniques—restatement, reflection, and clarification.

PROCEDURE 4-2   **Apply Feedback Techniques, Including Reflection, Restatement, and Clarification, to Obtain Patient Information**

Complete this procedure with another student playing the role of the patient. To make the experience more realistic, choose a student about whom you know very little. To maintain the student's privacy, he or she does not have to share any confidential information.

Goal: *To use restatement, reflection, and clarification to obtain patient information and document patient care accurately.*

EQUIPMENT and SUPPLIES

- History form or computer with the patient history window open
- If using a paper form, two pens: a red pen for recording the patient's allergies and a black pen to meet legal documentation guidelines
- Quiet, private area

PROCEDURAL STEPS

1. Greet the patient pleasantly, introduce yourself, and verify the person's ID and date of birth (DOB). Explain your role.
   PURPOSE: To make the patient feel comfortable and at ease.
2. Take the patient to a quiet, private area for the interview and explain why the information is needed.
   PURPOSE: A quiet, private area is necessary to protect confidentiality and prevent interruptions. An informed patient is more cooperative and therefore more likely to provide useful information.
3. Complete the history form by using therapeutic communication techniques, including restatement, reflection, and clarification. Make sure all medical terminology is adequately explained.
   PURPOSE: Therapeutic communication techniques help the medical assistant gather complete information.
4. Speak in a pleasant, distinct manner, remembering to maintain eye contact with your patient.
   PURPOSE: Positive nonverbal behaviors create a friendly, caring atmosphere.
5. Remain sensitive to the diverse needs of your patient throughout the interview process.
   PURPOSE: Maintaining awareness of your personal biases, treat all patients with respect despite their diverse backgrounds.

6. State the message to your patient. Demonstrate sensitivity appropriate to the message being delivered.
   PURPOSE: To send a clearly communicated message.
7. Allow your patient to respond to the sent message. Apply active listening skills.
   PURPOSE: To make sure your patient understood your message and to allow him or her to communicate a response.
8. Restate your patient's response.
   PURPOSE: To make sure you understand the patient's message and to give the patient the opportunity to expand on the information.
9. Use reflection as appropriate to communicate your acknowledgement of the patient's feelings.
   PURPOSE: Use a "feeling" word in your response to demonstrate to the patient that you are attending to his or her emotions and words.
10. Clarify any issues that are unclear.
    PURPOSE: To make sure the meaning of each message sent is understood. You can use clarification to summarize the information you learned. This could serve as a final check on the accuracy of the information you gathered from the patient.
11. Continue to communicate back and forth, using active listening techniques to make sure that your message is understood correctly.
12. Analyze communications in providing appropriate responses and feedback.
    PURPOSE: To continually improve the communication process between healthcare professionals, other staff members, and patients.
13. Thank the patient for sharing the information and direct him or her back to the reception area.
    PURPOSE: To demonstrate respectful patient care.

Open and Closed Questions or Statements

When you gather information from a patient, it is helpful to use a combination of open and closed questions or statements.

An *open* question or statement asks for general information or states the topic to be discussed, but only in general terms. Use this communication tool to begin a conversation with a patient, to introduce a new section of questions, or whenever the person introduces a new topic. It is a very effective method of gathering more details from the patient about his or her problem. Example questions include:

"Why do you need to make an appointment to see Dr. Neill?"
"How have you been getting along?"
"You mentioned having problems with your insurance. Tell me more about it."

This type of question or statement encourages patients to respond in a manner they find comfortable. It allows patients to express themselves fully and provide comprehensive information about their chief complaint.

Direct, or *closed,* questions ask for specific information. In many cases, this form of questioning limits the patient's answer to one or two words: yes or no. Use this form of question when you need confirmation of specific facts, such as when asking about demographic information. For example:

"What is the name of your insurance carrier?"
"What is your birth date?"
"What pharmacy do you prefer for prescription refills?"

COMMUNICATION ACROSS THE LIFE SPAN

The key to communicating effectively with patients is using an age-specific approach. Given the age and developmental level of your patient, how can you best interact with the person and with significant family members?

For example, Tasha, a 2-year-old patient, is scheduled for a physical examination. How can you best interact with her and her father to ensure that the history phase of the visit is complete and accurate? Therapeutic use of nonverbal language is essential to interacting with children of all ages. Getting down on the child's level, establishing eye contact, and using a gentle but firm voice are ways of gaining the child's confidence and cooperation. Children fear the unknown, so explaining all procedures in language the child understands is important. At the same time, the medical assistant must communicate with the child's caregiver so that he or she can contribute to the intake process. The following are some important guidelines for communicating with children and their caregivers.
- Make sure the environment is safe and attractive.
- Do not keep children and their caregivers waiting any longer than necessary because children become anxious and distracted quickly.
- Do not offer a choice unless the child can truly make one. If part of the treatment requires an injection, asking the child whether she'd like her shot now is most likely to get an automatic "No!" However, giving her a choice of stickers after the injection is appropriate.

- Praising the child during the examination helps reduce anxiety and increase self-esteem. When possible, direct questions to the child so that he or she feels like part of the process.
- Involving the child in procedures by permitting him or her to manipulate the equipment may help relieve anxiety. If possible, use your imagination and make a game of what needs to be done.
- A typical defense mechanism seen in sick or anxious children is regression. The child may refuse to leave the mother's lap or may want to hold a favorite toy during the procedure as a comfort measure. Look for signs of anxiety, such as thumb-sucking or rocking during the assessment, and encourage caregivers to be involved in the process to help make the child feel as safe as possible.
- Listen to parents' concerns and respond truthfully to questions.

Older children may also have difficulty during the health visit. To help school-aged children gain a sense of control, give them the opportunity to make certain decisions about treatment. For example, Heather, a 13-year-old patient with diabetes, could be given the choice of having her father present during the visit. Or, if she requires an insulin injection, she could choose the site of the injection or perhaps administer the medication herself. This gives the medical assistant an opportunity to observe her technique and allows Heather to exert her independence.

Privacy is an important issue to consider with older children, especially adolescents. Respect their privacy by keeping body exposure to a minimum and adequately preparing the child for procedures and positions. In addition, older children want to know what is going on, what to expect, and what the findings mean; therefore, keeping them informed in a language they can understand is important. Teen patients should always be encouraged to ask questions, which should be answered as completely and clearly as possible. Take every opportunity to teach your patients, regardless of their age, about their disease and to share information about related wellness factors.

Therapeutic communication is extremely important when interacting with adult patients (Figure 4-5). Using language the adult patient understands and involving the patient in treatment decisions as much as possible are essential to developing a helping relationship with your older patients. Adults are bombarded by multiple responsibilities, which means that stress-related health problems are not unusual in these patients. Get to know your adult patients and

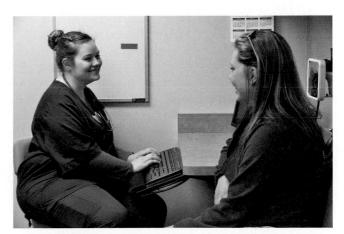

FIGURE 4-5 Medical assistant communicating with an adult patient.

emphasize preventive healthcare when possible. Coaching patients based on their cultural diversity, developmental age, and communication style is a key approach to effective communication and patient education (also see the chapter, Patient Education).

Suggestions for Effective Communication with Aging Patients

- Address the patient by Mr., Mrs., or Miss unless the patient has given you permission to use his or her first name.
- Introduce yourself and explain the purpose of a procedure before performing the procedure.
- Face the aging person and softly touch the individual to get his or her attention before beginning to speak.
- Use *expanded speech* by lowering the pitch or tone of your voice and speaking firmly, making sure to sound out each word clearly.
- Use gestures and demonstrations to clarify communication and print out instructions in block print using a larger font size to be sure aging individuals can read the information.
- If the message must be repeated, paraphrase or find other words to say the same thing.
- Observe the patient's nonverbal behavior for cues indicating whether he or she understands.
- Provide adequate lighting without glare.
- Allow patients time to process information and take care of themselves unless they ask for assistance.
- Conduct communication in a quiet room without distractions.
- Involve family members as needed for continuity of care.
- When leaving a telephone message, remember to speak slowly and clearly and repeat the message in the same manner. It is difficult to interpret a message, and even more difficult to write it down, if the message was delivered in a hurried manner.
- Use referrals and community resources for support.

MASLOW'S HIERARCHY OF NEEDS

Psychologist Abraham Maslow created what he called the "hierarchy of needs" (Figure 4-6). A *hierarchy* is defined as things arranged in order, rank, or a graded series. Maslow believed that our human needs can be categorized into five levels and that the needs on each level must be satisfied before we can move to the next level. These levels often are depicted as a triangle, with the most basic needs at the bottom and the highest potential for growth as a human being at the top.

The needs we have as humans, at the most basic level, are those that involve our physical well-being: food, rest, sleep, water, air, and sex. The second level includes issues related to our safety: we need to feel safe and secure in our homes, our environments, and the places where we work. The third level involves our social needs for love, a sense of belonging, and interaction with others. The fourth level relates to our self-esteem: we have an inner need to feel good about ourselves and to know that others view us in a positive manner. The highest level is the self-actualization stage, in which we maximize our potential. At this level, we attempt to be at our best and to live our lives to the fullest extent possible.

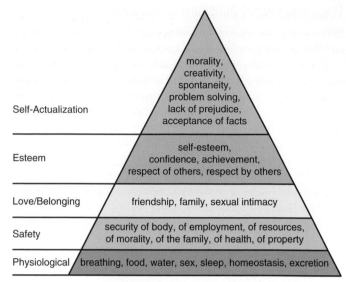

FIGURE 4-6 Maslow's hierarchy of needs.

People adapt to life based on their individual needs, and many factors influence that adaptation, including family history, culture, relationships, and socioeconomic status. The medical assistant should actively investigate the community resources available to help patients adapt to situations that affect their health status. Therapeutic communication techniques should be used to help gather information about current patient needs, especially those related to feeling safe in the healthcare environment. The medical assistant can play an important role in recognizing patient needs and helping to meet those needs in the ambulatory care center.

CLOSING COMMENTS

Developing therapeutic communication skills is critical to your success as a medical assistant. Communication is a part of all interactions throughout the day, and the better developed these skills are, the better the medical assistant can serve the patients in the facility and relate with co-workers. Every attempt should be made to enhance the interpersonal and human relations skills the medical assistant currently has and to strive continually to better these skills. This ensures that effective communication is part of the relationship with patients and with others with whom the medical assistant interacts.

Patient Education

The medical assistant has the opportunity to provide an educational service to every patient who enters the healthcare facility. Patients often have questions about their care or treatment, and the medical assistant with good communication skills can assist the patient in understanding a diagnosis and treatment protocol.

Patients must have a clear knowledge of the role they play in their own care. The medical assistant can communicate information to the patient in many ways other than verbally. Handouts and brochures can help patients understand their illness better and can educate them, but the medical assistant should always explain each piece of literature given to a patient. Never just hand out printed information and expect it to be read. Have the patient repeat instructions to clarify whether he or she understands.

Remember that physical care is not the only aspect of patient care; patients also have emotional needs. Often the very things we take for granted, such as food, shelter, or the ability to pay for healthcare, are a struggle for some patients. The resulting stress can worsen their physical condition. Ask questions and observe nonverbal behaviors to remain aware of what the patient is communicating to the staff and what is not being said. This helps the medical assistant to best serve the patient.

Legal and Ethical Issues

Patients see the medical assistant as an extension of the provider; therefore, it is important that all communication with the patient be professional and accurate. Never give a patient advice that is not approved by the provider, to prevent accusations of practicing medicine without a license. Always discuss with the provider any issues that might affect the patient's care. Never agree to withhold any information from the provider because even a small piece of information could completely change the plan of treatment. When you give instructions to patients, it is always best to have them in writing and to document the patient education intervention in the health record so that a record exists of what was communicated to the patient. Remember that all the patients in the facility deserve to be treated with respect and compassion. Help providers establish trust with the patient. An open, trusting relationship helps prevent legal issues in the future.

SUMMARY OF SCENARIO

Mrs. Cloyd and her daughter both face significant issues in dealing with Mrs. Cloyd's chronic heart condition. Both patients and their families need compassion and caring from the medical team. They want to feel as if they are being heard and that their opinions are important. Some of their needs are similar, but they also have differing needs. A gentle touch and laughter can brighten their day, and these nonverbal expressions are critical to a person experiencing a serious illness.

The medical assistant must ensure that Mrs. Cloyd understands her medications and treatments. She should assist Mrs. Cloyd and her daughter in finding community resources for which Mrs. Cloyd might be eligible. Be sure to directly interact with Mrs. Cloyd, but at the same time, make sure her daughter understands any directions her mother should follow. Even on the busiest of days, patients and their families deserve warmth from the staff and should be made as comfortable as possible when they seek medical care.

Although the ambulatory care center is always a busy place, medical assistants can take a moment to individualize the care they provide to patients. Establishing eye contact and genuinely asking how the person has been getting along demonstrate interest. Call patients by their name, and ask about their families. These techniques allow the medical assistant to develop rapport, which results in a more pleasant healthcare visit for the patient.

Listening is a skill that must be practiced and refined. Patients need to know that the medical assistant is focusing attention on them, listening to their concerns, and responding with restatement, reflection, and clarification to make sure the patient is understood correctly. Active listening is one of the most important skills the medical assistant can develop.

SUMMARY OF LEARNING OBJECTIVES

1. **Define, spell, and pronounce the terms listed in the vocabulary.**
   Spelling and pronouncing medical terms correctly reinforce the medical assistant's credibility. Knowing the definitions of these terms promotes confidence in communication with patients and co-workers.

2. **Discuss first impressions and patient-centered care.**
   First impressions are very important and are formed based on attitude, appearance, compassion, and therapeutic communication skills. Delivering patient-centered care is imperative for the professional medical assistant. To provide high-quality patient care, we must communicate effectively with the patient and provide a warm, caring environment. Good communication skills are vital to meeting the needs of the patient and his or her support system.

3. **Do the following related to communication paths:**
   - *Identify types of verbal communication.*
     When we are communicating verbally with our patients, we are using words to deliver the intended message. The two major forms of verbal communication are oral and written communication. Verbal communication is the expression of thoughts with words. When we put our thoughts to paper, such as writing down instructions for a patient, our oral words are now in written form.
   - *Identify types of nonverbal communication.*
     Much of what we communicate to our patients is conveyed through the use of conscious or unconscious body language. Our nonverbal actions, such as gestures, facial expressions, and mannerisms, are learned behaviors that are greatly influenced by our family and cultural backgrounds. The body naturally expresses our true feelings; in fact, experts say that more than 90% of communication is nonverbal. This means that, even though the verbal message is an important method of delivering information, the way we deliver those words is how the patient interprets them.
   - *Recognize and respond to verbal and nonverbal communication.*
     Procedure 4-1 presents an example of how to respond to nonverbal communication. The key to successful patient interaction is congruence between the words used and the body language observed. The medical assistant should use therapeutic communication skills to interpret the person's message and level of understanding.

Continued

SUMMARY OF LEARNING OBJECTIVES—*continued*

4. Recognize communication barriers.

Effective therapeutic communication requires the delivery of a clear message to the patient. However, along the way are many communication barriers that can create misunderstanding and misinterpretation of your message. Successful communication relies on knowing what barriers to communication exist and how to navigate around these roadblocks. By understanding what barriers may stand in the way of your attempts at effective communication, you can more successfully sidestep these challenges and engage in patient-centered communication. Communication barriers can occur with both medical assistants and patients.

5. Summarize factors that should be considered when communicating with diverse patient populations.

Practicing respectful patient care is extremely important when working with a diverse patient population. *Empathy* is the key to creating a caring, therapeutic environment. Empathy goes beyond sympathy. A medical assistant who is empathetic respects the individuality of the patient and attempts to see the person's health problem through his or her eyes, recognizing the effect of all holistic factors on the patient's well-being. Empathetic sensitivity to diversity first requires those interested in healthcare to examine their own values, beliefs, and actions; you cannot treat all patients with care and respect until you first recognize and evaluate your personal biases.

6. Identify techniques for overcoming communication barriers.

Most people who enter the medical field have a natural sense of caring and empathy, but the medical assistant can nurture communication skills by using patience, observation, and sensitivity to patient needs, in addition to therapeutic listening skills. If a patient has a physical impairment, being observant helps with communication issues. Often these patients want to be self-sufficient, so they may not appreciate help with simple tasks. Encourage these patients to bring an interpreter so that accurate, quality information can be placed in the health record. Prejudice can be overcome with facts about the source of the social bias, and the same is true for stereotyping. Even highly abrasive patients can be tolerated when the medical assistant wants to be an effective communicator with all patients.

7. Do the following related to communication during difficult times:

- *Recognize the elements of oral communication using the sender-receiver process.*

  The linear communication model describes communication as an interactive process involving the sender of the message, the receiver, and the crucial component of feedback to confirm reception of the message. The sender is the person who sends a message through a variety of different channels. Channels can be spoken words, written or e-mailed messages, and body language. The sender encodes the message, which simply means that he or she chooses a specific means of expression using words and other channels. The receiver decodes the message according to his or her understanding of what is being communicated. There is no way to confirm that the message was actually received unless the patient provides feedback about what he or she interpreted from the message.

- *Apply feedback techniques, including reflection, restatement, and clarification, to obtain information.*

  Three processes are involved in active listening: restatement, reflection, and clarification. Restatement is simply paraphrasing or repeating the patient's statements; reflection involves repeating the main idea of the conversation while also identifying the sender's feelings; clarification seeks to summarize or simplify the sender's thoughts and feelings and to resolve any confusion in the message (see Procedure 4-2).

- *Discuss open and closed questions or statements.*

  When gathering information from a patient, it is helpful to use a combination of open and closed questions or statements. Open questions ask for general information, whereas closed questions typically limit the patient's answer to yes or no.

8. Discuss important factors about therapeutic communication across the life span.

The key to communicating effectively with patients is using an age-specific approach. Therapeutic use of nonverbal language is essential to interacting with children of all ages. Getting down on the child's level, establishing eye contact, and using a gentle but firm voice are ways of gaining the child's confidence and cooperation. To help school-aged children gain a sense of control, give them the opportunity to make certain decisions about treatment. Privacy is an important issue to consider with older children, especially adolescents. In addition, older children want to know what is going on, what to expect, and what the findings mean; therefore, keeping them informed in a language they can understand is important. Using language the adult patient understands and involving the patient in treatment decisions as much as possible are essential to developing a helping relationship with your older patients.

9. List and explain the levels of Maslow's hierarchy of needs.

Psychologist Abraham Maslow created what he called the "hierarchy of needs." A *hierarchy* is defined as things arranged in order, rank, or a graded series. Maslow believed that our human needs can be categorized into five levels and that the needs on each level must be satisfied before we can move to the next level. These levels often are depicted as a triangle, with the most basic needs at the bottom and the highest potential for growth as a human being at the top.

CONNECTIONS

Study Guide Connection: Go to the Chapter 4 Study Guide. Read and complete the activities.

evolve Evolve Connection: Go to the Chapter 4 link at *evolve.elsevier.com/kinn* to complete the Chapter Review Quiz. Check out the other resources listed for this chapter to make the most of what you have learned from Therapeutic Communication.

PATIENT EDUCATION

5

SCENARIO

Taylor DiSalvo is a medical assistant in a busy family practice. He currently is working with a patient, Sam Ignatio, who is 62 years old and has been married for 30 years. Mr. Ignatio has just been diagnosed with diabetes mellitus (DM) type 2. Although his mother and sister developed DM type 2 in their 60s, he knows very little about the disease and nothing about the strides that have been made in its treatment. In addition, his diet is high in saturated fat and carbohydrates (especially simple sugars because he loves sweet treats), and he does not exercise regularly. Mr. Ignatio is 50 pounds overweight, has functional deafness in his left ear and decreased sound quality in his right ear, and shows early signs of diabetic-related vision loss. Taylor is responsible for assisting with Mr. Ignatio's patient teaching plan.

Mr. Ignatio is faced with a serious illness, and his future health depends on compliance with a wide range of lifestyle changes. The methods Taylor chooses to coach this patient in managing his disease can have a significant effect on his eventual health outcome.

While studying this chapter, think about the following questions:

- How should Taylor begin Mr. Ignatio's patient education?
- What are some of Mr. Ignatio's individual characteristics that may affect his ability to learn all the information required to manage his disease?
- How can Taylor coach Mr. Ignatio so that he understands the importance of following treatment and disease-monitoring guidelines?
- What teaching approaches and materials would best meet the needs of this patient?
- Are any community resources available that could help Mr. Ignatio learn how to manage his disease?

LEARNING OBJECTIVES

1. Discuss the holistic model of patient education related to health and illness; also, instruct patients according to their needs to promote health maintenance and disease prevention.
2. Summarize the stages of grief and suggest therapeutic interactions for grieving patients.
3. List at least five guidelines for patient education that can affect the patient's overall wellness.
4. Do the following related to patient factors that affect learning:
   - Define six patient factors that have an impact on learning.
   - Display respect for individual diversity.
   - Summarize educational approaches for patients with language barriers.
5. Do the following related to the teaching plan:
   - Determine possible barriers to patient learning.
   - Assess the patient's needs.
   - Determine the teaching priorities.
   - Decide on the appropriate teaching materials.
   - Develop a list of community resources related to patients' healthcare needs and facilitate referrals to community resources in the role of patient navigator.
   - Decide on the appropriate teaching methods.
   - Implement the teaching plan.
   - Demonstrate the ability to develop an appropriate and effective patient teaching plan.
6. Describe the role of the medical assistant in patient education.
7. Integrate the legal and ethical elements of patient teaching into the ambulatory care setting; also, discuss applications of the Health Insurance Portability and Accountability Act (HIPAA).

This chapter focuses on helping students recognize the individual learning needs of patients. It also provides guidelines for developing effective teaching approaches. The key to patient compliance with prescribed treatments is empowerment; that is, providing the patient with information and support that enable the person to take charge of his or her health problem. The concepts in this chapter are basic to all patient education interventions. Putting them into practice, as a medical assistant, can help you improve both a patient's understanding of the disease process and his or her willingness to comply with the disease management steps recommended by the provider.

PATIENT EDUCATION AND MODELS OF HEALTH AND ILLNESS

Patient education should begin with the first contact between the patient and the healthcare team. A well-informed patient is more likely to comply with treatment and adopt a healthy lifestyle. However, informing a patient about his or her disease is only part of the health teaching process. The key to successful health teaching is to empower the patient to accept the responsibility of his or her disease process and to become willing to implement teaching guidelines.

As a result of reductions in hospital admissions and shorter hospital stays, patients and families have had to assume responsibility for care that once was provided by the hospital staff. This means that those who work in ambulatory care settings have an even greater responsibility to meet the educational needs of their patients. To develop an effective teaching approach, we must implement a holistic model that considers not only the patient's physical state, but also his or her psychological, sociocultural, intellectual, and economic needs (Figure 5-1). The holistic model suggests that we look at patients and determine their needs based on a complete view of their lives rather than just as an analysis of their specific diseases. It is our responsibility not only to teach patients about disease processes, but also to help them implement related skills and changes in lifestyle to promote recovery and improve function. In the case of Mr. Ignatio, diabetes mellitus is a complicated disease that requires an in-depth understanding of the disease process, in addition to making significant lifestyle changes. When considering the impact of this diagnosis on the patient (in this case, Mr. Ignatio), the medical assistant should keep in mind the following factors, because they will affect the patient's response.

- *Psychological effect of the disease:* Is Mr. Ignatio in shock and denial? Is he angry or depressed? How will his emotional reaction to the diagnosis affect his response to patient education and coaching efforts?
- *Sociocultural impact:* How will his family and employer respond to the demands of the diagnosis? Does he have a support system that will assist him in making healthy lifestyle choices?

- *Intellectual impact:* Is Mr. Ignatio able to understand the complexities of the disease and treatment recommendations?
- *Economic impact:* Can he afford the treatment for diabetes? Does he have health insurance to cover the cost, or will he need assistance in paying for ongoing diagnostic and treatment recommendations?
- *Spiritual impact:* What is Mr. Ignatio's spiritual response to his diagnosis? How might his spiritual beliefs affect his compliance with treatment?

The health belief model may help you understand why some people do not follow recommended guidelines to maintain their health and prevent the development of disease.

The model focuses on individuals' attitudes toward and beliefs about themselves and their health. The model suggests that we first consider how the patient perceives his or her risk of developing a disease and the possible severity of the condition. For example, even though Mr. Ignatio's mother and sister developed diabetes type 2, he may believe he is not going to have the same problem. Therefore, even though wellness information recommends that he lose weight, exercise, and eat a healthy diet, he may not believe he is in danger of developing diabetes; consequently, he doesn't believe he needs to follow disease prevention recommendations. He may also believe that even if he does develop diabetes, the consequences of the disease are not that serious, so why bother altering his lifestyle to prevent it?

Another factor considered in the health belief model is the patient's perceived benefits of action; that is, whether the patient believes altering his or her health behaviors will prevent the person from developing the disease or from suffering serious complications. In this case, because Mr. Ignatio has a strong family history of the disease, he may have decided he was going to get diabetes anyway, so why should he bother exercising and watching his diet? Until the patient believes that teaching and health promotion guidelines affect him and are worth pursuing, he will not follow suggested health promotion tips or comply with treatment protocols.

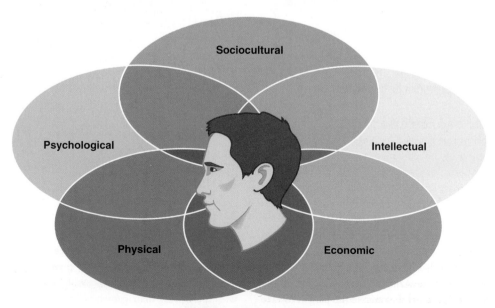

FIGURE 5-1 The holistic approach.

TABLE 5-1 Health Belief Model

PRINCIPLES	DEFINITION	PATIENT EDUCATION
Perceived susceptibility	Patient's opinion on the chances of developing a disorder	Supply information on the risk level; individual risk is based on the patient's health habits and family history.
Perceived severity	Patient's opinion on the seriousness of the condition and its health risks	Outline the potential complications of the disease.
Perceived benefits	Patient's belief in the value of altering lifestyle factors and complying with treatment	Emphasize the positive results that can be achieved if the patient complies with healthcare recommendations.
Perceived barriers	Patient's opinion on the financial and psychological costs of compliance	Identify patient barriers and work to reduce them through patient education, family outreach, and use of community resources.
Cues to action	Methods developed to activate patient compliance	Provide one-on-one education interventions; detailed handouts; family involvement in education efforts; follow-up at subsequent office visits; referral to community resources.
Self-efficacy	Patient has the confidence to take action to achieve a healthier state	Provide ongoing education and support.

Table 5-1 outlines the health belief model and suggests methods for applying the model in patient teaching and coaching efforts in the ambulatory care setting.

The five stages of grief, as defined by Dr. Elisabeth Kübler-Ross, are another model that may be helpful for understanding the way patients respond to health threats. When a patient faces a serious health threat, the grief process may delay the person in adjusting to the disease and starting to take control of his or her health. For example, Mr. Ignatio may respond to the news of his diagnosis with what is commonly the first stage of the grief process—denial. Both his father and sister suffered serious complications from diabetes, including blindness and leg amputation, and he may be using denial to deal psychologically with the burden of the diagnosis.

Each individual goes through the stages of grief in his or her own way and at his or her own pace. This process can take weeks to months; however, until the patient reaches the point of accepting the diagnosis and the possible ramifications of the disease, compliance with patient education will be very difficult to achieve.

The five stages of grief are:

- *Denial and isolation.* The patient denies the existence of the disease, may be unwilling to accept the reality of the situation, and refuses to discuss the health problem or remember health teaching interventions. For example, Mr. Ignatio refuses to meet with the dietitian because he says his diet is fine and there is no need to change it.
- *Anger.* The patient may be very angry and hostile when forced to discuss the condition. Mr. Ignatio may say, "Why did this happen to me? I am a good person, why did I get diabetes?"
- *Bargaining.* The patient tries to bargain for privileges or time. Mr. Ignatio may say, "Look, I know I'm supposed to start this new diet, but Christmas is coming. I'll meet with the dietitian after the holidays."
- *Depression.* The patient grieves the loss of health. Mr. Ignatio may be very sad about the diagnosis. He doesn't want to have to deal with the complexities of the disease, he just wants it to go away so he can live his life without the fear of diabetic complications.
- *Acceptance.* The patient finally gets to the point where he or she accepts the diagnosis and is ready to make the best of it. At this point, Mr. Ignatio may be willing to use community resources for education and support.

Therapeutic Interactions for Grieving Patients

Denial and isolation: Reinforce each education intervention with handouts that explain the disease and treatment. Encourage the patient's family to attend visits to the provider's office and to become involved in the patient's care. For example, if a patient has been diagnosed with diabetes, provide a list of approved online resources or YouTube videos so that the patient and/or family can learn more about diabetes privately at home.

Anger: Use therapeutic communication techniques, especially reflection, to acknowledge the patient's feelings about the diagnosis. Recognize the patient's need to use defense mechanisms as protection from the reality of the disease (these topics are addressed in more detail in the Patient Assessment chapter). Remember, the patient is not angry at you or the provider; he or she is angry about the diagnosis and its accompanying challenges.

Bargaining: Rely on the provider's recommendations regarding postponing certain treatments. Discuss the patient's bargaining requests with the provider and other staff members to work out a solution that promotes patient compliance with healthcare recommendations.

Depression: Use available community resources to provide support for the patient and family. The provider may recommend that the patient attend a support group, meet with a dietitian, or use professional counseling services to deal with depression.

Acceptance: Take advantage of this time to renew education efforts by providing multiple methods for learning about the disease, such as DVDs, professional websites, YouTube videos, and community support services.

Patient Factors That Affect Learning

Many factors or characteristics may affect the patient's ability to learn. Medical assistants must be aware of these factors to develop a coaching approach that best meets the needs of each patient.

Guidelines for Patient Education

- Provide knowledge and skills to promote recovery and health.
- Encourage patient ownership and participation in the teaching process.
- With the patient's approval, include the family and significant others in education interventions.
- Promote safe, appropriate use of medications and treatments.
- Encourage patient adaptation to healthy behaviors.
- Provide information about accessing community resources.

Perception of Disease Versus Actual State of Disease

Patients respond to a particular diagnosis in many different ways. One predictor of how a patient will respond, and therefore how he or she will react to health education, is the patient's perception of the disease. Previous life experiences may greatly influence the patient's knowledge base and/or desire to learn about the disease. Does the patient recognize and accept the seriousness of the diagnosis? Or, perhaps, does the patient overreact to potential disease risks? Both of these responses affect the patient's willingness to learn about the disease and his or her compliance with treatment recommendations.

How do you think Taylor's patient education efforts will be affected if Mr. Ignatio does not consider diabetes a serious disease?

Patient's Need for Information

The patient's perception of the impact of the disease on his or her general health also determines the need for information about the disease. Does the patient express a desire to learn all he or she can about the disease, or does the patient resist or act indifferent to teaching efforts? A vital part of patient education is encouraging patient ownership of the learning process. To accomplish this, you first may have to persuade the patient that he or she needs to understand the disease before an improvement in overall wellness can be achieved.

Mr. Ignatio tells Taylor that his father had diabetes and had to have both legs amputated; eventually he died of the disease. Mr. Ignatio says it doesn't matter whether he controls his blood sugar; he'll still have major health complications. What is the appropriate response?

Patient's Age and Developmental Level

Depending on the patient's age and ability to understand information about the disease, you may have to adapt the teaching plan to meet specific learning needs. For example, educating a 9-year-old patient with DM type 1 about disease management requires a different approach from one that would be used for Mr. Ignatio. You should be flexible and creative in providing learning opportunities that support the provider's attempt to educate the patient about disease prevention and health maintenance. Often the key to patient understanding and compliance is the involvement of family members.

During his assessment of Mr. Ignatio's diet, Taylor learns that his wife cooks all his meals and packs his lunch daily. He loves bread and desserts, and he tells Taylor he's too old to change his diet now. What should Taylor do to make sure Mr. Ignatio's diet complies with diabetic recommendations?

Patient's Mental and Emotional State

Even a well-planned teaching intervention can be ineffective if the patient is unable to pay attention because of anxiety, stress, anger, or denial (Figure 5-2). Frequently patients use defense mechanisms to protect themselves from the reality of a serious illness. It is important that the medical assistant be sensitive to the patient's mental state and adapt teaching interventions as needed. If a patient is overwhelmed by the diagnosis and his body language cues are defensive, limit the amount of information at this time to what he must know immediately about his disease, rather than trying to teach him detailed facts.

Mr. Ignatio has just been diagnosed with diabetes. He has already shared that his father died of diabetes. Do you think he is able to pay attention to coaching efforts about a diabetic diet? What should Taylor do to manage this problem?

Influence of Multicultural and Diversity Factors on Patient Education

Culture, family background, and religious beliefs influence patients' actions. Working with patients from diverse backgrounds is an exciting challenge; however, for your patient education to be successful, it is essential that you recognize and are sensitive to the impact of these factors on patient learning (Figure 5-3). Some questions you should consider when teaching a patient from another background include:

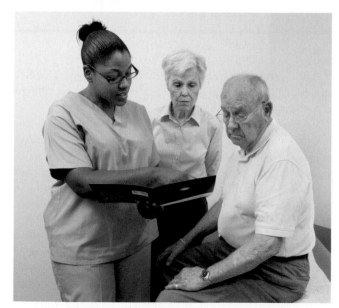

FIGURE 5-2 Demonstrating sensitivity to the patient's needs.

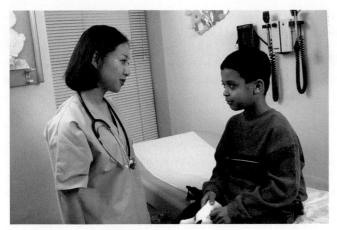

FIGURE 5-3 Considering diversity.

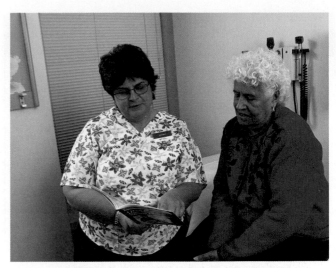

FIGURE 5-4 Using language-appropriate educational booklets.

- Is language an issue with your patient (Figure 5-4)? If the patient is unable to understand spoken English or to read it correctly, do you have an alternative method for getting the information across?
- Do the patient's culture, ethnic background, or religious beliefs influence the way he or she perceives disease and the role of healthcare workers?

Approaches for Language Barriers

- Determine whether the patient can read and/or understand English.
- Address the patient by his or her last name (e.g., Mrs. Martinez, Mr. Nugyen).
- Be courteous and use a formal approach to communication.
- Use gestures, tone of voice, facial expressions, and eye contact to emphasize appropriate parts of the discussion.
- Integrate pictures, handouts, models, and other aids that visually depict the material.
- Carefully observe the patient's body language, especially facial expression, for understanding or confusion.
- Use simple, everyday words as much as possible. If available, use a dictionary that translates as many words as possible for the patient.
- Demonstrate all procedures and have the patient return the demonstration to check for understanding.
- Implement the teaching plan in small, manageable steps.
- Give the patient written instructions for all procedures and treatments.
- If possible, have an interpreter present or have access to an online interpreter; if an interpreter is not available, a family member may be able to help with communication.
- If available, provide educational materials in the patient's native language. For example, vaccine information sheets (VIS) are available online in multiple languages from the Centers for Disease Control and Prevention (CDC); send materials home in English if a family member can interpret the material for the patient; refer the patient and family to online sources of educational materials in their native language.

- What strategies or techniques might minimize patient education problems?
- Are community resources available that could facilitate patient learning?

Patient Learning Style

All of us have a preferred way of learning; that is, methods that work best for us to learn new material. Patients also have a learning preference that reflects their individual learning style. Some patients learn best from discussion or lecture, whereas others must take time to think about the material before they understand it. Some patients can learn from observing; others must act or do something with the material to learn it. Start your teaching intervention by asking your patient how he or she prefers to learn new material, and pattern your teaching interventions along those lines.

Mr. Ignatio tells Taylor that he could never learn things by listening to someone tell him what to do. What approach to learning might best meet his needs?

Impact of Physical Disabilities

The patient first must be assessed to determine whether he or she can adequately hear instructions, see written material, and manipulate any required treatment equipment. All teaching efforts are lost if disabilities interfere with a patient's capacity to understand information or to handle equipment properly. A hearing or speech impairment may require the use of sign language with supplemental written instructions. If the patient is unable to manipulate equipment because of a physical disability or vision problem, family or adaptive equipment may be necessary for the patient to manage his or her care.

Mr. Ignatio's physical assessment revealed hearing and vision problems. Is he able to understand verbal instructions clearly? What can be done to adapt the teaching intervention to meet his needs?

Therapeutic Communication With Patients With Special Needs

Patients With Vision Loss

- Alert the patient that you are in the room and identify yourself; do not touch the patient without warning.
- The patient is unable to pick up on your body language; use clear, concise language and a normal tone of voice.
- Provide all written material in a large font or print size; large-print educational materials often can be ordered.
- Supply reliable Internet sources for information and provide audio material if possible.

Patients With Hearing Loss

- Stand in front of the patient or within the person's field of vision before you begin speaking; the patient may be able to lip-read.
- You may need to touch the patient lightly to get her or his attention.
- Use *expanded speech*; lower the tone of your voice and pronounce each syllable. Do not raise your voice or shout to be heard. The louder your voice, the higher the tone, and aging ears find high-pitched sounds the most difficult to interpret.
- Carefully observe the patient's body language for understanding or confusion.
- Use gestures or demonstration as needed to get the message across.
- Clearly print any information needed to clarify the patient teaching.
- If a patient is wearing a hearing aid, ask him or her whether it is on and working before starting the conversation; the patient may turn a hearing aid off to prevent annoying background noise.
- Provide written handouts that review the material being taught.
- Request family assistance in verifying that the patient received and understood the material.
- Refer patients and families to appropriate online resources

---

CRITICAL THINKING APPLICATION   5-1

Implement the holistic education model and the health belief model to determine and respond to Mr. Ignatio's individual learning needs.

THE TEACHING PLAN

What is it that patients need to know to manage a disease effectively? What is it about an individual patient that needs to be addressed for a teaching intervention to work? What are the immediate and long-term goals of patient education? What teaching materials or strategies should be used to meet the patient's learning needs and also effectively relay the information? How can the teaching plan be implemented successfully? How do you, as a medical assistant, manage the limited time available for patient coaching? How do you know the patient is learning and actually converting this knowledge into disease management? A vital aspect of patient teaching is to be flexible and to provide information about what patients want to know when patients want to know it. These and other guidelines for developing an appropriate and effective teaching plan follow.

Assess the Patient's Learning Needs

Developing a teaching plan that works for a particular individual first requires an assessment of the patient as a learner and consideration of any characteristics that might affect the learning process. Many of these factors already have been addressed, such as the patient's learning preference, perception of the illness, age, background, multicultural influences, language barriers, and disabilities. The medical assistant also must consider what the patient already knows about the diagnosis and whether that knowledge includes misconceptions about the disease.

The goal of the assessment process is to create a teaching plan that meets the patient's needs for understanding and managing his or her illness. Therefore, in the learning assessment, the medical assistant should consider what the patient needs to know, what the patient wants to know, and what can be done in the time available for learning.

Before developing a specific approach to patient education, you must consider potential barriers to learning other than those already presented, such as the presence of pain. A patient in acute distress is unable to concentrate on the information. In this case, the amount of material must be adjusted to meet the patient's immediate needs, and time should be planned in the future for a more in-depth teaching session.

Does Mr. Ignatio exhibit any potential barriers to learning about his disease?

Possible Barriers to Patient Learning

- Individual learning style
- Age and developmental level
- Use of defense mechanisms
- Language
- Motivation to learn
- Physical limitations or disabilities
- Emotional or mental state
- Cultural or ethnic background
- Pain
- Time limitations

Determine the Teaching Priorities

Once you have done an adequate assessment of your patient as a learner and you understand your patient's learning needs, the next question is, "Where do I start?" A patient such as Mr. Ignatio has a significant amount of information to learn before he can manage his disease completely. The volume of information might seem overwhelming unless priorities are established. How do you figure out what material should be first? The first question to ask is, "What is the patient's immediate versus long-term needs?" What must this patient learn today to be able to take care of himself, and what does he need to know overall about his illness to promote healthy behaviors?

Because the patient learning assessment told you what your patient knows about his or her disease, that is a good place to start. Confirm what the patient knows about the problem and attempt to correct any potential misconceptions. If you start with something the patient knows and understands, he or she will feel more competent and capable of managing new material. You then should go on to the new material that is causing the patient the most anxiety. If the patient is nervous or afraid about a particular aspect, he or she will be unable to pay attention to any other new material until that anxiety has been addressed.

For example, if Mr. Ignatio is most concerned about pricking his finger for a glucometer reading, that is the first skill he should learn. Once he is confident about that particular part of treatment, he will be able to pay attention to diet and exercise recommendations. You should always begin with the basic details about the disease and add more information during each patient visit.

Every interaction with the patient is an opportunity for health education. A major problem with delivering high-quality patient education in an ambulatory healthcare setting is the lack of time you have to spend with each patient. Therefore, you must take advantage of every "teaching moment"; that is, every time you interact with a patient, use it as an opportunity to assess the patient's current education needs and provide as much information or guidance about that specific learning need as possible during the time available.

Use the waiting room as a place for learning by providing up-to-date educational materials on a wide variety of health issues. Many facilities have DVD equipment in the waiting room for patient education while the patient is waiting to be seen. These can be specific to the type of practice or can provide general health information. Another good location for educational materials is in the examination rooms. The patient may be more likely to pick up brochures on sensitive topics such as types of contraceptives, the procedures for performing testicular or breast exams, or information about sexually transmitted infections in the privacy of a closed exam room.

Decide on the Appropriate Teaching Materials

What teaching materials would best meet the needs of your patient? A wide variety of patient education materials is available, and deciding which materials best meet your patient's needs depends on the patient's learning preference, individual characteristics, and lifestyle factors. Individualized instruction is the key to understanding and patient compliance; however, additional materials can help reinforce the information.

When possible, all patient instruction should include a handout or online reference that reinforces information and that the patient can use as a resource. Patient factors such as the use of defense mechanisms, emotional state, and language barriers can limit the patient's ability to comprehend and remember information. Printed information is needed to help the patient and the patient's family understand what is happening and what needs to be done to improve the patient's health (Figure 5-5). Informational flyers can be ordered from medical office suppliers, pharmaceutical company representatives, and health education companies. In addition, most electronic health record (EHR) systems include a package for printing out or e-mailing diagnose-specific educational materials. Many hospitals also offer free educational materials about diagnostic procedures, immunizations, and other disease-related topics. The ambulatory

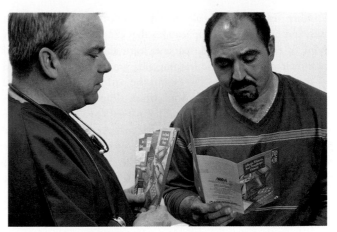

FIGURE 5-5 Reviewing printed information.

care setting where you are employed may develop its own educational materials.

Some guidelines to follow if you are responsible for developing or ordering educational supplies include the following:

- The material should be written in lay language at about a sixth grade level to promote general patient understanding.
- Information should be well organized and clearly described.
- All material should be checked for accuracy.
- Handouts should be attractive and professional.
- Copies should be available in other languages when possible and in large print for visually impaired clients.

Identifying Community Resources

One role of the medical assistant in ambulatory care settings is to assist patients and their families in finding and using community education and support services. The healthcare facility should keep an up-to-date file of area resources. The information should include the name of the group and the services provided; the contact person; a telephone number and address; meeting times and location if applicable; and a related website if available (see Procedure 5-1). This information can be found in a number of locations, such as the blue pages of the local phone book, through the community outreach or speakers bureau of area hospitals, or online by searching for area educational institutions at *.edu* sites or local chapters of national organizations at *.org* sites. For example, the American Cancer Society operates local branches throughout the United States, and information on local services can be found on the national home page (*www.cancer.org*).

An excellent comprehensive Internet site operated by the U.S. National Library of Medicine and the National Institutes of Health is MedlinePlus. Both health professionals and consumers can depend on it for accurate information that is updated frequently. The site provides a variety of information about health issues, an extensive list of diseases and conditions, a medical encyclopedia and dictionary, health information in Spanish, extensive details on prescription and nonprescription drugs, health information from the media, and links to thousands of clinical trials. It can be bookmarked at *medlineplus.gov*. Another excellent source of current information on diseases is the Centers for Disease Control and Prevention (CDC) website at *www.cdc.gov/*.

Other teaching materials include DVDs, approved YouTube links, and health-related applications that can be accessed by smart phone or computer to help patients learn about their disease and track their progress. These learning aids promote self-directed and self-paced learning. They also permit the patient to access material in a nonstressful environment, which improves the patient's learning potential. Depending on the patient's age or access to the appropriate technology, using media resources or referring the patient to provider-approved healthcare sites on the Internet can help develop patient ownership of the learning process and provide excellent resources for patient referral. However, using the Internet as a resource for patient education information has its drawbacks. It is important that the patient understand that there is no oversight or control over information posted on the Web; therefore, some sites may offer information that is erroneous, out of date, or misleading. Provide patients with accurate, well-researched sites and/or keep informed about what sites patients are accessing to make sure online recommendations support the provider's treatment protocol. The following website, posted by the National Institutes of Health, can help you learn how to assess Internet health information: *www.nlm.nih.gov/medlineplus/webeval/*

The Medical Assistant as a Patient Navigator

According to the American Medical Association, a patient navigator is a person who helps patients and families with insurance problems, explains treatment and care, communicates with the healthcare team, assists caregivers, and manages medical paperwork. This definition describes the role of the medical assistant as a patient advocate in ambulatory care settings.

The concept of patient navigation was pioneered in 1990 by Dr. Harold P. Freeman, a surgical oncologist at Harlem Hospital, for the purpose of eliminating barriers to timely cancer care for the indigent and underserved. In response to this need, the Patient Navigator Outreach and Chronic Disease Prevention Act of 2005 was passed to make grants available for the development of patient navigator programs. The original goal of patient navigation was to help people overcome barriers such as poverty, low literacy, or lack of health insurance that were preventing patients from gaining access to medical care. However, the care for illnesses such as cancer can be so complicated that patients, regardless of income or education level, can benefit from expert assistance. In fact, under a new requirement for accreditation by the American College of Surgeons Commission on Cancer, cancer centers must have started providing patient navigation services by 2015. Most recently, the Affordable Care Act required that "insurance navigators" be available to help consumers research and enroll in health insurance through the law's health insurance marketplace.

Because medical assistants are cross-trained in both administrative and clinical skills, they are in a unique position to serve as patient navigators in ambulatory care settings.

PROCEDURE 5-1   Develop a List of Community Resources for Patients' Healthcare Needs; also, Facilitate Referrals in the Role of Patient Navigator

As a medical assistant, one of your roles will be to help patients who need community health education or support services. To prepare for this role, you should collect a minimum of 25 community resources available in your area (e.g., support groups, educational workshops, dietary assistance, national organizations, medical equipment suppliers). In your directory, include the following information: name of the group; services provided; contact person; telephone number; address; meeting times and locations (if applicable); and a related website. As a patient navigator, apply what you have learned about community resources to assist the patient in the following scenario.

Goal: *To develop a list of community resources and perform the role of patient navigator by referring patients to resources.*

Scenario: Role-play the following scenario with your partner.

Mr. Tomás Garcia was admitted to the hospital last week for an acute myocardial infarction (MI). Mr. Garcia is 54 years old, overweight, smokes two packs of cigarettes a day, eats fast food almost daily, has a family history of heart disease, and works as a carpenter. The provider recommends that he lose weight; follow a diet high in fiber and low in saturated fat; and quit smoking. What community resources might help educate and support Mr. Garcia in making these complex lifestyle changes?

EQUIPMENT and SUPPLIES

- Patient's health record
- Educational handouts
- Computer with Internet connection and printer
- Quiet, private area

PROCEDURAL STEPS

1. Greet and identify the patient in a pleasant manner. Introduce yourself and explain your role.
   <u>PURPOSE</u>: To make the patient feel comfortable and at ease.

PROCEDURE 5-1 *—continued*

2. Take the patient to a quiet, private area that has computer access.
   <u>PURPOSE</u>: A quiet, private area is necessary to protect confidentiality and prevent interruptions.
3. Assess Mr. Garcia's needs, and identify factors that may limit his ability to learn and implement lifestyle changes. Use restatement, reflection, and clarification to verify the information.
   <u>PURPOSE</u>: Therapeutic communication techniques help you gather complete information and address the patient's immediate needs; it also improves the likelihood of success.
4. Speak in a pleasant, distinct manner, remembering to maintain eye contact with your patient.
   <u>PURPOSE</u>: Positive nonverbal behaviors create a friendly, caring atmosphere.
5. Remain sensitive to the individual needs of your patient throughout the interview process.

<u>PURPOSE</u>: Be aware of your personal biases, but do not let them affect the way you treat your patients; make sure to respect patients' diverse backgrounds.
6. Provide Mr. Garcia with appropriate handouts and a list of community resources that might be helpful. Print out this information or e-mail it to the patient for future use. One of the handouts could include a list of provider-approved websites the patient can consult.
   <u>PURPOSE</u>: Make sure the patient has all the handouts with him before he leaves the office; also make sure he has a list of appropriate online sites he can check out later for additional information and support.
7. Answer any questions the patient may have; use clarification and feedback methods to make sure all his questions have been addressed.
8. Document the patient education intervention in the health record.

Decide on the Appropriate Teaching Methods

A variety of methods may be used to get the message across to your patients. One of the best ways to manage a large amount of information within a short time is to use community resources to reinforce the message. Your local area provides a wide range of education services for your patients to help them better understand and manage their health problems, to promote wellness, and to provide support for treatment compliance. Hospitals and many community agencies and organizations provide patient education opportunities, support groups for specific problems or diseases, and learning materials. These same groups may help the patient by providing professional consultation for many topics, including diet, exercise, and emotional support. It is important that the medical assistant be aware of the various resources available in the community for patient education and referral.

Based on your evaluation of Mr. Ignatio's learning needs, what community resources would help him and his family better understand and manage his disease?

Teaching patients specific skills also is an important component of health education. The best way to coach a patient through the process of manipulating and operating medical equipment accurately is to use demonstration and return demonstration of the skill (Figure 5-6). Using the exact piece of equipment the patient will be using at home, you first should demonstrate to the patient how to perform the skill, ask for questions and explain further as needed, and then have the patient return the demonstration before leaving the facility. This gives you the opportunity to observe the patient performing the task and correct any mistakes or clarify any misconceptions before the patient has to use the equipment at home alone.

For some patients, an effective method of monitoring health education is to have the patient keep a journal of his or her activities and response to treatment. For example, a patient trying to adapt to a new diet could record daily intake to get a better idea of whether he or she is following through with dietary recommendations. Some excellent online applications (apps) are available, such as the *MyPlate.gov* site,

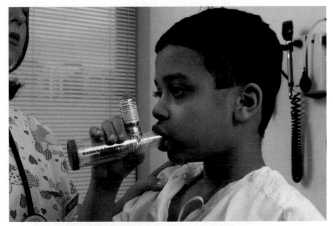

FIGURE 5-6 Demonstration and return demonstration.

that can help patients perform this task. In the case of Mr. Ignatio, referring to the memory log on his glucometer or tracking blood glucose levels with an app on his phone or computer could reinforce the results of his compliance with medication and diet therapies.

Another vital link to the success of patient education is family involvement. If the patient is being treated holistically, the family plays an integral role in patient wellness. Involving family members in patient education efforts provides support and understanding for the patient and manages family concerns about the patient's welfare. An educated family member can be an excellent resource for patient concerns and a vigilant reinforcer of healthy behaviors.

CRITICAL THINKING APPLICATION   **5-2**

The provider recommends that Mr. Ignatio start a 1,200-calorie diabetic diet for weight reduction and blood glucose control and that he take glucometer readings three times a day. After you consider various teaching methods, which strategies do you think would be most useful in helping Mr. Ignatio learn about his disease and follow the provider's recommendations?

Implement the Teaching Plan

After you have completed the patient assessment, decided on teaching materials and methods that match your patient's characteristics and learning needs, and adapted the material and your approach for any potential barriers to learning, it is time to implement the plan. Conduct the lesson in a quiet area away from distractions. Assemble the equipment the patient will need to follow through with treatment. The patient should learn to handle and practice on the same type of equipment that will be used at home so that no problem occurs in transferring the skill. Time is always an issue in the ambulatory care setting, so it is important to present only the material or skill it is possible for the patient to master before the end of the appointment. Throughout the lesson, remember to maintain an adequate pace for learning—not too fast and not too slow—to optimize the patient's understanding.

A crucial aspect of successful patient teaching is to consistently ask for feedback about the process (Figure 5-7). It also helps to restate, repeat, or rephrase the material to make sure the patient understands the process. As patients provide correct feedback about what they are learning or demonstrate skills correctly, it is important to be positive about their progress. It also helps to summarize the material learned or the skills mastered at the end of each teaching intervention, as a way of reviewing the material and clarifying important concepts.

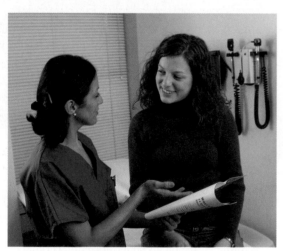

FIGURE 5-7 Patient feedback.

CRITICAL THINKING APPLICATION   5-3

Taylor has just completed the initial patient education session with Mr. Ignatio and his wife. He used demonstration–return demonstration to teach Mr. Ignatio how to check his blood glucose levels properly with the glucometer he will be using at home. Taylor answered Mrs. Ignatio's questions about diabetic diets, but the provider has also referred the couple to the dietitian at the hospital for further information on that topic. Taylor plans to review the skills practiced today at Mr. Ignatio's next appointment and to continue the teaching intervention, emphasizing the importance of Mr. Ignatio checking his feet daily for open areas or any signs of infection.

Accurately and completely document Taylor's initial coaching session with Mr. Ignatio.

The medical assistant should continue to evaluate the teaching plan throughout the process to make sure the time was adequate for learning and that the patient understood the information needed to follow through with care at home. In addition, plans should be made for the education intervention during the patient's next visit. All of this information needs to be included in the progress note about the lesson. Finally, the medical assistant must document details about the material covered, the patient's competency or level of skill in learning treatment techniques, and any referrals made for community and hospital experts or education groups (Procedure 5-2).

Summary of the Patient Teaching Plan

1. Perform an assessment.
   - Consider pertinent patient factors.
   - Identify barriers to learning.
   - Prioritize patient information.
2. Determine the patient's immediate and long-term needs.
   - Decide on the appropriate teaching materials and methods; prepare the teaching area; and assemble the necessary equipment and materials.
   - Demonstrate techniques and procedures using the supplies the patient will use at home.
   - Provide positive feedback when the patient performs skills correctly.
3. Maintain an adequate pace while teaching (not too fast).
4. Repeatedly ask for patient feedback to confirm understanding.
   - Barriers to learning are eliminated.
   - Immediate learning needs can be addressed.
   - Repetition and rephrasing promote understanding.
5. Summarize the material learned or skill mastered at the end of each teaching interaction.
6. Outline a plan for the next meeting.
7. Evaluate the teaching plan.
   - Was there enough time to complete the lesson?
   - Was the patient physically and psychologically ready for the information?
   - Were the goals for the session reached?
8. Document the teaching intervention in the patient's health record.
   - Material covered
   - Patient response or level of skill performance
   - Plans for next session
   - Community referrals

Role of the Medical Assistant as Patient Coach

- Reinforce provider instructions and information
- Encourage patients to take an active role in their health
- Use each patient interaction as an opportunity for health teaching
- Keep information relevant to the patient's needs
- Establish and maintain rapport with the patient
- Communicate clearly
- Be sensitive to the patient's learning factors
- Modify the teaching plan as needed to best meet the patient's needs

PROCEDURE 5-2	Coach Patients in Health Maintenance, Disease Prevention, and Following the Treatment Plan

Goal: *To consider patient factors, such as cultural diversity, developmental life stage, and communication barriers, when coaching patients in health maintenance, disease prevention, and following the treatment plan.*

Scenario: Role-play the following scenario with your partner.

Samuel Wu is a 74-year-old patient who was recently diagnosed with hypertension. The provider has designed a treatment plan for health maintenance and disease prevention that includes a low sodium diet, weight loss, and hypertensive medication. What patient education approaches should the medical assistant use that are age- and culturally appropriate? Should the medical assistant provide an educational brochure for Mr. Wu that he can take home for reinforcement of patient education? Include in your discussion the importance of following the provider's instructions for diet and weight loss.

EQUIPMENT and SUPPLIES

- Patient's health record
- Educational handouts and/or access to online resources that can be printed
- Quiet, private area

PROCEDURAL STEPS

1. Greet and identify the patient in a pleasant manner. Introduce yourself and explain your role.
   PURPOSE: To make the patient feel comfortable and at ease.
2. Take the patient to a quiet, private area. If this room has a computer with Internet access, you can help Mr. Wu research appropriate sites and print educational materials for his use at home.
   PURPOSE: A quiet, private area is necessary to protect confidentiality and prevent interruptions.
3. Identify factors that may limit the patient's ability to learn and implement lifestyle changes. Mr. Wu is of Chinese descent and is 74 years old. Will these patient factors affect learning?
   PURPOSE: You can promote patient learning if you identify and address the patient's primary concern and are sensitive to possible barriers to patient education, such as cultural influences, developmental stage, and possible communication barriers.
4. Prioritize the patient information and determine the patient's immediate and long-term needs. What does Mr. Wu need to know to maintain his health, prevent complications related to hypertension, and to follow the provider's treatment plan?
5. Prepare the teaching area and assemble necessary equipment and materials, making sure to use the same supplies and equipment the patient will use at home. Mr. Wu has a wrist blood pressure machine that he will use at home to monitor his blood pressure. Monitoring his blood pressure at home will help Mr. Wu determine if he is following diet restrictions and taking his medication as ordered.
   PURPOSE: Using the same equipment that the patient uses at home reinforces learning and limits the need to apply newly learned skills to a

different type of equipment. Taking his blood pressure routinely will help reinforce diet restrictions, and the need for taking his medication as ordered.
6. Use restatement, reflection, and clarification to promote understanding.
   PURPOSE: Therapeutic communication techniques help you gather complete information.
7. Remain sensitive to the individual needs of your patient throughout the interview process.
   PURPOSE: Consistently keep in mind the patient's cultural background, developmental stage, and possible communication barriers as you progress through the teaching intervention. Treat all patients with respect.
8. Summarize the material learned or the skill mastered at the end of each teaching interaction and outline a plan for the next meeting. Emphasize the importance of following the treatment plan to maintain health and prevent disease complications.
   PURPOSE: Summarizing the material covered helps clarify the information for the patient and also helps you determine where to start or what to review at the next appointment.
9. Give the patient appropriate handouts and/or conduct an online search of community resources that might be of benefit. Print out this information or e-mail it to the patient for future use.
   PURPOSE: Make sure the patient takes the handouts when leaving the office; include a list of online sites that can be checked for additional information and support.
10. Document the teaching intervention, including the material covered; the patient's response or level of skill performance; plans for the next session; and any community referrals.
    PURPOSE: Documentation in the health record of the teaching intervention and the patient's comprehension helps ensure consistency and appropriate follow-up for subsequent visits.

CLOSING COMMENTS

Legal and Ethical Issues

Providing adequate, correct, understandable information to patients is integral to the informed consent mandate in the Patients' Bill of Rights. All patients have the right to information before they agree to receive care. An extension of this concept is the right of patients to understand their disease process and to manage their health. Another consideration arising from the Patients' Bill of Rights is the issue of patient confidentiality as it relates to patient education. When developing and implementing the teaching plan, designing teaching interventions and strategies, and referring patients for community assistance, the medical assistant must protect the patient's confidentiality.

Essential factors in risk management for the ambulatory care setting include conducting adequate patient education and follow-up. Also integral to risk management is the importance of documenting each patient education intervention completely and accurately. The patient's health record should clearly describe the education intervention, methods and materials used, the patient's response to the intervention, the date of each session, and the individual who conducted each intervention. Each documentation entry should completely describe the material covered and the patient's feedback about the information so that no doubt exists that the patient understood the information and was able to perform any related skills properly and adequately.

Teaching interventions should demonstrate sensitivity to multicultural factors and diverse populations. Meeting the needs of all patients without evidence of prejudice is a key risk management step.

HIPAA Applications

- The patient has the right to restrict who can receive protected health information (PHI). At the first office visit, the patient should complete a release of information form, if he or she wants to do so. This form identifies a particular family member, close friend, or any other individual who the patient states can receive disclosures of health information.
- Only the person or persons identified on the HIPAA release form completed by the patient have the right to the patient's personal information. Therefore, if an individual requests information about the patient, the medical assistant first must check the release form to determine whether the individual was approved by the patient before discussing the patient's condition. This holds true regardless of the individual's relationship to the patient.
- If the provider believes that it is in the patient's best interest that family members be involved in patient health education, the medical assistant can contact the family only if the patient has given approval. This permission should be included in the patient's HIPAA information and should be documented in the medical record so that all employees can read evidence of the patient's approval.

Professional Behaviors

Medical assistants are members of a profession in which information about disease, treatment, diagnostics, and management of health problems is constantly changing. Keeping up with current medical information requires a commitment to lifelong learning from all members of the healthcare team. To be effective patient educators, we first must be sure to have adequate knowledge ourselves. Medical assistants are perfectly placed in the healthcare team to represent the patient; that is, to perform the duties of a patient navigator. Who else in the ambulatory care setting is better able to understand the complex administrative and clinical skills needed for patients to navigate their care? From understanding treatment protocols to helping patients with insurance issues, medical assistants can serve as intermediaries who represent and support the patient throughout the healthcare environment.

SUMMARY OF SCENARIO

After working with Mr. Ignatio, Taylor realizes the significance and complexity of educating patients in the ambulatory care setting. Despite the time constraints typical in this particular healthcare setting, patients still must learn how to manage their disease and follow treatment guidelines. Approaching each patient as an individual learner with particular needs and characteristics is crucial to the ultimate success of the teaching plan. By using a holistic approach and taking into account the health belief model, Taylor has considered the ramifications of diabetes mellitus for Mr. Ignatio's life and has made efforts to include family and community resources in the management of his disease.

SUMMARY OF LEARNING OBJECTIVES

1. **Discuss the holistic model of patient education related to health and illness; also, instruct patients according to their needs to promote health maintenance and disease prevention.**

The holistic model suggests that patient education should consider all aspects of the patient's life, including physical, sociocultural, intellectual, economic, and psychological needs. (See Table 5-1 and Figure 5-1.) The health belief model analyzes what people believe to be true about themselves and their health. This model suggests that healthcare practitioners consider how the patient perceives the risk of developing the disease and whether he or she believes that altering health behaviors will prevent the disease. Dr. Elisabeth Kübler-Ross's stages of grief may also help explain a patient's reaction to a particular diagnosis, especially if the disease requires a drastic change in lifestyle. Grief is an ongoing process, with patients moving through denial, anger, bargaining, depression, and finally resolution, at their own pace and in their own way.

Many factors or patient characteristics may affect the patient's ability to learn. Medical assistants must be aware of these factors to develop a patient education approach that best meets the needs of each patient.

2. **Summarize the stages of grief and suggest therapeutic interactions for grieving patients.**
   - *Denial and isolation:* Reinforce each education intervention and encourage family members to attend visits.
   - *Anger:* Use therapeutic communication techniques to acknowledge the patient's feelings about the diagnosis.
   - *Bargaining:* Discuss the patient's bargaining requests with the provider to work out a solution.
   - *Depression:* Use available community resources to provide support for the patient and family.
   - *Acceptance:* Renew education efforts by providing multiple methods for learning about the disease.

3. **List at least five guidelines for patient education that can affect the patient's overall wellness.**

The guidelines for patient education include providing knowledge and skills that promote recovery and health; including family in education interventions; encouraging patient ownership of the education process; promoting safe use of medications and treatments; encouraging healthy behaviors; and providing information on how to access community resources.

4. **Do the following related to patient factors that affect learning:**
   - *Define six patient factors that have an impact on learning.*
   Patient factors that have an impact on learning include the patient's perception of disease versus the actual state of disease; the need for information; age and developmental level; mental and emotional state; the influence of multicultural and diversity factors; individual learning style; and the impact of physical disabilities on the education process.
   - *Display respect for individual diversity.*
   Culture, family background, and religious beliefs influence a patient's actions. For patient education to be successful, it is essential that the medical assistant be aware of and sensitive to the impact of these factors on patient learning. Consider the patient's language, ability to understand English verbally or read it correctly, and cultural relationships to healthcare workers. Develop techniques to minimize the patient's education problems.
   - *Summarize educational approaches for patients with language barriers.*
   Educational approaches for patients with language barriers include addressing the patient formally and courteously; using nonverbal language to promote understanding; integrating pictures or models that illustrate the material; observing the patient for understanding or confusion; using simple lay language; demonstrating procedures; implementing teaching in small, manageable steps; providing written instructions; and using an interpreter when available.

5. **Do the following related to the teaching plan:**
   - *Determine possible barriers to patient learning.*
   Possible barriers to patient education include the patient's learning style, physical limitations, age, and developmental level; any emotional or mental state that interferes with learning; use of defense mechanisms; cultural or ethnic factors; language; the presence of pain; a patient's lack of motivation to learn; and limited time for teaching.
   - *Assess the patient's needs.*
   The goal of the assessment process is to create a teaching plan that meets the patient's needs for understanding and managing his or her illness.
   - *Determine the teaching priorities.*
   Every interaction with the patient is an opportunity for health education. Use the waiting room as a place for learning by providing up-to-date educational materials on a variety of issues.
   - *Decide on the appropriate teaching materials.*
   When possible, all patient information should include a handout or online reference that reinforces information and that can be used as a resource. Other teaching materials include DVDs, approved YouTube links, and health-related applications that can be accessed by smart phone or computer.
   - *Develop a list of community resources related to patients' healthcare needs and facilitate referrals to community resources in the role of a patient navigator.*
   The medical assistant should assist patients and their families in finding and using community education and support services when needed. The healthcare facility should maintain a current file of area resources that give the name of the group and the services provided; the contact person; a telephone number and address; meeting times and location if applicable; and a related website if available. Patients should be provided with accurate, well-researched sites to make sure that online recommendations support the provider's treatment protocol. A patient navigator is a person who helps patients and families with insurance problems, explains treatment and care, communicates with the healthcare team, assists caregivers, and manages medical paperwork. This definition describes the role of the medical assistant as an advocate for

Continued

SUMMARY OF LEARNING OBJECTIVES—*continued*

the patient in the ambulatory care setting. (Refer to Procedure 5-1.)

- *Decide on the appropriate teaching methods.*
  A variety of methods may be used to get the message across to patients. Some excellent apps are available that can help patients keep track of their progress. Family involvement is also important.

- *Implement the teaching plan.*
  The medical assistant should consistently ask for feedback about the process. It also helps to restate, repeat, or rephrase the material to make sure the patient understands.

- *Demonstrate the ability to develop an appropriate and effective patient teaching plan.*
  The parts of the teaching plan include assessing learning needs; eliminating learning barriers; determining teaching priorities; using appropriate teaching materials and methods; gathering feedback repeatedly to ensure that the patient understands; summarizing the material at the end of each education session; planning for the next meeting; evaluating the effectiveness of the session; and completely and accurately

documenting the details of the teaching intervention. (Refer to Procedure 5-2.)

6. **Describe the role of the medical assistant in patient education.**
   The role of the medical assistant in patient education is to reinforce the provider's instructions and information by encouraging patients to take an active part in their health; using teaching moments effectively; keeping information relevant to the patient; establishing and maintaining patient rapport; communicating clearly; remaining aware of learning factors; being flexible with the teaching plan; and using community resources for learning and support.

7. **Integrate the legal and ethical elements of patient teaching into the ambulatory care setting; also, discuss HIPAA applications.**
   Appropriate patient education reflects the emphasis of the Patients' Bill of Rights on patient confidentiality and informed consent. Risk management practices related to patient education include accurate and complete documentation of patient education sessions, sensitivity to the needs of the individual patient, and application of HIPAA rules.

CONNECTIONS

Study Guide Connection: Go to the Chapter 5 Study Guide. Read and complete the activities.

evolve Evolve Connection: Go to the Chapter 5 link at *evolve.elsevier.com/ kinn* to complete the Chapter Review Quiz. Check out the other resources listed for this chapter to make the most of what you have learned from Patient Education.

6

MEDICINE AND LAW

Barbara Johnson is the new office manager for two neurologists in an urban area. Recently she was subpoenaed to appear in court with medical records to testify about a patient. This particular patient was referred to one of the providers in the clinic, Dr. Rebecca Patrick. Dr. Patrick saw the patient several years ago, and the patient has brought a medical professional liability case against a surgeon in another city. Barbara is considered the custodian of medical records and will take them to court and answer questions about the information in them.

One of Barbara's first priorities at her new job is to make sure the office is operating in compliance with the legal regulations that affect the facility. She is knowledgeable about the requirements of the Health Insurance Portability and Accountability Act (HIPAA) and the Health Information Technology for Economic and Clinical Health Act (HITECH), in addition to other legal issues. Two of the employees Barbara supervises, Samantha and Lynda, are newly graduated from medical assisting school and are anxious to learn more about the statutes and laws that affect the providers' office. Barbara is more than happy to share what she has learned with them.

While studying this chapter, think about the following questions:

- How can the medical assistant comply with legal regulations in the ambulatory care facility?
- How can new graduates learn about the laws that affect them in their state?
- What are some risk management strategies that will help prevent medical liability suits?

LEARNING OBJECTIVES

1. Define, spell, and pronounce the terms listed in the vocabulary.
2. Compare criminal and civil law as they apply to the practicing medical assistant; also discuss contract law.
3. Summarize the anatomy of a medical professional liability lawsuit and explain the four essential elements of a valid contract.
4. Discuss the various parts of a medical professional liability lawsuit.
5. Discuss the advantages of mediation and arbitration.
6. Do the following related to medical liability and negligence:
   - Differentiate malfeasance, misfeasance, and nonfeasance.
   - Explain the four Ds of negligence.
   - Define the types of damages.
7. Discuss risk management and describe liability, malpractice, and personal injury insurances, including the importance of informed consent.
8. Define statutes of limitation and confidentiality.
9. Discuss compliance reporting, the Patient Self-Determination Act, the Uniform Anatomical Gift Act, and the Patients' Bill of Rights.
10. Describe the important features of the ADAA and GINA Acts.
11. Explain the components of the Health Insurance Portability and Accountability Act (HIPAA).
12. Identify HITECH and its impact on electronic transmission of patient records.
13. Summarize the primary features of the Affordable Care Act.

VOCABULARY

abandonment The withdrawal of protection or support; in medicine, to discontinue medical care without proper notice after accepting a patient.

act The formal action of a legislative body; a decision or determination of a sovereign state, a legislative council, or a court of justice.

arbitration (ar-buh-tra′-shun) A type of alternative dispute resolution that provides parties to a controversy with a choice other than going to court for resolution of a problem. Arbitration is either court ordered to resolve a conflict, or the two sides select an impartial third party, known as an *arbitrator*, and agree in advance to comply with the arbitrator's award. The arbitrator's decision is usually final.

assault An intentional attempt to cause bodily harm to another; a threat to cause harm is an assault if it is combined with a physical action (e.g., a raised fist) so that the victim could reasonably assume there would be an assault.

VOCABULARY—continued

battery An intentional act of contact with another that causes harm or offends the individual being touched or injured.

contributory negligence A law that recognizes there may be some instances in which the individual contributes to the injury or condition; the injury or condition is partly due to the individual's own unreasonable action.

damages Money awarded by a court to an individual who has been injured through the wrongful conduct of another party. Damages attempt to measure in financial terms the extent of harm the victim has suffered. Harm may be an actual physical injury but can also be damage to property or the individual's reputation.

defendant A person required to answer in a legal action or suit; in criminal cases, the person accused of a crime.

due process A fundamental constitutional guarantee that all legal proceedings will be fair; that one will be given notice of the proceedings and an opportunity to be heard before the government acts to take away life, liberty, or property; a constitutional guarantee that a law will not be unreasonable or arbitrary.

emancipated minor A person under the age of majority (usually 18) who has been legally separated from his or her parents by the courts. The person is responsible for his or her own care.

expert witnesses People who provide testimony to a court as experts in certain fields or subjects to verify facts presented by one or both sides in a lawsuit. They typically are compensated and used to refute or disprove the claims of one party.

guardian ad litem An individual who is assigned by the court to be legally responsible for protecting the well-being and interests of a ward, typically a minor or a person who has been declared legally incompetent.

healthcare clearinghouses Businesses that receive healthcare transactions from healthcare providers, translate the data from a given format into one acceptable to the intended payer, and forward the processed transaction to designated payers. They include billing services, community health information systems, and private network providers or "value-added" networks that facilitate electronic data interchanges.

implied contract A contract that lacks a written record or verbal agreement but is assumed to exist. For example, if a patient is being seen in a physician's office for the first time, it is assumed that the patient will provide a comprehensive and accurate health history and that the provider will diagnose and treat the patient in good faith to the best of his or her ability.

incompetent Refers to a person who is not able to manage his or her affairs because of mental deficiency low IQ, deterioration, illness, or psychosis) or sometimes physical disability. The individual cannot comprehend the complexities of a situation and therefore cannot provide informed consent.

informed consent Voluntary agreement, usually written, for treatment after being informed of its purpose, methods, procedures, benefits, and risks. The patient must understand the details of the procedure and give his or her consent without duress or undue influence, and the patient must have the right to refuse treatment or voluntarily withdraw from treatment at any time.

law A binding custom or practice of a community; a rule of conduct or action prescribed or formally recognized as binding or enforceable by a controlling authority.

liable (li'-uh-buhl) Obligated according to law or equity; responsible for an act or a circumstance.

libel A written remark that injures another's reputation or character.

litigious (luh-tih'-juhs) Prone to engage in lawsuits.

malpractice A type of negligence in which a licensed professional fails to provide the standard of care, causing harm to a person.

negligence (neh'-glih-jents) Conduct expected of a reasonably prudent person acting under similar circumstances; it falls below the standards of behavior established by law for the protection of others against unreasonable risk of harm.

ordinance (or'-dih-nens) An authoritative decree or direction; a law set forth by a governmental authority, specifically, municipal regulation.

perjured testimony The voluntary violation of an oath or vow, either by swearing to what is untrue or by omission to do what has been promised under oath; false testimony.

plaintiff The person or group bringing a case or legal action to court.

precedent (preh'-suh-dent) A person or thing that serves as a model; something done or said that may serve as an example or rule to authorize or justify a subsequent act of the same kind.

prudent Marked by wisdom or judiciousness; shrewd in the management of practical affairs.

relevant Having significant and demonstrable bearing on the matter at hand.

slander An oral defamation or insult; a harmful, false statement made about another person.

subpoena duces tecum A subpoena for the production of records or documents that pertain to a case as evidence.

verdict The finding or decision of a jury on a matter submitted to it in trial.

The **law** is a fascinating subject. When law is applied to medicine, it can provoke interesting case studies and complex decisions. In today's **litigious** society, medical assistants, in addition to providers and other staff members, must take steps to protect themselves from lawsuits. Legal issues underlie many aspects of the provision of healthcare in a provider's office. Although the wording of statutes and regulations often is long and complicated, medical assistants must stay abreast of the rules governing medical facilities and do everything possible to remain in compliance with the standards and regulations for all organizations that oversee the medical industry.

Generally, the law holds that every person is **liable** for the consequences of his or her own **negligence** when another person is injured as a result. In some situations, this liability also extends to the employer. Providers may be held responsible for the mistakes of those who work in their healthcare facility, and sometimes they must pay **damages** for the negligent acts of their employees.

Under the doctrine of *respondeat superior* (Latin for "let the master answer"), providers are legally responsible for employees acting within the scope of their employment duties. In healthcare, this principal states that the physician-employer is legally responsible for the actions of his or her employees, including medical assistants, when they are performing duties as outlined in their job descriptions. Medical assistants guilty of negligence are liable for their own actions, but the injured party generally sues the provider because the chance of collecting damages is greater. However, medical assistants, regardless of their financial worth, can be held liable for negligent acts; this fact illustrates the continuing importance of exercising extreme care in performing all duties in the healthcare environment.

JURISPRUDENCE AND THE CLASSIFICATIONS OF LAW

Jurisprudence is the science and philosophy of law. The term *jurisprudence* comes from the Latin words *juris,* which means "law, right, equity, or justice," and *prudentia,* which means "skill or good judgment."

Law is a custom or practice of a community. It is a rule of conduct or action prescribed or formally recognized as binding or enforceable by a controlling authority. Law is the system by which society gives order to our lives. The U.S. Constitution is the supreme law of the United States (Figure 6-1); the rules established by the Constitution take priority over federal statutes, court opinions, and state constitutions. The state constitution is the supreme law within the boundaries of each state unless it conflicts with the U.S. Constitution. States cannot pass laws that conflict with the U.S. Constitution, nor can local governments pass laws that conflict with the state constitution.

A law enacted at the federal level, which must be passed by Congress, is called an **act**. *Statutes* are laws that have been enacted by state legislatures. Local governments create and enact **ordinances**. Much of our law is based on previous judge and jury decisions, which are called **precedents**. Often judges and juries follow precedents when making a decision on a case. The two basic categories of jurisprudence are criminal law and civil law.

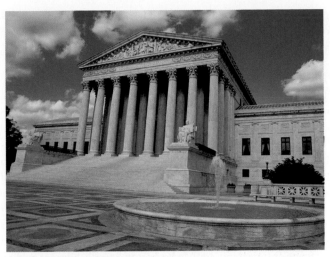

FIGURE 6-1 The U.S. Supreme Court. The Supreme Court decides cases that involve interpretation of the U.S. Constitution.

Criminal Law

Criminal law governs violations of the law punishable as offenses against the state or the federal government. Such offenses involve the welfare and safety of the public as a whole, rather than of one individual. A medical assistant can be prosecuted for criminal acts such as **assault** and **battery**, fraud, and abuse. Criminal offenses are classified into three basic categories: misdemeanors, felonies, and treason. To ensure fair treatment under the law, all individuals are entitled to **due process**, which guarantees that the accused will have an opportunity to defend himself or herself against any charges brought in opposition.

Misdemeanors

A minor crime is called a misdemeanor. Punishment for misdemeanors can include payment of a fine, probation, community service, and restitution. These cases are tried in the lowest local court, such as municipal, police, or justice courts. Typical misdemeanors include petty theft, disturbing the peace, simple assault and battery, and drunk driving without injury to others. If convicted of a misdemeanor, individuals may spend up to a year in jail. Some states have created a subcategory of misdemeanors for infractions, which often are called *violations*. Infractions are minor offenses, such as traffic tickets, which are punishable only by a fine.

Felonies

A *felony* is a major crime, such as murder, rape, or burglary. A felony charge can end with imprisonment for 1 or more years or even death for more serious crimes. An individual convicted of a felony may lose the right to vote, cannot be employed in certain professions (e.g., teachers and social workers), are not allowed certain types of licenses (e.g., medicine or nursing), and cannot buy or carry firearms. Felonies often are divided into subgroups, or degrees, such as first degree, second degree, and third degree. A first-degree offense is normally the most serious.

Civil Law

Civil law is concerned with acts that are not criminal in nature but involve relationships with other individuals, organizations, or government agencies. Many types of civil law exist to address numerous issues. The three that most directly affect the medical profession are tort law, contract law, and administrative law.

Tort Law

Tort law provides a remedy for a person or group that has been harmed by the wrongful acts of others. For example, a defamation case would be judged under tort law. *Defamation* is an intentional false statement, either written or spoken, that harms a person's reputation, diminishes the respect in which a person is held, or creates negative opinions toward another person. **Libel** (written) and **slander** (oral) are acts that fall into the category of defamation.

When a person is liable for an act, he or she is obligated or responsible according to the law. Professional and personal injuries are types of torts, meaning that a person or group has injured someone or something else. Medical professional liability, or medical **malpractice**, falls into this category. Providers carry professional liability insurance to help guard them from liability costs. Medical assistants can also invest in liability insurance. Remember, the terms *libel* and *liable* are defined differently, although they sound much the same.

CRITICAL THINKING APPLICATION   **6-1**

- What is the difference between libel and slander?
- Give an example of how a medical assistant might commit each of these actions against tort law?

Contract Law

A contract is an agreement that creates an obligation. Contract law touches our lives in many ways practically every day, but we usually do not give much thought to its influences. If a person parks a car in a parking garage for a monthly fee and signs a contract for a year, and then begins parking elsewhere and refuses to pay the fee, the person may be liable for the fees for the duration of the entire contract. If the person's vehicle is damaged while parked in the garage, the garage may be responsible for reimbursement if the contract does not specify otherwise.

A contract does not have to be formalized in writing to be binding on the parties involved. Oral contracts also are valid in many states in most situations. For example, an oral contract is created when the medical assistant makes an appointment for a new patient visit. Simply as a result of the scheduling of that first appointment, the patient and provider now are in an oral contract that requires the provider to care for the patient and the patient to comply with treatment protocols and payment of services. This is why most ambulatory care facilities require the medical assistant to gather payment information (e.g., the type of health insurance the patient has) before an appointment is scheduled.

ANATOMY OF A MEDICAL PROFESSIONAL LIABILITY LAWSUIT

A medical liability case often stems from a breach of trust or miscommunication between the provider and the patient. These cases fall into the category of tort law. Even when the provider has made an error, often the level of trust between the provider and patient determines whether a lawsuit is pursued. First, the provider-patient relationship must be formed. However, before this relationship can be discussed, you must understand the requirements for a valid, enforceable contract.

What Constitutes a Valid Contract?

A valid legal contract has four essential elements: agreement, legality, competence, and consideration.

1. The two parties must have a mutual understanding and *agreement* on the intent of the contract.
2. The contract must involve something that is *legal*.
3. Both parties must be legally *competent*.
4. *Consideration* must be involved; consideration is an exchange of something of value (e.g., money) for the provider's time.

CRITICAL THINKING APPLICATION   **6-2**

Barbara works for Dr. Rebecca Patrick, who saw the patient bringing the lawsuit against the surgeon as a referral patient. Does Dr. Patrick have a contract with the patient, based on a provider-patient relationship? Why or why not?

The provider-patient relationship is generally held by courts to be a contractual relationship that is the result of three steps:

1. The provider invites an offer by establishing availability (e.g., posting office hours).
2. The patient accepts the appointment and makes an offer by arriving for or requesting treatment.
3. The provider accepts the patient's offer by examining the patient and beginning treatment. Before accepting a patient, the provider is under no obligation, and no contract exists. However, once the provider has accepted the patient, an **implied contract** exists (Figure 6-2). An implied contract in this case assumes that the provider will treat the patient using reasonable care and that the provider has a degree of knowledge, skill, and judgment that might be expected of any other provider in the same locality and under similar circumstances.

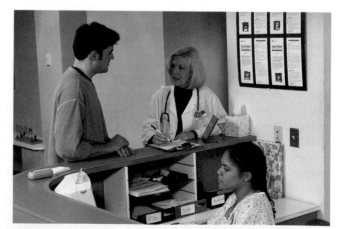

FIGURE 6-2 The provider-patient relationship is built on a strong foundation of trust, but it also is a contractual relationship.

It is extremely important that no express promise of a cure be made by anyone in the office, including the provider, because this would become a part of the contract.

The patient's responsibility in this agreement includes the liability of payment for services and a willingness to follow the advice of the provider. Most provider-patient contracts are implied contracts. Although the patient may complete many forms before he or she is accepted by the provider, these forms do not in most cases constitute a formal contract.

CRITICAL THINKING APPLICATION   **6-3**

- If the patient does not pay for the services rendered by the provider, does this negate the provider-patient contract?
- How might Barbara, Samantha, and Lynda ensure that patients understand that they are expected to follow the advice of the provider?

After the provider-patient relationship has been established, the provider is obligated to attend the patient as long as attention is required, unless the provider or patient terminates the contract. When a provider terminates the contract, the patient must be given notice of the provider's intentions so that the patient has sufficient time to arrange for another healthcare provider. The provider must write a letter of withdrawal from medical care of the patient, and it should be delivered by certified mail, return receipt requested. A copy of the letter and the return receipt should be included in the patient's health record. Reasonable time should be allowed for the patient to find other medical care.

To protect the provider against a lawsuit for **abandonment**, the details of the circumstances under which the provider is withdrawing from the case should be included in the patient's health record. To specify the withdrawal of care, a letter should be sent to the patient that includes a brief reason for the withdrawal of care, such as missing appointments or failing to comply with treatment orders. The letter should state the following:

- That professional care is being discontinued as of a particular date
- That the provider will supply copies of the patient's records to another provider on request
- That the patient should seek the attention of another provider as soon as possible

A patient who wants to terminate the provider-patient relationship simply no longer sees the provider for treatment. The patient does not have to inform the office; however, if she or he does so, the office manager or provider should follow up with a confirmation letter, stating that the patient has ended the relationship.

Breach of Contract

A breach of contract occurs if there is a failure to perform any term of a contract, written or oral, without a legitimate legal excuse. For example, if a plastic surgeon prepares an estimate for services and it states that the fee will be no more than $9,000, but then charges the patient $10,200, a breach of contract exists. Although most providers state that the document is just an estimate, this particular provider stated a clear amount that the surgery costs would not exceed.

CRITICAL THINKING APPLICATION   **6-4**

- For what reasons might a provider not want to accept a patient?
- Must the provider treat every patient who attempts to make an appointment?
- How might Barbara tactfully explain that the provider will not accept the patient into treatment?

---

responsibility

MEDICAL PROFESSIONAL LIABILITY LAWSUIT

Medical professional liability suits are far from rare, and every provider faces the probability of being sued at least once during his or her career. A medical assistant may be involved in preparing materials for court and scheduling or participating in depositions. The best advice for a medical assistant in this position is to remember to tell the truth. Attorneys help prepare the defense of the provider and the staff, but everyone should be truthful in answering in court to prevent the loss of his or her credibility in the trial and charges of perjury. Be especially careful to present a true, complete statement to the representing attorney. Unless he or she knows the whole truth, an appropriate defense cannot be prepared.

Interrogatories

Before the trial, the provider may be asked to complete an *interrogatory,* which is a list of questions from each party to the other in the lawsuit. Answers to the interrogatory must be provided within a specified time, and the answers are considered to be given under oath. Only the parties named in the lawsuit may be questioned through interrogatories.

Depositions

A *deposition* is an oral testimony of a party or witness in a civil or criminal proceeding taken before trial. A witness who is not a party to the lawsuit may be summoned by subpoena for a deposition. If you are called to be deposed in a case, the attorney will prepare you for questions from opposing attorneys and will be present during the process. A deposition is taken in the presence of a court reporter and under oath. The transcribed deposition is sent to the witness for review, and the witness has the right to request changes or corrections in the document before it goes into the record. Depositions are a discovery tool. *Discovery* is the pretrial disclosure of pertinent facts or documents by one or both parties to a legal action or proceeding. Many states have extensive discovery statutes that require each side to reveal to the other the facts that they "discover" while investigating the case.

Subpoenas

A *subpoena* is a document issued by a court that requires a person to be present at a specific time and place to testify as a witness in a lawsuit, either in a court proceeding or in a deposition (Figure 6-3). A **subpoena duces tecum** is a court order to produce identified documents or records. This type of subpoena does not require the person named in it to give testimony at a deposition or trial.

In medical practice, a subpoena duces tecum typically is ordered for patient records needed in a malpractice suit. The facility may charge a fee for the time spent in compiling the records and for

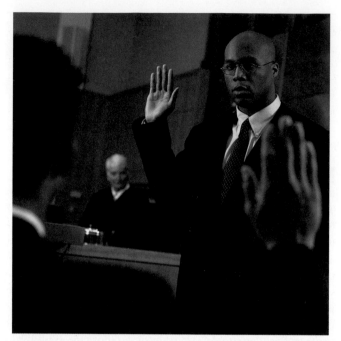

FIGURE 6-3 Witnesses must be credible and must tell the truth on the stand in court to avoid charges of perjury.

photocopying charges, but this fee must be requested at the time the subpoena duces tecum is served or it is considered to be waived. Original records should never be released under any circumstances. If an original record is demanded in the subpoena, it usually is taken to court or to mediation by the provider or an employee of the provider's office. Copies can be released in advance of the court date. Release only the information requested in the subpoena and provide only information that originated in the provider's office. Do not provide records sent from previous or consulting providers. Those records must be subpoenaed separately from the originating office.

Before responding to a subpoena, make sure it is valid. Although variances may occur from state to state, some general rules can be used to judge the validity of a subpoena:

- A subpoena issued in one state court generally is not valid in another state. Always verify the state in which the subpoena was issued.
- A subpoena issued by a federal court in one state generally is not valid in another state unless a federal statute authorizes nationwide service of process.
- Any duly authorized law officer may execute a valid subpoena anywhere in the same state. The officer notifies the issuing court once the subpoena has been served.
- Generally, the person or entity subpoenaed has 21 days to respond, but this period can differ from place to place.
- A subpoena duces tecum should be filed no less than 15 days before a trial. One served less than 15 days before a trial should not be honored.

Read the subpoena carefully to determine exactly what records are requested. The provider should always be notified of subpoenas served to the medical facility. Never copy records required in a subpoena without bringing the matter to the attention of the provider or office manager, or both. It also is advisable to keep a log of

subpoenas served to the office, what records were involved, and the disposition of the request, including when the records were presented to the court. Always inform the provider about the subpoena because he or she may want to present the document to an attorney for review before any information is released.

Inside the Courtroom

Knowing the role of each person in a court of law can be helpful. The person or body bringing the lawsuit to court is referred to by different terms, depending on the type of case. In a criminal court, the government brings the case and is represented by a prosecutor. In civil court, the person or group bringing the case to court is called the **plaintiff** (or *complainant* in some court systems), and the opposite party is called the **defendant**, or *respondent*. A judge presides over the case, giving instructions concerning the law to the jury, if a jury is present. If no jury is present, the judge decides the case; this is called a *bench trial*.

Burden of Proof

In a criminal case the burden of proof is on the prosecution, which must prove guilt beyond any reasonable doubt. *Reasonable doubt* is defined as the level of certainty a juror must have to find a defendant guilty of a crime. It is real doubt, based on reason and common sense after careful and impartial consideration of all the evidence, or lack of evidence, in a case.

Civil cases must be proven by a preponderance of the evidence. This means that the greater weight of evidence must point to the defendant or respondent as being responsible for the act involved in the case.

Outcome of the Case

Once both sides have presented their case to the judge or jury, they usually are given the opportunity to present a final summation of their case. The jury then retires to consider the **verdict**. This can take minutes, hours, days, or weeks. After the jury reaches a decision, the judge may enter it as a final verdict or may disregard it if the evidence does not support the jury's decision. The judge may also revise the verdict to comply with statutes, such as statutory limits on the amount of punitive damages. The final decision of the trial court is reflected in the judgment, signed by the judge.

MEDIATION AND ARBITRATION

Mediation and **arbitration** are two examples of alternative dispute resolutions that share the goal of avoiding litigation in court. In mediation, a neutral third party, the mediator, helps those involved in a dispute solve their own problems. The mediator facilities the parties' decisions by helping them communicate and move through the more difficult parts of their differences in search of a compromise that both parties can live with. Once the parties reach a resolution, a final settlement agreement is signed. Successful mediation enables the parties to design and retain control of the process at all times and, ideally, eventually strike their own bargain.

Arbitration is an alternative to trial in which a third party (an arbitrator) is chosen to hear evidence and make a decision about a case. The patient and the provider both have the opportunity to agree on who will arbitrate the case so that one side is not favored over the other. The arbitrator renders a legally binding decision based on very specific rules. Many providers and attorneys see mediation and arbitration as ways to solve the crisis of litigation in this country. Court battles can take years and can be extremely expensive, and much of the money reverts to the attorneys rather than the victors in the lawsuit.

MEDICAL LIABILITY AND NEGLIGENCE

When a patient is injured as a result of a provider's negligence, the patient may initiate a malpractice lawsuit to recover financial damages. However, experience has shown that the incidence of malpractice claims is directly related to the personal relationship and trust that exist between the provider and the patient. Deterioration of the provider-patient relationship is a common reason patients sue providers for malpractice, even when the patient has sustained no real injury.

Medical professional liability, commonly called *medical malpractice,* is governed by the law of torts. Medical malpractice occurs when a provider treats a patient in a way that does not meet the expected medical standard of care in the same medical community and because of this, the patient suffers harm. The medical standard of care is considered the type and level of care that a reasonably competent healthcare professional, in the same field and with similar training, would have provided in the same situation. Medical professional liability is much more easily prevented than defended.

To understand medical malpractice, the term *negligence* first must be understood. Negligence, in general, implies inattention to one's duty or business, or a lack of necessary diligence or care. In medicine, *negligence* is defined as the performance of an act that falls below the standards of behavior established by law, or the failure to perform an act that a reasonable and **prudent** provider would perform in a similar situation. The standard of prudent care and conduct is not defined by law; it is left to the determination of a judge or jury, usually with the help of **expert witnesses**. Expert witnesses are members of the profession involved (in this case, medicine). To be considered an expert witness, the individual has knowledge beyond that of the ordinary lay person, which enables him or her to give testimony that requires expertise to understand.

Professional negligence in medicine falls into one of three general classifications:

- *Malfeasance:* Intentionally doing something either dishonest or illegal. For example, a physician performs a surgical procedure for higher insurance payment when the patient could be treated with a nonsurgical method, such as medication. Another example would be if the wrong surgical procedure is performed on a patient.
- *Misfeasance:* Performing an act that is legal but not properly performed. For example, the surgeon performs abdominal surgery that is indicated and necessary to help the patient recover but does not do it properly, and the patient dies of complications that could have been avoided.
- *Nonfeasance:* Failure to perform an act that should have been performed. For example, diagnostic findings indicate that a patient has a tubal pregnancy, but the physician opts not to perform laparoscopic surgery to remove the tube.

A provider who performs an operation carelessly or fails to render care that should have been given may be found negligent. The doctrine of *res ipsa loquitur* (a Latin term meaning "the thing speaks for itself") presumes negligence if the individual or group being sued had exclusive control over whatever caused the injury, even though there is no specific evidence of negligence. For example, if a patient suffers an injury during surgery that is not connected to the actual surgical procedure (e.g., he has a reaction to the anesthetic or the provider amputated the left leg instead of the right leg). All those connected to the operation may be found negligent.

Although a medical assistant acts as an agent of the provider in carrying out most of his or her duties, the medical assistant may perform an act that can result in litigation. For instance, if the medical assistant gives a patient the wrong medication or the wrong dose of medication, both the provider and the medical assistant can be held liable for the error. Some states limit the scope of practice of medical assistants where medications are involved. However, if medical assistants are performing within the realm of duties for which they have received training, and the provider is accepting responsibility for the actions of those in the medical office, medical assistants usually are allowed to dispense and administer medications unless prohibited by state law. The medical assistant should always practice within the legal scope of practice of the state (see the chapter, The Medical Assistant and the Healthcare Team).

CRITICAL THINKING APPLICATION   **6-5**

Lynda asks Barbara whether a provider, as a medical professional, is liable if he or she makes a mistake in diagnosing a patient. When might this be considered malpractice and when might it not be considered malpractice?

What if the patient makes his or her own condition worse? Perhaps the patient does not take the medicine prescribed or refuses to schedule surgery as recommended by the physician. Is the provider responsible for the bad outcome? **Contributory negligence** exists when the patient contributes to his or her own condition, and it can lessen the damages that can be collected or even prevent them from being collected altogether. Some states have adopted a *comparative negligence* approach in which each party's negligence that resulted in an injury is considered when damages are determined.

The Four Ds of Negligence

Negligence is not presumed; it must be proven. The Committee on Medicolegal Problems of the American Medical Association (AMA) has determined that patients must present evidence of four elements before negligence has been proven. These elements have become known as the four Ds of negligence:

1. *Duty:* Duty exists when the provider-patient relationship has been established. Providers have a duty to provide the most accurate diagnosis and care and the duty to inform patients of potential problems they observe.
2. *Dereliction:* Dereliction refers to the failure of a provider to perform his or her duty; there must be proof that the provider somehow neglected the duty.

3. *Direct cause:* The patient must prove that the provider was aware of potential risks but did not inform the patient and as a result the patient was injured.
4. *Damages:* A physical, mental, emotional, or financial harm caused by the breach of duty.

If all four of these elements exist, the patient may obtain a judgment against the provider in a medical professional liability case.

Types of Damages

Five types of damages are common in tort cases: nominal, punitive, compensatory, general, and special damages.

- *Nominal damages* are small awards that are token compensations for the invasion of a legal right in which no actual injury was suffered. For instance, if an unauthorized medical facility employee accesses a patient's health record and is discovered but has not revealed any of the information in the record, the patient has not actually been harmed but may be awarded nominal damages in a lawsuit for the invasion of his or her privacy.
- *Punitive damages* are designed to punish the party who committed the wrong in such a way so as to deter repetition of the act; these are sometimes called *exemplary damages*. These damages historically were set so that the amounts would discourage intentional wrongdoing, misconduct, and outrageous behavior. The amount of damages awarded coincides in some percentage with the wealth of the defendant. Tort reform would cap the amount of money that could be collected during personal injury litigation, including medical malpractice cases. A specific monetary figure (e.g., $500,000) has been suggested as a limit on punitive damages; some believe that plaintiffs should be allowed to collect only up to three times the amount of compensatory damages. Some states have passed legislation that caps one or more of the categories of damages.

CRITICAL THINKING APPLICATION   **6-6**

Samantha and Lynda disagree on whether punitive damages should be awarded in medical professional liability cases. Samantha believes that nothing compensates for certain losses, but Lynda believes that monetary compensation is reasonable when a loss has been suffered. Discuss both sides of the issue.

- *Compensatory damages* are designed to compensate for any actual damages caused by the negligent person. They are intended to make the injured person "whole." Of course, nothing can substitute for the loss of an arm or a leg, for example, but compensatory damages help the patient or the family recover from the loss.
- *General damages* include compensation for pain and suffering, for loss of a bodily member or faculty, for disfigurement, or for other similar direct losses or injuries. The fact of the losses has to be proven, but the monetary value does not.
- *Special damages* are awarded for injuries or losses that are not a necessary consequence of the provider's negligent act or omission. These may include the loss of earnings or costs of travel. Both the fact of these losses and the monetary value must be proven.

RISK MANAGEMENT PRACTICES

Risk management practices are a combination of different approaches in the healthcare facility that reduces the likelihood that either an individual healthcare professional or the healthcare facility will be sued. The primary focus should be on delivering quality, safe patient care, but a secondary goal is to avoid the potential financial consequences of a malpractice suit. Each facility should have a plan for risk management that covers patient-specific risks. These plans might include the following features:

- Adequately trained providers and staff members.
- Open lines of communication among staff members regarding potential risky practices.
- Specific policies on how expired prescriptions are refilled to prevent prescription medication abuse.
- Policies on patient test results; making sure patients follow up with ordered diagnostic procedures; making sure the results are reviewed by the attending provider, and the patient is contacted with the results.
- Tracking missed appointments; implementing systems to follow-up with patients who miss appointments but fail to reschedule.
- Communication issues with patients; medical assistants can follow up with patients to make sure they understand information received from providers so that orders are not misinterpreted.
- Making sure that the facility is safe for patient use; this includes adequate lighting, grab bars, exit signs, assisting patients as needed, and a safe exterior area.
- Documentation procedures are strictly followed; all pertinent information is documented in the correct format in the patient's record.

LIABILITY, MALPRACTICE, AND PERSONAL INJURY INSURANCES

Individual providers and healthcare facilities typically purchase several different types of insurance. The administrative medical assistant may be involved in either researching or renewing these insurance policies for their employers. The following are types of insurance that are purchased by medical practices.

- *Liability insurance* protects the healthcare facility if there is an accident in the facility that causes bodily injury or property damage. For example, if a patient falls in the parking lot of the facility and suffers a broken arm, liability insurance covers this injury and protects the facility from financial loss.
- *Medical malpractice insurance* protects the provider and/or healthcare facility if there is a judgment against them for medical negligence, malfeasance, or malpractice. Most states require that providers have some form of medical malpractice insurance to protect them from a faulty or negligent action. The provider can either choose individual coverage or be part of a policy that incorporates the practice or institution where the provider is employed. The premiums for malpractice insurance are determined by the provider specialty. Each specialty area of practice has an insurance rate that is based on the probability of medical malpractice occurring. For example, orthopedic surgeons are more susceptible (because of the skill

required to perform surgery and the likelihood of patient complications) to negligent actions or mistakes, and as a result, are more likely to face a medical malpractice suit than a primary care provider (PCP). Therefore orthopedic surgeons have higher premiums for their medical malpractice insurance policies. Malpractice insurance rates also vary according to the location of the medical facility. For example, malpractice rates are higher in the Northeast than they are in the Midwest.

- *Personal injury insurance* covers both bodily harm and non-physical, noneconomic harm. Examples of nonphysical harm are libel or slander, discrimination, and invasion of privacy, which can cause psychological harm or damage the individual's reputation. Personal injury insurance is most commonly seen in auto insurance coverage for bodily injury if there is a car accident or in home owner's insurance if someone has an injury in or around personal property.

Consent

A provider must have consent to treat a patient, even though this consent usually is implied by the patient's appearance at the facility for treatment. This *implied consent* is sufficient for common or simple procedures generally understood to involve little risk. However, the medical assistant should always ask the patient's permission to perform procedures, even those as simple as taking vital signs. You can do this by using expressed consent. *Expressed consent,* sometimes known as general consent, is consent given after the patient is asked a question such as "Can I gather your health history?" If the patient replies, "Yes," you have been given expressed consent to perform that procedure.

When more complex procedures are involved, the provider must obtain the patient's **informed consent**. A provider who fails to secure consent could be charged with the crime of battery. A case for battery can be established if an individual is physically harmed or injured or if an illness occurs because of the contact. Battery may also occur if there is no physical harm but an act is considered offensive or insulting to the victim, such as touching a person without consent. If the patient refuses to consent to treatment and the treatment is performed anyway, the patient can sue for battery.

Informed consent involves a full explanation of the plan for treatment, including the potential for complications and the potential risks or side effects. Informed consent is not satisfied merely by having the patient sign a form. A discussion must occur during which the provider gives the patient or the patient's legal representative enough information to decide whether the patient will undergo the treatment or seek an alternative. The medical assistant cannot legally provide the information for the patient about informed consent. It is the provider's responsibility to make sure that each patient understands the treatment or procedure and has had all questions answered satisfactorily before the patient signs a consent form. However, the medical assistant can witness the document and ask the patient to sign the consent form. After consideration, the patient either consents to the proposed therapy and signs a consent form or refuses to consent. According to the AMA's standards for informed consent, the discussion about informed consent should include at least the following elements:

- Patient's diagnosis, if known
- Nature and purpose of the proposed treatment or procedure
- Risks and benefits of the proposed treatment or procedure
- Alternative treatments or procedures, regardless of the cost or the extent to which the treatment options are covered by health insurance
- Risks and benefits of the alternative treatment(s) or procedure(s)
- Risks and benefits of not receiving or undergoing a treatment or procedure

The discussion should be fully documented in the patient's health record, and a copy of the signed form should be placed in the record. Treatment may not exceed the scope of the consent that the patient has given. Often consent forms are lengthy and mention excessive possibilities and complications. Some language may attempt to be all inclusive (e.g., "included, but not limited to") when risks are listed. It is wise to have an attorney review the forms used for informed consent, because those that are too broad or too specific can be detrimental to the provider in a medical professional liability case.

Patients cannot be forced to undergo any type of medical treatment or care. The ultimate decision about care must be left to the patient or the legal guardian, and although medical professionals should disclose information to help the patient make a sound, informed decision, the patient should never be persuaded to act in any manner or accept any treatment with which he or she does not agree. Should the patient decide not to undergo treatment the provider feels is necessary, the patient should sign an informed refusal of treatment or care. This should be a statement similar to the informed consent, but it indicates that the patient has elected not to undergo treatment. Some providers discontinue all treatment if a patient does not participate in the care the provider recommends. This document, once signed, should be added to the patient's health record.

Each state has its own consent laws. Some states and insurance programs require a certain period to pass between the signing of the consent and the actual medical procedure; for instance, Medicaid sometimes requires a 30-day waiting period between the signing of consent for a tubal ligation and performance of the procedure. Medical assistants should be familiar with the laws in their own state that apply to their particular facility. Most of the laws can be found easily by searching on the Internet.

CRITICAL THINKING APPLICATION   6-7

Barbara stresses to Samantha and Lynda that at some time in their professional career, a patient will ask for their advice on whether the patient should undergo a certain procedure or treatment. Barbara explains that patients often consider advice from the medical assistants in the office to be an extension of the provider's opinions. How might they handle such questions from patients? Should a medical assistant offer any type of advice?

Giving Consent to Medical Procedures

Mentally competent adults (i.e., individuals capable of legally making their own decisions) can give consent to medical procedures. However, if an act is unlawful, the consent is invalid. For instance, a provider cannot prescribe medical marijuana for a patient who gives consent for the treatment unless it is legal to do so in that state.

Consent is also invalid if it is given by a person who is unauthorized to do so or if it is obtained by misrepresentation or fraud. For example, an adult child cannot give consent for a parent's treatment unless that individual has been declared **incompetent**. If a person is confused and unable to understand informed consent, a court of law can declare the individual mentally incompetent and appoint a guardian to give consent for treatment. If this is the case, the only care that can be given without the guardian's consent is emergency treatment. The patient's ability to give informed consent can also be compromised if the person is receiving pain medication or under the influence of alcohol or drugs. If the patient is not able to pay attention to the details of a procedure, or to understand those details or the need for care, or the risks of and alternatives to treatment, it is impossible for the patient to give informed consent.

Providers sometimes are reluctant to render aid in an emergency to someone who is not their patient for fear they will later be charged with negligence or abandonment. Under Good Samaritan laws, volunteers at the scene of an accident are given immunity to liability for any civil damages resulting from the rendering of emergency care. Most states now have either Good Samaritan or Volunteer Protection statutes. As long as the emergency care is given in good faith and without gross negligence, and the healthcare worker provides only emergency care that he or she has been trained to provide, the likelihood of a successful lawsuit against that individual is very slim.

Generally, when the patient is a minor, consent for surgery or treatment must be obtained from a parent, guardian, or **guardian ad litem**, except in an emergency requiring immediate treatment. If the parents are legally divorced or separated, consent should be obtained from the custodial parent, but if the child is visiting the second parent, consent may be obtained from that parent because in such a situation that parent has temporary custody.

Consent is not required for minors in the following circumstances:

- When consent may be assumed, such as in a life-threatening situation
- When a court order has been issued, as in a situation in which parents withhold consent for a necessary treatment because of religious reasons

In many states, treatment of sexually transmitted infections, drug abuse, alcohol dependency, pregnancy, or providing contraceptive methods does not require parental consent. Even if there are age of consent laws, providers can still treat minors with these issues.

An area of potential confusion regarding consent to treatment is the *mature minor doctrine,* which allows minors to give consent to medical procedures if they can show that they are mature enough to make a decision on their own. The mature minor doctrine is recognized in only a few states as law, but where it does exist it has been applied in cases where the minor is 16 years or older and demonstrates understanding of the consequences of the proposed surgical or medical treatment or procedure.

An exception to the need for parental consent is if the individual is an **emancipated minor**. Eligibility for emancipation varies, depending on state laws; however, it can be sought by those younger than the age of majority (usually 18 years of age) who meet one or more of the following conditions:

- Married
- In the armed forces

- Living separately and apart from parents or a legal guardian
- Self-supporting

Unless state law declares otherwise, an emancipated minor has the right to consent to treatment and the right to complete patient confidentiality, even from parents.

Statute of Limitations

A *statute of limitations* is a period after which a lawsuit cannot be filed. The statute of limitations for medical malpractice issues varies from state to state, ranging from 1 to 5 years. Most states have a separate deadline for minor children in medical malpractice cases. To research the limitations for minors in your state, see the National Conference of State Legislatures website: *www.ncsl.org/research/financial-services-and-commerce/medical-liability-malpractice-statutes-of-limitation.*

The statute of limitations may be extended because of a delay in the discovery of an injury. For example, a patient has surgery to replace a heart valve, and the surgery seems successful. One year later, the patient undergoes a routine echocardiogram, and the provider discovers that the valve was not implanted properly by the surgeon. Although it has been over a year since the surgery, the statute of limitations begins at the point of discovery of the injury; therefore the patient could now bring suit against the surgeon for the error.

Confidentiality

Confidentiality is one of the most sacred trusts the patient places in the hands of the provider and staff (Figure 6-4). Breach of patient confidentiality is grounds for immediate dismissal of a healthcare professional. The strictest care must be taken when handling patient records and discussing information about patients.

In special cases, patient confidentiality plays a vital role. A patient who tests positive for the human immunodeficiency virus (HIV) may face discrimination if the information surfaces. Providers who treat such patients may want to take extra care when leaving phone messages, texting, or sending e-mail or regular mail. Instead of leaving a message for a patient from "Dr. Watson's office," the medical assistant could say that the message is from "Terry Watson's office." This type of message does not identify the message as coming from a healthcare facility. Curious co-workers or relatives may not

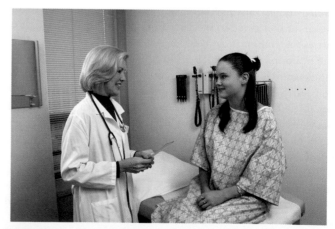

FIGURE 6-4 Patient confidentiality is the most important trust that exists between the provider and the patient.

grow as suspicious as they might if they were to encounter a message from a provider's office.

Patients receiving treatment for substance abuse are protected by federal statutes. Confidentiality also is of utmost importance to patients receiving treatment for mental health issues, sexually transmitted infections, sexual assault, and any type of abuse.

LAW AND MEDICAL PRACTICE

Law affects the provider's day-to-day practice. Some of the ways the medical assistant encounters legal issues in a healthcare setting are discussed in this section. Medical assistants must comply with both state and federal laws and regulations while performing the duties associated with their job.

Compliance Reporting

The provider is charged with safeguarding patient confidences within the constraints of the law, but according to state laws, which vary somewhat across the nation, certain disclosures must be made. Frequently the medical assistant is involved with the responsibility for compliance reporting.

Births and deaths must be reported. In some states, detailed information about stillbirths is required. Public health statutes also require compliance with wounds of violence reporting including gunshot wounds, knife injuries, or poisonings. Any death from accidental, suspicious, or unexplained causes must also be reported. In some states, occupational diseases and injuries must be reported within specific time limits.

Sexually transmitted infections are reportable in every state. All 50 states require that patients with confirmed cases of acquired immunodeficiency syndrome (AIDS) be reported by name to the local health department. Furthermore, most states require that patients who test positive for HIV be reported. Individuals are reported either by name or by unique identifiers. A continuing controversy exists as to whether the reporting prompts patients to receive care or deters individuals in high-risk groups from seeking care.

Child abuse is a leading cause of death among children younger than 5 years of age, and healthcare professionals are required by law to report any suspected cases of child abuse. The report should be made as soon as evidence is discovered that gives the provider "cause to believe" that abuse, neglect, or exploitation has occurred. Even if the evidence is uncertain, the provider should report it and allow the government to investigate and determine what action to take to protect the child. However, it is essential to make every attempt to ensure that the report is legitimate because it could lead to the child's being removed from the home and placed in foster care. Cases of spousal and elder abuse are difficult, because the person being abused often is reluctant to report the situation for fear of further mistreatment. The law requires that suspected cases of abuse of children, the elderly, or any others at risk be reported to the authorities.

Local health departments publish lists of reportable diseases and the method to use in reporting them. Reports are typically filed electronically to local public health officials or the state public health department. County and state health departments periodically issue bulletins that are sent to healthcare providers with information about disease outbreaks and various statistics. Local health departments should be consulted for specific procedures and reporting protocols.

Laws Having a Significant Impact on Healthcare
Patient Self-Determination Act

The Patient Self-Determination Act of 1990 brought the term *advance directive* to the forefront of medical care. This act requires healthcare facilities to develop and maintain written procedures that ensure that all adult patients receive information about advance directives and medical durable powers of attorney. Advance directives are legal documents that allow individuals to make decisions about end-of-life care ahead of time. They are a way for patients to communicate their wishes to family, friends, and healthcare professionals so that there is no confusion about what type of care they would like to receive or not receive when their condition is terminal. Advance directives specify which treatments you want if you are dying or permanently unconscious. Before completing an advance directive, patients should consider the following questions:

- What are your values about death and dying?
- Would you want treatment to extend your life by any means in any situation?
- If you are suffering from a terminal illness, would you want life-saving measures taken?

Patients can exert their right to accept or refuse treatment when they complete an advance directive form. Forms may be provided by healthcare facilities, hospitals, or long-term care facilities, but they can also be accessed online.

Advance directive forms ask patients to make decisions about a number of different treatment options, such as those in the following list. Patients may need assistance from medical personnel to understand the ramifications of each.

- The use of cardiopulmonary resuscitation (CPR) or a defibrillator; this means the heart has stopped and needs to be artificially stimulated with drugs and machines.
- Whether a mechanical ventilator or respirator should be used if breathing complications occur; this means the patient would have to have an airway put in place or be intubated.
- If, when, and for how long artificial feeding should be done; tube feeding supplies the body with nutrients and fluids intravenously or via a tube in the stomach.
- If, when, and for how long renal dialysis should be done to remove waste materials from the blood if the kidneys stop functioning.
- Antibiotics or antiviral medications can be used to treat infections. Many debilitated individuals develop pneumonia near the end of life. Should infections be treated aggressively, or should they be allowed to run their course?
- Decisions about palliative care measures to keep individuals comfortable and manage pain; these may include being allowed to die at home, pain medications, and avoiding invasive tests or treatments.
- Organ and tissue donations can be specified in a living will; if organs are removed for donation, the individual is kept on life-sustaining treatment temporarily until the procedure is complete.
- Donating the body for scientific study to a local medical school or university can be specified in the living will.

When completing an advance directive, the individual may also identify a *medical durable power of attorney* or a healthcare proxy; this is someone the person trusts to make health decisions for him or her if he or she is unable to do so. The patient may choose a spouse, family member, friend, or member of a faith community. This can be a different person from the one chosen to be the executor of a will. According to the American Bar Association, a person chosen as a medical durable power of attorney should:

- Meet your state's requirements for a healthcare agent
- Not be your doctor or a part of your medical care team
- Be willing and able to discuss medical care and end-of-life issues with you
- Be trusted to make decisions that follow your wishes and values
- Be trusted to be your advocate if disagreements arise about your care

Advance directives need to be in writing. Each state has different forms and requirements for creating legal documents. In some states the title of an advance directive can be different, such as a Living Will or an Advanced Health Care Directive. Depending on where you live, a form may need to be signed by a witness or notarized. A lawyer can assist with the process, but it is generally not necessary. Links to state-specific forms can be found on the National Hospice and Palliative Care Organization website: *www.caringinfo.org/i4a/pages/index.cfm?pageid=3289*. The American Bar Association also has a basic, easy to use advance directive form that can be used in most states. All adults should prepare an advance directive because unexpected end-of-life situations can develop at any age.

After completing the form, the patient should share it with his or her healthcare provider. A copy should be given to all providers involved in the patient's care, and this copy should be included in the patient's health record. An advance directive can be changed at any time. However, a new form must be created and witnessed as required by the state of residence, and revisions must be shared with family members and healthcare providers.

In most states, a Physicians Orders for Life Sustaining Treatment (POLST) form can also be completed to plan for the type of care desired if the patient has a medical emergency, such as respiratory or cardiac failure. POLST forms are created by the patient and physician to inform emergency care providers, such as emergency medical technicians (EMTs) and ambulance workers, what treatments you want and don't want in a medical emergency. The form must be signed by a physician and must instruct emergency medical personnel whether to perform CPR or an intubation, administer antibiotics, or start a feeding tube.

Uniform Anatomical Gift Act

The Uniform Anatomical Gift Act was developed to make sure that all states have the same laws about organ donation. The law states:

- A competent individual who is 18 years of age or older may donate all or any part of his or her body after death for research, transplantation, or placement in a tissue bank.
- A donor's valid statement of organ or tissue donation is enacted except when an autopsy is required by law or requested by the family.

- The donor's family can give permission for organ or tissue donation after the individual dies, even if the person did not do so.
- Providers who accept organs or tissues for transplant are protected from lawsuits.
- The time of death must be determined by a provider who is not part of a transplant team.
- The donor may change his or her mind about organ or tissue donation at any time.

The most important clause of the act permits the donation to be made by a written or witnessed document, such as an advance directive, organ donor identification on a driver's license, and/or possession of a donor card (Figure 6-5). This allows for immediate donation of the organs and/or tissues. The Uniform Donor Card is considered a legal document in all 50 states but must be signed by two witnesses.

The provisions of the Uniform Anatomical Gift Act are designed so that the donation occurs only after death. Therefore, donors should reveal their intentions to as many of their relatives and friends as possible and to their providers. Because the human body and its parts are not commodities in commerce, no money can be exchanged in making an anatomic donation itself. Fees are charged for performing the transplant and various procedures, but organs cannot be bought and sold. It also is important to note that family members should be prepared to receive the body of the person who has donated his or her entire body to research once the research facility has completed its study. This can often be a traumatic experience that rekindles the grief process, so the procedures and final disposition of the body should be decided at the time of the donation to avoid this difficult situation.

Patients' Bill of Rights

The Consumer Bill of Rights and Responsibilities, more commonly known as the Patients' Bill of Rights, outlines the relationship patients should have with their insurers, health plans, and care providers. The Patients' Bill of Rights was designed to strengthen confidence in the healthcare system, to encourage the development of quality provider-patient relationships, and to clarify that healthcare consumers also have a responsibility to participate in their care. Most healthcare facilities have adopted a Patients' Bill of Rights that is a condensed version of the entire bill. This information typically is

DONOR   DONOR CARD

I _____, have spoken to my family about organ and tissue donation. I wish to donate:
__ any needed organs and tissue
__ only the following organs and tissue: _____
The following people have witnessed my commitment to be a donor.
donor signature _____ date _____
witness_____
witness_____
next of kin _____ ph _____

FIGURE 6-5 Organ donation card.

shared with patients when they are admitted to healthcare facilities, or it may be posted in a prominent place in the facility. For medical assistants, every time you interact with a patient, you should keep the Patients' Bill of Rights in mind. For example, you should explain procedures to patients and make sure they understand treatments. Printed information about the facility should contain details about how and where a patient can make a complaint about the care received. Policies and procedures should honor the provisions of the Patients' Bill of Rights that apply in that particular medical facility (Procedure 6-1).

CRITICAL THINKING APPLICATION   **6-8**

Summarize how the medical assistant can apply the Patients' Bill of Rights to everyday practice in the healthcare setting.

Patients' Bill of Rights

I. Information Disclosure
You have the right to receive accurate and easily understood information about your health plan, healthcare professionals, and healthcare facilities. If you speak another language, have a physical or mental disability, or just don't understand something, assistance will be provided so you can make informed healthcare decisions.

II. Choice of Providers and Plans
You have the right to a choice of healthcare providers that is sufficient to provide you with access to appropriate high-quality healthcare.

III. Access to Emergency Services
If you have severe pain, an injury, or a sudden illness that convinces you your health is in serious jeopardy, you have the right to receive screening and stabilization emergency services whenever and wherever needed, without prior authorization or financial penalty.

IV. Participation in Treatment Decisions
You have the right to know all your treatment options and to participate in decisions about your care. Parents, guardians, family members, or other individuals whom you designate can represent you if you cannot make your own decisions.

V. Respect and Nondiscrimination
You have the right to considerate, respectful, and nondiscriminatory care from your doctors, health plan representatives, and other healthcare providers.

VI. Confidentiality of Health Information
You have the right to talk in confidence with healthcare providers and to have your healthcare information protected. You also have the right to review and copy your own medical record and request that your provider amend your record if it is not accurate, **relevant**, or complete.

VII. Complaints and Appeals
You have the right to a fair, fast, and objective review of any complaint you have against your health plan, doctors, hospitals, or other healthcare personnel. This includes complaints about waiting times, operating hours, the conduct of healthcare personnel, and the adequacy of healthcare facilities.

VIII. Consumer Responsibilities
In a healthcare system that protects consumer rights, it is reasonable to expect and encourage consumers to assume reasonable responsibilities. Greater individual involvement by consumers in their care increases the likelihood of achieving the best outcomes and helps support a quality-improvement, cost-conscious environment.

PROCEDURE 6-1   **Apply the Patients' Bill of Rights in Choice of Treatment, Consent for Treatment, and Refusal of Treatment**

Goal: *To ensure that the patient's rights are honored in the daily procedures performed and policies enacted in the ambulatory healthcare setting.*

Case Study: *With a partner, role-play the following case study, which requires the application of the Patients' Bill of Rights to treatment choices, consent for treatment, and refusal of treatment.*

Dr. Patrick recommends that Mr. Tim Shields start taking Lipitor for his elevated blood cholesterol levels. She provides informed consent to Mr. Shields about the risks and benefits of Lipitor, including a decrease in total blood cholesterol levels, an increase in his "good" cholesterol and a decrease in his "bad" cholesterol. She also informs him of the possible side effects of the drug, including liver complications, leg cramps, and photosensitivity (increased risk of sunburn). Mr. Shields states he understands the information but is hesitating to give consent because he has a history of elevated liver enzymes and he works outside most of the year. Mr. Shields opts to refuse the Lipitor treatment. Dr. Patrick tells him that he might be able to lower his blood cholesterol by reducing saturated fat in his diet and exercising (aerobic exercise at least 4 or 5 days a week). Although Mr. Shields admits he may have trouble sticking to those recommendations, he chooses to try diet and exercise rather than medication at this time. Based on your knowledge of the Patients' Bill of Rights, has Dr. Patrick complied with the provider part of the agreement? Does Mr. Shields have the right to refuse the recommended medication? Because he has refused it, is it important to document his refusal of the recommended treatment in his health record? How can the medical assistant help both the provider and the patient in this situation?

PROCEDURE 6-1 *—continued*

EQUIPMENT and SUPPLIES

* Copy of the Patients' Bill of Rights
* Notice of Privacy Practices form

PROCEDURAL STEPS

1. Review the eight points of the Patients' Bill of Rights.
   PURPOSE: To become familiar with the points and content of the document.

2. The patient has the right to receive information about his health plan, professionals, facilities, and personal care. Role-play the information the physician gave Mr. Shields about his treatment choices.
   PURPOSE: To comply with the first article of the Patients' Bill of Rights.

3. Patients have the right to choose a healthcare provider, but their insurance plans may restrict those choices. Role-play the fact that Dr. Patrick's services are covered by Mr. Shields' insurance.
   PURPOSE: To comply with the second article of the Patients' Bill of Rights.

4. The patient has the right to receive emergency treatment and to be informed about the procedures for referral to emergency facilities and for emergency treatment in the office. Role-play a discussion with Mr. Shields about how he can contact the facility or Dr. Patrick if he has a medical emergency.
   PURPOSE: To comply with the third article of the Patients' Bill of Rights.

5. The patient has the right to know all treatment options and to participate in decisions about care. Role-play the information that Dr. Patrick gave Mr. Shields about his care and treatment choices.
   PURPOSE: To comply with the fourth article of the Patients' Bill of Rights.

6. The patient has the right to considerate, respectful, and nondiscriminatory care by all healthcare staff. Role-play respectful care for Mr. Shields.
   PURPOSE: To comply with the fifth article of the Patients' Bill of Rights.

7. Patients have the right to review their records and to expect confidential treatment of their healthcare information. Review methods of enforcing patient confidentiality in the facility. Role-play the patient completing a Notice of Privacy Practices form. Role-play a scenario in which Mr. Shields' girlfriend calls and asks you to tell her what Dr. Patrick suggested for treatment. She is not identified on the patient's Notice of Privacy Practices form. Can you give her that information?
   PURPOSE: To comply with the sixth article of the Patients' Bill of Rights.

8. The patient has the right to a fair and objective review of complaints. During your interaction with Mr. Shields, he complains about how long he had to wait for his appointment and that the receptionist was rude. Role-play how you should manage Mr. Shields' complaints.
   PURPOSE: To comply with the seventh article of the Patients' Bill of Rights.

9. The patient has the responsibility to be involved in care. Mr. Shields has opted to try exercise and dietary changes to manage his elevated cholesterol. Does he have a responsibility to follow through with this care plan? Role-play your interaction with Mr. Shields about his responsibilities.
   PURPOSE: To comply with the eighth article of the Patients' Bill of Rights.

10. Demonstrate sensitivity to patients' rights through empathy, use of therapeutic communications, and respect for individual diversity.
    PURPOSE: To reassure patients so that they know healthcare professionals are sensitive to their needs and desires.

Americans with Disabilities Act

In 1990 the Americans with Disabilities Act (ADA) was signed into law with the intent of eliminating discrimination against individuals with disabilities. The act addressed many areas in which a person might experience discrimination, including telecommunications, housing, public transportation, air carrier access, voting accessibility, education, and rehabilitation.

In 2008, Congress passed the ADA Amendments (ADAA) Act to broaden the definition of disability, which had been narrowed by U.S. Supreme Court decisions. The ADAA Act emphasizes that the definition of disability should be interpreted broadly to include any individual with a physical or mental impairment that substantially limits one or more of his/her major life activities; the individual has a record of such an impairment; or is thought to have an impairment. All individuals meeting this broad definition of disability should be provided the rights associated with the ADAA Act. To clarify the public accommodations requirement, the ADAA Act requires that all new construction and building modifications must be accessible to individuals with disabilities. For existing facilities, barriers that make services inaccessible must be removed if possible. Healthcare facilities fall under the category of public accommodations that must comply with specific requirements related to architectural standards for new and altered buildings; reasonable modifications to policies, practices, and procedures; effective communication with people with hearing, vision, or speech disabilities; and other access requirements.

Individuals with disabilities must be able to enter and exit the facility without difficulty. This means that individuals in wheelchairs need a ramp to enter and exit the building. They also must be able to navigate throughout the facility without major barriers. The law requires that public medical facilities must allow people with disabilities to easily and safely:

* Reach door handles for opening and closing
* Enter and exit buildings
* Move through doors and hallways
* Use drinking fountains, phones, and restrooms
* Move from floor to floor (elevators are required for multilevel buildings)
* Do everything the general public can do in a public place
* Have access to communication devices if they have a problem with vision, hearing, reading, or comprehension.

Genetic Information Nondiscrimination Act

The Genetic Information Nondiscrimination Act (GINA) of 2008 prohibits discrimination in health coverage and employment based on genetic information. Regardless of family history or personal genetic studies, individuals cannot be denied health insurance and employers cannot make job-related decisions based on an individual's genetic history. For example, if genetic testing reveals that an individual carries the gene for Huntington's disease (HD), an inherited neurologic illness that causes involuntary movements, severe emotional disturbance, and cognitive decline and ultimately leads to the need for complete care and an early death, statutes in GINA prevent insurance companies from cancelling coverage and employers from firing the affected individual. Many states already have laws that protect against genetic discrimination in health insurance and employment situations; however, the degree of protection varies widely. All entities subject to GINA must, at minimum, comply with all applicable GINA requirements, and they may also need to comply with more protective state laws.

CRITICAL THINKING APPLICATION   **6-9**
How do the ADAA and GINA acts affect the physical structure of a healthcare facility and the release of patient information to health insurance companies?

Health Insurance Portability and Accountability Act

The original Health Insurance Portability and Accountability Act (HIPAA) was signed into law in 1996. HIPAA sets national standards for how healthcare plans, **healthcare clearinghouses**, and most healthcare providers protect the privacy of a patient's health information. The law has two provisions: Title I (Insurance Reform) and Title II (Administration Simplification). HIPAA's primary purpose was to limit the administrative costs of healthcare, protect patient privacy, and prevent medical fraud and abuse in the Medicare and Medicaid systems.

Notice of Privacy Practices. The HIPAA Privacy Rule requires healthcare providers to distribute a notice that provides a clear, user-friendly explanation of individual personal health information rights. The law requires that patients sign a statement acknowledging they have received the Notice of Privacy Practices (NPP) (Figure 6-6). This document must be filed in the patient's health record. Signing the statement does not mean that patients have agreed to disclosure of health information. The signed statement simply means that the patient has been informed of the privacy practices of that particular facility. Even though patients have the right to refuse to sign the facility's NPP, the practice can use or disclose the patient's health information as long as the Privacy Rule is followed. However, if the patient does refuse to sign the form, that refusal must be documented in the patient's health record. The NPP describes the ways the practice will use and disclose protected health information. It must also explain that the practice will obtain the patient's permission before using individual health records for any other reason. The notice must include information about the patient's right to complain to the Department of Health and Human Services (HHS) and to the healthcare facility if privacy rights are violated. Most healthcare providers give the NPP to patients at their first service encounter (usually at the first appointment). The notice must also be posted in an easy to find location in the facility. If the practice has a website, the privacy notice must be included there.

Title I, which deals with insurance reform, includes several provisions that protect individuals and their insured dependents if they change jobs or lose a job. Individuals can no longer be prevented from getting insurance coverage because of their previous health history. However, most of the regulations in Title I consider the Privacy Rule, which protects all health information that can identify a specific individual and that is held by a covered entity or an entity's business associate. Covered entities must follow strict procedures to keep all patient information confidential. *Covered entities* include health insurance plans that provide or pay the cost of medical care, providers, healthcare facilities, pharmacies, home health agencies, healthcare clearinghouses, and so on.

A *business associate* is a person or an organization that uses or discloses individually identifiable health information in the process of filing insurance claims, billing, or performing business-related functions for the covered entity. Business associates include insurance claim processors, accounting or legal firms whose service includes access to protected health information, utilization review consultants for a hospital, medical transcriptionists, and a healthcare clearinghouse that performs insurance functions. A written agreement or contract must be in place addressing how the business associates will protect patient information before confidential information can be given to the business associate. This includes information about a patient's health history, the patient's diagnosis, the care provided, and payment information.

The Privacy Rule also defines how covered entities use individually identifiable health information, or personal health information (PHI). PHI is also referred to as protected health information, which includes the patient's demographic information (e.g., name, Social Security number, age, gender, and address), medical history, test and laboratory results, insurance information, and other items collected to identify a patient and determine appropriate care. A major purpose of the Privacy Rule is to define and limit the circumstances in which an individual's PHI may be used or disclosed by covered entities. A covered entity can disclose protected health information only if the Privacy Rule permits or requires it or if the patient authorizes its release in writing. PHI must be protected in all forms of communication, including telephone, fax, e-mail, text, and others.

However, according to the Centers for Disease Control and Prevention (CDC), the Privacy Rule allows covered entities to disclose PHI to public health authorities when required by federal, tribal, state, or local laws. This includes state laws for reporting certain diseases or infections, reportable injuries (e.g., gunshot wounds, child abuse), births, or deaths. PHI may also be used to perform public health studies or treatments. This process may include procedures to de-identify PHI through two different methods:

1. Removal of all information that could lead to the identification of the individual, including address, birth or death date, telephone numbers, e-mail addresses, medical record numbers, health plan account numbers, and so on, so that no reasonable method remains of identifying the person.

PATIENT HIPAA ACKNOWLEDGEMENT

I.   **Acknowledgement of Practice's *Notice of Privacy Practices*:**
By subscribing my name below, I acknowledge that I was provided a copy of the Notice of Privacy Practices and that I have read (or had the opportunity to read if I so chose) and understand the Notice of Privacy Practices and agree to its terms.

_____   _____   _____   _____
Name of Patient   Date of Birth   Signature of Patient/Parent/Guardian   Date

II.   **Designation of Certain Relatives, Close Friends and other Caregivers as my Personal Representative:**
I agree that the practice may disclose certain pieces of my health information to a Personal Representative of my choosing, since such person is involved with my healthcare or payment relating to my healthcare. In that case, the Physician Practice will disclose only information that is directly relevant to the person's involvement with my healthcare or payment relating to my health care.

Print Name: _____ Last four digits of SSN or other identifier: _____
Print Name: _____ Last four digits of SSN or other identifier: _____
Print Name: _____ Last four digits of SSN or other identifier: _____

III. **Request to Receive Confidential Communications by Alternative Means:**
As provided by Privacy Rule Section 164.522(b), I hereby request that the Practice make all communications to me by the alternative means that I have listed below.

Home or Cell Telephone Number: **Written Communication Address:**
_____   _____
____ OK to leave message with detailed information   ____ OK to mail to address listed above
____ Leave message with call back numbers only   ____ E-mail me at:
Work Telephone Number: **Email Communication:**
_____   _____
____ OK to leave message with detailed information   ____ OK to text at the number listed above
____ Leave message with call back numbers only   ____ E-mail me at:
Other:
_____

IV.   **The following person(s) are not authorized to receive my Patient Health Information (PHI):**
Print Name: _____ **Print Name:**_____
Print Name: _____ **Print Name:**_____

V.   **The HIPAA Privacy rule requires healthcare providers to take reasonable steps to limit the use** or disclosure of, and requests for PHI. I understand that this accounting will not reflect disclosures that are made in the course of the Practice's ordinary health care activities related to providing patient treatment, obtaining payment for its services or its internal operations. Also, the Practice does not have to account for disclosures for which I have executed an Authorization permitting disclosures of my PHI.

Date of disclosure request	Disclosed to whom: address/email	Description of disclosure	Purpose of disclosure	Dates of service of disclosure	Person completing request	Date completed

1. The above authorizations are voluntary and I may refuse to agree to their terms without affecting any of my rights to receive healthcare at the Practice.

2. These Authorizations may be revoked at any time by notifying the Practice in writing at the Practices mailing address marked to the attention of "HIPAA Compliance Officer."

3. The revocation of this authorization will not have any effect on disclosures occurring prior to the execution of any revocation.

4. I may see and copy the information described in this form, if I ask for it, and I will get a copy of this form after I sign it.

5. This form was completely filled in before I signed it and I acknowledge that all of my questions were answered to my satisfaction, that I fully understand this authorization form, and have received an executed copy.

6. This authorization is valid as of the date I have signed below and shall remain valid until changed or revoked.

Name of Patient (Printed) _____Signature of Patient _____Date _____

FIGURE 6-6 Example of a privacy practices acknowledgment form. (Department of Health and Human Services. *http://www.hhs.gov/ocr/privacy/hipaa.* Accessed June 28, 2015.)

2. Determination by an expert with knowledge of statistical and scientific principles that the risk is very small that the information could be used to identify an individual.

Definitions of HIPAA Terms

Covered transactions: A transaction is covered under the regulations of the Health Insurance Portability and Accountability Act (HIPAA) if it involves the processing of healthcare claims, such as a request for payment by a healthcare provider to a health plan; an inquiry about the patient's benefit plan; a request for authorization for patient referrals; or any electronic communication about a patient's healthcare claim status. The enrollment or termination of health plan coverage is also a covered transaction.

Minimum necessary standard: The minimum necessary standard requires covered entities to take reasonable steps to limit unnecessary access to and disclosure of protected health information (PHI). The amount of personal information released should be the minimum amount necessary to accomplish the intended purpose.

State's preemption of HIPAA regulations: The HIPAA Privacy Rule provides federal privacy protections for PHI with covered entities or business associates. The federal Privacy Rule takes precedence over state laws unless the state law provides greater privacy protections; the information involves reporting of disease or injury, child abuse, birth, death, or data for public health purposes; or, if the reported information is to be used for financial audits.

TPO: HIPAA permits use and disclosure of PHI for treatment, payment, and healthcare operations (TPO). Treatment is the care provided to patients; payment includes billing and collection activities; and healthcare operations include administrative and business activities.

Medical assistants must be aware of the rights of individual patients regarding the use of and access to PHI. These include the following (for complete details you can refer to the CDC site at *www.cdc.gov/mmwr/preview/mmwrhtml/m2e411a1.htm*):

- Individuals have the right to access their own PHI. As long as the healthcare facility maintains the patient's records, individuals can request those records and receive copies of them. The only exceptions are psychotherapy notes and records that have been gathered for legal action. Psychotherapy notes are those recorded by a mental health professional that document conversations that occur during counseling sessions. The only time a provider can disclose psychotherapy notes without the express authorization of the patient is if the information can prevent serious harm to another person. Psychotherapy notes are kept in a separate record from the patient's health record. Covered entities must also release PHI if requested by patients, but only the part of the patient record that is requested, nothing more.
- Individuals can request changes or amendments to PHI and the covered entity must inform individuals if PHI changes have been made.
- Individuals have the right to be notified about the uses and disclosures of their PHI by a covered entity.

- Individuals have the right to know who the covered entity shared their PHI with and a brief description of the information disclosed.
- Individuals have the right to request restrictions on the use of PHI by covered entities.

Limited Data Sets

With the controls established by the Health Insurance Portability and Accountability Act (HIPAA) and the rules that apply to protected health information (PHI), medical researchers must follow specific protection guidelines to use patient data. A *limited data set* is a limited set of identifiable patient information that may be disclosed to an outside party without a patient's authorization. Before the patient data is released, all identifiers must be removed. These include the patient's name and address; any identifiable numbers (e.g., phone, fax, and medical record and account numbers, and also the Social Security number); e-mail addresses; and all biometric identifiers, including full face photos.

The reason for the disclosure may be only for research or public health purposes, and the person receiving the information must sign a data use agreement that must be kept on file. It is important to note that this information is still PHI under HIPAA rules; it is not just de-identified information, and it is still subject to the requirements of the Privacy Rule.

The HIPAA Security Rule (SR) covers the use and transmission of electronic protected health information (ePHI). The Security Rule requires three types of safeguards for protection of ePHI:

1. *Administrative safeguards:* Actions, policies, and procedures put into place to manage and maintain security measures to protect ePHI at both the healthcare facility and at the covered entity.
2. *Physical safeguards:* Actions, policies, and procedures taken to protect a covered entity's electronic information systems from natural and environmental hazards and unauthorized access.
3. *Technical safeguards:* The use of technology to secure PHI and limit its access. Covered entities are required to provide each individual who has access to PHI a Unique User Identification name and/or number that identifies and tracks that individual each time he or she accesses patient PHI.

Covered entities must also have in place procedures for obtaining ePHI during an emergency for healthcare employees with the authority to access the information. For example, if there is a natural disaster, healthcare workers who need individual PHI must know how to access it. The Security Rule recommends automatic log-off to prevent unauthorized access of ePHI. Another recommendation is to have encryption and decryption systems in place to protect ePHI.

Anyone can file a health information privacy complaint through the complaint portal of the Office for Civil Rights at the HHS: *https://ocrportal.hhs.gov/ocr/cp/wizard_cp.jsf*. The complaint also can be filed in writing by mail, fax, or e-mail. The complaint must include the name of the covered entity or business associate involved and describe the act or omission that violated HIPAA regulations. Under HIPAA an entity cannot retaliate against the individual filing a complaint.

Overview of the HIPAA Privacy Rule

- Gives patients control over the use of their health information
- Defines rules that covered entities must follow either to use or to disclose patients' health records
- Establishes national standards for safeguarding protected health information (PHI)
- Establishes limits to the use of PHI and minimizes the chance of its inappropriate disclosure
- Strictly investigates compliance-related issues and holds violators accountable with civil or criminal penalties for violating the privacy of an individual's PHI

Title II of HIPAA details the process of administrative simplification. Standardization of the exchange of healthcare data is one way HIPAA promotes computer-to-computer transactions. Standard 1 reduces the number of forms and methods used in insurance claim processing, including electronic transactions and standard code sets (e.g., diagnosis, procedure, and supply codes). Standard 4 provides for national identifiers for providers, employers, health plans, and patients. Medical professionals who access medical information must use log-in and password systems that prevent unauthorized individuals from accessing PHI. HIPAA standards have increased the use of electronic data interchange. All healthcare organizations that transmit any health information electronically must comply with HIPAA; fines and prison terms can be imposed on those who do not comply with the regulations (Procedure 6-2).

CRITICAL THINKING APPLICATION   6-10

What parts of the HIPAA Privacy Rule will the medical assistant have to practice? Give four examples of how the management of patient information must comply with HIPAA rules.

PROCEDURE 6-2   **Apply HIPAA Rules on Privacy and Release of Information and Report Illegal Activity in the Healthcare Setting**

Goal: *To be aware of HIPAA privacy and release of information rules and apply them in the ambulatory care center.*

Although not specifically required by HIPAA, a medical practice may want to use a routine Patient Consent form that specifies methods by which a patient agrees to let the practice notify the patient of routine treatment, payment, and healthcare operations (TPO) purposes. Figure 1 is an example of a routine consent form.

With a partner, role-play the following case study, which requires the application of the HIPAA privacy and release of information rules.

You recently graduated from a CAAHEP-accredited medical assisting program and just passed the certification exam to earn the CMA (AAMA) credential. You learned a great deal about HIPAA applications in your medical assisting program and are confident that you can apply these regulations in the family practice where you work. A patient comes to the office today very upset because a message about her laboratory test results was left on her home answering machine, even though she specifically requested in her disclosure consent form that messages be left only on her cell phone. Her mother then called the facility and requested information about her diagnosis. How should this situation be handled? The office manager does nothing to correct this error. Can the patient and/or the medical assistant report this infraction of the Privacy Rule to the Office for Civil Rights (OCR)? How can this be done? The patient decides to switch physicians because of her dissatisfaction with the management of her personal health information. Role-play the completion of a release of medical records form.

EQUIPMENT and SUPPLIES

- Computer with Internet access
- Copy of facility's protected health information (PHI) consent form
- Notice of Privacy Practices form
- Authorization for Release of Medical Records form

PROCEDURAL STEPS

1. Consistently review and apply HIPAA regulations that apply to the facility.
   <u>PURPOSE</u>: To ensure compliance with the law.
2. Identify the ramifications of noncompliance with HIPAA's Privacy Rule. Role-play the scenario presented. Did the facility comply with the Privacy Rule and the proper release of information?
   <u>PURPOSE</u>: To ensure full compliance in the medical facility.
3. Routinely apply Privacy Rule regulations to all operations in the medical office. Role-play how the patient's confidentiality and privacy should have been maintained.
   <u>PURPOSE</u>: To be in compliance with HIPAA regulations and to safeguard patients' health information.
4. Follow patient-directed methods of contact when TPO information must be left on an answering machine, mailed, or e-mailed. Role-play the correct way of contacting the patient about personal health information.
   <u>PURPOSE</u>: To be in compliance with HIPAA regulations and to safeguard patient health information.
5. Always follow office policy when performing any action that is covered under HIPAA rules.
   <u>PURPOSE</u>: To ensure full compliance in the medical facility.
6. Report HIPAA violations as you see fit to the appropriate supervisor in the medical facility. Role-play the methods for reporting HIPAA violations in the facility.

PROCEDURE 6-2   —*continued*

PURPOSE: To follow the chain of command in the medical facility and incorporate new regulations or changes into the office policy manual.

7. If appropriate, report HIPAA violations to the Office for Civil Rights at the Department of Health and Human Services (*https://ocrportal.hhs.gov/ocr/cp/wizard_cp.jsf*) or file a complaint in writing by mail, fax, or e-mail. Role-play how you could assist the patient in reporting a privacy violation.

PURPOSE: To ensure full compliance with laws and regulations that affect patient privacy issues.

8. The patient decides to switch providers because of her dissatisfaction with the care provided in the facility. Role-play the completion of an Authorization for Release of Medical Records form.

PURPOSE: To comply with the legal requirements for release of medical information.

9. Demonstrate sensitivity to patients' rights through empathy, use of therapeutic communication, and respect for individual diversity.

PURPOSE: To demonstrate your support of the patient's privacy issues and to act as a patient advocate/navigator in a complicated situation.

Kennedy Family Practice
414 Jacksonia St., Armandale, VA. 26004

Patient Consent for Use and Disclosure
of Protected Health Information

I hereby give my consent for Kennedy Family Practice to use and disclose protected health information (PHI) about me to carry out treatment, payment and health care operations (TPO).

I have the right to review the Notice of Privacy Practices prior to signing this consent. Kennedy Family Practice reserves the right to revise its Notice of Privacy Practices at any time. A revised Notice of Privacy Practices may be obtained by forwarding a written request to Sophia Viero, 414 Jacksonia St., Armandale, VA. 26004.

With this consent, a representative of Kennedy Family Practice may call my home or other alternative location and leave a message on voice mail or in person; may e-mail me on my approved email site; and/or may mail to my home or other alternative location any items that assists the practice in carrying out TPO such as appointment reminders, insurance items and any calls pertaining to my clinical care, including laboratory test results.

I have the right to request that Kennedy Family Practice restrict how it uses or discloses my PHI to carry out TPO. By signing this form, I am consenting to allow Kennedy Family Practice to use and disclose my PHI to carry out TPO.

I may revoke my consent in writing however previous disclosures are considered valid based on my prior consent.

_____
Signature of Patient or Legal Guardian

_____   _____
Print Patient's Name   Date

_____   _____
Patient Approved Telephone number   Patient Approved Email address

1

HITECH Act

The Health Information Technology for Economic and Clinical Health Act (HITECH) was signed into law in 2009 to promote the adoption and meaningful use of health information technology. The law encourages providers and healthcare entities to comply with HIPAA regulations by enacting stiff penalties for noncompliance. According to this law, providers who do not adopt electronic medical records in their practices will be penalized in Medicare payments.

The HITECH Act also requires that patients be notified if there is a breach that exposes their PHI. The HITECH Act allocated funds through the Medicare and Medicaid reimbursement systems as incentives for hospitals and providers who are "meaningful users" of EHR systems.

Under HITECH, mandatory penalties are imposed for "willful neglect" of the HIPAA Privacy Rule. Medical assistants who do not comply with HITECH guidelines can be fined. Civil penalties can be as high as $250,000, with repeated violations costing up to $1.5 million. In addition, HITECH requires the HHS to conduct periodic audits of covered entities and business associates.

Affordable Care Act of 2010

The Affordable Care Act (ACA), signed into law in March, 2010, was designed to provide better health security by enacting comprehensive health insurance reforms that hold insurance companies accountable, lower healthcare costs, guarantee more choice, and enhance the quality of care for all Americans. The law restricts the use of annual limits and bans lifetime limits on healthcare benefits. For example, if a patient has cancer, the insurance company cannot put a limit on the amount of coverage provided to that patient, even if it is a catastrophic amount.

Health insurers and employers are required to provide clear and consistent information about health plans, including an easy-to-understand Summary of Benefits and Coverage and a uniform Glossary of terms commonly used in health insurance coverage. Benefits from the act have taken effect over the last 5 years.

Healthcare Changes Resulting From the Affordable Care Act

2010: Stopped denial of healthcare insurance coverage based on pre-existing conditions; eliminated lifetime limits on insurance coverage; provided free preventive care, including mammograms and colonoscopies; allowed young adults to stay on their parents' plan until they turn 26 years old unless offered insurance at work; allowed states to cover more people on Medicaid.

2011: Made changes to Medicare, including free preventive services and a 50% discount on brand-name drugs; provided older adults with community care transition programs; increased access to services for disabled individuals through Medicaid.

2012: Established Accountable Care Organizations and other programs to help physicians and healthcare providers work together to deliver better care.

2013: Started open enrollment in the Health Insurance Marketplace.

2014: Implemented tax credits for middle- and low-income families that covered a significant portion of the cost of healthcare coverage; expanded the Medicaid program to cover more low-income Americans; prevented insurance companies from charging higher rates because of gender or health status.

2015: Modified provider payments so that practitioners who provide higher-value care receive higher payments.

CRITICAL THINKING APPLICATION   **6-11**

Summarize five details of the Affordable Care Act that have changed access to healthcare for all Americans.

CLOSING COMMENTS

Most patients never entertain the thought of taking legal action against their providers, and a medical assistant should not develop an attitude of skepticism. However, a medical assistant can play an important role in risk management in the healthcare setting.

- Give scrupulous attention to the needs of each patient and do not leave patients alone for long periods. This especially applies to young children and elderly patients. Do not criticize other providers or healthcare facilities. Never give out any information about the patient without the patient's written consent.
- Use discretion in phone and office conversations. One never knows who may be standing nearby. Be aware of tone of voice and attitude during spoken conversations. Communicate office policies and procedures to patients clearly before treatment whenever possible.
- Keep accurate records that show exactly what was done to the patient and when it was done. The medical assistant must never make any promises as to the outcome of treatment. Record cancelled and no-show appointments and record the facts if a patient discontinues treatment.
- Perform only the tasks for which you are trained and keep abreast of new findings and procedures in healthcare. Correctly follow all federal and state regulations.

Patient Education

Perhaps the most important detail to remember with regard to patient education and the law is patience. Many medical forms are complicated, and regulations change often. Patients usually are not as well educated as the medical assistant on matters concerning legal policies and procedures. Often patients become frustrated with the number of changes they have to deal with, and they unintentionally may project this frustration onto the medical assistant. Remain calm and answer questions, offering as much assistance to the patient as possible.

Legal and Ethical Issues

Generally, the law holds that every person is liable for the consequences of his or her own negligence when another person is injured as a result. In some situations, this liability extends to the employer. Providers may be held responsible for the mistakes of those who work in their healthcare facility, and sometimes they must pay damages for the negligent acts of their employees.

Under the doctrine of *respondeat superior,* providers are legally responsible for the acts of their employees when they are acting within the scope of their duties or employment. Providers also are responsible for the acts of assistants who are not their own employees if they commit acts of negligence in the presence of the provider while under the provider's immediate supervision. When providers practice as partners, they are liable not only for their own acts and those of their partners, but also for the negligent acts of any agent or employee of the partnership.

Medical assistants guilty of negligence are liable for their own actions, but the injured party generally sues the provider because the chances of collecting damages are better. However, even assistants with no money can be held liable for any negligent action, and liens can be placed on their property in anticipation of its sale and potential profit. This fact illustrates the continuing importance of exercising extreme care in performing all duties accurately and professionally in the healthcare facility.

Professional Behaviors

As professionals, medical assistants are responsible for their own actions and must adhere to the laws that guide healthcare practice. Medical assistants typically make the first appointment for new patients. In doing so, they initiate an unspoken contract between a new patient and the providers in the healthcare facility. Therefore, office policy must be strictly followed when establishing new patients. Most facilities want basic demographic information before accepting the patient into the practice, including insurance information and/or proof of the individual's ability to pay. As an agent of the provider, medical assistants are the first employee to interact with patients and must always present themselves as knowledgeable and caring individuals.

Medical assistants may work for a facility that occasionally uses temporary staff. The Latin term *locum tenens* means "to hold a place." *Locum tenens* physicians, nurse practitioners, and physician assistants are examples of professional staff that may be employed by a facility to temporarily fill open positions. The medical assistant is responsible for providing assistance to these individuals so that quality patient care is delivered seamlessly and professionally.

SUMMARY OF SCENARIO

Barbara is enthusiastic about her new job and duties. She is confident about appearing in court to represent Dr. Patrick and discuss the contents of the medical record of the patient suing his surgeon. Dr. Patrick is not a party to the lawsuit but has a provider-patient relationship with the patient just the same. An offer existed, as did the acceptance of that offer. The relationship was based on legal subject matter, and the provider and the patient had the legal capacity to enter into a contract. Consideration also existed, because the patient paid for services and the provider treated the patient. Both received something of value. Samantha and Lynda would like to accompany Barbara to the court proceedings to watch and learn.

Even if a patient does not pay for treatment, a contract still exists. The provider may elect to terminate the provider-patient relationship if the patient does not pay, but the trust that the patient places in the provider can be considered a thing of value.

Patients should understand their role in treatment and their responsibilities to the provider. Often this information is communicated in the patient policy brochure, or it may be discussed orally with the patient. Providers are not required to accept all patients; for instance, not all providers deliver babies. Some providers do not treat patients with workers' compensation claims. Providers have the right to see the types of patients they want to and are competent to treat, but they should never discriminate on the basis of race, gender, or any other protected status.

A provider may not always be correct in his or her diagnoses, but this does not mean that the provider has committed malpractice. However, if expert witnesses feel that the provider should have made a different diagnosis based on the case, the provider might be held liable for negligence. If an employee has information about a case that is damaging to the provider, he or she is ethically obligated to report the information, but rarely legally liable to speak up unless a law has been broken.

Medical assistants can help the provider comply with legal regulations in the office by making sure that they understand the policies and procedures required by the facility. Rules are made to ensure compliance so that both patients and employees are kept safe and risks in the office are kept to a minimum. Patient confidentiality is one of the most important rules to remember. New graduates can learn about the laws that affect medical facilities in their area by discussing them with their supervisors and by attending seminars and training. Much information is available on the Internet regarding legal issues.

Trust is a critical factor in avoiding medical professional liability lawsuits. When the patient trusts the provider, he or she is much more likely to work through issues that otherwise might lead to legal action. Keeping accurate patient records and documenting all information required helps prove that the provider adequately cared for the patient. Clearly, legible handwriting is vital in this process.

The medical assistant may find that the provider is not in compliance with certain rules and regulations. Never jump to conclusions and assume that the provider has no intention of complying. There are various reasons for noncompliance, and any issues should be brought to the attention of the office manager or the provider for clarification. It is the medical assistant's responsibility to question noncompliance and make every effort to bring the facility into compliance with the cooperation of supervisors, co-workers, and providers. As a team, medical professionals can remain in compliance and deliver excellent care to all patients.

SUMMARY OF LEARNING OBJECTIVES

1. **Define, spell, and pronounce the terms listed in the vocabulary.**
   Spelling and pronouncing medical terms correctly reinforce the medical assistant's credibility. Knowing the definitions of these terms promotes confidence in communication with patients and co-workers.

2. **Compare criminal and civil law as they apply to the practicing medical assistant; also discuss contract law.**
   Criminal law governs violations of the law punishable as offenses against the state or the federal government. A medical assistant can be prosecuted for criminal acts such as assault and battery, fraud, and abuse. Misdemeanors are minor crimes and include simple assault and battery or drunk driving without injury to others. If convicted of a misdemeanor, individuals may spend up to a year in jail. Felonies are major crimes that can result in imprisonment for one or more years or even death for more serious crimes. An individual convicted of a felony loses many rights including the ability to work in healthcare. Civil law is concerned with acts that are not criminal but involve relationships between individuals and other individuals, groups, or government agencies. Tort law is the division of civil law that deals with medical professional liability. Contract law involves contracts and a contract is an agreement that creates an obligation.

3. **Summarize the anatomy of a medical professional liability lawsuit and explain the four essential elements of a valid contract.**
   Four elements are essential to a valid legal contract: (1) Mutual understanding and agreement; (2) the contract must involve legal subject matter; (3) the parties to the contract must be legally competent; and (4) some type of consideration must be involved.

   A medical assistant may be involved in preparing materials for court including completing interrogatories and scheduling or participating in depositions. Discovery is the pretrial disclosure of pertinent facts or documents by one or both parties to a legal action or proceeding. Attorneys help prepare the defense of the provider and the staff.

4. **Discuss the various parts of a medical professional liability lawsuit.**
   Medical professional liability suits are far from rare, and they involve interrogatories, depositions, and subpoenas. Knowing the role of everyone inside the courtroom is imperative, and, in a criminal case, the burden of proof must prove guilt beyond any reasonable doubt. The final decision of the trial court is reflected in the judgment, signed by the judge.

5. **Discuss the advantages of mediation and arbitration.**
   Mediation and arbitration are two examples of Alternative Dispute Resolutions that share the goal of avoiding litigation in court. In mediation a neutral third party, the mediator, helps those involved in a dispute solve their own problems. Arbitration involves the use of a third party familiar with law or the issues at hand. The arbitrator renders a legally binding decision based on very specific rules. Many providers and attorneys see mediation and arbitration as a way to solve the crisis of litigation in this country.

6. **Do the following related to medical liability and negligence:**
   • **Differentiate malfeasance, misfeasance, and nonfeasance.**
     Malfeasance, misfeasance, and nonfeasance are types of negligence often involved in medical professional liability cases. *Malfeasance* is performing an act that is completely wrong or unlawful. *Misfeasance*, comparable to a mistake, is the improper performance of a lawful act. *Nonfeasance* is the failure to perform some act that should have been performed.
   • **Explain the four Ds of negligence.**
     The four Ds of negligence are (1) the duty to care for the patient; (2) dereliction, or failure to perform that duty; (3) proof that this failure was the direct cause of a patient's injury; and (4) proof that the patient suffered damages from the injury.
   • **Define the types of damages.**
     Nominal damages are token compensations for invasion of a legal right. Punitive damages are designed to punish an offender and discourage repetition of an act. Compensatory damages are designed to compensate for the actual damages suffered, whereas general damages include compensation for pain and suffering, loss of a body member, disfigurement, and other similar losses. Special damages can include such losses as earnings or travel costs.

7. **Discuss risk management and describe liability, malpractice, and personal injury insurances, including the importance of informed consent.**
   Risk management practices are a combination of different approaches in the healthcare facility that reduces the likelihood that either an individual healthcare professional or the healthcare facility will be sued.

   General liability insurance protects the healthcare facility if there is an accident in the facility that causes bodily injury or property damage. Medical malpractice insurance protects the provider and/or healthcare facility if there is a judgment against them for medical negligence, malfeasance, or general malpractice. Personal injury insurance covers both bodily harm and nonphysical, noneconomic harm.

   Informed consent gives the patient a full understanding of the condition that has been diagnosed, including what could happen if the patient undergoes treatment, refuses treatment, or delays treatment. It provides the patient with information on the advantages and risks of a medical procedure and alternative treatments the patient may want to consider. Informed consent places control in the hands of the patient, who is given the opportunity to make the decisions about his or her healthcare.

8. **Define statutes of limitation and confidentiality.**
   A statute of limitations is a period after which a lawsuit cannot be filed. Confidentiality is one of the most sacred trusts the patient places in the hands of the provider and staff. It is of the utmost importance to patients receiving treatment for mental health issues, sexually transmitted infections, sexual assault, and any type of abuse.

9. Discuss compliance reporting, the Patient Self-Determination Act, the Uniform Anatomical Gift Act, and the Patients' Bill of Rights.

The provider is charged with safeguarding patient confidences with the constraints of the law, but according to state laws, which vary somewhat across the nation, certain disclosures must be made, like births and deaths, sexually transmitted diseases, and child abuse.

The Patient Self-Determination Act of 1990 brought the term "advance directives" to the forefront of medical care. This act requires healthcare facilities to develop and maintain written procedures that ensure that all adult patients receive information about advance directives and medical durable powers of attorney.

The Uniform Anatomical Gift Act was developed to make sure that all states have the same laws regarding organ donation.

The Patients' Bill of Rights was designed to (1) strengthen consumer confidence by ensuring that the healthcare system is fair and responsive to consumers' needs; (2) provide consumers with credible and effective mechanisms to address their concerns; (3) encourage consumers to take an active role in improving and ensuring their health; (4) affirm the importance of a strong relationship between patients and their healthcare professionals; and (5) affirm the critical role consumers play in safeguarding their health by establishing rights and responsibilities for all participants in improving patients' health.

10. Describe the important features of the ADAA and GINA Acts.

The ADAA Act broadens the definition of disability and emphasizes that the definition of disability should be interpreted broadly to include any individual with a physical or mental impairment that substantially limits one or more of his/her major life activities, the individual has a record of such an impairment, or is thought to have an impairment. GINA is a federal law that prohibits discrimination in health coverage and employment based on genetic information. Regardless of family history or personal genetic studies, individuals cannot be denied health insurance and employers cannot make job-related decisions based on individual genetic history.

11. Explain the components of the Health Insurance Portability and Accountability Act (HIPAA).

HIPAA is a federal law that sets national standards for how healthcare plans, healthcare clearinghouses, and most healthcare providers protect the privacy of a patient's health information. The law has two provisions: Title I (Insurance Reform) and Title II (Administration Simplification). HIPAA's primary purpose was to limit the administrative costs of healthcare, protect patient privacy, and prevent medical fraud and abuse in the Medicare and Medicaid systems.

12. Identify HITECH and its impact on electronic transmission of patient records.

The Health Information Technology for Economic and Clinical Health Act (HITECH) was signed into law in 2009 to promote the adoption and meaningful use of health information technology. Providers who do not adopt electronic medical records in their practices will be penalized in Medicare payments. The HITECH Act also requires that patients be notified if there is a breach that exposes their PHI. The HITECH Act allocated funds through the Medicare and Medicaid reimbursement systems as incentives for hospitals and providers who are "meaningful users" of EHR systems.

13. Summarize the primary features of the Affordable Care Act.

The Affordable Care Act, signed into law in March of 2010, was designed to provide better health security by enacting comprehensive health insurance reforms that hold insurance companies accountable, lower healthcare costs, guarantee more choice, and enhance the quality of care for all Americans. The law restricts the use of annual limits and bans lifetime limits on healthcare benefits. Health insurers and employers are required to provide clear and consistent information about health plans, including an easy-to-understand summary of benefits and coverage and a uniform glossary of terms commonly used in health insurance coverage. Benefits from the Act have taken effect over the last 5 years.

CONNECTIONS

Study Guide Connection: Go to the Chapter 6 Study Guide. Read and complete the activities.

evolve Evolve Connection: Go to the Chapter 6 link at *evolve.elsevier.com/kinn* to complete the Chapter Review Quiz. Check out the other resources listed for this chapter to make the most of what you have learned from Medicine and Law.

7

MEDICINE AND ETHICS

Monica Johnson has been employed for 6 months as a medical assistant in a primary care practice. She works as the clinical medical assistant for Dr. Richard Wray. One of Dr. Wray's patients, Anna Walsh, recently adopted a baby after 8 years of trying to conceive a child. The baby, Delaney Gracelia, was born to a single mother, Susan, who participated in an open adoption in which she and the Walshes met and got to know each other during her pregnancy. Susan dated the baby's father for about 6 months before discovering that she was pregnant, and they are no longer dating. Susan wanted to make a good decision for the baby and decided to place her for adoption. Dr. Wray performed some genetic testing on Delaney, and the adoptive parents were involved throughout the pregnancy, even meeting Delaney's birth mother for physician appointments from time to time. Monica observed both Susan and the Walshes and saw many benefits from the arrangement, noticing that everyone was primarily concerned with Delaney and her happiness and well-being. However, some periods were difficult for both sides. This prompted Monica to give some thought to her own feelings and ideas about many different ethical situations and issues and how she would react in the face of having to make ethical decisions.

While studying this chapter, think about the following questions:

- How can personal values affect an ethical relationship with diverse patients?
- How can the medical assistant separate her personal beliefs from her professional behaviors?
- Should the medical assistant discuss personal beliefs about ethical situations with patients?

LEARNING OBJECTIVES

1. Define, spell, and pronounce the terms listed in the vocabulary.
2. Do the following related to medicine and ethics:
   - Define ethics and morals.
   - Identify the effect of personal morals and values on professional performance.
   - Differentiate between personal and professional ethics.
   - Recognize the effect personal ethics and morals have on the delivery of healthcare.
   - Develop a plan for separation of personal and professional ethics.
   - Demonstrate appropriate responses to ethical issues.
3. Discuss the history of ethics in medicine.
4. Do the following related to making ethical decisions:
   - List and define three general elements of ethics.
   - List and define the four types of ethical problems.
   - Discuss the five-step process used to make an ethical decision.
5. Summarize the ethical opinions reached by the Council on Ethical and Judicial Affairs (CEJA).
6. Describe the process of compliance reporting of conflicts of interest.

VOCABULARY

advocate (ad'-vuh-kat) A person who pleads the cause of another; one who defends or maintains a cause or proposal.

procurement (pro-kuhr'-ment) The act of getting possession of, obtaining, or acquiring; in medicine, this term relates to obtaining organs for transplant.

public domain A classification of information that indicates the information is open for public review; information or technology that is not protected by a patent or copyright and is available to the public for use without charge.

ramifications (ra-muh-fuh-ka'-shuns) Consequences produced by a cause or following from a set of conditions.

reparations (reh-puh-ra'-shuns) Acts of atonement for a wrong or injury.

sociologic Oriented or directed toward social needs and problems.

upcoding A fraudulent practice in which provider services are billed for higher procedural codes than were actually performed, resulting in a higher payment.

veracity (vuh-ra'-suh-te) A devotion to or conformity with the truth.

Ethics can be defined as the thoughts, judgments, and actions on issues that have implications of moral right and wrong. Ethics guides society's moral principles, which govern a person's or group's behavior. Various beliefs exist about what is and is not ethical in everyday life and in the medical profession. The decisions that people make based on ethical beliefs can quite possibly alter the course of human existence.

Ethics are different from legal issues mainly because something that is legal is not necessarily ethical. Ethics is considered a higher authority than legality. The American Medical Association's Council on Ethical and Judicial Affairs (CEJA) clarifies the relationship between law and ethics as follows: "Ethical values and legal principles are usually closely related, but ethical obligations typically exceed legal duties." In some cases, the law mandates unethical conduct. In general, when healthcare professionals believe a law is unjust, they should work to change the law. In exceptional circumstances of unjust laws, ethical responsibilities should supersede legal obligations. Ethics and morals are more closely related, although ethics often are attributed to professional interactions, whereas morals and values are usually personal in nature. An individual's morals are defined as his or her standards for behavior or beliefs about what is right and what is wrong. Individual morals are closely tied with value systems and help us judge others and conflict situations as being either acceptable or unacceptable. Medical assistants not only must have a strong knowledge base about ethical issues they might face throughout their careers, they also must come to terms with some of the deeply rooted morals and value systems that have been a part of their lives since youth.

To be able to treat all people ethically, you first must examine your own values, beliefs, and actions; you cannot treat all patients with care and respect until you first recognize and evaluate your personal biases. We think and act a certain way for many reasons. The first step in understanding the process is to evaluate your individual value system. Why do you have certain attitudes or beliefs about the worth of individuals or things?

Many different factors influence the development of a value system. Value systems begin as learned beliefs and behaviors. Families and cultural influences shape the way we respond to a diverse society. Other factors that influence reactions include socioeconomic and educational backgrounds. To develop ethical behaviors and therapeutic relationships, you first must recognize your own value system to determine whether it could affect how you interact or treat others. Preconceived ideas about people because of their race, religion, income level, ethnic origin, sexual orientation, or gender can act as barriers to the development of ethical behaviors. You will not be able to provide nonjudgmental, ethical treatment to your patients unless you can connect with them in some way. Personal biases or prejudices are monumental barriers to the development of ethical behaviors.

CRITICAL THINKING APPLICATION   **7-2**

Honestly evaluate your personal biases. What do you find unacceptable in people? Do you prejudge an individual based on his or her affiliation with a particular group or because of a certain lifestyle decision? Do these biases create barriers to ethical care? If so, how can you get beyond these barriers?

Personal, professional, and organizational ethics all contribute to the way the medical assistant approaches the patient. For instance, if a medical assistant personally believes that each child should receive immunizations, he or she must understand that, professionally, this decision must be left to the child's caregivers. The medical assistant must not force his or her personal ethical beliefs on the patient or family members. Personal and professional ethics must be kept separate so that patients can make their own decisions about their healthcare (Procedure 7-1). Professional organizations offer ethical guidelines; for example, each medical assistant is required to maintain patient confidentiality. This practice reflects the ethical belief that all patients have the right to confidentiality of their information and records (Procedure 7-2).

CRITICAL THINKING APPLICATION   **7-1**

What do you value most in life? What is important to you? What influences you to act in a certain way? Make a list of five things you value the most and share them with the class. Try to determine why you feel so strongly about those particular things.

| PROCEDURE 7-1 | Develop a Plan for Separating Personal and Professional Ethics: Recognize the Impact Personal Ethics and Morals Have on the Delivery of Healthcare |

Goal: *To determine one's ethical and moral views before having to confront an ethical decision.*

Using the following case studies, role-play with your partner issues of personal and professional ethical behavior and how personal ethics and morals can affect the delivery of healthcare.

(1) While you are gathering information from a new patient, he informs you he is HIV positive. Do you think this will affect your therapeutic relationship?

(2) You are responsible for performing an in-depth diabetic education intervention with an individual with very poor hygiene. Will this cause a problem with your professional manner?

(3) You are told by your office manager that an inmate of the county prison is scheduled for an appointment this afternoon. Do you think his status will affect your reaction to this patient?

(4) You are attempting to gather insurance information from a 20-year-old patient who brought her two young children with her to the office today. She is a single mother who is pregnant with her third child and receives public assistance. What do you think? Will you have difficulty being empathetic?

PROCEDURE 7-1   —continued

EQUIPMENT and SUPPLIES

- Pen and paper
- Copy of the AAMA's Medical Assisting Code of Ethics

PROCEDURAL STEPS

1. Set aside time to study and consider the ethical issues outlined in this chapter.
   PURPOSE: To make any ethical decision, research the subject and give thought to each issue so that the decision is credible.

2. For each issue, make notes on your personal thoughts, paying particular attention to whether you agree with the AAMA's Medical Assisting Code of Ethics.
   PURPOSE: To examine the impact that personal ethics and morals may have on your practice.

3. Look at each issue as a separate ethical problem and apply the ethical decision-making process to each.
   PURPOSE: To consider each issue in an organized way.

4. Gather relevant information by researching each problem.
   PURPOSE: To make sure that you consider all facts in determining your personal views about each issue.

5. Identify the type of ethical problem each issue represents.
   PURPOSE: By accumulating information about the issue and matching it with an ethical problem, you will be able to apply knowledge and determine your personal views more easily.

6. Determine your personal view on each issue.
   PURPOSE: To recognize how personal ethics and morals can affect the delivery of quality patient care.

7. Determine the ethical approach to use.
   PURPOSE: Knowing the type of problem that each ethical issue represents helps you determine the best approach to each decision.

8. Explore practical alternatives.
   PURPOSE: Considering all practical alternatives helps you make the best ethical decisions.

9. Decide your personal stand on each issue.
   PURPOSE: By gathering information, identifying the problem and the best ethical approach to use, and then considering all practical alternatives, you can arrive at a sound ethical decision about your personal stand on each issue.

10. Determine the position of the Medical Assisting Code of Ethics on each issue.
    PURPOSE: By determining your personal stance and learning the professional position on each ethical issue, you will not be faced with having to make a decision on the spot.

11. Continue the process until each ethical issue has been addressed.

12. Refrain from inflicting personal ethical views on any patient.
    PURPOSE: To ensure that patients determine their own ethical views and make medical decisions based on their own views rather than those of the medical staff.

13. Interact with patients in a professional way, regardless of their or your ethical views.
    PURPOSE: All patients must be treated in a professional way, regardless of their ethical views or healthcare choices.

14. Re-evaluate personal ethical views periodically and apply new knowledge and experience to determine whether ethical views have changed.
    PURPOSE: To be open to change based on experience in the medical field and new discoveries or technology. Healthcare is an ever-changing profession; therefore, you must develop the attitude of being a lifelong learner. New trends or experiences may change your position on ethical issues.

PROCEDURE 7-2   Respond to Issues of Confidentiality

Goal: *To ensure that medical assistants treat all information on patient care as completely confidential.*

EQUIPMENT and SUPPLIES

- Patient's health record
- Copy of the Medical Assisting Code of Ethics
- Copy of the Medical Assisting Creed
- Copy of the Oath of Hippocrates (see the chapter, The Medical Assistant and the Healthcare Team)
- Copy of HIPAA guidelines (see the chapter, Medicine and Law)
- Notepad and pen
  Using the following case studies, role-play issues of patient confidentiality with your partner.
  (1) You work for a local OB/GYN. Your best friend tells you her brother's wife is having an affair, and your friend wants you to find out if she

is pregnant. You saw the woman in the office today and know that her pregnancy test was positive. How would you manage this situation?

(2) An attorney calls the office today and requests you send copies of a patient's health records to her office ASAP for a liability case. The patient has not signed a release form, but the attorney tells you she doesn't need one because this is a legal matter. What would you do?

(3) The mother of an 18-year-old patient calls and asks you to release her son's laboratory test results. The son lives with her and is covered by her medical insurance. Does the mother have the right to this information?

PROCEDURE 7-2   *—continued*

PROCEDURAL STEPS

1. Read through each document, paying particular attention to the references to confidentiality.
   PURPOSE: To gain insight into documents that stress confidentiality as a critical aspect of the healthcare process, to reinforce the importance of patient confidentiality, and to understand the roots of ethical behavior.
2. Select a student with whom to role-play as a patient. The patient should present with a situation or an illness he or she wants to keep confidential.
   PURPOSE: Apply ethical behaviors, including honesty and integrity, in medical assisting practice.
3. Identify each patient by name and date of birth.
4. Take the patient to a private exam room or other area suitable for a private conversation and attend to his or her needs and questions.
   PURPOSE: To restrict the conversation to medical personnel and the patient.
5. Listen carefully to what the patient says, taking notes if necessary, asking clarifying questions, and using restatement to clear up any misunderstandings.
   PURPOSE: To demonstrate to patients an interest in what they say and to make sure all their concerns are addressed and answered.

6. Assure the patient that his or her concerns and health issues are confidential.
   PURPOSE: To put the patient at ease, so that he or she feels comfortable in sharing each detail of the condition or of the concerns that need to be discussed.
7. Explain to the patient that information shared with you cannot be kept from the provider.
   PURPOSE: To make sure you will not be asked to withhold information from the provider.
8. Discuss the information with the practitioner or ask the provider to speak personally with the patient, depending on which is appropriate to the circumstances.
   PURPOSE: To act only with authorization from the provider.
9. Instruct the patient according to the provider's orders, if necessary.
10. Document the patient's concerns, information given by the patient, and the provider's orders in the health record.
    PURPOSE: To provide a record of the conversation and the circumstances of the patient's concerns and the provider's plan for resolution.
11. Do not share information about the patient with anyone not directly related to the patient's care.
    PURPOSE: To ensure complete patient confidentiality.

HISTORY OF ETHICS IN MEDICINE

From earliest recorded history, humans have pondered ethics, or the judgment of right and wrong. Ethics should not be confused with etiquette. Etiquette refers to courtesy, customs, and manners, whereas ethics explores the moral right or wrong of an issue. It is not surprising that for centuries, the field of medicine has set for itself a rigid standard of ethical conduct toward patients and professional colleagues.

The earliest written code of ethical conduct for medical practice was devised in approximately 2250 BC by the Babylonians. It was called the *Code of Hammurabi.* It elaborated on the conduct expected of a physician and even set the fees a physician could charge. The code was quite lengthy and detailed, which is probably the reason it did not survive the ages. In approximately 400 BC, Hippocrates developed a brief statement of principles that remains an inspiration to the physicians of today. The most significant contribution to medical ethics after Hippocrates was made by Thomas Percival, an English physician, philosopher, and writer. In 1803 he published his Code of Medical Ethics. Percival was very concerned about **sociologic** matters and took great interest in the study of ethical concepts as they related to the medical profession.

In 1846, as the American Medical Association (AMA) was being organized in New York City, medical education and medical ethics already were considered important aspects of the profession. At the first annual AMA meeting in 1847, a Code of Ethics was formulated and adopted. It specifically acknowledged Percival's code as its foundation, and this document became a part of the fundamental standards of the AMA and its components. Even today, sections of the AMA Code of Ethics stem from Percival's writings.

The medical assisting profession has followed suit. The American Association of Medical Assistants (AAMA) has published the Medical Assisting Code of Ethics, which identifies ethical and moral principles as they relate to the practice of medical assisting (Figure 7-1).

Medical Assisting Code of Ethics

Members of AAMA dedicated to the conscientious pursuit of their profession, and thus desiring to merit the high regard of the entire medical profession and the respect of the general public which they serve, do pledge themselves to strive always to:

1. Render service with full respect for the dignity of humanity.

2. Respect confidential information obtained through employment unless legally authorized or required by responsible performance of duty to divulge such information.

3. Uphold the honor and high principles of the profession and accept its disciplines.

4. Seek to continually improve the knowledge and skills of medical assistants for the benefit of patients and professional colleagues.

5. Participate in additional service activities aimed toward improving the health and well-being of the community.

FIGURE 7-1 Medical Assisting Code of Ethics of the AAMA. (http://www.aama-ntl.org/about/overview#.VY2at_m6e7Q. Accessed 6/26/2015.)

Medical assistants are agents of the physicians who employ them and therefore should follow a code of ethics similar to that established by the AMA. Medical assistants facing ethical issues, such as managing confidential patient information, can use the AAMA code of ethics as a guide to help them make ethical decisions.

The AAMA has also written a Medical Assisting Creed, which can be used as a guideline for medical assistants facing complex ethical and moral issues in the course of their work. The Medical Assisting Creed supports the code of ethics by asking members to abide by ethical statements of belief. These include:

- I believe in the principles and purposes of the profession of medical assisting.
- I endeavor to be more effective.
- I aspire to render greater service.
- I protect the confidence entrusted to me.
- I am dedicated to the care and well-being of all people.
- I am loyal to my employer.
- I am true to the ethics of my profession.
- I am strengthened by compassion, courage, and faith.

To promote professionalism and ethical behaviors in those seeking the AAMA certification, individuals who are applying to or who have earned the CMA (AAMA) credential are expected to follow a Code of Conduct for CMAs (AAMA), which can be found on the AAMA website: *www.aama-ntl.org*. The following are provisions of the code:

- Act with integrity and adhere to the highest standards for personal and professional conduct.
- Accept responsibility for your actions.
- Continually seek to enhance your professional capabilities.
- Practice with fairness and honesty.
- Abide by all federal, state, and local laws and regulations.
- Encourage other medical assistants to act in a professional manner consistent with the certification standards and responsibilities of your profession.

CRITICAL THINKING APPLICATION   **7-3**

As you can see, a number of documents support ethical decision making and behaviors in those pursuing a career in medical assisting. How can you apply these statutes to your practice? Consider the following scenarios and discuss with the class how they can be ethically managed.

1. You discover a co-worker taking a controlled substance from the locked medicine cabinet. She begs you not to report her and promises never to do it again. She tells you she is having horrible back pain and has to continue to work to support her two young children.
2. You are working in the practice's billing department and realize that one of the providers is routinely **upcoding** office visits and patient procedures. There is no documentation in patient health records to support these coding charges.

MAKING ETHICAL DECISIONS

An understanding of a few of the elements of ethics, the different types of ethical problems, and how an ethical decision is made can help when entry-level medical assistants are faced with complicated issues in the workplace. This section enables the medical assistant to recognize the types of ethical problems that might arise in the ambulatory care center and provides a pattern to follow in making an ethical decision.

Elements of Ethics

Dr. Ruth Purtilo is an authority on ethics in medicine and has written a book on the subject, *Ethical Dimensions in the Health Professions*. She presents three general elements of ethics: duties, rights, and character traits. A *duty* is an obligation a person has or perceives himself or herself to have. For example, a daughter may feel the obligation to care for her elderly parents, or a husband who has hurt his spouse may feel an obligation to somehow make up for his act.

Purtilo mentions several types of duties related to the medical profession. *Nonmaleficence* is a principle of bioethics that states that healthcare professionals have an obligation not to inflict harm intentionally. *Beneficence* is a moral obligation to act for the benefit of others. In the case of healthcare professionals, the principle of beneficence asserts that those who pursue a profession in healthcare have an obligation to help others and that it furthers their interests to do so. *Fidelity* is the duty to follow through with obligations and keep promises, and **veracity** is the duty to tell the truth. In the practice of medical ethics, *justice* is the fair distribution of benefits to those who have legitimate claims on them. When a person has wronged another, he or she has a duty to make **reparations**, or right the wrong. Last, a person should feel grateful if he or she is a beneficiary of someone else's goodness; this also is a type of duty.

Rights are defined as claims made on society, a group, or an individual. The Bill of Rights appended to the U.S. Constitution guarantees certain liberties that we enjoy as American citizens. For instance, Americans have the "right" to vote, regardless of whether they choose to exercise that right. A *right* applies to all people within a group, without prejudice.

Purtilo defines *character traits* as a tendency to act a certain way. A person who values honesty as an important character trait usually can be trusted to speak the truth. One who feels comfortable with taking small items from work for use at home may not be able to resist an opportunity to take something more valuable. Character traits certainly do not always indicate how a person will react in all situations. No human being is perfect, and we sometimes are unpredictable. Stress also can interfere with our normal reactions, and other factors, such as depression or anger, influence how we act. The phrase that someone is acting "out of character" usually means that the person is deviating from his or her normal behavior patterns.

With an understanding of these basic elements of ethics, we have a good foundation to help us look more objectively at ethical problems and solve them to the best of our ability.

Types of Ethical Problems

Purtilo presents four basic types of ethical problems:

- Ethical distress
- Ethical dilemmas
- Dilemmas of justice
- Locus of authority issues

Ethical distress is a problem in which a certain course of action is indicated, but some type of problem or barrier prevents that action. A professional in ethical distress knows the right thing to do but for some reason cannot do it.

An *ethical dilemma* is a situation in which an individual must make a decision about two or more acceptable choices; however, choosing one course of action means that the person cannot follow the other course of action. A choice must be made, and something of value may be lost if a second choice is eliminated. This could be viewed as the saying, "being caught between a rock and a hard place," when the effect of a choice made may be greater than is immediately obvious.

The third type of ethical problem is the *dilemma of justice.* This problem focuses on the fair distribution of benefits to those who are entitled to them. Choices must be made about who receives these benefits and in what proportion. Examples include organ donation and distribution of scarce or costly medications.

In *locus of authority issues,* two or more authority figures have their own ideas about how a situation should be handled, but only one of those authorities can prevail. If one physician feels that a patient should have surgery and another does not, how does the patient decide?

Recognizing the type of ethical problem is not always easy. Sometimes an issue is a mixture of one or more types of ethical problems. When possible, it is wise to take time to weigh the courses of action before making an important decision. Unfortunately, with the fast pace of the medical profession, this is not always possible. Some decisions must be made in a split second; therefore, having a thorough grasp of ethical decision making before the need arises is important.

The Ethical Decision-Making Process

Purtilo proposes a five-step process for ethical decision making:
1. Gathering relevant information
2. Identifying the type of ethical problem
3. Determining the ethical approach to use
4. Exploring the practical alternatives
5. Completing the action

To gather information, a medical professional should ask questions, review records, talk to the patient and other professionals, and search for other data so that the entire situation is available for review. Once the information has been gathered, the medical professional must decide which ethical problem or problems are presented. In determining the ethical approach to use, we must consider the duties, rights, and character traits of all the individuals involved, paying close attention to the **ramifications** of all possible decisions. All of the alternatives must be considered and evaluated, after which an action should be taken.

Although taking time to give these areas some thought is best, it may not be possible. Therefore, those entering the medical profession should take stock of their core beliefs. Scan the newspapers and search professional journals for ethical situations, think about the facts, then decide how you would react to each one. This is excellent preparation for the day you are faced with making a quick ethical decision.

CRITICAL THINKING APPLICATION   **7-4**
- What are the ramifications of an open adoption, such as occurred with Delaney? What problems might occur during the first year of her life?
- How might these problems be prevented?
- What are the positive aspects of the adoption?

THE COUNCIL ON ETHICAL AND JUDICIAL AFFAIRS

The Council on Ethical and Judicial Affairs (CEJA) develops ethics policy for the AMA by analyzing and addressing ethical issues that confront physicians and the medical profession. The recommendations from the council ultimately are used to update the AMA's Code of Medical Ethics, which can be found at *http://www. ama-assn.org/ama/pub/physician-resources/medical-ethics/code-medical-ethics.page*. The part of the code that is perhaps most pertinent to medical assistants is the section that deals with allied health professions. An excerpt follows:

> When physicians practice medicine with allied health professionals, they should be guided by the following principles:
> 1. It is ethical for a physician to employ allied health professionals, as long as they are trained to perform the assigned activities.
> 2. Physicians have an ethical obligation to the patients for whom they are responsible to ensure that medical and surgical conditions are evaluated and treated appropriately.
> 3. The physician should not substitute the services of an allied health professional for those of a physician when the allied health professional is not adequately trained.

What do these principles mean to the medical assistant working in a healthcare facility? As the physician's agent, the medical assistant must be trained to perform assigned tasks. The entry-level medical assistant who has earned a nationally recognized credential, such as the CMA (AAMA) or the RMA, has proven that she or he has met national standards of medical assisting excellence, and healthcare facilities can be assured that these individuals have entry-level competency in all identified areas.

The AMA's Code of Ethics consists of nine separate categories of ethical concerns. The medical assistant can refer to these categories for guidance if he or she faces an ethical dilemma in the workplace. This chapter provides a short summary of AMA ethical policies with applications to the field of medical assisting.

Opinions on Social Policy Issues
Preventing, Identifying, and Treating Violence and Abuse
All patients may be at risk of interpersonal violence and abuse, regardless of socioeconomic issues. Therefore, providers should routinely inquire about physical, sexual, and psychological abuse as part of the medical history. These questions are often part of the initial intake form that is completed either by the patient or the medical assistant during the patient interview process. If the medical assistant suspects that a patient may be a victim of abuse, he or she should report this concern to the provider immediately. In addition, the clinic should keep a current list of community and health care resources available to abused or vulnerable individuals and share this information with suspected victims. The clinic also should follow up with whatever the state requirements are for reporting violence or abuse.

Healthcare professionals should do the following to address acts of violence and abuse:
- Providers must treat the immediate symptoms and results of violence and abuse and provide continued care to affected patients.

- Providers should be aware of cultural differences in response to abuse and public health measures that are effective in preventing violence and abuse.
- The practice should have policies and procedures in place for dealing with a suspected or confirmed abuse case.

HIV Testing

Providers must protect individual patient's rights while at the same time safeguarding the public's welfare. The AMA recommends the following ethical and legal guidelines on HIV testing. For a complete summary of AMA guidelines refer to *www.ama-assn.org/ama/pub/physician-resources/medical-ethics/code-medical-ethics/opinion 223.page*.

1. Physicians should promote routine HIV screening for all adult patients.
2. Written consent for HIV testing is not required in most states. However, when considering the ethics of testing, providers should ask patients for consent before testing is done. This conversation should be documented in the patient's record, even if the patient refuses testing.
3. If a healthcare worker has an accidental exposure, such as a needlestick, HIV testing can be done on the patient without informed consent.
4. Providers must help HIV-positive patients access suitable follow-up care and counseling.
5. Providers must comply with state and federal reporting guidelines for infectious diseases while at the same time ensuring patient confidentiality.
6. Providers must attempt to prevent HIV-positive individuals from infecting third parties. If an HIV-positive individual is not compliant with infection control guidelines, the provider should:
   a. Notify local public health officials
   b. Counsel the HIV-positive patient about the risks of exposing others to the disease
   c. If permitted by state law, contact any third party who is in danger of infection while still maintaining patient confidentiality

---

CRITICAL THINKING APPLICATION   **7-5**

You have just had an accidental needlestick exposure. Does the source patient have to give legal consent to have a test done for the human immunodeficiency virus (HIV)? How should HIV information be managed in a busy healthcare practice?

Withholding or Withdrawing Life-Prolonging Treatment

A physician is committed to saving life and relieving suffering. Sometimes these two goals are incompatible, and a choice between them must be made. If possible, the patient should decide what treatment is given. Often the patient makes his or her wishes known to a responsible relative or other representative in case the patient becomes incapacitated. Some patients want a "do not resuscitate" (DNR) or "no code" order added to their health records. Usually such an order is established so that no heroic measures are taken in

a situation in which a patient would be unable or incompetent to make a decision. The decision to withdraw life support should be made before any mention of organ donation is made by the medical professionals tending the patient. In the best situation, the patient has formally completed an advance directive.

Organ Donation

Organ donation is not only considered ethical by the AMA, it is encouraged. However, it is considered unethical to participate in proceedings in which the donor receives payment, except reimbursement of expenses directly incurred in the removal of the donated organ. The rights of the patient and the donor must be protected equally. If the donor is deceased, the death must be certified by a physician other than the recipient's physician.

Because the need for donated organs is so extreme, protocols have been established by healthcare facilities to determine when it is proper to harvest organs. Organ **procurement** may be performed immediately after a person has died, or it may be done after a patient has been kept alive artificially for a time. Hospitals also have specific guidelines for the donation of organs from living donors, such as a kidney donation. When donations are made from one living person to another, both patients must have an **advocate** team that includes a physician so that the interests and well-being of each patient are addressed. Blood donations probably are the most common form of organ donation.

CRITICAL THINKING APPLICATION   **7-6**

- Monica has often thought about being an organ donor. Her parents are very opposed to the idea because of their religious beliefs. How can Monica deal with this conflict within her family?
- If Monica dies before her parents do, how can she ensure that her wishes are carried out?

Allocation of Health Resources

Sometimes society must decide who receives care when serving all who need care is not possible. Decisions must be made fairly and should be weighed carefully. The criteria to consider when allocating health resources include urgency of need, likelihood of benefit, duration of benefit, amount of resources required for successful treatment, and potential for change in the quality of life. Nonmedical criteria should not be considered; these include the ability to pay, the social worth of the individual, age, obstacles to treatment, and the patient's contribution to the illness. The provider must remain the patient's advocate and should not be involved in making allocation decisions for that patient. For example, individual providers do not decide who receives an organ donation. There are established national protocols for matching needy patients with available organs that help determine the potential success of the transplant rather than someone deciding which patient is more worthy.

Opinions on Confidentiality, Advertising, and Communications

Confidentiality is one of the cardinal rules of the medical profession. It is completely unethical to divulge any information about a patient to any other person not directly related to the patient's care. The places where confidentiality often is breached are elevators, hallways, waiting or reception areas, break rooms, and lunch rooms. A relative may be standing behind the medical assistant, listening to conversations that are inappropriate for those not personally involved in the patient's care to hear. Breach of patient confidentiality is grounds for immediate termination from a healthcare facility.

Confidentiality restrictions apply to information documented in a patient's record and also to anything the medical assistant is told by the patient or the patient's family. Never investigate a patient's record strictly for curiosity. All information in the record must be kept in confidence. Never share information about patients with anyone outside the medical facility or office, including your own immediate family (Figure 7-2).

Individuals accompanying the patient to the healthcare facility should be in the examination room only if the patient gives approval. In addition, students should not be permitted to observe in patient examination rooms unless the patient gives permission. Never discuss one patient's case with another patient. If curious patients ask questions about others, simply explain that medical assistants are obligated to keep all patient information confidential. Patients who ask questions of a medical nature about their own case should be referred to the provider for information and instructions unless the medical assistant is authorized to provide this information. When minors request confidential services and the law does not require otherwise, providers should allow competent minors to consent to medical care and should not notify the parents without the minor's consent.

Remember that the Health Insurance Portability and Accountability Act (HIPAA) has established strict regulations for patient confidentiality and disclosure of private health information. Make sure the healthcare facility is abiding by its own privacy policy and that all patients have been given a chance to review that policy. A document stating that the patient has read and understands the privacy policy or that he or she has refused to sign should be part of the patient's record.

Patients may not always understand the ethical standards to which providers and medical assistants adhere. They may ask questions about their own health or the health of a fellow patient.

Medical assistants must educate patients about the issues of confidentiality in such a way that they are not offended; they should explain that all patients deserve to have their medical and personal information kept private. Now more than ever, the medical assistant's obligation to keep information private is not only an ethical but also a legal responsibility. All patients should understand that they are entitled to confidential treatment of their records and that the facility is dedicated to that principle.

CRITICAL THINKING APPLICATION 7-7
Patient confidentiality must be safeguarded at all times in the healthcare setting. You are working in an infectious disease facility, and your sister calls you very upset; she just heard a rumor that her daughter's boyfriend is HIV positive. She thought you might be able to find out for her. How should you manage this situation? Is there anything that the provider can do to safeguard others who may be infected by an HIV-positive person?

Advertising and Publicity
Advertising. There are no restrictions on advertising by physicians; the key issue is whether advertising or publicity is true and not misleading. The advertisement should be free of medical terminology so that the public can readily understand the message. Testimonials of patients should not be used in advertising because they are difficult to verify or measure by objective standards. Statements regarding the quality of medical services are highly subjective and difficult to verify. All advertised claims must be supported by actual data and facts.

Communication with the Media. Although information about some patients, such as celebrities and politicians, may be considered news, the provider cannot discuss any patient's condition with the press without authorization from the patient or the patient's legal representative. The provider may release only authorized information or that which is public knowledge. Certain kinds of news are part of public records; such news in the **public domain** includes births, deaths, accident reports, and police cases.

A medical assistant must be aware that only the provider is authorized to release information, and under no circumstances should the medical assistant violate the confidential nature of the provider-patient relationship. It is unethical to even verify that a patient is under the provider's care without the patient's permission. A policy must be in place for every medical office on how media inquiries should be handled and to whom they should be referred. Communication with the media falls under the HIPAA guidelines. Do not release a patient's health information without written permission.

Opinions on Practice Matters
Fees and Charges
Charging or collecting an illegal or excessive fee is unethical. The medical assistant is responsible for keeping informed about current billing regulations and for seeing that these regulations are followed conscientiously. However, requesting payment at the time of treatment is appropriate and very common in today's medical offices.

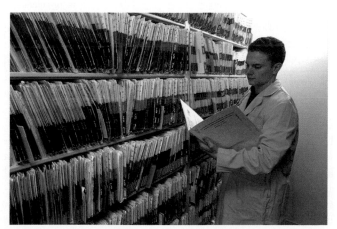
FIGURE 7-2 Confidentiality applies to all information about the patient, including what is documented and what is said between the patient and the medical assistant.

Often, managed care patients are asked to remit their co-payment before seeing the provider on the day of the visit. If the patient is notified in advance, adding interest or other reasonable charges to delinquent accounts also is considered ethical. In addition, a reasonable fee may be charged for duplicating patients' records. Most facilities use a patient information booklet which provides a written reference for all policies.

Providers should never base decisions about whether to order a diagnostic test or a procedure on the patient's insurance coverage. If an expensive diagnostic test is needed, such as a magnetic resonance imaging (MRI) scan, the provider cannot withhold it because of financial reasons. However, if the physician is aware of a way the patient could obtain financial assistance with the test, he or she should relay that information to the patient.

Fee Splitting and Contingent Fees

According to the AMA's Code of Ethics, "Payment by or to a physician solely for the referral of a patient is fee splitting and is unethical." This practice is unethical whether it involves another physician, a clinic, a laboratory, or a drug company.

Although attorneys often accept a case on a contingency fee basis, it is unethical for a provider to engage in this practice. The fee in this case is contingent on a successful outcome, but a provider should never set his or her fee on the successful outcome of medical treatment. A provider's fee must always be based on the value of service provided to the patient.

Waiver of Insurance Co-Payments

Providers may opt to write off or waive co-payments to help a patient who cannot afford care. If access to care is directly threatened because the patient cannot make the co-payment, the provider may forgive the payment. However, routine waiver of co-payments may violate the policies of some insurance companies. Providers need to make sure that their policies about co-payments follow applicable laws and are within the legal boundaries of their contracts with insurers. To avoid conflicts, providers may discount the entire service and all related fees to avoid potential legal conflicts with co-payment collection.

Professional Courtesy

Providers may opt not to charge or may offer a reduced rate for care given to other physicians, staff, or family members. This practice is called *professional courtesy.* This is a long-standing tradition but certainly not an ethical requirement. Providers make the decision as to who receives professional courtesy in their offices, and this should be written into the office policy manual. In some cases, extending professional courtesy is contrary to insurance and/or managed care contracts. In addition, some providers have stopped offering professional courtesy because of the rising costs of healthcare and shrinking reimbursements.

Conflicts of Interest

Questions about healthcare professionals and conflicts of interest can occur when providers or their employees accept gifts, including meals and drug samples, from pharmaceutical representatives; when the provider acts as a spokesperson on behalf of medical device companies; or when the professional has a financial interest in a medical product company whose products they prescribe, use, or recommend. The AMA recommends that physicians not meet with pharmaceutical and medical device sales representatives except by documented appointment and at the physician's express invitation. It also recommends that physicians not accept drug samples except in specified situations for patients who lack financial access to medications.

If you work in a medical office, you soon learn that gifts from pharmaceutical and medical device representatives are commonplace. These gifts range from free drug samples to lunch for all employees, in addition to pens, notebooks, and other giveaways. A recent national survey revealed that more than 90% of physicians had received free drug samples and more than 60% had received meals, tickets to entertainment events, or free travel. What does that mean for the medical assistants working in the facility? It is always nice to get a free lunch, and it certainly helps patients to have access to free drug samples when approved by the physician. However, all employees must make sure that decisions on patient care are based on ethical matters, rather than as a result of gifts.

CRITICAL THINKING APPLICATION   7-8

A pharmaceutical representative who frequently requests appointments with the providers in your office to discuss new products brings lunch for the staff every Wednesday. Is this a conflict of interest? Is it more likely that the staff will treat this individual differently and make sure the provider blocks off time to meet with the sales rep?

Compliance With Conflicts of Interest Standards

The American College of Physicians recommends the following for all physicians:

Do not accept items of material value from pharmaceutical, medical device, and biotechnology companies unless it is part of a payment for a legitimate service.

Do not make educational presentations or publish scientific articles that are controlled by the industry.

Do not act as a consultant unless you are being paid for your expertise.

Do not meet with pharmaceutical and medical device sales representatives unless you have invited them and the appointment is documented.

Do not accept drug samples except in specified situations for patients who lack financial access to medications.

http://www.ncbi.nlm.nih.gov/books/NBK22944/. Accessed February 5, 2016.

Unethical Conduct by Members of the Health Professions

In rare instances, a medical assistant is faced with a situation in which the physician-employer's conduct appears to violate established ethical standards. Before making any judgments, the medical assistant must be absolutely sure of all the information and circumstances. If unethical conduct occurs, the medical assistant must then make his or her own decision about continued employment in the facility and whether the unethical behavior should be reported to a law enforcement agency or the local medical society. Would it be wise to remain in the practice under the circumstances? Would it be better to seek other employment? Would remaining adversely affect future opportunities for employment in another facility?

These decisions are difficult, especially if the relationship and employment conditions have been favorable and congenial. An ethical medical assistant does not want to participate in known substandard or unlawful practices, especially those that might be harmful to patients. In addition, the medical assistant must never make inaccurate reports about unethical behavior and should realize that some states can prosecute individuals who file a false report. Be absolutely certain of the facts before making such accusations against any health professional. When the provider's ethical standards conflict with those of the medical assistant, the medical assistant must decide whether staying with the provider is the best option. However, if the medical assistant believes that patient safety is at risk, he or she is ethically compelled to report provider actions to the local authorities and the state Medical Board.

CLOSING COMMENTS

Medical assistants have an ethical obligation to keep up with current developments that affect the practice of medicine and the care of patients. Membership in a professional organization provides access to continuing education to help you keep current in your knowledge and skills in medical assisting and to stay up-to-date on the latest ethical topics.

The study of ethics requires considerable thought and honest appraisal of what the medical assistant believes. Sometimes reflection at this level is difficult. Often our beliefs are a result of our environment, upbringing, and other factors that have influenced our thinking and actions from the time we were small children. It is important that our belief system is one that we developed personally, not just a set of beliefs and values that we learned from our families or were influenced by our friends. Medical assistants should take a serious look at the thoughts and concepts that make up their own ethical beliefs. With personal insight into how we feel about complex ethical issues, we are better prepared to recognize the difference between professional and personal ethics.

Patient Education

Patients may not always understand the ethical standards to which providers and medical assistants adhere. They may ask medical assistants questions about the health of a fellow patient or a friend or family member who are also patients at the facility. Medical assistants must educate patients about confidentiality in such a way that the patient does not take offense, explaining that all patients deserve to have their medical and personal information kept private. Now more than ever, ethical obligations for privacy, in addition to legal ones, are imperative. A medical assistant must make sure that all patients understand that they are entitled to confidential treatment of their records and that the facility is dedicated to that principle.

Legal and Ethical Issues

The prime objective of the healthcare profession is to render service and provide quality care to all individuals, regardless of race, gender, age, sexual orientation, or socioeconomic status. The importance of respecting the confidentiality of information learned from or about patients in the course of employment cannot be overemphasized. It is unethical to reveal the patient's identity or information to anyone, including family members, a spouse, best friends, and other medical assistants.

This chapter summarized a wide range of potential ethical conflicts. Regardless of the situation, the medical assistant is bound by ethical standards to treat all patients with respect and to make ethical decisions based on principles rather than personal beliefs and values. As members of the healthcare team, medical assistants are also responsible for reporting ethical infractions to their supervisors. In addition, legal requirements may exist for the reporting of ethical issues to local or state authorities. One of the roles of each medical assistant is to serve as the patient's advocate. In this role, it may be necessary to use legal means to protect the rights of patients in the practice.

Professional Behaviors

Ethics guides society's moral principles. The decisions that medical assistants make based on ethical beliefs can drastically alter how they treat individual patients. Ethics is considered a higher authority than legality since something that is legal may not necessarily be ethical. It is crucial that each person working in healthcare take the time to evaluate his or her own belief system and core values. Regardless of how we believe a particular situation should be handled, we must always provide our patients with respectful patient care. The AAMA Code of Ethics serves as a guide for the ethical responsibilities of the professional medical assistant.

SUMMARY OF SCENARIO

Pregnancy usually is a joyous time, but Monica has learned that even such an anticipated event can bring ethical issues to light. She has realized that every situation has two or more sides and that she must be open and willing to look at all sides when making an ethical decision.

Medical assisting is a rewarding career, but sometimes the decisions medical professionals face are quite difficult. Monica must learn to be nonjudgmental and not to inflict her opinions on her patients. They must make their own decisions about their health and emotional well-being, and the medical assistant should not influence their thinking unfairly.

Monica must continue to evaluate her own ideas and beliefs throughout her career as a medical assistant. Periodic self-evaluation is good for everyone, and she will grow both personally and professionally by always providing her patients ethical care.

SUMMARY OF LEARNING OBJECTIVES

1. **Define, spell, and pronounce the terms listed in the vocabulary.**
Spelling and pronouncing medical terms correctly reinforce the medical assistant's credibility. Knowing the definitions of these terms promotes confidence in communication with patients and co-workers.

2. **Do the following related to medicine and ethics:**
   - *Define ethics and morals.*
   Ethical issues are not as strict as laws and vary from person to person, but most physicians follow the ethical guidelines set forth by the AMA. *Moral* issues are related to a person's concept of right and wrong. An individual's morals are defined as their standards for behavior or their beliefs about what is right and what is wrong.
   - *Identify the effect of personal morals and values on professional performance.*
   Morals and values are usually personal in nature. Medical assistants not only must have a strong knowledge base about ethical issues they might face throughout their careers, they also must come to terms with some of the deeply rooted morals and value systems that have been a part of their lives since childhood. Interacting ethically requires you to examine your own values, beliefs, and actions; you cannot treat all patients with care and respect until you first recognize and evaluate personal biases.
   - *Differentiate between personal and professional ethics.*
   Personal ethics are the beliefs or values held by an individual. *Professional* ethics are the beliefs or values generally held by most people in a profession; they typically are guided by established codes of ethics.
   - *Recognize the effect personal ethics and morals have on the delivery of healthcare.*
   Medical assistants must avoid judging a situation or a patient based on the values they learned as a child or in their personal lives. If a patient makes a decision or performs in a way we do not approve, we still must treat him or her with respect and deliver the highest quality patient care.
   - *Develop a plan for separation of personal and professional ethics.*
   Using the case studies in Procedure 7-1, role-play with your partner issues of personal and professional ethical behavior and how personal ethics and morals can affect the delivery of healthcare.
   - *Demonstrate appropriate responses to ethical issues.*
   Using the case studies in Procedure 7-2, role-play with your partner issues of patient confidentiality.

3. **Discuss the history of ethics in medicine.**
The earliest written code of ethical conduct for medical practice was created in approximately 2250 BC by the Babylonians. It was called the Code of Hammurabi. In 1846, the American Medical Association (AMA) was organized, and a Code of Ethics was formulated at its first meeting in 1847. The American Association of Medical Assistants (AAMA) has published its own version of a Code of Ethics for Medical Assistants and has also created a Medical Assisting Creed that can be used as a guideline by medical assistants.

4. **Do the following related to making ethical decisions:**
   - *List and define three general elements of ethics.*
   The three general elements of ethics, according to Dr. Ruth Purtilo, are duties, rights, and character traits. A duty is an obligation a person has or perceives himself or herself to have; rights are defined as claims made on society, a group, or an individual; character traits are a tendency to act a certain way.
   - *List and define the four types of ethical problems.*
   Purtilo presents four basic types of ethical problems. *Ethical distress* is a situation in which an individual knows what should be done, but for some reason the action cannot be accomplished. An *ethical dilemma* exists when a situation can be handled in different ways, but only one way can be chosen, regardless of the benefit of the others. A *dilemma of justice* exists when a conflict arises over how limited resources can be distributed fairly. A *locus of authority* problem occurs when authority figures differ in their opinions on how a medical problem should be managed.
   - *Discuss the five-step process used to make an ethical decision.*
   Making an ethical decision is a five-step process that begins with gathering information about the situation; determining which ethical problem or problems are presented; considering the duties, rights, and character traits of all the individuals involved; paying close attention to the ramifications of all possible decisions; and then making a decision to act in a particular way.

5. **Summarize the ethical opinions reached by the Council on Ethical and Judicial Affairs (CEJA).**
The CEJA develops ethics policy for the AMA by analyzing and addressing ethical issues that confront physicians and the medical profession. The recommendations from the council ultimately are used to update the AMA's Code of Medical Ethics, which can be found at *www.ama-assn.org/ama/ pub/physician-resources/medical-ethics/code-medical-ethics.page*. AMA ethical opinions have been published to address social policy issues (e.g., preventing, identifying, and treating violence and abuse; HIV testing; withholding or withdrawing life-prolonging treatment; organ donation; and allocation of health resources), confidentiality, advertising, and communication (e.g., advertising and publicity), and public matters (e.g., fees and charges, fee splitting and contingent fees, waiver of insurance co-payments, professional courtesy, conflict of interest, and unethical conduct by members of the health professions).

6. **Describe the process of compliance reporting of conflicts of interest.**
The American College of Physicians has made specific recommendations for physicians regarding conflicts of interest. If the physician's ethical standards conflict with those of the medical assistant, the medical assistant must decide whether staying with the physician is the best option. However, if the medical assistant believes that patient safety is at risk, he or she is ethically compelled to report the physician's actions to the local authorities and the state medical board.

CONNECTIONS

Study Guide Connection: Go to the Chapter 7 Study Guide. Read and complete the activities.

evolve Evolve Connection: Go to the Chapter 7 link at *evolve.elsevier.com/ kinn* to complete the Chapter Review Quiz. Check out the other resources listed for this chapter to make the most of what you have learned from Medicine and Ethics.

TECHNOLOGY AND WRITTEN COMMUNICATION

Christiana has been a medical assistant in Dr. Zachary Brown's family practice clinic for 5 years. She had been working as a clinical medical assistant, helping with diagnostic tests and treatment procedures. Christiana enjoyed providing patient care, but she wanted to use more of the administrative skills she learned in college 5 years ago. She is organized and enjoys challenges and technology. When a front office position opened up, Christiana transitioned into the administrative role. She is now the lead administrative medical assistant. Her role entails answering phones, scheduling appointments, greeting patients,

and processing correspondence to patients. She also is responsible for reviewing the clinic's e-mails. Patients are encouraged to use e-mail to communicate with Dr. Brown. Christiana has seen the number of daily e-mails increase. She answers those that pertain to appointments, and the others are forwarded to Dr. Brown or to his clinical medical assistant. Besides performing her administrative duties, Christiana is now responsible for the clinic's computer system. She is excited to continue to learn the administrative role and the computer system.

While studying this chapter, think about the following questions:

- How does a computer system help with efficiency and accuracy in the ambulatory care center?
- What steps can a medical assistant take to ensure that written communication is professional?
- What are the benefits of providing professional communication to patients, whether by letter or e-mail?
- How can a medical assistant safeguard the privacy of medical records when using electronic health records?

LEARNING OBJECTIVES

1. Define, spell, and pronounce the terms listed in the vocabulary.
2. Explain what a personal computer is, and identify input and output hardware for personal computers.
3. Identify internal computer components, secondary storage devices, and network and Internet access devices.
4. Explain how to maintain computer hardware.
5. Identify principles of ergonomics that apply to a computer workstation.
6. Differentiate between:
   - System software and application software.
   - Electronic medical records (EMRs) and a practice management system.

7. Explain the importance of data backup and other computer network security activities performed in the healthcare setting.
8. Discuss applications of electronic technology.
9. Recognize the elements of fundamental writing skills.
10. Explain the guidelines for using capitalization, numbers, and punctuation in business communication.
11. Describe each component of a professional business letter.
12. Summarize the formats for business letters and memorandums.
13. Compose professional correspondence using electronic technology.

VOCABULARY

audit trail A record of computer activity used to monitor users' actions within software, including additions, deletions, and viewing of electronic records.

back up The process of copying and archiving computer data so that the duplicate files can be used to restore the original data if a compromise occurs.

computer network A system that links personal computers and peripheral devices to share information and resources.

computer on wheels (COW) Wireless mobile workstation; also called workstation on wheels (WOW).

data server Computer hardware and software that perform data analysis, storage, and archiving; also called a *database server.*

decryption The computer process of changing encrypted text to readable or plain text after a user enters a secret key or password.

dumb terminal A personal computer that doesn't contain a hard drive and allows the user only limited functions, including access to software, the network, and/or the Internet.

electronic health record (EHR) An electronic record of health-related information about a patient that conforms to nationally recognized interoperability standards and that can be created, managed, and consulted by authorized clinicians and staff members from more than one healthcare organization.

electronic medical record (EMR) An electronic record of health-related information about an individual that can be

VOCABULARY—continued

created, gathered, managed, and consulted by authorized clinicians and staff members within a single healthcare organization. An EMR is an electronic version of a paper record.

e-prescribing The use of electronic software to communicate with pharmacies and send prescribing information. It takes the place of writing a prescription by hand and giving it to a patient; most new or refill prescriptions can be submitted electronically, cutting down on fraud and errors.

ethernet A communication system for connecting several computers so information can be shared.

firewall A program or hardware that acts as a filter between the network and the Internet.

magnetism The attraction of materials to magnets; strong magnets can damage magnetic storage devices, such as hard drives.

Meaningful use requirements Requirements established by the Centers for Medicare and Medicaid Services (CMS) as part of the Electronic Health Records (EHR) Incentives Program. The program provides financial incentives for healthcare organizations that "meaningfully used" their certified EHR technology. The requirements include implementing security measures to ensure the privacy of patients' EHRs.

media A type of communication (e.g., social media sites); with computers, the term refers to data storage devices.

modem Peripheral computer hardware that connects to the router to provide Internet access to the network or computer.

operating system Software that acts as the computer's administrator by managing, integrating, and controlling application software and hardware.

output device Computer hardware that displays the processed data from the computer (e.g., monitors and printers).

point of care Something designed to be used at or near where the patient is seen; point-of-care tools and apps are resources for the provider to use when working directly with the patient.

portrait orientation The most common layout for a printed page; the height of the paper is greater than its width.

practice management software Computer programs used to run business operations, including scheduling, billing, and accounting tasks.

privacy filters Devices attached to the monitor that allow visualization of the screen contents only if the user is directly in front of the screen; also called *monitor filters* or *privacy screens.*

secondary storage devices Media (e.g., jump drive, hard drive) capable of permanently storing data until it is replaced or deleted by the user.

security risk analysis Identification of potential threats of computer network breaches, for which action plans are devised.

software A set of electronic instructions to operate and perform different computer tasks.

stylus A pen-shaped device with a variety of tips that is used on touch screens to write, draw, or input commands.

USB port The most common type of connector device that allows hardware to be plugged into the computer.

Zip Software that compresses a file or folder, making it smaller.

The uses for technology in healthcare facilities are growing. Technology was first introduced in the ambulatory care setting to help promote efficiency and accuracy in business functions. Many healthcare facilities used computer software to help with billing and accounting procedures. Registration and scheduling software were implemented to help limit the number of times patient information was collected and entered into computer programs. As technology advanced, the federal government provided incentives for healthcare organizations to use electronic health records instead of paper medical records to increase accuracy and efficiency, which in turn helped reduce the cost of healthcare. More recently, healthcare workers have been using "smart" devices for quicker access to information to help provide better patient care.

The format of communication also has changed over the years. Many people have moved from letter writing to sending e-mails and text messages. Social **media** sites have gained in popularity. Many of these changes have affected the ambulatory care center environment. Patients are communicating with their providers via e-mails and text messages instead of phone calls. To help ensure confidentiality, administrators have instituted tighter network security procedures and restrictions on employee social media postings.

Medical assistants in today's healthcare facilities must be more computer savvy than ever before to meet these technologic demands.

They must follow procedures to safeguard the privacy and security of patients' records. The need for correct grammar, punctuation, and word use is greater than ever as medical assistants communicate using letters and electronic technology.

CRITICAL THINKING APPLICATION   **8-1**

Christiana answers e-mails from patients. How might her response differ from her personal e-mails to her family and friends?

ELECTRONIC TECHNOLOGY IN THE AMBULATORY CARE CENTER

For many clinics, technology was first used in administrative departments for scheduling and billing procedures. This helped increase the efficiency and accuracy of those activities. Processes that previously had taken hours to perform now took minutes with technology. Information was entered once and then used for many purposes.

Today, many clinics use electronic technology in both administrative and patient care areas. Most clinics have replaced paper medical charts with electronic health records (EHRs). Technology has increased the efficiency of the office environment and has made patient information and resources quickly accessible to healthcare staff. Regardless of the medical assistant's duties, knowledge about computers is crucial in today's healthcare environment.

Personal Computer Hardware

A personal computer (PC) is a relatively inexpensive piece of hardware that is used by a single person. A personal computer is considered a *system unit*, and all other pieces of hardware used are considered *peripheral devices*. The personal computer is an electronic data processing device that accepts, stores, and processes data. After processing the information, it generates the data output in a specific form.

A personal computer can be a desktop, laptop, or tablet computer. A desktop computer is designed for use on a desk. In the ambulatory care center, desktop computers are typically used for employees who primarily perform word processing, data entry, and business tasks, such as scheduling, bookkeeping, and billing (Figure 8-1). Laptop computers have evolved over the years into thinner, lighter weight models with more functionality (Figure 8-2). Many laptop and tablet computers have a touch screen panel (Figure 8-3). Users can enter data on the touch screen panel or use the keyboard. Laptop and tablet computers are portable, allowing healthcare staff to be more mobile while accessing technology.

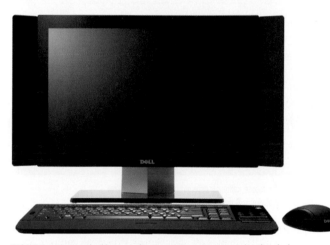

FIGURE 8-1 Many healthcare employees, including receptionists, clinical medical assistants, and providers, use desktop computers. (Courtesy Dell, Round Rock, Texas.)

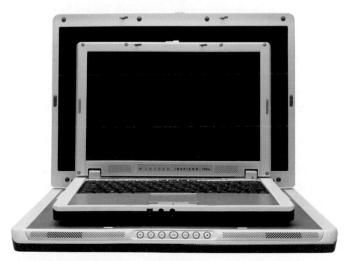

FIGURE 8-2 Laptop computers are available in thinner, lighter weight models with more functionality than older models. (Courtesy Dell, Round Rock, Texas.)

The hardware of a computer system includes the physical equipment required for communication and data processing functions. Computer hardware can be divided into the following categories: input devices, **output devices**, internal components, secondary storage devices, and network and Internet access devices.

CRITICAL THINKING APPLICATION	8-2

When Christiana transitioned into the administrative role, Dr. Brown hired Michaela as the new clinical medical assistant. Recently the medical practice switched from using desktop computers to tablet computers when working with patients in the exam rooms. How might Christiana's experience using the desktop computer in the exam rooms be different from Michaela's use of the tablet computer? Thinking of the patient's perception, which technology might a patient prefer the medical assistant to use? Why?

Input Devices

An *input device* is any peripheral hardware that allows the user to provide data to the computer. Many types of input devices are available on the market, but this discussion focuses on those typically used in the ambulatory care setting. Common input devices include keyboards, mice and other pointing devices, touch screens, webcams, microphones, scanners, and signature pads.

Keyboards are the most common input devices. The QWERTY keyboard is the standard keyboard for computers. (Q-W-E-R-T-Y are the first six letters, from left to right, just below the number keys on the keyboard.) A wide variety of keyboards is available, including standard, Internet, wireless, and ergonomic. Keyboards may have special keys that perform the same functionality as the buttons on Web pages. Numeric keypads are also a feature on many keyboards. Ergonomic keyboards help reduce repetitive strain injuries by minimizing muscle strain; these keyboards allow the user's hands to be in a natural position when typing. The two most common ergonomic keyboards are the split-key models and the "waved" or "curved" key layout (Figure 8-4).

CRITICAL THINKING APPLICATION	8-3

Christiana's keyboard looks different from Dr. Brown's keyboard in his office. Why might Christiana have a different keyboard?

FIGURE 8-3 Tablet computers and other new computers have touch screen panels that allow users to easily enter data.

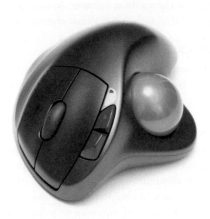

FIGURE 8-4 Ergonomic keyboards have different appearances, yet they all help reduce repetitive strain injuries.

FIGURE 8-5 A trackball mouse uses a large ball to control the movement of the cursor/pointer.

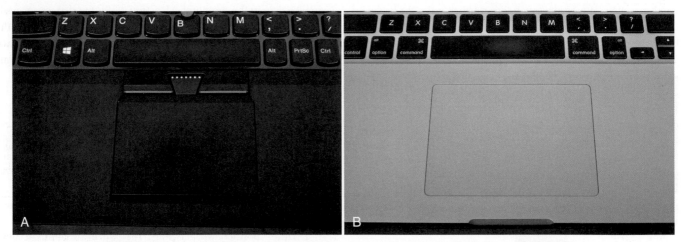

FIGURE 8-6 A touch pad is built into a computer, and its functions are similar to those of a mouse, although different touch pads may have different functions. For example, the device in **A** has a left and right click button, whereas the device in **B** does not.

Keyboards typically have the following categories of keys: typing, numeric, function, control, and special purpose keys. Typing keys include the numeric and alphabetic keys used for typing. Numeric keypads have the numeric keys in the same position as calculators. The twelve keys at the top of the keyboard are function keys, and each key has a specific purpose. Some software allows the function keys to be programmed by the user. When these programmed function keys are used, a specific task is performed by the computer. Control keys move the cursor and the screen. They include the following keys: Home, End, Insert, Delete, Page Up, Page Down, Control, Escape, Alternate, and four arrow keys. Special purpose keys include Enter, Shift, Caps Lock, Num Lock, Space Bar, Print Screen, and Tab.

The mouse is one of the most common input devices, making screen navigation much simpler than using the keyboard. A mouse is a palm-sized box with a laser sensor that tracks the user's movement of the mouse and sends those messages back to the computer. The mouse is used to move the pointer (cursor) on the screen. Many mice have a left and right button with a wheel between to help with cursor/pointer navigation and functionality. With a trackball mouse,

the user moves the enlarged ball on the top of the mouse to control the pointer (Figure 8-5).

Touch pads are becoming more popular on laptops because they are portable and compact. Touch pads are touch sensitive; they move the pointer based on the user's finger movements on the touch pad. Touch pads' functionality can vary, but many include a left and right click button similar to a mouse (Figure 8-6).

A touch screen is different from a touch pad. A touch screen allows a person to interact with the computer by touching the display screen with a finger or **stylus**. The touch screens on computers and other electronic devices can vary, which means the compatible stylus can vary.

- Resistive Touch Screen: Responds to the touch of almost anything that can generate pressure (e.g., finger, plastic stylus, rubber-tip stylus). These screens are found in many handheld electronic devices.
- Capacitive Touch Screen: Responds to the electrical characteristics of a finger and is found in smart phones and other electronic devices. It requires a specialized stylus that has more surface area in the point.

- Surface Acoustic Wave Touch Screen: Responds to an inaudible wave of sound that is created on the screen from a finger. Like the resistive touch screen, it is very common and can be found in kiosks and ordering screens. A stylus with a rubber or soft tip the size of a pencil eraser is required.

Wireless webcams and microphones are becoming more popular. To see patients who are not able to come to the healthcare agency, providers can use webcams, microphones, and Internet video chat software. Webcams and microphones are also used for meetings and continuing education opportunities. Microphones can be used for dictating notes into a patient's health record.

CRITICAL THINKING APPLICATION   **8-4**

Dr. Brown works with a home health agency. Patients and nurses can communicate with him using the Internet, microphones, and webcams. How does this technology benefit the patients?

Scanners convert images to digital text through a process called *optical character recognition* (OCR). Handheld, sheet-fed, and flatbed scanners are available. Handheld scanners are used to scan bar codes. Sheet-fed scanners may be stand-alone units or include other features such as duplicating and faxing. Flatbed scanners have a glass panel on which the documents are placed for scanning. Scanners in the healthcare setting have become more popular since the use of electronic health records (EHRs) has increased. Old medical records are scanned, and the images are uploaded into the patient's new EHR. Receptionists use small, sheet-fed scanners to scan insurance cards when patients check in for appointments. The insurance card images are then uploaded into the patient's record and are referenced for billing activities.

In the ambulatory care setting, signature pads are used in the reception area. Patients need to sign a number of documents, including release forms, consent forms, and the Notice of Privacy Practices. Patients sign the signature pad, and the signatures are imported into the EHR as part of the patient's permanent health record (Figure 8-7).

Output Devices

The data entered into the computer with the input devices are processed by the computer. The processed data are displayed using

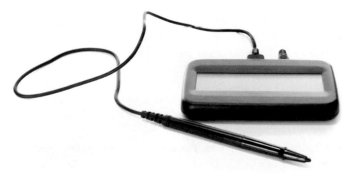

FIGURE 8-7 Signature pads allow patients' signatures to be imported into the electronic health record or practice management software.

output devices. Common output devices in the healthcare setting include monitors, printers, and speakers.

Monitors display the output as images, which are created by tiny dots called *pixels*. The higher the number of pixels used in the monitor, the sharper the image. The most common monitor in the healthcare setting is the liquid crystal display (LCD) monitor. These monitors are easier on the eyes and use less electricity, and they are smaller and lighter than older monitors. Some clinics use LCD monitors in the reception area so that patients can read documents before signing the signature pad.

Printers produce the output on paper. The two most common types of printers used in the ambulatory care center are inkjet and laser printers. Inkjet printers create images by spraying small drops of ink on the paper. Inkjet printers can create high-quality printing but are slower to print a document. Inkjet printers are inexpensive to purchase, but the maintenance costs are high because of the need for frequent ink cartridge changes. A laser printer uses a laser, electrical charges, and toner to produce images on paper. The advantages of laser printers include high-speed printing, high-quality output, quality graphics, and support of many fonts and font sizes. The initial cost of a laser printer is higher than that of an inkjet printer, but the maintenance costs may be less because the toner cartridges are changed less often compared to inkjet printers.

CRITICAL THINKING APPLICATION   **8-5**

Christiana frequently prints documents, including billing statements, appointment reminders, and receipts for payment. What type of printer might be the most economical to use in the reception area? Why?

Speakers for electronic devices come in all shapes and sizes. Typically in the ambulatory care center, speakers are built into the devices used (e.g., monitor, laptop, tablet).

Internal Components

For a desktop personal computer, the internal components are found in the tower or case. The central processing unit (CPU), or processor, is the "brains" of the computer. It is responsible for interpreting and executing commands from the software or the program. The CPU sits on the motherboard. The motherboard is a platform where all the internal computer parts attach, including the primary memory, hard drive, optical drive, sound and video cards, and ports.

The primary memory is accessed directly by the CPU and includes read-only memory (ROM), cache memory, and random access memory (RAM). ROM contains hardwired instructions that are used when the computer boots up or starts. The cache memory contains data and instructions for opened programs. When the computer needs to read memory or instructions, it first scans the cache memory to see if the data exist there before looking at the RAM or main memory. If the data exist in the cache memory, the computer doesn't look at the RAM. The cache memory is quicker than the main memory and allows programs to operate more quickly and efficiently. The limitations of cache memory include limited size and expense, and it provides only temporary use of information.

RAM is the working memory of the computer, which is needed for the computer to operate. It holds the data that are currently being used. When a program is opened, the instructions are stored temporarily in RAM for easy access. The main memory has limited capacity and can be lost if the power is turned off. Before installing new software, make sure the computer has the required RAM. If there is not enough RAM for the program, the computer must go to the hard drive to read the data, which is a slower process.

The hard disk drive (HDD) is often referred to as the "hard drive." The HDD reads and writes on the hard disk, which provides the largest amount of permanent storage for the computer. Because the HDD and the hard disk are packaged together, "HDD" or "hard drive" is used to reference the entire unit. The hard drive is considered a secondary storage device and is not required to operate the computer. When you save a file on the computer, the file is saved on the C drive, which is the internal hard drive of the computer. Because of their low cost, hard drives are found in most desktop and laptop computers. A solid-state drive (SSD) can replace a hard drive in a computer, but an SSD is more expensive than an HDD. However, compared to an HDD, an SSD has faster access speed and better performance and reliability, and it is not affected by **magnetism**.

Optical drives can read or read and save data on optical discs, such as compact discs (CDs), digital versatile/video discs (DVDs), and Blu-Ray discs (BDs), which are removable storage devices. The sound card, also called the *audio card* or *audio adapter,* allows audio information to be sent to speakers or headphones. The video card is also called a *graphic card* or *video adapter.* It allows the computer to send graphic information to output devices, such as projectors or monitors. On many computers the sound and video card features are integrated into the motherboard; this limits the sound and graphic systems but lowers the overall computer cost. Most desktop computers and laptops have a number of **USB ports** that allow hardware (e.g., printers, mice, keyboards, and external hard drives) to connect to the computer.

Secondary Storage Devices

A **secondary storage device**, or **medium**, is capable of permanently storing data until it is replaced or deleted by the user. These devices can be considered removable, internal (such as the hard drive previously discussed), or external. The computer needs a secondary storage device to allow the user to save data. Without a storage device, the computer would be considered a **dumb terminal**. Dumb terminals provide the user access to software, the network, and/or the Internet but don't allow the user to save data to the C drive of the computer.

CRITICAL THINKING APPLICATION   8-6

Christiana would like to have a small patient education space in the reception area. She would like to have a computer with Internet access for patients so they can access health information. Christiana knows that cost is a factor in a small practice. The computer would have to be reasonable and reliable. What might be some technology options she could propose to Dr. Brown?

The types of computer storage devices are categorized as magnetic, optical, and flash (Table 8-1). One of the oldest types of storage is magnetic storage, which uses magnetic technology to read and write data to the device. Optical drives use lasers and lights to read and write data onto optical storage devices. Some optical devices are just recordable; for example, a CD-R disc allows only one opportunity to save data to the device. Other optical devices allow Read/Write (RW), which means discs allow data to be written and erased multiple times. Flash memory devices, which are becoming cheaper and have larger storage capacity, are replacing the older magnetic media. The jump drive is a portable device that connects to the USB port in the computer (Figure 8-8).

Besides storage hardware, the use of cloud storage is becoming more popular. Cloud storage, also known as *file sharing* or *online storage,* allows individuals to store computer files using the Internet and a third-party service. To get started, an individual signs up with a cloud storage service. Many companies allow free minimal storage, while others charge monthly fees or fees based on storage size. After signing up, individuals use the Internet to send computer files to the service company's **data servers**. The files are copied onto many servers in various locations. This is called redundancy and allows the information to be accessible even if one site goes down and needs repairs. With Internet access and a password, an individual has access to the files anytime and can share the files with others.

TABLE 8-1	Data Storage Devices
DEVICE	**EXAMPLES**
Magnetic storage device	Internal hard drive, portable hard drive
Optical storage device	Blu-Ray Disc (BD), Compact Disc (CD), Digital Versatile/Video Disc (DVD)
Flash memory device	Jump drive (also called USB flash, data stick, pen drive, keychain drive, travel drive, or thumb drive), memory card, memory stick, solid-state disk or drive (SSD)

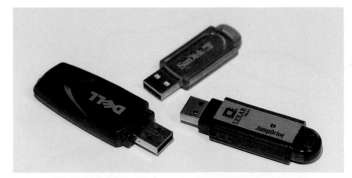

FIGURE 8-8 Jump drives, known by many different names, allow users to store documents and files for use on other computers.

TABLE 8-2   Terms for Data Storage Capacity on Electronic Devices

1 kilobyte (KB)	1,024 bytes
1 megabyte (MB)	1,024 KB (about 1 million bytes)
1 gigabyte (GB)	1,024 MB (about 1 billion bytes)
1 terabyte (TB)	1,024 GB (about 1 trillion bytes)

The capacity of storage devices also must be considered. The storage capacity of such devices is measured in bytes. Most computers consider a byte to be a character, such as a number, letter, or symbol. To simplify communication, the storage size often is estimated. For instance, 1,024 bytes might be stated as 1,000 bytes. Over the years, the size of storage devices has increased, and the cost of additional storage has decreased (Table 8-2). Flash drives range in size, and some now can hold more than 250 gigabytes (GB), or 268,435,456,000 bytes.

Network and Internet Access Devices

The computers and output devices in a healthcare facility are usually all connected to the clinic's network, which can also be called the *local area network* (LAN). The local area network can span one building or multiple buildings. Some healthcare facilities that have clinics at a distance may have wide area network (WAN) technology, which consists of two or more LANs. LAN and WAN technology can use telephone lines or fiberoptic cables that increase the speed of transmission.

A router must be used to allow multiple devices to be on the same network. Most routers used today have wireless connectivity. This peripheral hardware is a small box that may have antennas, and it uses the **ethernet**, a standard communication protocol for hardware and software. The router allows multiple computers and other devices (e.g., smart devices) to use the same network to send and receive information.

For the **computer network** to have Internet access, the medical office must subscribe with an Internet services provider (ISP) and the facility's router must be connected to a **modem**. A modem provides access to the Internet. Most routers have a specific port that is designed to connect to the ethernet port of a cable or digital subscriber line (DSL) modem. DSL is a high-speed Internet service that uses a modem to translate the computer's digital signals into voltage that is then sent over telephone lines.

Maintaining Computer Hardware

The medical assistant must maintain the computer hardware. The maintenance level will depend on the size of the ambulatory care center and whether the ambulatory care center has information technology (IT) internal or external support. The medical assistant should always do a quick check of the malfunctioning hardware before calling IT support. A quick check to see that the cables and electric cords are securely plugged in can help reduce additional downtime. Primarily, the medical assistant's role is to prevent issues from arising and to do routine cleaning.

CRITICAL THINKING APPLICATION   8-7

Christiana works with an information technology (IT) company that provides hardware, software, and services to the medical practice. How might her role with her agency's computer network differ if the practice had its own IT department?

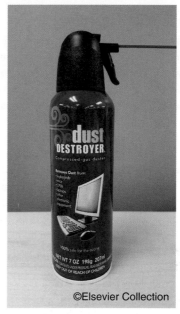

©Elsevier Collection

FIGURE 8-9 Compressed air dusters provide an efficient means of removing the dust and dirt from keyboards.

To prevent problems, the computer and all peripheral devices should be located on a stable, even surface away from heat sources. Ventilation slots should be clear, allowing air to flow into the computer to cool the components. Liquids and food should be kept away from the devices. If liquids spill on the keyboard, unplug the keyboard and tip the keyboard upside down to drain out the liquid. Let the keyboard dry overnight. Sticky liquids are more apt to damage the keyboard.

Before cleaning the computer or peripheral components, turn off and unplug the device. To remove the grime and dirt, use a damp lint-free cloth to wipe the hardware's casing. All vents and air holes should be wiped clean. For glass monitor screens, spray a household glass cleaner on a lint-free cloth and then wipe the monitor. Do not spray liquid directly on a component as the liquid may drip into the device. For nonglare monitors or antiglare screens, just use a lint-free cloth dampened with water. The keyboard usually contains a lot of bacteria. To disinfect the keyboard, spray a disinfectant on a lint-free cloth or use a disinfectant cloth and wipe each key. Avoid spraying or dripping liquids into the keyboard. To remove the dirt from the keyboard some people turn the keyboard upside down and gently shake it to remove dirt. Using compressed air dusters (i.e., pressurized air in a can) is a more efficient way to blow the dirt out of the keyboard (Figure 8-9). Air dusters can be purchased at many office supply stores. To clean the hardware, disconnect the cords and cables. Attach the extension tube to the duster and apply pressure on the trigger. Quick little bursts of air are enough to blow the dirt and dust from the hardware. Keeping the hardware clean and preventing complications help increase its useful life.

A disc should be handled with care; grasp its outer edges or center hole. Keep discs clean and dust free and store them in cases. Use a clean lint-free cloth to clean a disc, wiping in a straight line from the center of the disc toward the outer edge. Keep discs and flash drives out of sunlight and extreme heat or high-humidity environments. To prevent flash drive data loss, make sure you never unplug the flash drive while it is writing or reading data.

Computer Workstation Ergonomics

For people working on computers, it is important to arrange the workstation correctly to avoid the risk of repetitive stress injuries. Poor posture and straining can cause physical stress and injury to the body. Ergonomics is the field of study that involves reducing strain and injuries by improving the workstation design.

When you sit at a workstation, your torso and neck should be vertical and in line. The chair should be adjusted so that your feet are flat on the floor or a footrest (Figure 8-10, *A*) and your legs are comfortably below the workstation. The backrest lumbar support area should be fitted to the small of your back (Figure 8-10, *B*). The backrest should help support the upper body in the upright position. The seat pan should be the appropriate size and height to accommodate your body build so that there is no added pressure on the back of the knees or thighs. The armrest should support the forearms with the shoulders in a relaxed position (Figure 8-10, *C*). For standing workstations, your legs, torso, head, and neck should be vertical and in line. One foot can be elevated on a step.

The top of the monitor should be at or just below eye level, to prevent bending of the head or neck. The monitor should be directly in front of you and tilted to avoid glare. Use a document holder, so documents are placed at the same distance and height of the monitor, to prevent continual movement of the head as you look at the document and then at the monitor (see Figure 8-10, *D*). The keyboard should be an ergonomic split-key or waved model if possible and placed at a height and an angle that allow the wrists to be in a neutral position. The work surface and mouse should be at elbow level for typing. Your wrist should be supported by a foam wrist rest (see Figure 8-10, *E*). Headsets should be used for those answering frequent phone calls to prevent muscle strain. Laptop computers and tablets are not ergonomically designed for prolonged use.

Whether you are standing or sitting at a workstation, it is important to change positions every 30 minutes. If you are sitting, adjustments can be made to chairs or backrests. Stretching your fingers, arms, and torso is important. Frequently look away from the computer to a distant object to prevent eye strain. Stand up and walk around for a few minutes. Preventing repetitive stress injuries is important for all computer users.

Software Used in the Ambulatory Care Center

For hardware to work, the computer must have **software**, or a set of electronic instructions to operate and perform different tasks. The terms "software" and "program" are mostly synonymous. Programs existed before software. A program is a sequence of instructions, written in a language understood by the computer that directs the computer to perform a specific task. Software contains several programs that together perform a function; Web browser, e-mail, games, spreadsheet, and word processor are all types of software.

The two main categories of software are system software and application software. System software is a collection of programs that operate and control the computer. **Operating systems** and utility software are two types of system software. Operating systems, such as Windows, act as the computer's software administrator by managing, integrating, and controlling application software and hardware. Utility software helps the computer function and can include file managers, screensavers, backup software, and clipboard managers. The system software loads on the computer and operates in the background while other application software is used.

Application software (also called an *application, app,* or *application program*) allows the user or other application programs to perform specific tasks. Application software may consist of a single program or a collection of programs, called a *software package* or

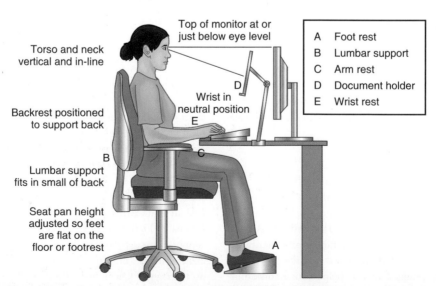

FIGURE 8-10 Medical assistants should use an ergonomically correct workstation to prevent repetitive stress injuries. Equipment that helps create this type of workstation includes a foot rest **(A)**, lumbar support **(B)**, arm rest **(C)**, document holder **(D)**, and wrist rest **(E).**

system. In the ambulatory care center, several types of application software are used. Word processing software (e.g., Microsoft Word) is used to compose letters and documents. Spreadsheet software (e.g., Microsoft Excel) is used to manage numbers, data, and expenses. Telecommunication software allows employees to e-mail patients and vendors. Antimalware software is used to protect computers against viruses (malware), which are programs that can damage the computer. (Additional security applications are discussed later in the chapter.) Database software allows the user to work with large amounts of data stored in the program. Microsoft Access, **practice management software** systems, and EHR software are examples of database software. Practice management software can include programs for scheduling, registering, billing, coding, and managing finances. Practice management software features can include appointment reminder e-mail or letter tools, bookkeeping programs, and financial analysis tools. Managers use practice management software for running their business, making processes more efficient.

The terms **electronic medical record (EMR)** and **electronic health record (EHR)** are used interchangeably by many people. However, there is a significant difference between these two types of software. When patients' records became electronic (or computerized), they were called *electronic medical records.* The EMR software contains limited information, usually related to medical treatment for one healthcare facility. The EMR was a digital version of the paper medical record. The *electronic health record* has advantages over the EMR. The EHR allows sharing of information with other providers outside the facility, including medical laboratories, nursing homes, hospitals, and specialists. The information from all types of healthcare providers can be managed in the EHR, making the EHR more of a health record than just a medical record.

It is important for the medical assistant to be aware of the differences between the practice management software and the EHR. You may use both during your day as a medical assistant, but the EHR contains a record of patient interactions and health history, whereas the practice management software allows the facility to operate the business side of the practice by maintaining schedules and financial information.

Computer Network Security

Electronic security is becoming more important in today's society as we store vast quantities of confidential and personal information in computer files. Several hospitals and clinics have had their network computer systems compromised by hackers and malware, potentially exposing patient and employee confidential information, which can lead to identity theft and other criminal actions. The Privacy Rule under the Health Insurance Portability and Accountability Act (HIPAA) and the Health Information Technology for Economic and Clinical Health Act (HITECH) require privacy and confidentiality of patient records. These acts mandate training and policies and procedures to be implemented in healthcare facilities to keep electronic records safe. Employers must provide medical record privacy and security training to new employees and periodic refreshers for current staff. Most clinics also need to comply with the **Meaningful use requirements**, which include developing a security risk analysis process to monitor for potential threats to privacy of the EHR and network files. (This process is explained in more detail later in the chapter.) Administrators and employees must work together to keep the computer network safe.

Common network security procedures used by employees include authentication, frequent password changes, and logging out of the network when leaving a workstation. Authentication means that each employee with network access must log in using a unique password. Strong passwords have more than eight characters and use a random combination of upper and lower case letters, numbers, and symbols. It is important to use different passwords and to change them frequently. Employees need to log out of the computer programs when leaving their workstation to prevent unauthorized users from viewing confidential information. Leaving the EHR open and unsupervised can allow others to document in the patient's health record using someone else's electronic signature. To prevent others from seeing the information on the screen, computer users can apply **privacy filters** to the monitor. These filters diminish the viewing angle and require the user to be directly in front of the monitor to see the content on the screen.

Administrators have additional security responsibilities. To help manage these responsibilities, many medical clinics appoint an information technology (IT) employee to oversee the security and privacy of the network. This person, who is considered the "security officer," helps the facility meet federal regulations related to electronic technology security and monitors the network for suspected breaches. Many clinics have banned employees from downloading files, which can lead to malware being introduced into the network. Some of the software and procedures used to uphold the security include encryption, firewalls, virus protection, security risk analysis, audit trails, monitoring of log-in activity, automatic log-off, and access restrictions.

Encryption software is used to encode or change the information into nonreadable or encrypted data. Another name for encrypted data is *cipher text.* This prevents unauthorized users from reading the information. An authorized user must enter a password for **decryption** to occur and make the text readable again. A **firewall** is a program or hardware device that acts as a barrier or filter between the network and the Internet. Data coming from the Internet must pass through the firewall. Data that do not meet the firewall criteria are not allowed into the network. Virus protection software (also called *antivirus* or *antimalware software*) is used in the clinic to protect against malware. This software detects and removes malicious programs. Many types of virus protection software are available, including Norton and AVG Anti-Virus.

Healthcare agencies' IT departments manage **audit trails** to track the activity of users in the software (e.g., practice management and EHRs). They can identify who has been looking at a specific patient's record or what files a person looked at while on the computer. IT also performs **security risk analysis**, which means potential threats of network breaches are identified and action plans are instituted to prevent the breaches. Log-in activity is monitored, and multiple incorrect log-in attempts are flagged. With just a few incorrect log-in attempts, some systems lock out the user. This is to prevent hackers, unauthorized users that attempt to break into networks, from cracking passwords. The security officer is responsible for managing passwords, reminding staff to change passwords, and providing staff with the adequate access levels needed for each job. Automatic log-offs are also used in the healthcare facility to safeguard records. After a period of inactivity, the workstation logs off. *Access restrictions* limit what staff members can see on the computer. The information a receptionist can view would be different from that accessible to the medical assistant, who assists the provider. Not all staff members have the same access in software programs, such as EHRs and practice management software. Those with more responsibilities typically have more access.

CRITICAL THINKING APPLICATION   8-8

Like many small healthcare facilities without an IT department, Christiana must assume a leadership role with the EHRs. She has administrator rights, which means she can assign different levels of access for the various staff members. In such a small practice, what other security measures should she consider using to ensure the privacy of EHRs? What resources might she use to implement the security measures identified?

Another important role in securing the network is to perform data backup procedures. Depending on the size of the medical facility, the network may be backed up once to several times a day. **Back up** is a process in which the network files are copied and the copy is stored in a secure off-site location. Many healthcare facilities contract with cloud backup services, which back up all the data on the network to protect against data loss. Cloud backup services are similar to cloud storage services with regard to the access of the data anytime, anywhere, but file sharing is not a typical service provided by the backup companies. When computer data are compromised, either by errors, natural causes (e.g., floods, storm damage), or human causes (e.g., fires, hackers, and malware), the data can be restored using the backup copy.

CRITICAL THINKING APPLICATION   8-9

Some healthcare facilities store network backup copies in fireproof safes on site. Why is it important to store the backup copy off site? What would be the advantage of using a data backup Internet service that has several data storage locations around the country?

Technology Advances in Healthcare

Patients are seeing more technology in healthcare settings today compared to 10 years ago. Receptionists are wearing Bluetooth headsets, which allow them to be more mobile when answering phone calls (Figure 8-11). Bluetooth is a short-range wireless communication technology that uses short-wave radio frequencies to interconnect wireless electronic devices, such as phones and headsets.

Some of the technology changes in the reception area have been instituted for HIPAA compliance. Sign-in sheets are being replaced by sign-in kiosks. Some clinics have patients enter health information using the kiosk or a tablet computer. This information is then incorporated into the EHR. For copayment collection, receptionists have card readers for credit and debit cards. The card reader machines can be mounted on the computer monitor or stand-alone units. Many have a printer feature, allowing the receptionist to print a receipt for the patient.

Clinics are using the common hospital procedure of providing patients with wristbands with bar codes. Before diagnostic tests and

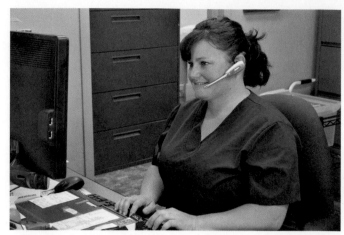

FIGURE 8-11 Bluetooth headsets are helpful for receptionists and other healthcare employees who frequently answer or make phone calls.

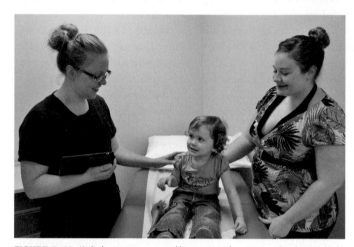

FIGURE 8-12 Medical assistants can use tablets to enter information into the electronic health record.

administration of medications, the patient's bar code is scanned, along with codes for the test or medications. This scanning process creates an automatic entry or note in the patient's EHR. This process is another step in ensuring patient safety and accuracy in billing.

Medical laboratories, ambulatory surgery centers, walk-in clinics and urgent-care centers are using patient tracking systems in both the reception area and the patient care area. Patients sign in or are signed into the system and their names go into the queue. For confidentiality purposes, patients may be given a unique number. As patients move from one area of the clinic to another, their progress shows on monitors in the reception area so family members can keep informed of their progress. Patients awaiting appointments or laboratory services can easily identify when their number moves up in the queue and/or current wait times. These tracking systems provide cost-effective ways to promote patient satisfaction while improving flow and efficiency.

In the exam room, healthcare workers are using more technology to help provide better patient care. Some clinics use wireless mobile workstations, such as **computers on wheels (COWs)** and workstations on wheels (WOWs). Providers and medical assistants use tablets, smart devices, and wearable computing devices to access EHRs and online resources (Figure 8-12). **Point-of-care** tools and apps are available for providers to use in the exam room with the patients. This technology gives providers the latest clinical information on diagnostic test results and treatments. Apps are available to help provide patients with visuals of surgical procedures, disease processes, and anatomic structures. Wearable computing devices allow healthcare employees to access medical records and information while moving around and providing patient care. Mobile devices and apps are helping providers make quicker decisions with a lower rate of error and improved patient care outcomes. With advances in Bluetooth smart technology, more medical equipment can work with apps on smart devices.

With advancements in EHR software and practice management software, new features and programs are being used. **E-prescribing** allows providers to send prescriptions to the pharmacy electronically (Figure 8-13). With voice recognition software, providers can dictate notes directly into the patient's EHR. Computerized provider/physician order entry (CPOE) is software that allows orders for medical laboratory tests, diagnostic tests, and medications to be entered into the computer. In many healthcare facilities, physicians, licensed healthcare providers, or credentialed medical assistants are able to use CPOE, which improves the efficiency of ordering tests and medications. Some healthcare agencies are hiring scribes, healthcare employees that enter data into the EHR for providers who are examining and treating patients. With all the advances in technology, medical assistants need to remain flexible and willing to adapt to changes in the workplace, while ensuring the privacy and confidentiality of patient records.

CRITICAL THINKING APPLICATION   8-10

Christiana had considered applying for a scribe position at a local healthcare facility before she was promoted to the lead administrative medical assistant. Why would a strong background in EHR be important for a scribe position?

FUNDAMENTALS OF WRITTEN COMMUNICATION

Whether electronic or paper, written communication from an ambulatory care center is a reflection of the provider and the clinic. Medical assistants commonly compose e-mails and letters to patients and vendors. A poorly worded message or incorrect punctuation in a letter or e-mail gives the reader a negative impression of the sender and thus the clinic. A medical assistant needs to know how to correctly write a letter or message to others. It is important that the sentence structure and tone of the message are professional.

Parts of Speech

A noun is a word or phrase for a person, place, thing, or idea (Table 8-3). A common noun is a general group of people, places, things, and ideas (e.g., desk, office) and a proper noun names a specific person, place or thing (e.g., Zachary, Boston). A proper noun should start with a capital letter. A pronoun is a word that takes the place of a noun (e.g., I, he, she, it, and they).

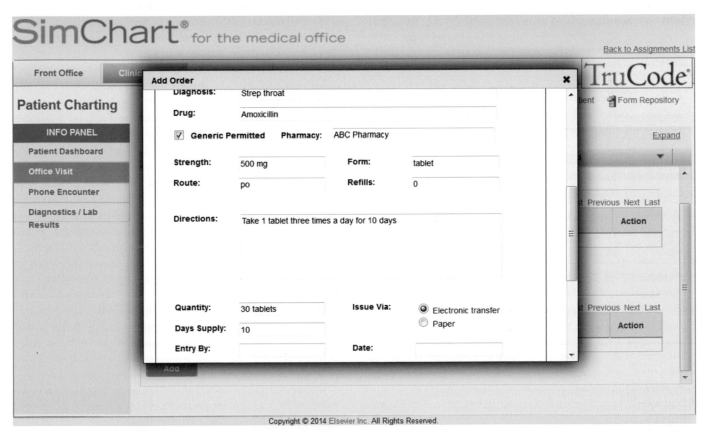

FIGURE 8-13 With e-prescribing, providers can enter the prescription information into the EHR and send it to the pharmacy. The pharmacist can easily read the information, which reduces the chance of errors.

A verb is a word or a phrase that shows action or a state of being (e.g., talks, walks, is, and are) (see Table 8-3). In a sentence the subject is a noun, pronoun, or set of words that performs the verb action (see Table 8-3). A sentence requires at least one main clause, which contains an independent subject and verb that expresses a complete thought. A fragment is a phrase without a main clause and is a major error in writing (Table 8-4). When the medical assistant composes written communication, it is important to make sure the subject and verb agree. A singular subject (e.g., provider, patient) must be matched with a singular verb (e.g., is, reads, goes). A plural subject (e.g., providers, patients) must be paired with a plural verb (e.g., are, read, go) (Table 8-4).

Many sentences also include dependent clauses, phrases, adjectives, adverbs, and prepositions. Dependent clauses often begin with words such as although, since, when, because, and if. Dependent clauses need an independent clause (e.g., subject and verb) to be a complete sentence (see Table 8-3). A phrase is a group of words without a subject or verb (see Table 8-3). An adjective is a word or group of words that describes a noun or pronoun. Adjectives come before or after the noun or pronoun they describe (see Table 8-3). An adverb is a word or group of words that answers how, where, when, or to what extent, thus further describing a verb, adjective, or other adverbs (see Table 8-3). A preposition is a word that indicates a relationship or a location between a noun or pronoun and the rest of the sentence. Examples of prepositions include near, beside, about, to, with, by, after, and in. A preposition must be accompanied by a related pronoun or noun (see Table 8-3).

CRITICAL THINKING APPLICATION   **8-11**

Christiana needs to compose a letter. How can she be sure she doesn't have any incomplete sentences in her letter? What parts of speech are required for a complete sentence?

Appropriate Use of Words

When you compose professional communications in the ambulatory care center, it is important to use language the reader will understand. Refrain from slang, generational terms, and abbreviations used with electronic communication. These can cause miscommunication with the reader. The medical assistant should know the proper use of commonly confused words and misspelled phrases (Table 8-5). Homonyms (i.e., words that sound alike) can lead to mistakes and may not always be identified by word processing software's spell-checker (Table 8-6).

A common mistake when communicating is a mismatch between the noun and pronoun number. When referring to plural nouns, use plural pronouns, such as *we, us, you, they,* and *them*. Singular pronouns, such as *I, me, you, she, her, he, him,* and *it,* should be used when referring to a singular noun. For example, "When the receptionist answers the phone, they need to be polite." The *receptionist* is a singular noun, but *they* is a plural pronoun. The noun and pronouns should agree in number, as in this example: "When receptionists answer the phones, they need to be polite."

To ensure that the message is clear to the reader, refrain from using two negatives in the same sentence. Refrain from using vague expressions or overusing the same words within a paragraph. Avoid using run-on sentences, which contain several independent clauses together without the required punctuation. Proper spelling, use of words, and sentence structure are important because they reflect on the writer and the healthcare practice.

Capitalization, Numbers, and Punctuation

Part of composing written communication is using correct capitalization and punctuation. As mentioned earlier, errors can reflect

---

TABLE 8-3   Parts of Speech

PART	EXAMPLE	USE
Noun	computer	The medical assistant used the *computer*.
Verb	greeted	The receptionist *greeted* the patient.
Subject	receptionist	The *receptionist* of the Orthopedic and Pediatric departments answers the phone.
Dependent clause	because the patient felt sick	The receptionist immediately notified the clinical medical assistant *because the patient felt sick*.
Phrase	warm exam room	A *warm exam room* helps keep the patient comfortable during a physical exam.
Adjective	warm	The *warm* room was full of patients.
Adverb	softly	The patient spoke *softly*.
Preposition	beside	The student sat *beside* the receptionist.

TABLE 8-4   Common Grammatical Errors

ERROR	INCORRECT	CORRECT
Fragment or incomplete sentence	*Greeted patients before she updating their information.*	*The receptionist always* greeted patients before she updated their information.
Nonagreement of subject and verb	The medical assistant talk to the patient. The patients is waiting for the doctor.	The medical assistant *talks* to the patient. The patients *are* waiting for the doctor.

Commonly Misspelled Words and Phrases

Anyway (not *anyways*)	Toward (not *towards*)
Supposed to (not *suppose to*)	Used to (not *use to*)

TABLE 8-5   Commonly Confused Words

WORDS	EXAMPLES
As: used in comparisons Has: to possess, own, or experience	She is *as* fast as he is on the keyboard. The medical assistant *has* increased his keyboarding speed by using the computer every day.
Lie: to recline or rest on a surface Lay: to put or place	I *lie* down to sleep. I *lay* down the book.
Set: to put or place Sit: to be seated	She *set* the gown on the table for the patient. *Sit* on the table when you have changed into a gown.
Who: refers to people; he or she did an action Whom: refers to him or her	*Who* placed the order for supplies? Mike saw *whom* yesterday?
That: refers to people, things, and groups of people Which: refers to things or groups	The letters *that* are on the printer need to be signed. The letters, *which* are on the printer, need to be signed.
Like: means "similar to" As: means "in the same manner" and requires a verb	The child is *like* her mother. He works *as* a phlebotomist.
Farther: refers to a measurable distance Further: refers to an abstract length	The clinic is *farther* away than I thought. *Further* research is needed before we purchase a new computer.

TABLE 8-6   Meanings of Common Homonyms

HOMONYMS	EXAMPLES
Affect (verb): to influence or transform Effect (noun): a result, outcome, consequence, or appearance	The outbreak of influenza will *affect* our patients. The *effect* of influenza was devastating to the city.
Accept (verb): to receive Except (preposition): excluding	Will you *accept* this certified letter? She mailed all the envelopes, *except* the certified letter.
Than (conjunction): used to compare Then (adverb): tells when	The receptionist was busier *than* the clinical medical assistant. The receptionist finished registering the patient and *then* she scheduled the appointment.
There (adverb): indicates place Their (pronoun): indicates possession They're (contraction): they are	*There* were 25 chairs in the reception area. *Their* children remained in the reception area. *They're* the only patients in the reception area.
Your (pronoun): indicates possession You're (contraction): you are	*Your* new job is in Pediatrics. *You're* working in Pediatrics today.
To (preposition): indicates direction, action, or condition Too (adverb): means "also" Two (noun): number	She went *to* answer the phone. The medical assistant's phone was ringing, *too*. Her phone has *two* lines.
Where: to, at, or in what place Were (verb): past tense plural of "be" Wear (verb): to have something on your body	*Where* did the patient go? *Were* you finished? *Wear* the gown, please.

poorly on the writer and the ambulatory care center. Professional documents should contain correct capitalization, appropriate punctuation, and the right number format.

The first letter of the first word in a sentence or question should be capitalized. The pronoun "I" should be capitalized. The first letter of proper nouns, including names of people, months, institutions, organizations, countries, and national nouns and adjectives (e.g., French, British) should be capitalized. Common nouns (e.g., girls, women, boys, men) should not be capitalized unless the word is the first word of a sentence.

A few rules apply to writing numbers. Spell out all numbers at the beginning of a sentence. Hyphenate all compound numbers from 21 to 99 (e.g., twenty-three) and all written-out fractions (e.g., two-thirds). Use commas for figures with four or more digits (e.g., 1,234). It is not advised to include a decimal point or a dollar sign when writing out sums less than a dollar (e.g., 23¢). Use noon and midnight, instead of 12:00 PM and 12:00 AM. The format for AM and PM can vary: a.m. and p.m., am and pm, AM and PM, and with or without a space between the time and AM or PM.

A sentence can end with one of three types of punctuation, a period (.), a question mark (?), or an exclamation point (!). For a sentence that makes a statement, use a period. A period goes inside a closing quotation mark (e.g., "Thank you for coming in today."). Use a question mark after a direct question. For sentences that express strong emotion, use an exclamation point. An exclamation point is rarely used in professional written communication.

Commas are frequently used in written communication (Table 8-7). A semicolon (;) is a common punctuation mark used in professional letters and documentation. The semicolon is used before certain words (however, therefore, for example) and when separating phrases in a series (e.g., "The provider is running late; however, our first two patients cancelled this morning."). A colon (:) is used to introduce a series of items either in the sentence or bulleted. A colon is also used after the greeting or salutation in a professional letter. Quotation marks (" ") are used to set off direct quotes. These are used frequently when documenting a patient's chief complaint, the main reason for the patient's visit. When using quotation marks, the periods and commas go inside the quotation marks. An apostrophe (') is used to show ownership. To show plural possession, the apostrophe is placed after the "s" (e.g., patients'). These are the most common punctuation marks used in professional correspondence and in charting in a patient's health record.

Using the correct words and punctuation marks is important when composing written correspondence. To reduce the risk of errors, the medical assistant should also perform a spelling and grammar check and proofread the document before sending it out to the recipient. Many times the reader develops an impression of the writer, the employer, and the agency based solely on written correspondence.

WRITTEN CORRESPONDENCE

Medical assistants are responsible for communicating with vendors or supply companies. They are also required to send written communication to patients and other providers as directed by their provider-employers. Knowing how to compose a professional letter is an important skill for medical assistants. To compose a letter, you must know the correct content and location for the parts of the letter. Creating an e-mail requires the writer to follow business etiquette while composing the e-mail.

TABLE 8-7   Use of Commas

RULE	EXAMPLE
Use before a coordinator (*and, but, yet, nor, for, or, so*) that links two main clauses. Do not use a comma before a coordinator that links two names, words, or phrases.	The last patient left, and the receptionist locked the door.
Use to separate items in a list.	The medical assistant escorted the mother, the father, and the child to the exam room.
Use to separate two interchangeable adjectives.	The patient was a strong, healthy child.
Use after certain words at the start of a sentence (i.e., yes, no, hello).	Yes, the bill was correct.
Use to set off the name or title or an expression that interrupts the flow of the sentence.	Will you, Michaela, want an appointment in two weeks? I am, by the way, very excited about the job opportunity.
Use after a dependent clause that starts a sentence.	If you have any questions, let me know.
Use to separate the day from the year.	May 24, 20—
Use to separate the city from its state. (*This rule does not apply when addressing envelopes.*)	Madison, Wisconsin
Can be used to separate Sr. or Jr. from the person's name, but this is not mandatory.	Bob Smith, Sr. or Bob Smith Sr. Bob Smith, Sr., has arrived for his appointment.
Use after a degree or title and to enclose the degree or title if it appears in a sentence.	John Williams, M.D. John Williams, M.D., will be the speaker for the event.
Use to set off nonessential words or phrases.	Catherine, the newest secretary, has arrived. My brother, Keith, has an appointment to see Dr. Smith.
Use with direct quotations.	She stated, "I have waited too long." "Why," I asked, "do you want tomorrow off?"

Parts of a Professional Letter

A professional letter is produced on 8.5 × 11-inch paper or letterhead paper. The letter typically has 1-inch margins on all four sides. The entire letter should be written using single line spacing. Consistency in line spacing is important for a professional appearance. The font should be a simple, easy to read one, such as Times New Roman or Arial, in a 10- or 12-point size. Limit the use of boldface and italics in the letter.

Sender's Address

The sender's address is usually located in the letterhead (Figure 8-14). Most facilities use letterhead, either preprinted or created at the top of the document using the word processing software's header tool. Depending on the ambulatory care center, the letterhead may or may not include the provider's name. It should have the clinic's name, street address or post office box, city, state, and ZIP code. Some letterheads have additional clinic contact information, such as phone numbers, website address, and an e-mail address. If letterhead is not used for a professional letter, the sender's address is placed at the left margin, 1 inch from the top of the document. Use single spacing and include the facility's address, but not the sender's name because that is located in the closing section of the letter.

Date

All professional letters must include a date. The date location is either at the left or right margin or starts at the center point of the document (see Figure 8-14). The location depends on the type of letter format used (this is discussed later in the chapter). When using letterhead, the date line starts on the second line after the letterhead. If letterhead is not used, the date line starts on the second line below the sender's address. In either situation, there should be one blank line between the date and the last line of the letterhead or sender's address.

When typing the date, write out the name of the month, then the number of the day, followed by a comma and the four-digit year. Make sure to have a blank space between the month and the day and after the comma (e.g., May 14, 20–). Do not use "th" or "st" after the day (e.g., May 14th, 20–).

Inside Address

The inside address starts between the second to the tenth line below the date line, depending on the length of the letter (see Figure 8-14). If the body of the letter is long, leave one blank line between the date and the inside address. If the body is short, add up to nine blank lines between the date line and the first line of the inside address. The goal is to have the body of the letter centered vertically on the page.

The inside address is always left-justified, regardless of your letter style. It includes the recipient's name and title on the first line, department and agency follow, and the last lines include the street address, followed by the city, state, and ZIP code. Always address the letter to a specific person. If the letter relates to a minor patient, address the letter to the guardian of the patient. When writing out the person's name, include the person's personal title (e.g., Miss, Ms., Mrs., Mr., or Dr.). If you are unsure of a woman's title preference, use Ms. Use the U.S. Postal Service format and abbreviations for the address (Table 8-8). No comma is needed between the city and state.

TABLE 8-8   U.S. Postal Service Standard Street Suffix Abbreviations

Alley	ALY	Drive	DR
Avenue	AVE	Estate	EST
Boulevard	BLVD	Highway	HWY
Bridge	BRG	Parkway	PKWY
Bypass	BYP	Road	RD
Center	CTR	Route	RTE
Circle	CIR	Street	ST
Court	CT	Terrace	TER
Crossing	XING	Way	WAY

Use the two-letter abbreviations for the states. For all other abbreviations in the address, use only approved abbreviations. For international addresses, type the name of the country in capital letters on the last line.

Reference Line

The reference line may be used occasionally. It starts on the second line below the inside address at the left margin. The salutation then is placed on the second line below the reference line. The purpose of the reference line is to refer to a specific item, such as a file, case number, or product number, and provides easy reference for the reader and sender (e.g., Reference: Invoice #44549).

Salutation

The salutation is the greeting. It starts on the second line below the inside address and is always left-justified (see Figure 8-14). For business letters, the salutation should be formal. "Dear" is followed by the person's title and name and then ends with a colon (e.g., Dear Mr. Smith:). Some clinics, when addressing patient letters, also include the person's first name (e.g., Dear Mr. Ted Smith:). If the person's gender is not known, use the first and last name without the title (e.g., Dear Chris Smith:). The phrase "To Whom It May Concern" can also be used if a person's name is not known.

Subject Line

This notation, which is not used very often, would be left-justified and placed on the second line below the salutation. The body of the letter starts on the second line below the subject line. The purpose of the subject line is to state the main subject of the letter. The subject line should be composed using bold face, underlining, or all capital letters because this would draw the reader's attention (SUBJECT: ORDER NO. 45677-93).

Body of the Letter

The body of the letter starts on the second line below the salutation (see Figure 8-14). Depending on the type of letter, the body may be either left-justified or left-justified with each paragraph indented. There should be one blank line between paragraphs. The body of the

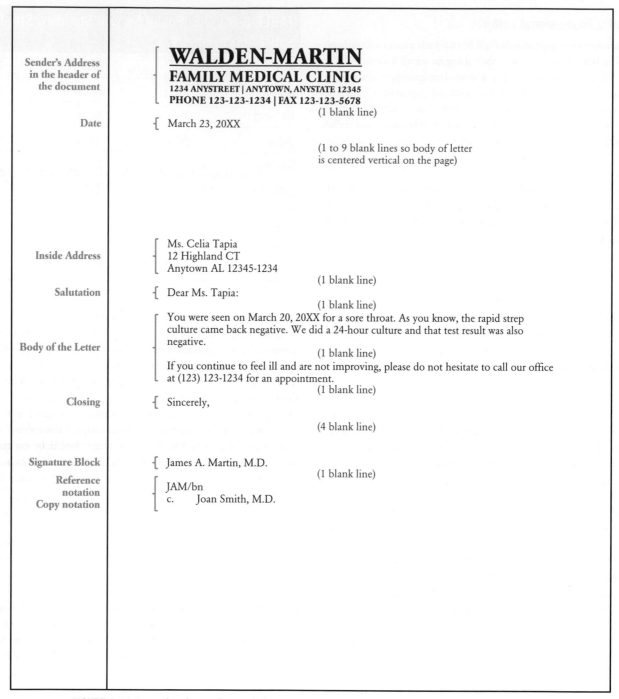

FIGURE 8-14 Business letter format. When a medical assistant types a letter for a provider, the letter must be signed by that provider after it has been printed.

letter should be vertically in the middle of the page. Depending on the size of the letter, additional blank lines may be added after the date and before the inside address to move the body to the center of the page.

The body of the letter contains the content of the letter. The first paragraph is a friendly opening and states the purpose of the letter. The remaining paragraphs support the purpose of the letter and should be concise. The final paragraph may give a request for a specific action.

Closing

The closing is positioned vertically in the same position as the date (see Figure 8-14). There should be one blank line between the last line of the body of the letter and the closing. The first word should include a capital letter, although remaining words in the closing should be in lower case. Typically, "Sincerely" is used; more formal closings include "Yours truly" or "Very truly yours." The word or phrase is followed by a comma.

Signature Block

The signature block includes the signature, typed name, and title of the sender. There should be four blank lines between the closing and the typed name and credentials of the sender. This space allows the person to sign the letter. The person's title is capitalized and on the line directly below the typed name (e.g., Director of Walden-Martin Family Medicine Clinic). If the medical assistant typed the letter for a provider, the letter must be signed by that individual after it has been printed (see Figure 8-14).

CRITICAL THINKING APPLICATION   **8-12**

Christiana is composing several letters. Who would sign each letter?
- A letter to a patient indicating her test results.
- A letter to a vendor asking for specific pricing for a new computer.
- A letter to a referring physician, thanking him for the patient referral.

End Notations

Several items may be noted on the letter after the signature block. This may vary from agency to agency.

- The reference notation notes the initials of the person who composed the letter (e.g., MR) followed by the initials of the person who typed the letter (e.g., bn) (see Figure 8-14). A colon (:) or a forward slash (/) divides the two sets of initials (e.g., MR:bn, MR/bn). This notation should be left-justified on the second line below the last line of the signature block.
- The enclosure/attachment notation indicates the number of documents or attachments that accompany the letter. The enclosure notation is left-justified and starts on the second line below the reference notation. If the reference notation is not present, the enclosure notation is placed on the second line below the last line of the signature block. The enclosure notation can be typed in several ways. It can be indicated with either "Enclosure" or "Enc." If more than one enclosure is sent, the number of enclosures or the names of the enclosures should be indicated.
- The copy notation (c.) is used to notify the letter's recipient who also received a copy of the letter. The "c" is left-justified and goes on the line immediately following the last notation. It is then followed by a period. Use the tab tool to move ½ inch before typing the person's name (e.g., c. John Smith). Additional names should be aligned vertically on the document. You may still see letters that have "cc:," which means carbon copy or courtesy copy. Before computers and copy machines, duplicate letters were created by using carbon sheets placed between papers, thus creating carbon copies. With computers, "c." means "copy."
- Blind copy (bc.) is used if the sender does not want the recipient to know a copy was sent to another person. The format is the same as "c.," but the "bc." is added only to the office copy of the letter, not to the letter going to the recipient.

CRITICAL THINKING APPLICATION   **8-13**

For the letters that Christiana will sign, should she include a reference notation at the bottom of the letter? Why or why not? For the letters prepared by Christiana and signed by Dr. Brown, should she add the reference notation? Why or why not?

Suggested Styles for an Enclosure Notation

Any of the following three formats can be used to indicate that an enclosure is included with the letter:

Enclosures: 2

Enclosures (2)

Enclosures:
1. Draft of the policy statement
2. Invoice #45433

Continuation Pages

If the letter requires more than one page, the subsequent pages should be on paper that matches the letter but does not have the letterhead printing. Usually, letterhead paper is 20 to 24 lb bond paper (e.g., the thicker the paper, the larger the lb bond number). Each sheet after the letterhead must have a heading that includes these elements on separate lines: the recipient's name, the page number, and the date. The name should be on the first line below the top margin, and all three elements should be left-justified.

Ms. Celia Tapia
Page 2
March 23, 20–

Business Letter Formats

Three main formats are used to compose a business letter. The formats vary slightly in the position of certain elements of the letter. Although the location of the elements may change, the spacing between the elements remains the same (Table 8-9). It is important for a medical assistant to be able to compose a professional letter (Procedure 8-1).

Full Block Letter Format

The full block format is the most common type of business letter (Figure 8-15). All elements are left-justified, meaning the elements start at the left margin of the document. Typically for business letters, "closed" punctuation is used. Closed punctuation means the document is typed using the punctuation marks described earlier in this chapter. Closed punctuation gives the letter a professional appearance.

Informal full block–formatted letters can use open punctuation, which means minimal punctuation is used in the letter. The body is the only part of the letter that contains the normal grammatical punctuation. No punctuation appears in the sender's or inside addresses, date, salutation, and the closing. This is a current

TABLE 8-9 Business Letter Formats

LETTER TYPE	FORMAT WITH VARIATIONS
Full block format	• Left-justified: All elements • Professional business letters use "closed" punctuation • Informal letters can use "open" punctuation
Modified block format	• Left-justified: Sender's address (if not using letterhead) and inside address • Center point or right-justified: Date, closing, and signature block start
Semi-block format (or modified block with indented paragraphs)	• Left-justified: Sender's address (if not using letterhead) and inside address • Center point or right-justified: Date, closing, and signature block start • Indented paragraphs 5 spaces

trend with electronic technology and letters produced by word processing, although it should not be used with professional letters.

Modified Block Letter Format

With the modified block format, the body and the inside address are left-justified. If letterhead is not used, the sender's address is also left-justified. The date, closing, and the signature block start either at the center point of the document or are right justified. If the center point is used, all three elements must start at that point (Figure 8-16). The text flows toward the right margin, and the three elements vertically line up in the document. When you use the right justified technique, the text for these three elements finish in a vertical line at the right margin (Figure 8-17).

Semi–Block Letter Format

The semi–block letter format can also be called the modified block with indented paragraphs (see Figure 8-17). The semi–block format resembles the modified block format with the three elements (i.e.,

---

PROCEDURE 8-1 | Compose Professional Correspondence Using Electronic Technology: Compose a Professional Business Letter

Goal: *To compose a professional letter using technology.*

Scenario: *Create a letter for the following scenario: Jean Burke, NP, has requested that you compose a letter to Janine Butler (DOB 04/25/1968) and let her know that her mammogram from last Wednesday was negative. She should make a follow-up appointment in 6 months. If she has any questions, she should call the office. Janine's address is: 37 Park West Avenue, Anytown, AL 12345-1234. You are working at Walden-Martin Family Medical Clinic. The practice's address is: 1234 Anystreet, Anytown, AL 12345. The phone number is 123-123-1234 and the fax number is 123-123-5678.*

EQUIPMENT and SUPPLIES

- Patient's health record
- Computer with word processing software and printer
- Paper or letterhead paper
- #10 envelope

PROCEDURAL STEPS

1. Obtain the intended recipient's contact information and determine the message to convey to the recipient.
   <u>PURPOSE</u>: This gives you a focus when composing the letter. You will need the recipient's information to create the letter.
2. Using the computer and word processing software, compose the letter using one of the three business letter formats. If using blank paper, create a letterhead in the header of the document and include the clinic's name, street address or Post Office box, city, state, and ZIP code.
   <u>PURPOSE</u>: The information in the letterhead provides the reader contact information for the clinic.
3. Type the date in the correct location using the correct format. Have one blank line between the date line and the last line of the letterhead.
   <u>PURPOSE</u>: All letters require a date for legal purposes.
4. Type the inside address using the correct spelling, punctuation, and location for the information. Leave 1 to 9 blank lines between the date and the inside address, depending on the location of the body of the letter.
   <u>PURPOSE</u>: The body of the letter must be centered vertically from the top to the bottom of the document. More blank lines can be added to move the body to the correct location (see Figure 8-14).
5. Starting on the second line below the inside address, type the salutation, using the correct format.
   <u>PURPOSE</u>: A proper greeting helps set the tone of the letter.
6. Use your critical thinking skills to compose a concise, accurate message. Type the message in the body of the letter using the proper location and format. There should be a blank line after the salutation and between each paragraph. The message should be clear, concise, and professional. Use proper grammar, punctuation, capitalization, and sentence structure.
   <u>PURPOSE</u>: Proper grammar helps convey the message accurately and professionally.
7. Type a proper closing, leaving one blank line between the last line of the body and the closing. Use the correct format and location.
   <u>PURPOSE</u>: The closing helps end the message with a professional tone.

PROCEDURE 8-1   *—continued*

8. Type the signature block using the correct format and location. If a typist is preparing the letter for a provider, he or she must include a reference notation. There should be four blank lines between the closing and the signature block.
   <u>PURPOSE</u>: The signature block provides the reader with the name of the sender of the letter. The reference notation identifies who typed the letter.

9. Spell-check and proofread the document. Check for proper tone, grammar, punctuation, capitalization and sentence structure. Check for proper spacing between the parts of the letter.
   <u>PURPOSE</u>: The spell-checker identifies only certain errors; proofreading helps you find incorrect word use, improper tone, and errors in formatting.

10. Make any final corrections. Print the document on letterhead or on regular paper on which you have inserted the letterhead.

11. Address the envelope, using either the computer and word processing software or a pen and following the correct format. After addressing the envelope, give the letter with the envelope
   <u>PURPOSE</u>: Following the Post Office guidelines on format helps prevent a delay in delivery of the letter. The provider is the sender of the letter and should have the opportunity to review it before it is mailed to the patient.

12. File a copy of the letter in the paper medical record or upload an electronic copy of the letter to the electronic health record (EHR).
   <u>PURPOSE</u>: A copy of all correspondence should be kept in the patient's health record.

13. Fold the letter using the correct technique and place it in the envelope.

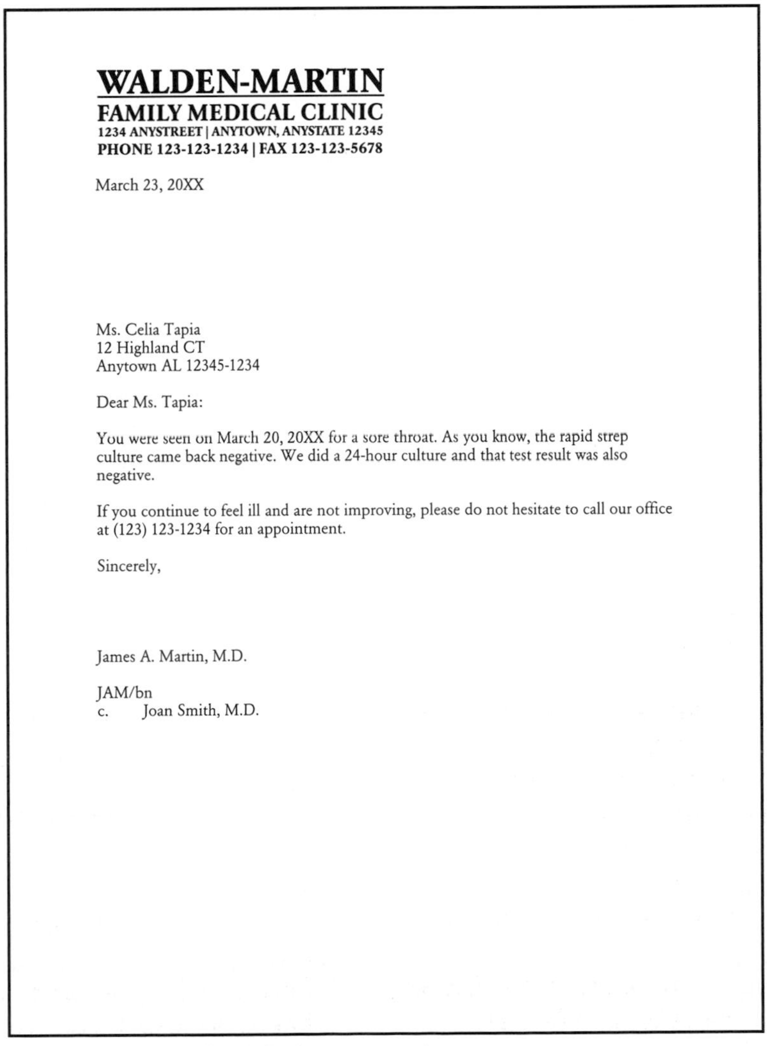

WALDEN-MARTIN
FAMILY MEDICAL CLINIC
1234 ANYSTREET | ANYTOWN, ANYSTATE 12345
PHONE 123-123-1234 | FAX 123-123-5678

March 23, 20XX

Ms. Celia Tapia
12 Highland CT
Anytown AL 12345-1234

Dear Ms. Tapia:

You were seen on March 20, 20XX for a sore throat. As you know, the rapid strep culture came back negative. We did a 24-hour culture and that test result was also negative.

If you continue to feel ill and are not improving, please do not hesitate to call our office at (123) 123-1234 for an appointment.

Sincerely,

James A. Martin, M.D.

JAM/bn
c.   Joan Smith, M.D.

FIGURE 8-15 Full block letter format.

WALDEN-MARTIN
FAMILY MEDICAL CLINIC
1234 ANYSTREET | ANYTOWN, ANYSTATE 12345
PHONE 123-123-1234 | FAX 123-123-5678
(1 blank line)
March 23, 20XX

(1 to 9 blank lines so body of letter
is centered vertical on the page)

Ms. Celia Tapia
12 Highland CT
Anytown AL 12345-1234
(1 blank line)
Dear Ms. Tapia:
(1 blank line)
You were seen on March 20, 20XX for a sore throat. As you know, the rapid strep
culture came back negative. We did a 24-hour culture and that test result was also
negative.
(1 blank line)
If you continue to feel ill and are not improving, please do not hesitate to call our office
at (123) 123-1234 for an appointment.
(1 blank line)
Sincerely,

(4 blank line)

James A. Martin, M.D.
(1 blank line)
JAM/bn
c.   Joan Smith, M.D.

FIGURE 8-16 Modified block letter format, showing the date, closing, and signature block starting at the center point of the document.

date, closing, and signature block) right-justified or starting at the center point of the document. The difference with the semi–block format is the indented paragraph or paragraphs in the body of the letter. The paragraphs should be indented five spaces.

Letter Templates

Using one of the business letter formats, a medical assistant can design a letter template, which is a sample letter that can be personalized for the patient. For routine communication with patients (e.g., normal laboratory results or appointment reminders), a letter template can be created. You can use the practice management software, EHR, or word processing software to merge the patient data into the letter template, creating an individualized letter for the patient. This is an efficient method of providing a customer-friendly document for a patient.

Preparing the Letter for Delivery

Business letters should be enclosed in business-sized envelopes, the standard #10 envelope, which is 4.125 × 9.5 inches. Business envelopes are available with a few variations, including the type of flap, preprinted return address, and a window envelope. The window envelope and the #6¾ envelope may be used for statements to patients. The envelopes can be white, manila, or made of recycled paper.

When the automated mail processing machine at the post office reads the envelope, it reads the bottom line of the recipient's address (i.e., city, state and ZIP code) before moving up and reading the next line. To ensure timely delivery, use the following tips when addressing mail:

- Type the envelope using a simple black font of at least 10-point size. Use all capital letters and no punctuation marks (Figure 8-18).
- Put one space between the city and state and two spaces between the state and ZIP code.
- If you can't fit the suite or apartment number on the same line as the delivery address, put it on the line above the delivery address, not below it.
- Use ZIP code + 4 code (e.g., 55555-1111) as often as possible. This allows the piece of mail to be directed to a more precise location than when just using the ZIP code.
- Do not put anything (e.g., logo, slogan, attention line) below the last line of the delivery address. The machine will read that and your letter may get misrouted or delayed.
- Use only approved U.S. Postal Service abbreviations.

WALDEN-MARTIN
FAMILY MEDICAL CLINIC
1234 ANYSTREET | ANYTOWN, ANYSTATE 12345
PHONE 123-123-1234 | FAX 123-123-5678

March 23, 20XX

Ms. Celia Tapia
12 Highland CT
Anytown AL 12345-1234

Dear Ms. Tapia:

You were seen on March 20, 20XX for a sore throat. As you know, the rapid strep culture came back negative. We did a 24-hour culture and that test result was also negative.

If you continue to feel ill and are not improving, please do not hesitate to call our office at (123) 123-1234 for an appointment.

Sincerely,

James A. Martin, M.D.

JAM/bn
c.   Joan Smith, M.D.

FIGURE 8-17 Semi–block letter format (also called modified block with indented paragraph letter format). This letter uses right justification for the date, closing, and signature block.

The medical assistant should fold the letter by pulling up the bottom end of the letter until it reaches just below the inside address or two-thirds of the way up the letter. Crease the paper. Then fold the top of the letter down so it is flush with the bottom fold and crease the paper. For windowed business envelopes, fold the letter in a Z pattern. With the letter's print side facing up, place the envelope over the top third of the letter. Fold the bottom edge of the paper up to the bottom edge of the envelope and crease the paper. Then remove the envelope and flip the letter over so the backside of the document is facing up. Fold the top of the letter down to the prior crease line and crease the paper. The letterhead and recipient's addresses should then be visible. Place the letter in the envelope so that the recipient's address shows through the window.

Memorandums

Memorandums, or memos, are communication documents within an agency. They address one topic and provide a message to the reader. Use the **portrait orientation** for the document and 1-inch margins. Memorandums typically have four headings:

- **To**: Include the name of the recipient or recipients and omit the titles (e.g., Mr., Mrs.). For a number of recipients, each name can be followed by a comma, or each name can be on its own line.
- **From**: Include the name of the sender of the memo. It is optional if the sender initials the memo before it is sent.
- **Date**: Spell out the month and follow it with the day and year (e.g., May 23, 20–).
- **Subject**: Include the topic of the memo.

The headings are left-justified (Figure 8-19). Boldface and capital letters are used for the headings, and a colon (:) follows the heading. The information should be in regular font, with a mix of capital and small letters. The information should be aligned vertically down the page, using the tab tool in the word processing software. The date should be written out as indicated for professional letters.

The headings may be separated from the body of the memo by a centered black line that extends from 2 inches to the entire width of the page. Regardless if the line is used or not, there should be two to three blank lines separating the headers from the body of the memo. The body of the memo should be single-spaced and

Return Address
Use same format as the
delivery address

WALDEN-MARTIN FAMILY MEDICAL CLINIC
1234 ANYSTREET
ANYTOWN AL 12345-1235

Postage

CELIA TAPIA
12 HIGHLAND CT
ANYTOWN AL 12345-1234

Delivery Address
1st line: Recipient's Name
2nd line: Company name
3rd line: Post Office box or street address, including Apartment or Suite number
4th line: City, State (2 letter abbreviation), zip code

FIGURE 8-18 Address format for an envelope.

TO:	Staff
FROM:	James Martin, M.D.
DATE:	December 15, 20XX
SUBJECT:	Holiday Office Hours

The office will be closed at noon on December 24, 20XX through December 26th. We will reopen at our normal time on December 27, 20XX. We will then close at 3 p.m. on December 31st for the holiday and will reopen at our normal time on January 2, 20XX.

FIGURE 8-19 Format for a memorandum.

left-justified. If it consists of multiple paragraphs, skip a single line between paragraphs. The content in the body of the letter should be clear, concise, and informative. The writer does not need to add a closing or signature. Special notations, including reference, copy, and enclosures, can be added to the bottom of the memo and are formatted as indicated in the End Notations section.

Professional E-Mails

The use of electronic communication between the ambulatory care center staff and patients is increasing, and medical assistants need to know how to compose a professional e-mail (Procedure 8-2). Following e-mail etiquette is important for maintaining a customer-friendly environment. Tips on writing customer-friendly e-mails include:

- If you are sending the e-mail to several people, separate each e-mail address by a semicolon (;).
- Add an e-mail address to the cc line if another person needs to receive a courtesy copy of the e-mail.
- Make sure to include a subject on the subject line. Delete any messy FWD: or RE: RE: strings.
- Start with a greeting (salutation), which includes a formal greeting followed by the person's title and name (e.g., "Good morning, Mr. Jones," "Dear Mr. Jones,").
- Be courteous, polite, and respectful in your words and tone. Maintain the appropriate level of formality in the e-mail. Be gracious, using expressions such as "please" and "thank you."
- Refrain from using all capital letters because many people consider that to be "shouting" in e-mails.

PROCEDURE 8-2	Compose Professional Correspondence Utilizing Electronic Technology: Compose a Professional E-Mail

Goal: *To compose a professional e-mail that conveys the message to the reader clearly, concisely, and accurately.*

Scenario: *Create an e-mail for the following scenario: Johnny Parker (DOB 06/15/2010) has an appointment at 10:00 AM. next Tuesday. Send his guardian an appointment reminder via e-mail. Johnny will be seeing Jean Burke, NP. The guardian should bring in any medications Johnny is currently taking. You are working at Walden-Martin Family Medical Clinic. The practice's address is: 1234 Anystreet, Anytown, AL 12345. The phone number is 123-123-1234 and the fax number is 123-123-5678. Your instructor will supply you with the guardian's name and e-mail address.*

EQUIPMENT and SUPPLIES

- Patient's health record
- Computer with e-mail software

PROCEDURAL STEPS

1. Obtain the intended recipient's contact information and determine the message to convey to the recipient.
   PURPOSE: This gives you a focus when composing the e-mail. You will need the recipient's information to create the e-mail.

2. Using the computer and e-mail software, type in the recipient's e-mail address. If the e-mail has two recipients, use a semicolon (;) after the name of the first recipient. Double-check the e-mail addresses for accuracy.
   PURPOSE: If the e-mail address is incorrect, the e-mail will not get to the recipient.

3. Type in a subject, keeping it simple but focused on the contents of the e-mail.
   PURPOSE: In many e-mail software packages, the user can search for e-mails using the subject field. Keeping the subject simple and focused makes it easier for the user to find the message.

4. Type a formal greeting, using correct punctuation.
   PURPOSE: A proper greeting helps set the tone of the letter.

5. Type the message in the body of the e-mail using proper grammar, punctuation, capitalization, and sentence structure. Avoid abbreviations. The message should be clear, concise, and professional.
   PURPOSE: Using proper grammar and avoiding abbreviations help convey the message accurately and professionally.

6. Finish the e-mail with closing remarks.
   PURPOSE: In the closing, you can thank the recipient or encourage him or her to follow up with concerns or questions. This gives the e-mail a professional tone.

7. Type a closing, followed by your name and title on the next line. Include the clinic's name and contact information below your name.
   PURPOSE: The e-mail clearly states who is sending it.

8. Spell-check and proofread the e-mail. Check for proper tone, grammar, punctuation, capitalization, and sentence structure. Check for proper spacing between the parts of the e-mail.
   PURPOSE: White space or spacing between the elements of an e-mail helps separate the parts of the e-mail, making it easier to read.

9. Make any final revisions, select any features to apply to the e-mail, and then send it.
   PURPOSE: If the e-mail is urgent (!), that feature should be selected before you send the e-mail. If you require a confirmation e-mail when the e-mail is opened, this can also be selected.

10. Print a copy of the e-mail to be filed in the paper medical record or upload an electronic copy of the e-mail to the patient's electronic health record (EHR).
    PURPOSE: A copy of all correspondence should be kept in the patient's health record.

- Write out the entire word and refrain from using abbreviations and emoticons.
- Use proper capitalization, grammar, sentence structure, and punctuation. Check the spelling of the e-mail before sending it. Most e-mail software has a spell-checker.
- Be concise, accurate, and clear in your message.
- Always end your e-mail with "Thank you" or "Sincerely" and your complete name. For business e-mails, include contact information after your name, including the agency's address, phone number, and fax number.
- Leave white space (i.e., one blank line) between the salutation, paragraphs, and your complete name.
- Zip large attachments before sending the files. **Zip** is a computer program that compresses a file or folder, making it smaller and easier to send. The receiver uses an unzip program to extract the contents.
- Many e-mail programs have features such as (!) urgent or a response box that sends an e-mail back to the sender when the e-mail is opened by the recipient. Use the urgent feature only for crucial e-mails.

CRITICAL THINKING APPLICATION   **8-14**

Christiana receives an e-mail from a patient that is in all capital letters. How might she perceive the situation with the patient? How could she verify her perceptions? How should she handle this situation?

Some healthcare facilities may also include language in e-mails related to confidentiality and whom to contact if the e-mail was sent to the wrong address. Medical assistants must adhere to the facility's confidentiality rules when communicating with or about patients. Copies of e-mail communications should be uploaded to the patient's EHR for a permanent record of the electronic communication.

EHR software frequently contains clinical messaging or clinical e-mail features. This feature is an e-mail within the EHR. The clinical messaging feature provides secure communication for healthcare employees to converse about the patient. For instance, the message may be sent from the receptionist to the medical assistant regarding a patient who called requesting a refill. The medical assistant can then follow up with the provider regarding the refill.

Faxed Communication

Fax (short for facsimile) machines send and receive documents using the phone lines. In the healthcare facility, the fax machine may be part of a copy machine, or the computers may have software that allows faxes to be sent and received. As communications technology has advanced, the use of fax machines has decreased, but they are still an important piece of equipment in the ambulatory care center.

When sending a fax, you must adhere to HIPAA and HITECH rules. Healthcare facilities usually have a required face sheet (the first sheet) that includes confidentiality language, which instructs the recipient, if he or she is not the intended party, to destroy the fax and contact the medical facility. Besides the confidentiality statement, the face sheet should include the contact information for sender and recipient, the date, and the total number of pages.

CLOSING COMMENTS

Patient Education

If the medical assistant is responsible for preparing patient education materials using the computer's word processing program, it is important that these materials contain correct grammar, spelling, punctuation, and sentence structure. The appearance of brochures and documents created by the ambulatory care center staff reflects on the medical practice. The medical assistant should proofread all documents carefully before printing them.

Legal and Ethical Issues

The medical assistant should keep a copy of all documents produced using word processing. A copy of any document sent to a patient must also be uploaded into the patient's EHR. All patient-related documents are confidential, and the medical assistant must ensure the security and privacy of the information.

Professional Behaviors

Written communication in any form requires the medical assistant to be respectful, polite, and professional. It is important to proofread all written communication before it is sent to the recipient. Spell-checker tools can help identify misspelled words and sometimes incorrect usage of grammar and punctuation. However, these tools cannot always identify a word used incorrectly; only proofreading can capture those errors. Proofreading also allows the reader to reassess the tone of the communication, making sure it is appropriate. Finally, the medical assistant should recheck the spelling of the person's name and address for accuracy. A well-composed message gives the reader a reassuring sense of the accuracy and professionalism of the healthcare facility's staff.

SUMMARY OF SCENARIO

Since her promotion, Christiana has learned many helpful administrative and computer procedures. She also has been implementing changes in the administrative area. Her first change was to e-mail, rather than mail, appointment reminders. She uses the appointment reminder feature of the practice management software when e-mailing the notifications to patients. Not only does this save time for the practice, but it also saves postage costs. Christiana also has learned how to create letter and memo templates. She uses templates to notify patients about laboratory and diagnostic test results. She continues to create custom letters for patients, yet saves time by using predesigned templates.

Christiana has learned a great deal about the medical practice's computer network, and she is implementing more security measures. For example, she is training staff members to log out of their workstations before leaving the computer. She also is working with a local IT company to beef up the network's protection against unauthorized users. She has contracted with an online backup service to protect the network files.

Christiana enjoys her new position and knows that she will need to stay up to date on technologic changes and privacy mandates. She plans to do this by reading online articles and attending continuing education events. She realizes that learning is an ongoing process that can help her become the professional she strives to be every day.

SUMMARY OF LEARNING OBJECTIVES

1. **Define, spell, and pronounce the terms listed in the vocabulary.**
   Spelling and pronouncing medical terms correctly reinforce the medical assistant's credibility. Knowing the definitions of these terms promotes confidence in communication with patients and co-workers.

2. **Explain what a personal computer is, and identify input and output hardware for personal computers.**
   A personal computer (PC) is a relatively inexpensive piece of hardware that is used by a single person. It can be a desktop, laptop, or tablet computer. The medical assistant should be knowledgeable about input and output hardware used in the healthcare environment. As technology advances, more input devices will be used in ambulatory care facilities. Medical assistants may need to help coach patients in the use of such devices if the healthcare agency has patients electronically enter personal data.

3. **Identify internal computer components, secondary storage devices, and network and Internet access devices.**
   Because medical assistants can have a variety of roles in ambulatory care centers, they must understand important computer features. Learning the names and functions of the internal components better equips medical assistants to purchase computers or deal with computer issues. Learning about secondary storage devices helps them identify what is needed by the ambulatory care practice. The computers and output devices in a healthcare facility are usually all connected to the clinic's network, which can be called the local area network (LAN). A router is used to allow multiple devices to be used on the same network. For the computer network to have Internet access, the ambulatory care center must subscribe to an Internet services provider and be connected to a modem.

4. **Explain how to maintain computer hardware.**
   Computer hardware should be located on a stable, even surface away from heat sources. Keep ventilation slots clear. Before cleaning the computer or peripheral components, turn off and unplug the device. To remove the grime and dirt, use a damp, lint-free cloth to wipe the hardware's casing. All vents and air holes should be wiped clean. For glass monitor screens, spray a household glass cleaner on a lint-free cloth and then wipe the monitor. For nonglare monitors or antiglare screens, just use a lint-free cloth dampened with water. To disinfect the keyboard, spray a disinfectant on a lint-free cloth or use a disinfectant cloth and wipe each key. To remove the dirt from the keyboard, turn the keyboard upside down and gently shake it to remove dirt or use compressed air dusters.

5. **Identify principles of ergonomics that apply to a computer workstation.**
   When sitting at a workstation, your torso and neck should be vertical and in line. The chair should be adjusted so that your feet are flat on the floor or a footrest and your legs are comfortably below the workstation. The backrest lumbar support area should be fitted to the small of your back, and it should help support the upper body in the upright position. The seat pan should be the appropriate size and height to accommodate your body build so that there is no added pressure on the back of the knees or thighs. The armrest should support the forearms with the shoulders in a relaxed position. For standing workstations, your legs, torso, head, and neck should be vertical and in line. One foot can be elevated on a step.

   The monitor should be directly in front of you and tilted to avoid glare. The top of the monitor should be at or just below eye level, to prevent bending of the head or neck. Use a document holder to prevent continual movement of the head. The keyboard should be an ergonomic split-key or waved model if possible and placed at a height and an angle that allow the wrists to be in a neutral position. The work surface and mouse should be at elbow level for typing. The wrists should be supported by a foam wrist rest. Headsets should be used for those answering frequent phone calls to prevent muscle strain.

6. **Differentiate between:**
   - *System software and application software.*
     System software is a collection of programs that operate and control the computer. Operating systems and utility software are two types

Continued

SUMMARY OF LEARNING OBJECTIVES—*continued*

of system software. The system software loads on the computer and operates in the background while other application software is used. Application software allows the user or other application programs to perform specific tasks. Application software may consist of a single program or a collection of programs. Examples of application software include word processing, spreadsheets, telecommunication, antimalware, and databases.

- *Electronic medical records (EMRs) and a practice management system.* As more ambulatory care facilities move to EMRs, electronic health records (EHRs), and practice management software, the medical assistant should be able to distinguish between the EMR and the practice management system. The EMR is used to document patient-related information, whereas the practice management software is used to run the "business." Scheduling, billing, and coding programs are part of the practice management software typically used in the healthcare agency.

7. **Explain the importance of data backup and other computer network security activities performed in the healthcare setting.**
   To abide by HIPAA rules and the meaningful use requirement, healthcare agencies must ensure that their computer networks are secure. Data backup procedures can help prevent problems if the network files are compromised by a hacker or an environmental situation (e.g., fire or flood).

8. **Discuss applications of electronic technology.**
   With the advances in technology, the healthcare environment has seen many changes, including portable devices in the exam room, improved procedural equipment, and increased efficiencies in the workday through the use of computers. More changes in technology will occur over the next few years; some will help healthcare institutions stay compliant with HIPAA, whereas others will support quicker and more accurate treatment of patients. Being flexible and willing to use new technology will be critical for medical assistants in the future.

9. **Recognize the elements of fundamental writing skills.**
   Medical assistants need to compose correspondence to patients and other businesses. They also need to create memos, meeting minutes, and other documents. Knowing the parts of speech helps medical assistants create complete sentences, which are crucial for professional written communications. It is also imperative to understand the appropriate use of words.

10. **Explain the guidelines for using capitalization, numbers, and punctuation in business communication.**
    Knowing the guidelines for using capitalization, numbers, and punctuation in business communication is crucial when composing professional documents. Correct word usage and spelling also are critical. The medical assistant should use the spell-checker in the word processing software when creating documents. Proofreading as a final step is also important to catch any incorrect words or incomplete sentences.

11. **Describe each component of a professional business letter.**
    Medical assistants should be familiar with the components or elements of a professional business letter. They must include the appropriate information and punctuation in each section of the letter to achieve professional results. Proper and consistent spacing in the letter provides the polished, professional appearance for which medical assistants should strive when creating letters through word processing.

12. **Summarize the formats for business letters and memorandums.**
    Written communication from a healthcare facility is a reflection on that facility. Using the proper format for business letters and e-mails is crucial for professional results. There are three main types of business letters: full block letter format, modified block letter format, and semi–block letter format. Procedure 8-1 provides guidance for composing a professional letter. Even though memos are internal documents, the medical assistant must use the correct format so that the reader obtains a clear message. A poorly created memo is a reflection on the writer.

13. **Compose professional correspondence using electronic technology.**
    With more patients communicating by e-mail with the ambulatory care staff, medical assistants must be able to write professional e-mails. E-mails must send a clear message to the recipient in a professional and respectful manner. The process of composing a professional e-mail is outlined in Procedure 8-2. When sending a fax, the medical assistant must follow HIPAA and HITECH rules.

CONNECTIONS

📖 Study Guide Connection: Go to the Chapter 8 Study Guide. Read and complete the activities.

evolve Evolve Connection: Go to the Chapter 8 link at *evolve.elsevier.com/kinn* to complete the Chapter Review Quiz. Check out the other resources listed for this chapter to make the most of what you have learned from Technology and Written Communication.

9

TELEPHONE TECHNIQUES

Ashlynn McDowell, a recent graduate of a medical assisting program, has begun her first position as a receptionist in an obstetrician's office. Ashlynn's lifelong goal has been to work in obstetrics, and she is determined to perform to the best of her abilities. However, she has never held a job in a professional office. She knows that she needs to practice all the skills she learned in school to be an effective receptionist.

Ashlynn works for Dr. Stella Frank, who is customer service—oriented and wants her patients to feel cared for and special. She insists that all their concerns be taken seriously. Ashlynn is anxious to build trust with the patients and offer them help with the problems they encounter that fall within her realm of responsibility.

Dr. Frank recently purchased computer software that allows Ashlynn to record telephone messages on the computer, and these messages are automatically routed both to an inbox for the provider and as an entry in the patient's health record. Although the system is new to everyone in the office, Ashlynn is determined to become proficient in its use as quickly as possible.

She knows that she must speak clearly and distinctly and must be adept at follow-up skills. She plans to dress professionally each day so that she projects the right image to the patients with whom she comes in contact. Ashlynn will strive to be the type of employee who has a willingness to learn, an ability to adapt, and a heart full of compassion for the patient. She is a team player who sincerely wants to cooperate with other staff members who might need her help.

Dr. Frank is pleased that she has found such an eager person to add to her staff and will assist and guide Ashlynn as she learns how to make the patients feel like part of the clinic family. Ashlynn's self-esteem has increased because she feels she is making a great contribution to healthcare.

While studying this chapter, think about the following questions:
- Why does tone of voice play an important role in patient perception?
- What can a medical assistant do to promote a positive image of the healthcare facility when using the telephone with patients?
- How can the medical assistant reduce patients' frustration with telephone issues?

LEARNING OBJECTIVES

1. Define, spell, and pronounce the terms listed in the vocabulary.
2. Identify and explain the features of a multiple-line telephone system, and also explain how each can be used effectively in a healthcare facility.
3. Do the following related to effective use of the telephone:
   - Discuss the telephone equipment needed by a healthcare facility.
   - Summarize active listening skills.
   - Demonstrate effective and professional telephone techniques.
   - Consider the importance of tone of voice and enunciation.
4. Explain the importance of thinking ahead when managing telephone calls; also, describe the correct way to answer the telephone in the office.
5. Discuss the screening of incoming calls, and list several questions to ask when handling an emergency call.
6. Do the following related to taking a message:
   - Document telephone messages accurately.
   - List the seven elements of a correctly handled telephone message.
   - Report relevant information concisely and accurately.
7. Discuss various types of common incoming calls and how to deal with each.
8. Discuss various types of special incoming calls and how to deal with each.
9. Discuss how the medical assistant should handle various types of difficult calls.
10. Discuss typical outgoing calls, including why knowledge of time zones and long distance calling is necessary.
11. Discuss the use of a telephone directory, and describe how answering services and automatic call routing systems are used in a healthcare facility.
12. Discuss the legal and ethical issues related to telephone techniques.

VOCABULARY

answering service A commercial service that answers telephone calls for its clients.

automatic call routing A system that distributes incoming calls to a specific group or person based on customer need; for example, the customer presses 1 for appointments, 2 for billing questions, and so on.

call forwarding A telephone feature that allows calls made to one number to be forwarded to another specified number.

caller ID A feature that identifies and displays the telephone numbers of incoming calls made to a particular line.

conference call A telephone call in which a caller can speak with several people at the same time.

emergency An unexpected, life-threatening situation that requires immediate action.

enunciation The use of articulate, clear sounds when speaking.

headset A set of headphones with a microphone attached, used especially in telephone communication.

intercom A two-way communication system with a microphone and loudspeaker at each station; often a feature of business telephones.

jargon The technical terminology or characteristic idioms of a particular group or special activity, as opposed to common, everyday terms.

monotone A succession of syllables, words, or sentences spoken in an unvaried key or pitch.

multiple-line telephone system A business telephone system that allows for more than one telephone line.

participating provider A physician or other healthcare provider who enters into a contract with a specific insurance company or program and by doing so agrees to abide by certain rules and regulations set forth by that particular third-party payer.

pitch The depth of a tone or sound; a distinctive quality of sound.

provider An individual or company that provides medical care and services to a patient or the public.

screen Something that shields, protects, or hides; to select or eliminate through a screening process.

speakerphone A telephone with a loudspeaker and a microphone; it can be used without having to pick up and hold the handset.

speed dialing A telephone function in which a selected stored number can be dialed by pressing only one key.

STAT The medical abbreviation for the Latin term *statum,* meaning immediately; at this moment.

tactful The quality of having a keen sense of what to do or say to maintain good relations with others or to prevent offense.

triage The process of assigning degrees of urgency to patients' conditions.

urgent An acute situation that requires immediate attention but is not life-threatening.

voice mail An electronic system that allows messages from telephone callers to be recorded and stored.

The telephone is one of the most important pieces of equipment used in a healthcare facility (Figure 9-1). It is used to communicate with patients, other healthcare organizations, and suppliers. It would be difficult to run an office without a telephone. It is often the first point of contact with patients, and this is an opportunity to make an outstanding first impression. Developing good telephone techniques will make you a valuable asset to your employer.

TELEPHONE EQUIPMENT

Multiple-Line Telephone

Familiarity with a **multiple-line telephone system** (Figure 9-2) is a must for the medical assistant. Even the smallest healthcare facility has at least two telephone lines so that patients rarely get a busy signal when they try to contact the office. The multiple-line telephone has a button for each line, and the button flashes when a call comes in on that line. The button also flashes, although in a different rhythm, when a caller is on hold on that line; this can serve as a reminder for the medical assistant to check back with the caller to see whether he or she would like to remain on hold or leave a message.

The multiple-line telephone also allows you to transfer calls and possibly to set up conference calls, which involve two or more callers. You should familiarize yourself with the multiple-line telephone system used in your healthcare practice.

Headset

Most business telephones have a handset that can be used to answer the telephone. However, the medical assistant who most frequently is responsible for answering the telephone may want to consider using a **headset** instead (Figure 9-3). Use of a headset can improve your ergonomics and help prevent neck strain. Also, having a headset frees your hands to use the computer or take a message.

A headset is a combination earphone and microphone that is attached to the telephone by a cord or is wireless. You can adjust the volume in the earpiece, and you may be able to adjust the volume of your voice through the microphone for callers who may have difficulty hearing. Bluetooth, a type of short-range wireless technology, allows you to be more mobile while on the telephone. Because this type of headset is not as visible, people may not be aware that you are on the telephone and may start a conversation with you. You should politely indicate that you are on the telephone and you will respond to the person when you can. Some healthcare facilities have a light system that indicates to a patient that you are on the phone and you will be with them when the call is complete. Many headsets can be muted so that you can speak with someone without the caller hearing you.

Features

Most multiple-line business telephones have many features that allow you to perform a number of different tasks in the healthcare facility.

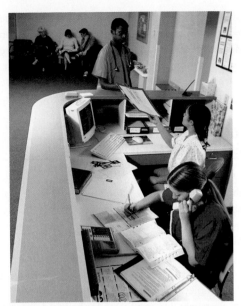

FIGURE 9-1 The telephone plays a vital role in the success of a medical practice.

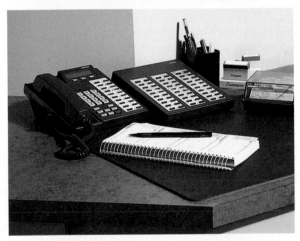

FIGURE 9-2 Multiple-line telephones allow numerous calls to come into the office at once. Each call deserves the same kind of attention and care from the medical assistant.

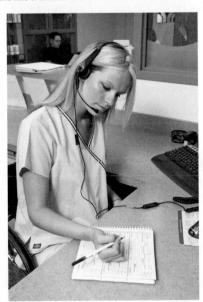

FIGURE 9-3 A headset allows the medical assistant to keep the hands free while using the telephone and is better ergonomically.

Speakerphone

The **speakerphone** function allows you to hear and speak to the caller without using the handset or a headset. Generally, a button on the telephone is labeled "speaker" (or is indicated with an icon), and once you push it, you can hang up the handset. This can be useful if you need to have more than two people on the call using the same phone.

You should always inform the caller that you will be putting him or her on speakerphone, and let the person know who else will be listening in. You must also be conscious of protecting patient information when using a speakerphone. The speakerphone function should not be used in areas such as the patient check-in area or anywhere a conversation can be overheard. The door or reception window should be closed so that no one just walking by can overhear the conversation.

Conference Calls

As mentioned, many multiple-line telephones allow you to set up **a conference call**, in which you can have multiple people on the call from different locations. The person initiating the call calls one person, puts that person on hold, and continues the sequence until all parties are on the call. Conference calls can be used when the healthcare facility has more than one location and people from all the locations must be involved in a conversation. For example, a committee may want to discuss policies and procedures for the practice. It is a much better use of time to set up a conference call than to have many people travel to one location.

Caller ID

Caller ID allows the user to see who is calling before he or she picks up the handset to answer the telephone. The caller's telephone number and name appear on a screen, and the user can decide whether to take the call. If the user subscribes to call-waiting services, another benefit, called *call-waiting caller ID,* is often available. This function allows the user to see who is calling even when the user is already on the telephone.

Voice Mail

Voice mail is widely used in today's business offices because it affords an around-the-clock method for receiving patient messages. Unfortunately, it can prove frustrating to those who find themselves speaking to an electronic device more often than a human being. Voice mail allows the caller to hear a recorded message that may also provide information about what to do in case of an emergency. Similar to an answering machine, voice mail records a caller's message, which can later be retrieved, and allows special temporary greetings when the user is away from the office. You can keep patients happy by answering voice mail messages promptly.

Call Forwarding

Call forwarding allows the user to forward calls to another designated number, such as an answering service. Usually a code is entered, then the telephone number to which the calls should be forwarded. If the medical assistant is going to be busy with a patient, the calls can be forwarded to another employee until the task is completed. This prevents the user from missing important calls when away from the main telephone.

Intercom

The business telephone in the healthcare facility may also have **intercom** capabilities. This feature allows for two-way communication, but it does not require you to pick up the handset or use a headset. This type of communication is not confidential, but it can be used to notify staff members of an emergency or to ask the provider to come out of the exam room.

CRITICAL THINKING APPLICATION   9-1

Ashlynn hears an employee using the speakerphone function to talk about a patient with another employee. How should she handle this situation? To whom, if anyone, should Ashlynn report this activity? What problems might be caused if this type of conversation is overheard?

Call Hold

The multiple-line business telephone has a hold button that allows you to interrupt a call temporarily. This often is used when you have answered an incoming call and then another line rings. You can put the first call on hold, answer the second call and put that person on hold, and then return to the first call. It is very important to be courteous and respectful of the caller. You should always ask if you can put the caller on hold and wait for a response before you push the hold button. You can also use this feature if you need to retrieve some information or speak to someone else to get some information.

Speed Dialing

Speed dialing allows you to program keys on the telephone keypad to automatically call a stored telephone number by just pressing one key. For example, if the healthcare facility uses a particular laboratory for specimen testing, the telephone number for that laboratory can be programmed for the numeral 1 on the telephone keypad; then, when you want to call that laboratory, you only need to press 1 and the call will be made. Speed dialing can be a time-saver; however, all staff members must know which telephone numbers have been programmed into particular keypad numbers.

Cell Phones

Considered a luxury item only 10 years ago, cell (or cellular) phones have become commonplace. Many people no longer have a landline because of the expenses of having two phones, and the cell phone usually is the better buy for the money. Several of the more popular cell phone companies offer free long distance calls in the United States and may provide users free night and weekend minutes. Most of today's smart phones even allow the user to access the Internet and check e-mail on their telephone. Cell phone companies usually offer a text messaging service, which allows the user to enter a message with cell phone keys, usually one that is a full QWERTY keyboard, which then is sent directly to a cell phone number.

Many people have a personal cell phone or smart phone. It is a great way to be accessible at all times, but it also can present some issues in a healthcare facility, particularly in regard to patient confidentiality. Most cell phones have a camera that could be used to take pictures of confidential information, and that information can be transmitted quickly to someone else or put on the Internet. Calls can be made or taken at inopportune times and may affect the care of patients. Most healthcare facilities have a policy that prohibits employees from having their personal cell phones with them during working hours.

TELEPHONE EQUIPMENT NEEDS OF A HEALTHCARE FACILITY

Number and Placement of Telephones

Few healthcare facilities can get along with just one telephone line. Two incoming lines, along with a private outgoing line with a separate number for the **provider's** exclusive use, is the minimum recommended number of lines.

One medical assistant can handle no more than two incoming lines; therefore, the addition of more lines may involve additional staffing. If a staff member is assigned solely to dealing with insurance and billing, a separate line and listing in the telephone directory for this service may considerably lessen the load on the main incoming lines.

Telephones should be placed where they are accessible but private. Each provider, in addition to the office manager, requires a telephone at his or her desk. A telephone should be available in the laboratory area and the clinical area, and multiple phones should be present in reception and business office areas. Many healthcare facilities also have a telephone available for patients to use. This telephone often has a separate line so that patient use does not interfere with the staff members' work.

EFFECTIVE USE OF THE TELEPHONE

Active Listening

It may seem odd to start out discussing listening instead of speaking in the Telephone Techniques chapter, but listening well while on the telephone is just as important as speaking well when it comes to communicating on the telephone. When you are on the telephone, you have fewer nonverbal cues to help you determine the message; therefore, it is very important that you use good listening skills. When you use active listening skills, your patients realize that you think they are important and that you respect the message they are communicating to you, whether you are on the telephone or face-to-face.

Active Listening

- Be present in the moment.
- Focus solely on the conversation.
- Don't interrupt.
- Don't start forming your response before the person has finished speaking.
- Confirm what the speaker has said, and ask if your interpretation is correct.
- Always be respectful and professional.

Active listening involves listening to what the speaker is saying, interpreting what the message is, and restating the message to make sure that you have received the intended message. For example, you receive a telephone call from a distraught mother. Using active listening skills, you pick up on the nonverbal cues, such as her tone of voice and rate of speech, and you can tell she is upset. The mother states that her child has been very sick for the past several days, and nothing she has done has helped with the fever her child has had for 2 days. Your response should be to restate what you have heard: the child has been ill with a fever for the past 2 days, and nothing she has tried has brought the fever down. This gives the caller the opportunity to correct any misinformation or to confirm that the information is correct. If it is correct, you should follow the healthcare practice's procedures for handling this situation; most likely, you will schedule an appointment for that same day.

Developing a Pleasing Telephone Personality

Each time a medical assistant answers the telephone, he or she is representing the healthcare practice (Procedure 9-1). The manner in which the telephone is answered can influence the caller's impression of the whole office and whether the person wants to be seen there. When patients call the healthcare facility, they should hear a friendly yet professional voice. Just as active listening is an important skill to receive the message being sent, a pleasing telephone personality facilitates the sending of the message.

Although it may seem silly, you should always smile when you answer the telephone. The physical act of smiling affects how your words sound. It is as if your caller can hear you smile, and you have created a positive impression.

It is also important to be aware of nonverbal communication that occurs during a telephone conversation. Be aware of your tone of voice. Is it helping to send the message that you want to send? Your callers can tell if you are preoccupied and not focused on the current conversation. You should vary the **pitch** of your voice and avoid speaking in a **monotone**.

Nonvisual/Nonverbal Communication

- Tone of voice
- Speed of speech
- Pitch
- Volume
- Enunciation
- Pausing or hesitation

Enunciation is crucial when speaking on the telephone. You should speak very clearly and distinctly so that the caller can understand what you are saying. Many letters of the alphabet sound very

similar on the telephone, such as B, P, T, and F and S. You may need to clarify with the caller by saying, "That is B as in bravo."

Phonetic Alphabet

A	Alpha	N	November
B	Bravo	O	Oscar
C	Charlie	P	Papa
D	Delta	Q	Quebec
E	Echo	R	Romeo
F	Foxtrot	S	Sierra
G	Golf	T	Tango
H	Hotel	U	Uniform
I	India	V	Victor
J	Juliet	W	Whiskey
K	Kilo	X	X-ray
L	Lima	Y	Yankee
M	Mike	Z	Zulu

It is important to always be courteous and **tactful**. Think about the words you will be using before actually speaking them. For those of us working in a healthcare facility, it is easy to integrate medical terminology into our conversations. However, we must be careful not to use medical **jargon** when speaking with patients because this makes the message more difficult for them to understand. For example, if you are giving a male patient preprocedural instructions, advise him that he must not eat or drink anything for 12 hours before the procedure; do not tell him he should "stay NPO" (nothing by mouth).

To create a pleasant, friendly, and professional image of the healthcare facility, you must give the caller your full attention. Do not become distracted by other things going on around you. In addition, you should never eat, chew gum, or drink when on the telephone. Use a normal volume and tone of voice, and speak directly into the mouthpiece. Be sure to speak at a moderate rate of speed because speaking too quickly makes it difficult for the caller to understand you.

CRITICAL THINKING APPLICATION 9-2

Ashlynn has a tendency to speak a little fast in her normal conversations. How will she need to adjust as she is answering phones in the healthcare facility? She also is a friendly person and enjoys talking on the phone. What precautions should she take so that this does not become an issue on the job?

PROCEDURE 9-1   Demonstrate Professional Telephone Techniques

Goal: *To answer the telephone in a provider's office in a professional manner and respond to a request for action.*

Case Study: *Charles Johnson, DOB 3/3/1958, an established patient of Dr. Martin, has called to schedule an appointment to have his blood pressure checked. This will be a follow-up appointment that is 15 minutes long. He is requesting that the appointment be on a Friday during his lunchtime between 11:00 and 12:00.*

EQUIPMENT and SUPPLIES

- Telephone
- Pen or pencil
- Appointment book or EHR with appointment scheduling abilities
- Computer
- Notepad

PROCEDURAL STEPS

1. Demonstrate telephone techniques by answering the telephone by the third ring.
   PURPOSE: To convey interest in the caller by answering promptly. This makes a positive impression on the caller.
2. Speak distinctly with a pleasant tone and expression, at a moderate rate, and with sufficient volume for the person to understand every word.
3. Identify the office and/or provider and yourself.
   PURPOSE: To assure the caller that the correct number has been reached and to identify the staff member.
4. Verify the identity of the caller, and if using an electronic health record, bring the patient's health record to the active screen of the computer.
   PURPOSE: To confirm the origin of the call.
5. Screen the call if necessary.

PURPOSE: To determine whether the caller has an emergency and needs immediate attention or referral to a hospital emergency department.

6. Apply active listening skills to assess whether the caller is distressed or agitated and to determine the concern to be addressed.
   PURPOSE: To make sure the medical assistant hears and understands the message being sent by the patient and to show that the patient has the medical assistant's full attention.
7. Determine the needs of the caller and provide the requested information or service if possible. Provide the caller with excellent customer service. Be as helpful as possible. Check the appointment schedule and determine the first Friday that would have an open appointment between 11:00 and 12:00.
   PURPOSE: To allow the medical assistant to handle many calls and conserve the provider's and staff members' time and energy.
8. Obtain sufficient patient information to schedule the appointment, including the patient's full name, DOB, insurance information, and preferred contact method. Repeat the date and time of the appointment to ensure that the patient has the correct information.
9. Terminate the call in a pleasant manner and replace the receiver gently, always allowing the caller to hang up first.
   PURPOSE: To promote good public relations, provide excellent customer service, and ensure that the caller has no further questions.

MANAGING TELEPHONE CALLS

Thinking Ahead

Whether you are answering incoming calls or placing outgoing calls, it is important to be completely prepared. Before you start answering calls, make sure you have all the supplies needed to do your job. For example, for taking messages, you should have access to a computer (if your office documents telephone messages electronically) or a paper message form, in addition to working pens and a watch or clock to record the time. Many offices also keep a list of commonly used telephone numbers. Such a list includes poison control, other emergency numbers, community resources to which patients can be referred, and so on.

For outgoing calls, have all the information you need, such as the patient's health record, the telephone number of the person you will be calling, a list of questions, and a pad and a pen to make notes during the conversation.

Confidentiality

All communication in a healthcare facility must maintain patient confidentiality. When using the telephone, you must be aware of what is going on around you and who may be able to overhear your conversation. If patient-sensitive information will be discussed, place the call in an area where others cannot hear, especially other patients. Be careful when using a speakerphone because the sound can travel farther than you might think, and someone might overhear private medical information—this is a violation of the law, specifically the Health Insurance Portability and Accountability Act (HIPAA).

Answering Promptly

As mentioned earlier, telephone contact is often the first interaction with a patient. If the person's call is not answered promptly, this can create a negative impression before he or she even talks to someone. It is important that a call be answered within three rings. To accomplish this, you may need to do the following: (1) interrupt the call you are on by asking if you can place the person on hold for a moment; (2) answer the second call; if it is not an emergency, ask that person if you may place him or her on hold; and (3) return to the first caller.

An incoming call should never be answered with "Please hold." You should always find out the nature of the call before placing the person on hold. If it is an emergency, the second call is handled promptly, before you return to the first call. If it is not an emergency, you should always ask if you can place the person on hold and wait for an answer before pushing the hold button. If the person refuses to be placed on hold, determine the reason why and assure them that you will return to his or her call quickly.

The medical assistant who routinely answers the telephone should know how to activate emergency medical services (EMS) in his or her area. Generally, this means dialing 911. You may need to make this call for a patient who has called the healthcare facility and is now unable to contact EMS on her own. If your phone system allows it, you can set up a conference call that includes the patient, EMS, and yourself. It is important to get a telephone number where the caller can be reached if you get disconnected. It also is important to keep the patient and/or caregivers on the line while contacting EMS.

Identifying the Facility

When answering incoming telephone calls, the medical assistant should identify the facility first, state his or her name, and then follow with an offer of help. For example: "Good morning, Walden-Martin Family Medical Clinic. This is Ashlynn. How may I help you?" Medical assistants must always follow the policy of the healthcare facility when answering incoming calls. Speaking slowly and smoothly, with good enunciation, ensures that your callers understand whom they have reached.

CRITICAL THINKING APPLICATION   9-3

Most offices dictate how the phone is to be answered. What should Ashlynn do if she is very uncomfortable with the way she is asked to answer the phone? Who ultimately should decide how the phone is answered?

Identifying the Caller

If the caller does not offer a name, the medical assistant should ask, "May I ask who is calling?" It can be helpful to write down the caller's name and try to use it at least three times during the conversation, if it does not compromise patient confidentiality. This helps make a strong connection with the patient and assures the person that he or she has been identified correctly.

Occasionally callers refuse to identify themselves to the medical assistant and insist that they speak with the provider. You must be clear, in a professional manner, that you cannot connect the caller to the provider without knowing who the caller is. The caller may be a sales representative who knows that if she identifies herself, she will not get the opportunity to talk with the provider. When it becomes clear that the caller will not give a name but still insists on speaking with the provider, you can tell the person that the provider is busy with patients and has asked that messages be taken; if the caller cannot leave a name for the message, then he or she may want to write a letter and mark it Personal. Most people do not want to wait for a response to a letter and will then give you their names so that a message can be taken.

Screening Incoming Calls

Most healthcare facilities expect the medical assistant answering the telephone to **screen** the calls. You must determine which calls should be routed directly to the provider, which to the **triage** area, or which to the billing office. The provider, office manager, and staff members who will be answering the telephone should work together to develop policies for screening calls.

The first step in screening calls is to determine who the caller is and the nature of the call. If the call is from a patient with a question about a statement he or she just received in the mail, the call can be transferred to the appropriate area. If the call involves determining whether a patient should be seen that day, it can be transferred to the triage area. If the caller asks to speak directly to the provider, the situation can become more complicated, and healthcare facility policies should be created to address these cases.

Healthcare facility policies often state that calls from other providers are put through immediately. If that is not possible, assure the caller that the provider will return the call as soon as possible. Some providers may also ask that calls be put through immediately for certain family members. If the provider does not want to take the calls, the medical assistant must tactfully tell the caller that the provider cannot be disturbed at this time.

Screening policies also should address how calls should be handled when the provider is out of the office. If the provider is to be out of the office for an extended period (e.g., for a conference or vacation), another provider usually is designated to handle calls. It should be explained to the patient that the provider that he or she asked for is out of the office, but another provider is taking the calls. If the call is not an emergency, take a message, and the designated provider can return the call.

If a call is an **emergency**, the policies for handling emergency calls apply. Many emergency calls require judgment on the part of the person answering the telephone in the medical practice. Good judgment comes from experience and proper training by the provider with regard to what constitutes a real emergency in each type of practice and how such calls should be handled. The person answering the telephone first should determine whether the call is truly urgent. If so, never hang up the telephone until an ambulance reaches the patient or other help arrives. When necessary, ask another staff member to call 911 while remaining on the line with the patient. Emergency calls may include such conditions and/or symptoms as chest pain, profuse bleeding, severe allergic reactions, cessation of breathing, injuries resulting in loss of consciousness, and broken bones. An **urgent** call may be an adult patient with a fever over 102° F (38.9° C), an animal bite, or an increasingly painful ear infection. Emergency calls are life-threatening, whereas an urgent call requires prompt attention but is not life-threatening. In the case of emergencies, often the provider instructs the patient to go straight to the closest hospital emergency department instead of the office. Policies and procedures manuals should indicate the action to take in emergency situations. When in doubt, always ask the office manager and/or the provider.

If the provider is in, the call may need to be transferred to him or her immediately. All offices should have a written plan of action for the times the provider is not physically present in the office. These policies should include typical questions to ask the caller to determine the validity and disposition of an emergency. Some examples of questions to ask include:

- At what telephone number can you be reached?
- Where are you located?

- What are the chief symptoms?
- When did they start?
- Has this happened before?
- Are you alone?
- Do you have transportation?

Screening Guidelines

In a facility with multiple employees, the provider may designate one individual, such as a nurse or an experienced and trained medical assistant, as the telephone screener. Every healthcare facility would be wise to have a written telephone protocol for handling urgent situations and emergencies. The protocol should state that employees are bound by the written guidelines and that unauthorized personnel may give no advice. If advice is given, it may be grounds for dismissal.

A special sheet of instructions listing specific medical emergencies (e.g., chest pain, heavy bleeding, fainting, seizure, and poisoning) should be posted by each telephone. The telephone numbers for the nearest poison control center, hospital, and ambulance should be listed.

Emergency calls should be routed to a provider immediately. Additional instructions should include what action to take if no provider is available (e.g., sending the patient to an emergency department or calling for an ambulance). Most offices have some means of constant contact with the provider, whether by pager, cell phone, or another method.

Getting the Information the Provider Needs

As the medical assistant gains experience and knows the provider better, he or she begins to have a sense of the questions the provider will have for patients who call the facility. For example, the provider is interested in how long the patient has had symptoms, what makes the symptoms better or worse, what remedies have been tried, what has worked and not worked, and other specifics about the condition. If the patient complains of painful urination, the medical assistant learns to ask about pain in the back or blood in the urine. One way to learn about questions to ask is to listen to the provider carefully as he or she questions patients about their symptoms. This can help you learn more about signs and symptoms and enable you to be a better assistant to the provider.

Remember to always be "patient with your patients." Those who call the healthcare facility for help are almost never at their best. When feeling ill, people often are short tempered and even display poor manners. Some can be verbally abusive. Care for patients as if they were family members, and they will feel care and compassion in the medical facility.

If the provider is unavailable for only part of the day, take a message and inform the caller that the provider currently is out of the office but will return calls when he or she returns. It is important to give the caller the time frame in which the provider will be returning those calls so that the patient's time is not wasted in sitting by the phone, waiting for the call. It should be stressed that the time frame is approximate because emergencies cannot be predicted. If the caller is unavailable when the provider usually returns calls, ask what would be a convenient time and let the caller know you will try to work with that time frame.

Screening calls is an important task for medical assistants who answer the telephone. It can keep the healthcare facility running on schedule and ensure that calls that need to get to the provider do so immediately.

Placing Callers on Hold

The medical assistant should always ask before placing a caller on hold. If it has been determined through the screening process that this is a call that does not need to be put through to the provider right away, or if the call needs to be transferred to someone else in the healthcare facility and that person is not immediately available, you should ask if the caller would like to be put on hold, or if he or she would prefer to be called back. If you know that the person with whom the caller needs to speak may be busy for quite a while, inform the caller of that. The caller may still want to wait. You should check back periodically to make sure the caller still wants to remain on hold. No longer than 1 minute should pass before you check back with the caller. When you return to the call, you can use a statement such as, "Thank you for waiting. Would you like to continue to hold, or should I take a message?"

Minimizing the wait for the caller shows concern, and freeing up the telephone lines is important for other people trying to contact the healthcare facility.

Transferring a Call

During the screening process, the medical assistant may determine that the call should be transferred to the provider or to another person in the facility. Consider the following example: Ms. Fields calls your office because she has a billing question. You should ask Ms. Fields' permission before placing her on hold, and wait for a response. It is also helpful to give Ms. Fields the name and extension of the person to whom you will be transferring her call (if it is not the provider); this way, if Ms. Fields' call happens to get disconnected, she will have that information when she calls back. Once you have Ms. Fields' permission to put her on hold, you should contact the person to whom the call is being transferred; in this case, that is Mr. Lewis in the billing department. Tell Mr. Lewis who is calling and the reason for the call; this allows Mr. Lewis to be prepared to help Ms. Fields when the connection is made. Mr. Lewis may ask for a moment to pull up information before you put Ms. Fields' call through. You should stay on the line to introduce Ms. Fields to Mr. Lewis and to make sure the connection is made. If Mr. Lewis is unavailable, you should ask Ms. Fields if she would like to be connected to his voice mail. Some callers may prefer that you take a message in written form and bring it to the proper person.

Medical assistants who answer telephone calls must know who does what in the healthcare facility. An organizational chart with telephone extensions can be helpful, but it must be kept up to date so that calls can be transferred successfully.

Taking a Message

Telephone messages, whether taken in a handwritten or an electronic format, are an important part of patient care (Procedure 9-2). The patient relies on the medical assistant to get the message to the appropriate person. Taking messages allows information to be delivered to a provider or an appropriate person, who can make a decision (then or later), which can be communicated back to the patient without interrupting the flow of patients through the healthcare facility. You should be sure to let the caller know when to expect a call back; for example, explain that the provider usually returns calls between 3 and 4 PM.

Whether the message is taken in a handwritten or an electronic format, the information needed for a complete message is the same:

1. The name of the person calling
2. The name of the person to whom the call is directed
3. The caller's daytime, evening, and/or cell phone number
4. The reason for the call, including the telephone number of the caller's pharmacy if a medication is requested
5. The action to be taken
6. The date and time of the call
7. The initials of the person who took the call

PROCEDURE 9-2	Document Telephone Messages and Report Relevant Information Concisely and Accurately

Goal: *To take an accurate telephone message and follow up on the requests made by the caller.*

Case Study: *Norma Washington, DOB 8/1/1944, an established patient of Dr. Martin, has called to report her blood pressure readings that she has been taking at home. Dr. Martin had made a recent change in her medication and wanted her to monitor her BP at home for 3 days and call in with the results. She has taken her blood pressure in the morning and in the evening for the past three days, with the following results:*

Day 1 : 144/92 in the AM, 156/94 in the PM
Day 2: 136/84 in the AM, 142/86 in the PM
Day 3: 132/80 in the AM, 138/82 in the PM

EQUIPMENT and SUPPLIES

- Telephone
- Computer
- Message pad
- Pen or pencil
- Notepad Health record

PROCEDURAL STEPS

1. Demonstrate telephone techniques by answering the telephone using the guidelines in Procedure 9-1.
   PURPOSE: To answer promptly and courteously, which conveys interest in the caller and promotes good customer service.
2. Using a message pad or the computer, take the phone message (either on paper or by data entry into the computer) and obtain the following information:
   - Name of the person to whom the call is directed
   - Name of the person calling
   - Caller's telephone number
   - Reason for the call
   - Action to be taken
   - Date and time of the call
   - Initials of the person taking the call
   PURPOSE: To have accurate information, which allows the staff member or provider to address the caller's issues quickly and efficiently.
3. Apply active listening skills and repeat the information back to the caller after recording the message.
   PURPOSE: To verify that all the information was recorded accurately.
4. End the call and wait for the caller to hang up first.
5. Document the telephone call with all pertinent information in the patient's health record.
   PURPOSE: To ensure that the patient's health record is kept up to date.
6. Deliver the phone message to the appropriate person.
7. Follow up on important messages.
   PURPOSE: To make sure important issues are addressed in a timely manner.
8. If using paper messaging, keep old message books for future reference. Carbonless copies allow the facility to keep a permanent record of phone messages. If using an electronic system, the message will be saved to the patient's record automatically.
   PURPOSE: To have a permanent source of messages in case the information is needed after the paper message has been discarded. This can also serve as a telephone log.
9. File pertinent phone messages in the patient's health record. Make sure the computer record is closed after the documentation has been done.
   PURPOSE: To keep a permanent record of important information in the patient's chart.

Messages Taken on Paper

Many types of message pads or books are available (Figure 9-4). Many are pressure-sensitive, making a copy of the message and serving as a telephone call log. The original is given to the person the message is for and the medical assistant will have a copy to use for follow-up. Having legible handwriting is a must when taking a manual, handwritten message.

Messages Recorded Electronically

Most electronic health record (EHR) systems can record telephone messages (Figure 9-5). The EHR automatically saves a copy of the message to the patient's health record and sends the message to the provider, who can either call the patient directly or give the medical assistant directions to respond to the patient. The electronic system may also be able to flag a message, to indicate its urgency, or that it requires a call back, or that a prescription refill is requested.

Taking Action on Telephone Messages

The message process is not complete until the necessary action has been taken. If a handwritten system is used, use an identifying mark to indicate a message that requires action. If an electronic system is used, check periodically during the day to be sure you do not have to complete the response to the message, such as calling the patient back or contacting the pharmacy. For risk management purposes, the healthcare facility should have a policy on the documentation of telephone messages and the specific information that must be included. Medical assistants should become familiar with that policy.

Retaining Records of Telephone Messages

If a handwritten system is used for recording telephone messages, the healthcare facility must establish a policy on the retention of telephone message records. If the message relates to patient care, a copy of the message should be added to the patient's health record. If the health record is electronic, this may mean scanning in a copy of the paper message and attaching it to the EHR. The copy in the

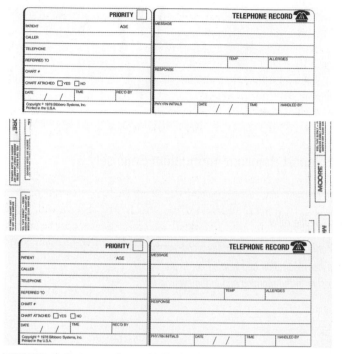

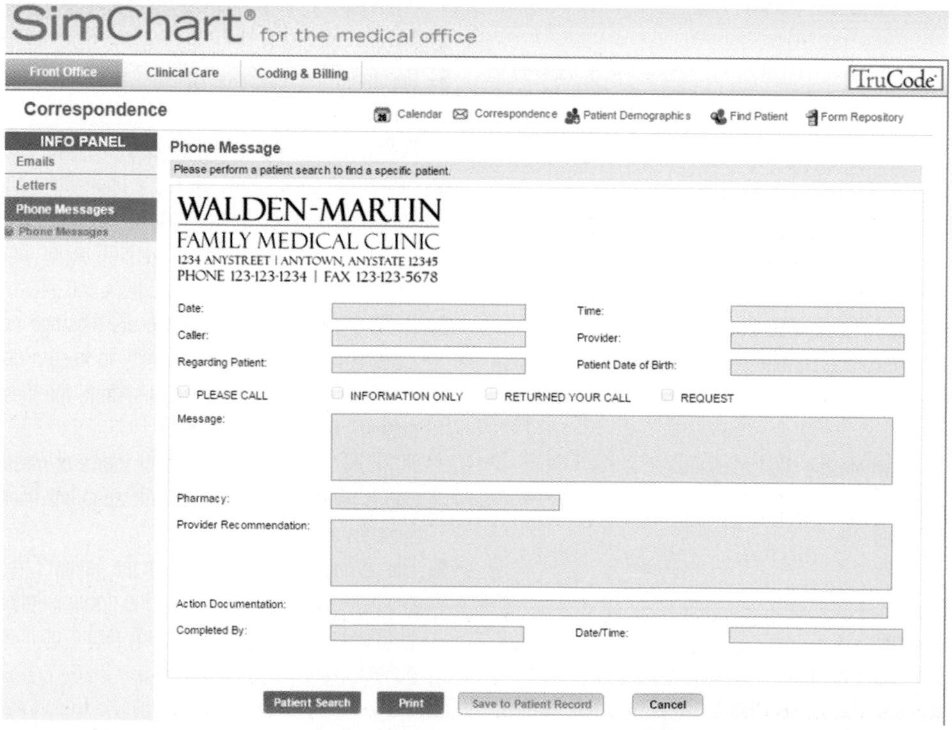

FIGURE 9-4 Phone message forms with self-adhesive backing make charting calls easier and more time efficient. (Courtesy Bibbero Systems, Petaluma, Calif.)

FIGURE 9-5 Phone message screen in an electronic health record system. (Elsevier: SimChart for the Medical Office, St Louis, 2015, Elsevier.)

message book usually is retained for the same period that the statute of limitations runs for medical professional liability cases.

If an electronic system is used, the message is automatically saved to the patient's record, along with the response to the message. The message record can show whether the patient contacted the office, if the office responded to that contact, and what the response was. All of these are key points if a medical professional liability case is brought against the provider. In addition, accurate telephone records can ensure quality patient care and customer service.

TYPICAL INCOMING CALLS

Handling incoming calls is often the responsibility of the medical assistant. You can handle many calls directly, but some will require the assistance of others. Knowing how to respond to the different types of calls will make you a valuable asset to the healthcare facility.

Requests for Directions

Each office should have a clear set of written directions that can be read to a caller who wants to know how to get to the office. Prepare the directions from various points in the area; for instance, one set for a patient coming from the north, and another for a patient coming from the south. Place these directions close to the telephone so that all employees can find them easily. Not all employees live close to the clinic or are familiar with the area; therefore, the written set of directions will be helpful both to staff members and to patients. Put a map on the office website and direct patients there for printable directions. Never simply suggest that callers refer to an Internet map when they ask for directions.

Inquiries About Bills

A patient may ask to speak with the provider about a recent bill. Ask the caller to hold for a moment while the ledger is obtained from the computer or files. If nothing irregular is found in the ledger, return to the telephone and say, "I have your account in front of me now. Perhaps I can answer your question." Most likely the caller will have some simple inquiry (e.g., whether the insurance company has paid its portion), or the person may want to delay making a payment until the next month. Not all patients realize that the medical assistant usually makes such decisions and is the best person with whom to discuss these matters. If the healthcare facility uses an external billing service, you may need to provide the caller with that agency's telephone number. When an external billing service is used, that telephone number is often shown on the patient's statement. When necessary, post a note in the EHR or to the physical ledger card about the patient's call, such as a promise to pay on a certain date.

A patient may have questions about a statement that came in the mail. If billing matters are handled by another employee, tell the patient that the call will be transferred to the billing office. If you are responsible for billing, politely ask the patient to hold the line while you obtain the patient ledger. On returning to the line, thank the patient for waiting and explain the charges carefully. If an error has occurred, apologize and say that a corrected statement will be sent out at once. Always remember to thank the patient for calling. If patients are properly advised about charges at the time services are rendered, the number of these calls can be reduced considerably.

Inquiries About Fees

Fees vary widely in each healthcare facility, and quoting an exact fee before the provider sees the patient can be difficult. However, a good estimate should be given to patients as to what they can expect to pay, especially on the first visit. Asking a patient to just appear at the office without having any idea of the cost is unreasonable. Discuss with the provider or office manager what range should be quoted to the patient, and then follow your quote with the statement that the fees vary, depending on the patient's condition and tests the provider orders. Most healthcare facilities require patients to pay the health insurance co-payment (or co-pay) on the day service is provided, and the caller should be informed of this. If fees are regularly discussed on the telephone, a suggested script should be included in the policies and procedures manual. Do not be evasive; have a list of fees available you can discuss with patients.

Questions About Participating Providers

Patients may call the office to inquire whether the provider is a **participating provider** with their particular insurance plan or managed care organization. A list of the insurance plans with which the provider has a contract should be readily available to the medical assistant who answers the telephone. This is important because insurance benefits vary widely for patients based on whether they see a participating provider or a nonparticipating provider. A claim may even be denied if the provider is not a provider for the patient's insurance company.

Requests for Assistance With Insurance

In the ever-changing world of health insurance, patients often are confused about their coverage, how payment is determined, and what they are actually financially responsible for when it comes to their bill from the healthcare facility. A solid understanding of the basics of health insurance, including managed care, allows you to answer patient questions about insurance. If the question is beyond your knowledge, you should know to whom to transfer the call so that the patient can get an answer.

Radiology and Laboratory Reports

Because of the increased use of EHRs, radiology and laboratory results often are available to providers as soon as the technician has completed the test. When the patient calls for those results, a message is taken, and the provider decides whether the medical assistant can relay the results or the provider needs to speak to the patient directly.

When tests are done at a facility that is not linked to the healthcare facility's EHR, the findings usually are delivered by mail to the provider's office. If the test has been marked **STAT**, which means the provider wants the results immediately, reports may be telephoned, faxed, or e-mailed to the provider's office and an original report delivered by mail.

It is helpful to have blank laboratory results forms available that list the various tests, with their normal values, so that you can easily and accurately document results telephoned to the healthcare facility. This can save time, and you can be assured that the test name is spelled correctly. You should repeat the results you have been given to make sure you have written them down correctly. This report must be documented in the patient's health record and sent to the provider for review.

Satisfactory Progress Reports from Patients

Providers sometimes ask patients to telephone the office to report on their condition a few days after the office visit. The medical assistant can take such calls and relay the information to the provider if the report is satisfactory. Assure the patient that you will inform the provider of the call. The report should be documented in the health record. The provider should always be informed immediately about unsatisfactory progress reports, and he or she should give instructions for the patient to follow in such situations. The provider may discuss this directly with the patient, or the medical assistant may be instructed to relay the information to the patient. All instructions given should also be documented in the health record.

Routine Reports from Hospitals and Other Sources

Routine calls may be received from hospitals and other sources reporting a patient's progress. Take the message carefully and make sure the provider sees it. The message should be placed in the patient's health record after the provider has reviewed and initialed it.

Requests for Referrals

Well-respected providers, especially primary care providers, are often asked for recommendations for referrals to other specialists. If the provider has furnished the medical assistant with a list of practitioners for this purpose, these inquiries may be handled without consulting the provider, unless the patient's insurance plan requires a written referral. However, the provider should always be informed of such requests. Referrals should also be documented in the patient's health record.

Some managed care organizations require a provider referral before a patient may see a specialist; this referral should come from the provider unless he or she has authorized automatic referrals. Most providers require the patient to come in for an office visit to discuss the referral. Afterward, a staff member calls the referral provider and notifies the office staff of the referral. This process may also be done electronically. A managed care organization may offer the option of using its website to enter the referral information and then electronically forwarding the information to the new provider. Handle these calls as quickly as possible so that the patient may make an appointment to see the referral provider.

Office Administration Matters

Not all calls concern patients. Calls may come from the accountant or the auditor or about banking procedures, office supplies, or office maintenance, most of which the medical assistant can handle or refer to the appropriate person. For some of these calls, the medical assistant may need to gather additional information and return the call.

SPECIAL INCOMING CALLS

Patients Refusing to Discuss Symptoms

Occasionally patients call and want to talk with the provider about symptoms they are reluctant to discuss with a medical assistant. Patients have the right to privacy, but the provider cannot be expected to take numerous calls from patients who do not want to speak to the medical assistant. If the patient refuses to discuss any symptoms, follow the healthcare facility's procedures, which may

include suggesting that the patient make an appointment with the provider to discuss the problem in person.

Unsatisfactory Progress Reports

If a patient under treatment reports that he or she is still not feeling well or that the prescription the provider provided is not helping, do not practice medicine illegally by giving the patient medical advice. Make detailed notes about the patient's comments and then give your notes to the provider. He or she may make a medication change or may decide that the patient should return to the office. Follow up with the patient and convey the provider's instructions.

CRITICAL THINKING APPLICATION   **9-4**

A patient calls the healthcare facility to report that she has been taking her prescribed antibiotic for 3 days and still isn't feeling any better. She says she might even be feeling worse than before she started taking the pills. She asks Ashlynn if she should stop taking the pills.
- How should Ashlynn respond to this patient?
- What actions should Ashlynn take in response to this telephone call?
- What should Ashlynn document in the patient's record?

Requests for Test Results

When the provider orders special tests, the patient may be told to call the office in a couple of days for the results. It is ultimately the responsibility of the provider to notify the patient of test results, especially if they are abnormal. When a patient calls for the results, make sure the provider has seen them and has given permission before sharing the results with the patient. If specified in the office policy, the medical assistant can give test results to the patient. Patients do not always understand that the medical assistant cannot give out information without the provider's permission. If the results are unfavorable, the provider should be the one to inform the patient and give further instructions. This call must be handled tactfully; otherwise, the patient may feel as if the staff is concealing information.

Most providers prefer that medical assistants give only normal test results to patients. However, the medical assistant may give abnormal test results if authorized by the provider. For example, when a patient has an abnormal Pap test result, the medical assistant usually is the person who calls the patient with the result and further instructions from the provider. If the patient has any questions about the test result, she must be referred to the provider. The medical assistant needs good communication skills to relay information such as this without crossing the line of practicing medicine without a license.

The best policy for dealing with more serious abnormal test results is to schedule an appointment for the patient to see the provider. These results are best relayed in person instead of on the telephone.

Patients who call the office for test results must be appropriately identified before the results are given. Some offices use a special code that is written in the patient's health record, and knowledge of this code or password gives the person access to the information. Other offices may use the patient's date of birth or other information that is known only to the patient and has been shared with the healthcare facility. You should always use at least two different methods of identifying patients.

Medical assistants must know and follow federal regulations and the laws in their state regarding the release of any information to someone other than the patient; this includes information about a minor. Make sure the right individual is on the line before offering results by verifying name and date of birth. It is considered a breach of confidentiality and of the Privacy Rules of the Health Insurance Portability and Accountability Act (HIPAA) if the patient is not identified correctly and information is released to the wrong individual.

Requests for Information from Third Parties

The patient must give permission before any member of the provider's staff can give information to third-party callers; this includes insurance companies, attorneys, relatives, neighbors, employers, and any other third party. HIPAA is very specific about the information that should be included in the release of information form. The patient must specify who can receive the information and exactly what information can be released. The release of information form also must include an expiration date. The medical assistant must carefully review the patient's form before releasing any information to third parties.

Complaints About Care or Fees

A medical assistant may be able to offer a satisfactory explanation to a patient who complains about the care he or she received or the fee charged. Often the patient simply does not understand a charge, and the medical assistant can provide assistance by reviewing the bill. If a patient seems angry, offer to pull the health record, research the problem and if needed, discuss it with the provider. Four magic words often calm the angry patient: "Let me help you." This reassures the patient that someone is willing to talk about the problem. However, if you are unable to appease the patient easily, the provider or office manager may prefer to talk directly to the patient.

When callers complain, do not attempt to blame someone else, and never argue with the patient. Find the source of the problem, and then present options to the caller as to how the situation can be resolved. Remember to treat callers in the same manner that you would wish to be treated. A complaint may seem small and insignificant to the office staff, but to the patient it may be a serious issue. Provide good customer service to patients, and complaints will be few and far between.

Calls from Staff Members' Families or Friends

The telephone lines should never be burdened with an excess of personal calls to the staff. A call is necessary in emergencies, but staff members should never monopolize the telephone for personal business and conversations. Emergency calls could be coming through, and the lines must be clear. Keep personal calls and texting to an absolute minimum.

HANDLING DIFFICULT CALLS

Angry Callers

No matter how efficient the medical assistant is on the telephone or how well liked the provider might be, sooner or later an angry caller will be on the line. The anger may have a legitimate cause, or the caller's irritation may have resulted from a misunderstanding. Handling such calls is a real challenge. First, take the required actions, even if it is to say that the matter will be discussed with the provider as soon as possible and the patient will be called back later. If answers are not readily available, a friendly assurance that the situation is important and that every attempt will be made to find the answer quickly usually calms the angry feelings.

The medical assistant may find that lowering his or her tone of voice and volume of speech may force the angry caller to do the same. This method does not always work, but it usually is true that when dealing with an angry person, calm promotes calm. Some patients may misread this method and become even angrier, thinking that their complaint is not being taken seriously. Interpersonal skills are critical when dealing with other individuals because the more skilled the medical assistant becomes, the better able he or she is to deal with multiple types of personalities.

Always avoid getting angry or defensive in response to an angry caller, and try to get to the root of the real problem. Express interest and understanding, take careful notes, and follow through with the problem to the most appropriate resolution. Never "pass the buck" by saying, "That's not my job," or "I am not the person who filed that insurance claim." No matter whose fault the problem is, it is best to deal with it and find a solution instead of placing blame. It is important to respond to the patient when you said you would, even if the call is to tell him or her that you need a bit more time to work on the problem. Keeping the patient in the loop shows that you want to come up with a solution.

CRITICAL THINKING APPLICATION   **9-5**

An angry caller raises his voice at Ashlynn over an issue that happened before she began to work at the facility. She suggests that he speak with the office manager, but he refuses and continues to berate Ashlynn.
- What choices does Ashlynn have in this situation?
- Should she simply hang up on the patient?
- How can the call be handled diplomatically?

Aggressive Callers

Aggressive callers insist that they receive whatever action they feel is necessary, and they usually insist on action immediately. Treat these callers with a calm, poised attitude, but do not allow the caller's aggression to initiate inappropriate action. Reassure the caller that his or her concern is valid and will receive the full attention of the right person. Explain when the caller can expect a response from the office, and be sure to follow up with the patient.

Unauthorized Inquiry Calls

Some individuals call the provider's office requesting information to which they are not entitled. These callers must be told politely but firmly that such information cannot be provided to them because of privacy laws. Insistent callers should be referred to the office manager or provider.

Sales Calls

Sales calls often are thought of as an interruption to the provider's busy day, but some salespersons may have important information on products, equipment, or services the office uses regularly. Do not completely disregard salespeople, but do not allow them to monopolize time or telephone lines, either. Keep these calls quick and to the point. Most professional salespeople realize that the provider's and staff's time is extremely valuable and respect this. It may be the healthcare facility policy to give the salesperson an appointment, possibly over the lunch hour, to discuss the new product or service with the provider and/or office manager. Developing a rapport with representatives of the companies whose products the practice uses frequently may result in a discounted price and first news of sales and promotions. In turn, these professionals rarely waste the time of office personnel.

CRITICAL THINKING APPLICATION   9-6

Ashlynn answers the phone; the caller is a pharmaceutical representative who has been visiting the clinic for several months. She cheerfully greets him and asks if he is calling to make an appointment. He states that he wants to make an appointment with Ashlynn—for a date. How should she handle this call? What problems could arise if this were a patient and Ashlynn were to accept the date?

Callers With Difficulty Communicating

Occasionally calls come into the office from patients or family members who have difficulty with the English language. In some cases English is not the caller's primary language, so the medical assistant must use listening skills to ensure understanding. If a certain language is predominant in the area, the healthcare facility should consider hiring a medical assistant who is bilingual. Some patients speak English but have a heavy accent, so you should listen carefully and ask questions to be sure you have understood the person correctly. Many resources are available to assist with translation. The healthcare facility may contract with a translator who would be available to help with telephone calls and patient visits in the office. Many online services also offer translation. If the healthcare facility has a number of patients who speak a specific language other than English, it would be helpful to have commonly used phrases available in that language, especially the phrase that would refer the patient to the specific translation service used by the healthcare facility.

Some providers may have a number of patients who are deaf or hard of hearing. These patients may use a relay system to communicate with healthcare facilities over the telephone. Some relay systems have the patient use a keyboard to enter the information to an operator, who calls the office and reads the information to you; your response is then typed back to the patient. Newer technology uses an online captioned telephone service, much like closed captioning for television. Many smart phones can use a translation app to assist the caller. You should be familiar with the way this system works so that you can engage in these conversations in a professional manner.

TYPICAL OUTGOING CALLS

Most outgoing calls in the healthcare facility are responses to incoming calls. The same rules for courtesy and diction apply to calls made from the office to patients, other individuals, and businesses.

It is helpful to plan outgoing calls in advance. For instance, if the medical assistant is placing an order for office supplies, a list should be made that includes the product, the price, the quantity needed, and a catalog page number, if applicable. Questions about the various products ordered should be noted so that they can be asked while the sales representative is on the telephone.

Some medical assistants find it helpful to make all outgoing calls at once, when possible. This way the calls can be made one after another, and if a call back is necessary, the medical assistant is likely to still be by the telephone. Organizing calls helps increase office efficiency.

Never be rude to an individual on the telephone. Remember to treat those on the other end of the telephone as you would wish to be treated. Do not forget that you are a representative of the provider and that you must behave in a professional manner at all times.

Time Zones

When making outgoing calls, it is important to keep time zones in mind, especially when calling patients. If you are trying to contact a patient who is spending the winter somewhere else, you should place that call at an appropriate time for the patient. If you are trying to get information from an insurance company, you should call when someone is available to answer your questions. The continental United States is divided into four standard time zones: Pacific, Mountain, Central, and Eastern (Figure 9-6). When it is noon Pacific time, it is 3 PM Eastern time. If you will be calling from San Francisco to a business or professional office in New York, plan to make the call no later than 1 PM. When it is 2 PM on the West Coast, it is 5 PM on the East Coast.

Long Distance Calling

Long distance calls are simple to place, usually inexpensive, and efficient. When information is needed in a hurry, telephoning is much more expedient than written communication. Before placing a long distance call, have the correct number ready. If you do not have the number, you may access directory assistance by dialing 1, then the area code of the party you want to call, followed by 555-1212. In some areas, numbers are available by calling 1-411. Directory assistance is now an automated service in many regions, and you will be asked for the name of the city and person you are calling. Often a fee is charged for using directory assistance, so look for the telephone number using free sources whenever possible.

Some Internet services, such as Skype, Jajah, or magicJack, allow the user to call long distance, and sometimes even internationally, through the computer with no long distance charges.

USING A TELEPHONE DIRECTORY

The primary purpose of a telephone directory is to provide lists of those who have telephones, their telephone numbers and, in most cases, their addresses. In addition, the directory is an aid in checking the spelling of names and in locating certain types of businesses through the Yellow Pages. Directories are found on the Internet and in print format.

The Internet makes searching for telephone numbers much easier. Try to find telephone numbers through websites such as *www.yellowpages.com* or *www.whitepages.com,* or use a printed telephone

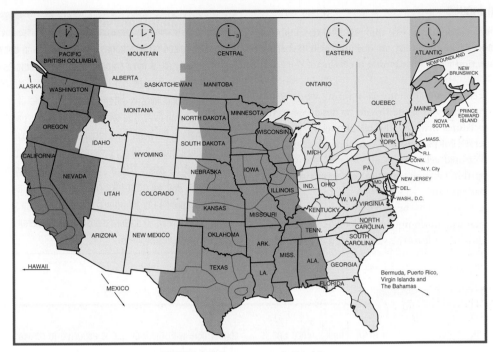

FIGURE 9-6 Time zones across the United States.

book to avoid directory assistance charges on the monthly phone bill. A Web search for the business or provider needed may yield the information. Companies with websites usually have a "Contact Us" page that directs the user to the individual departments.

In a print telephone directory, color coding is often used to differentiate between residence listings and business listings. Governmental offices usually have their own section (commonly blue). Some directories include ZIP code maps for the local area.

TELEPHONE SERVICES
Answering Services

Patients expect to be able to contact their provider if an emergency arises. This means that the telephone in the healthcare facility must be answered at all times, day and night, weekends and holidays. During normal office hours, the medical assistant is available to answer the telephone. After office hours, most healthcare facilities use an **answering service** or an answering machine that directs the caller to the answering service if there is an urgent issue.

With an answering service, an actual person answers the call, which can be comforting for patients. The staff at the answering service can act as a buffer for the provider after hours by screening the calls. By following the criteria given to them by the healthcare facility, they can determine whether the provider (or on-call person) should be contacted or the patient directed to the hospital emergency department, or whether a message can be taken and relayed to the healthcare facility in the morning.

It is common courtesy to call the answering service in the morning to let them know that you will be answering the calls and also to retrieve any messages taken overnight or over the weekend. You should also call the answering service when you are leaving for the day. Answering services also can be used to cover the telephone if all staff members need to be away from the telephones at the same time.

Automatic Call Routing

Many healthcare facilities have started using an **automatic call routing** system. The caller is given a menu of choices; he or she then presses a number on the telephone keypad to direct the call to the correct department. This can be an efficient way to handle a large volume of calls, but it can also be frustrating for some patients, especially elderly adults who may have trouble hearing and remembering the options. Some of the frustration can be minimized by providing a number option that connects the caller with a person (e.g., "Press 0"), who can then transfer the call to the appropriate department.

CRITICAL THINKING APPLICATION   9-7

Ashlynn has had many complaints from patients about the new call routing system because it takes so long to "get to a human being." How can she help make modern call routing systems easier for her patients?

CLOSING COMMENTS
Patient Education

Today's telephone systems allow providers to educate patients while they are on hold; recordings may be played that offer health information on subjects from A to Z. These messages can be professionally recorded and/or custom designed by the provider and staff. Special events may be announced, with the option to press a certain number for more information about the event.

Legal and Ethical Issues

The guidelines for medical confidentiality apply equally to telephone conversations; therefore, take care that no one overhears sensitive information. Use discretion when mentioning the name of the caller or patient.

Do not place or receive personal phone calls during work hours. Time limitations for personal phone use should be described in the office policies and procedures manual. The telephone is a business line and should be reserved for patients and others conducting business with the office. Personal cell phones also should not be used during working hours; this takes the medical assistant's time and attention away from patient care.

Telephone message records may be brought into court as evidence; make sure all messages are complete and legible. Most offices should keep these records for at least the same period as the statute of limitations in that state.

Professional Behaviors

We have talked on telephones and cell phones in our own lives, and most of us have used at least some of the special features on our phones. It is important to recognize that the way we present ourselves on the phone in our professional lives is different from the style of communication we use in our personal lives. The way we speak in our personal lives may not be appropriate in the healthcare facility. We must maintain a professional tone in communications with our patients and other contacts. For example, slang should not be used; "Hello" is not a proper way to answer a business telephone; and we must take care how we use medical terminology when on the telephone (jargon should not be used when speaking with patients). The goal is always to present a positive professional image of the healthcare facility we represent.

SUMMARY OF SCENARIO

Ashlynn is quickly becoming a part of the team at Dr. Frank's office and is developing into a well-liked asset to the staff. She has learned to slow down when speaking on the phone and to adjust her volume and pitch, depending on the patient with whom she is speaking. Although she tends to be quite talkative, she is balancing just the right amount of friendly chatter with the business at hand. She does this by offering a friendly greeting to callers, getting to the point of the call, then being affable before ending the call. By expressing her concern and asking how she can be of help to the patients, Ashlynn shows them that she sincerely cares about their problems. She is careful about her tone of voice, realizing that patients may take her comments the wrong way if she does not treat them in a cordial manner. Dr. Frank is very pleased with her performance.

Ashlynn takes care when she speaks to patients and others on the phone so that she does not breach confidentiality in any way. She has become comfortable with the way she is expected to answer the telephone. The pace of her speech and the wording are now a habit. Ashlynn is determined to maintain a professional relationship with all the people related to her work environment. She is adept now at handling calls from angry patients and can maintain control with even the most aggressive callers. She leaves callers on hold for a minimum time and reassures them frequently that she is attending to their situation. By treating callers as she would want to be treated, Ashlynn reduces frustration, and she feels that the office is more efficient at handling the large volume of calls that come in each day. She shows much promise for a long and rewarding career in the medical field and is satisfied with the current track of her career. As she continues to settle into her position, she looks forward to learning more about efficiency and time management. Her positive attitude and desire to learn will only enhance her performance at work, making her a valuable employee and one worth promoting.

SUMMARY OF LEARNING OBJECTIVES

1. **Define, spell, and pronounce the terms listed in the vocabulary.**
   Spelling and pronouncing medical terms correctly reinforce the medical assistant's credibility. Knowing the definitions of these terms promotes confidence in communication with patients and co-workers.

2. **Identify and explain the features of a multiple-line telephone system, and also explain how each can be used effectively in a healthcare facility.**
   A multiple-line telephone system has many features; most obviously, more than one telephone line comes into the office. This means that callers are less likely to get a busy signal when calling the healthcare facility. Additional features, such as speed dial, voice mail, and call forwarding, can increase efficiency.

   Medical assistants must understand how each feature of the telephone system works. For example, knowing when to use the speakerphone function and when not to helps protect patient confidentiality.

   Knowing how to use the conference call feature helps facilitate telephone meetings with satellite offices. Understanding how the voice mail system works is crucial to the medical assistant's work life.

3. **Do the following related to effective use of the telephone:**
   - *Discuss the telephone equipment needed by a healthcare facility.*
     Two incoming lines is the minimum recommended number of lines for a healthcare facility. Telephones should be placed where they are accessible but private. One medical assistant can handle no more than two incoming lines; this means that the addition of more lines may involve the need for more employees.
   - *Summarize active listening skills.*
     A big part of communication is being able to listen. Honing your active listening skills also will increase your communication skills. Focus on the conversation by being present in the moment. Not only is interrupting rude, it also shows that you were not listening, truly listening,

because you were coming up with your response. Part of active listening is confirming what you heard to be sure that you have received the intended message.

- *Demonstrate effective and professional telephone techniques.*
  Medical assistants should answer the telephone promptly and professionally. A pleasing telephone personality conveys a favorable impression of the healthcare facility. Enunciate, pronouncing words clearly and distinctly. Vary the pitch of your voice, and avoid a monotonous or droning manner. Courtesy to patients and other callers is vital. First impressions are important, and a medical assistant's telephone manner sets the tone for the caller's perception of the healthcare facility. Be courteous and polite to all callers. (Refer to Procedure 9-1.)

- *Consider the importance of tone of voice and enunciation.*
  Tone of voice can completely change the message sent. Make sure you use the correct tone of voice so that the message is not misunderstood. Enunciation also ensures that your message is not misunderstood. Communicating over the telephone has its own issues, and enunciation is crucial. Speaking clearly helps your caller to hear your message.

4. **Explain the importance of thinking ahead when managing telephone calls; also, describe the correct way to answer the telephone in the office.**
   Before you start answering calls, make sure you have all of the supplies you need to do your job. Confidentiality in a healthcare facility must always be a priority.

   Medical assistants should answer the telephone promptly and professionally. The provider's image is affected by the way telephone calls are handled. Be courteous and polite to all callers. The medical assistant should identify the facility first when picking up the phone, followed by his or her name, followed by an offer of help. If the caller does not offer a name, the medical assistant should ask who is calling.

5. **Discuss the screening of incoming calls, and list several questions to ask when handling an emergency call.**
   Most healthcare facilities expect the medical assistant answering the telephone to screen the calls; this is an important task. The facility's screening policies should address how calls should be handled when the provider is out of the office, and the medical assistant should always ask before placing a caller on hold or transferring a call.

   If a phone call is an emergency, the policies for handling emergency calls apply. Ask for a phone number where the caller can be reached in case of a sudden disconnection. Ask about the chief symptoms and when they started. Find out whether the patient has had similar symptoms in the past and what happened in that situation. Determine whether the patient is alone, has transportation, or needs an ambulance. In severe cases, do not hang up the phone until the ambulance or police arrive. A special sheet of instructions listing specific medical emergencies (e.g., chest pain, heavy bleeding, seizure, fainting, poisoning) should be posted by each telephone.

6. **Do the following related to taking a message:**
   - *Document telephone messages accurately.*
     When taking a telephone message, either in a handwritten or electronic format, strive for accuracy. Be sure to get all the information the provider will need to act. Repeat any words or numbers that are not heard clearly. (Refer to Procedure 9-2.)

   - *List the seven elements of a correctly handled telephone message.*
     The seven elements of a correctly handled phone message are (1) the name of the person to whom the call should be directed; (2) the name of the person calling; (3) the caller's telephone number; (4) the reason for the call; (5) the medical assistant's description of the action to be taken; (6) the date and time of the call; and (7) the initials of the person taking the call, so that if any question arises that person can be consulted.

   - *Report relevant information concisely and accurately.*
     If a handwritten system is used for recording telephone messages, a policy must be developed on the retention of the telephone message records. Accurate records can ensure quality patient care and customer service. (Refer to Procedure 9-2.)

7. **Discuss various types of common incoming calls and how to deal with each.**
   Knowing how to respond to the different types of calls received will make you a valuable asset to the healthcare facility. Common types of incoming calls include the following: requests for directions; inquiries about bills; inquiries about fees; inquiries about participating providers; requests for assistance with insurance; inquiries about radiology and laboratory reports; progress reports; routine report calls from hospitals or other sources; requests for a referral; and questions about office administration matters.

8. **Discuss various types of special incoming calls and how to deal with each.**
   If a patient refuses to discuss symptoms with a medical assistant, follow the healthcare facility's policies and procedures, which may suggest that the patient make an appointment with the provider to discuss the problem in person. Other types of special calls a medical assistant must know how to handle include unsatisfactory progress reports, requests for test results, requests for information from third parties, complaints about care or fees, and calls from a staff member's family or friends.

9. **Discuss how the medical assistant should handle various types of difficult calls.**
   With angry callers, never return the anger. Remain calm and speak in tones that are perhaps slightly quieter than those of the caller. This often prompts the caller to lower his or her tone of voice. Offer to help the angry person and ask questions to gain control of the conversation, moving it toward resolution. Do not argue with angry callers.

   Callers who have a complaint should be handled in a manner similar to that for angry callers. Remain calm and offer to help. Take a serious interest in what the caller has to say. Let the caller know that his or her

Continued

SUMMARY OF LEARNING OBJECTIVES—*continued*

concerns are important to the staff and the provider. Find the source of the problem and determine exactly what the caller wants or expects as a resolution. Always follow up on complaints and make sure they were resolved as much to the caller's satisfaction as possible.

Other types of difficult callers that medical assistants must know how to handle include aggressive callers, unauthorized inquiry calls, sales calls, and callers with difficulty communicating.

10. **Discuss typical outgoing calls, including why knowledge of time zones and long distance calling is necessary.**

Most outgoing calls in the healthcare facility are made in response to incoming calls. It is helpful to plan outgoing calls in advance. Organizing calls helps increase office efficiency.

The continental United States is divided into four standard time zones. Long distance calls are simple to place, usually inexpensive, and efficient. Knowledge of both concepts are important for a medical assistant handling the telephone.

11. **Discuss the use of a telephone directory, and describe how answering services and automatic call routing systems are used in a healthcare facility.**

The primary purpose of a telephone directory is to provide lists of those who have telephones, their telephone numbers and, in most cases, their addresses. The Internet makes searching for telephone numbers much easier.

Answering services are used to answer the telephone in the healthcare facility when the staff is not available. This could be during the overnight hours or during regular office hours when the staff is at lunch or in a meeting. Automatic call routing systems allow the patient to select a number from a menu to reach specific departments in the healthcare facility. The system should have an option that allows patients to choose to speak to a person if they are not sure what number to press.

12. **Discuss the legal and ethical issues related to telephone techniques.**

The guidelines for medical confidentiality apply equally to telephone conversations; therefore, take care that no one overhears sensitive information. Telephone records may be brought to court as evidence.

CONNECTIONS

Study Guide Connection: Go to the Chapter 9 Study Guide. Read and complete the activities.

evolve Evolve Connection: Go to the Chapter 9 link at *evolve.elsevier.com/kinn* to complete the Chapter Review Quiz. Check out the other resources listed for this chapter to make the most of what you have learned from Telephone Techniques.

SCHEDULING APPOINTMENTS AND PATIENT PROCESSING

10

SCENARIO

Ramona West is the medical assistant in charge of scheduling appointments and patient processing for Dr. Charlotte Brown. Ramona is an extremely organized person who thinks quickly and creatively. Two of her professional goals are to ensure that the healthcare facility remains on schedule throughout the day with minimal wait time for the patients and that patient flow through the office is done in an efficient manner. She is fortunate that Dr. Brown is cooperative and time oriented, and they work well together to reach these common goals.

Ramona usually arrives at work at least 15 minutes early to begin her preparations for the day. She reviews the electronic health record for each patient to make sure test results from previous visits are available to the provider and that the medical record is complete. She pays special attention to the

patients who arrive in the healthcare facility as she completes her daily tasks, remembering the importance of providing patients with good customer service. Ramona greets each patient by name and carries on a brief but cordial conversation. Patients appreciate that she goes the extra mile to remember something about them, and this promotes excellent patient relations.

Ramona leaves a little time in the morning and afternoon for emergency appointments. The healthcare facility uses an automatic call routing system to contact patients to confirm appointments in advance, which increases her show rate. She is always pleasant to the patients as they go through the check-in and checkout procedures. Her friendly, caring attitude makes her a favorite among the patients, and Dr. Brown is pleased with the relationship-building skills Ramona has developed.

While studying this chapter, think about the following questions:

- How can the medical assistant contribute to an efficient daily routine?
- How does the medical assistant contribute to keeping the daily schedule on track?
- How can the schedule be put back on track when emergencies disrupt the day?

- How does the flexibility of the medical assistant contribute to office efficiency?
- What are some ways to develop good rapport with patients?
- Why is the sign-in register a potential breach of patient confidentiality?
- What is the value of knowing some information about patients' personal lives?

LEARNING OBJECTIVES

1. Define, spell, and pronounce the terms listed in the vocabulary.
2. Describe guidelines to establishing an appointment schedule and creating an appointment matrix.
3. Discuss the advantages of computerized appointment scheduling.
4. Discuss appointment book scheduling and explain how self-scheduling can reduce the number of calls to the healthcare facility.
5. Discuss the legality of the appointment scheduling system.
6. Discuss pros and cons of various types of appointment management systems.
7. Discuss telephone scheduling and identify critical information required for scheduling appointments for new patients.
8. Discuss scheduling appointments for established patients.
9. Discuss how the medical assistant should handle scheduling other types of appointments.
10. Do the following related to special circumstances in scheduling:
    - Discuss several methods of dealing with patients who consistently arrive late.

- Recognize office policies and protocols for rescheduling appointments.
- Discuss how to deal with emergencies, provider referrals, and patients without appointments.
11. Discuss how to handle failed appointments and no-shows, as well as methods to increase appointment show rates.
12. Discuss how to handle cancellations and delays.
13. Discuss patient processing, including the importance of the reception area.
14. Describe how to prepare for patient arrival, including patient check-in procedures.
15. Explain why using the patient's name as often as possible is important, as well as how the medical assistant can make patients feel at ease.
16. Describe registration procedures, including obtaining a patient history.

LEARNING OBJECTIVES—*continued*

17. Do the following related to patient reception and processing:
    * Show consideration for patients' time.
    * Properly treat patients with special needs.
    * Escort and instruct the patient.
    * Describe where health records should be placed.

18. Describe how the medical assistant should deal with challenging situations, such as talkative patients, children, angry patients, and patients' relatives and friends.
19. Discuss the friendly farewell, patient checkout, and planning for the next day.
20. Discuss patient education, as well as legal and ethical issues, for scheduling appointments and patient processing.

VOCABULARY

amenity (uh-me′-nih-te) Something conducive to comfort, convenience, or enjoyment.

automatic call routing A software system that answers phones automatically and routes calls to staff after the caller responds to prompts; also used to call a large number of patients to remind them of appointments or make announcements.

demographics Statistical data of a population. In healthcare this includes patient name, address, date of birth, employment, and other details.

disruption An unexpected event that throws a plan into disorder; an interruption that prevents a system or process from continuing as usual or as expected.

established patients Patients who are returning to the office who have previously been seen by the provider.

expediency (ek-spe′-de-en-se) A means of achieving a particular end, as in a situation requiring haste or caution.

follow-up appointment An appointment type used when a patient needs to see the provider after a condition should have been resolved or to monitor an ongoing condition, such as hypertension. Also known as a recheck appointment.

harmonious Marked by accord in sentiment or action; having the parts agreeably related.

incidental disclosure A secondary use or disclosure that cannot reasonably be prevented, is limited in nature, and occurs because of another use or disclosure that is permitted.

intercom A two-way communication system with a microphone and loudspeaker at each station for localized use.

integral (in′-tih-grul) Essential; being an indispensable part of a whole.

interaction A two-way communication; mutual or reciprocal action or influence.

interval Space of time between events.

matrix Something in which a thing originates, develops, takes shape, or is contained; a base on which to build.

no-show When a patient fails to keep an appointment without giving advance notice.

Notice of Privacy Practices (NPP) A written document describing the healthcare facility's privacy practices. The patient must be provided with the NPP and sign an acknowledgment of receipt.

perception A quick, acute, and intuitive cognition; a capacity for comprehension.

phonetic (fuh-neh′-tik) Constituting an alteration of ordinary spelling that better represents the spoken language, uses only characters of the regular alphabet, and is used in a context of conventional spelling.

practice management software A type of software that allows the user to enter demographic information, schedule appointments, maintain lists of insurance payers, perform billing tasks, and generate reports.

preauthorization A process required by some insurance carriers in which the provider obtains permission to perform certain procedures or services or refers a patient to a specialist.

precertification A process required by some insurance carriers in which the provider must prove medical necessity before performing a procedure.

prerequisite (pre-reh′-kwih-zut) Something that is necessary to an end or to carry out a function.

proficiency (pruh-fih′-shun-se) Competency as a result of training or practice.

progress notes Notes used in the medical record to track the patient's progress and condition.

recheck appointment An appointment type used when a patient needs to see the provider after a condition should have been resolved or to monitor an ongoing condition, such as hypertension. Also known as a follow-up appointment.

screening A system for examining and separating into different groups; in the medical office, it means determining the severity of illness that patients experience and prioritizing appointments based on that severity.

sequentially (se-kwen′-shuh-le) Of, relating to, or arranged in a sequence.

The provider's time is the most valuable asset of a medical practice. The person responsible for scheduling this time must understand the practice, be familiar with the working habits and preferences of the provider (or providers), and have clear guidelines for time management in the practice.

Appointment scheduling is the process that determines which patients the provider sees, the dates and times of appointments, and how much time is allotted to each patient based on the complaint and the provider's availability. Time management involves the realization that unforeseen interruptions and delays always occur and must be handled appropriately. In addition, the medical assistant must assign the appropriate appointment time length for the complaint along with ensuring that the appointments are scheduled so that there are minimal gaps in the schedule. Most healthcare providers find that efficient appointment scheduling is one of the most important factors in the success of the practice. Scheduling can be done in a number of ways, and each facility must find the way that suits it best.

ESTABLISHING THE APPOINTMENT SCHEDULE

Developing a schedule that meets the needs of both the providers and the patients is key to keeping the office running smoothly and efficiently. The scheduling team, along with the provider, should come up with scheduling parameters to both meet the needs of the patient population and keep the providers' preferences and habits in mind.

Patient Needs

Consider the **demographics** of the patients that are being served when determining office hours and appointment times. The staff should answer the following questions:

- Is the office in a busy metropolitan area or a rural agricultural community?
- What type of patients are seen? Are they of a specific age or gender? Do they have common diagnoses? Is the provider a general practitioner?
- Are evening and weekend appointments essential for most of the patients served?

Knowing when the providers need to be available for patients is one of the factors in creating the patient schedule.

Provider Preferences and Habits

Consider the preferences and habits of the providers in the practice before establishing and implementing a scheduling plan. Ask the following questions:

- Does the provider become restless if the reception room is not packed with waiting patients?
- Does the provider worry if even one patient is kept waiting?
- Is the provider methodic and careful about being in the facility when patient appointments are scheduled to begin?
- Is the provider habitually late?
- Does the provider move easily from one patient to another?
- Does the provider require a "break time" after a few patients?

- Would the provider rather see fewer patients and spend more time with each one or schedule more patients each day?

All of these preferences and habits become an **integral** part of the scheduling process. Keep in mind that the provider cannot spend every moment of the day with patients. The provider also has telephone calls to make and receive, reports to examine and dictate, meetings to attend, mail to answer, and many other business responsibilities. An experienced staff can handle many but not all of these tasks.

Next the office hours and the length of appointment time **intervals** need to be determined. Keeping in mind patients' needs and the provider's preferences and habits, decide what would be the shortest time possible for an appointment. Most healthcare facilities use 10- or 15-minute time intervals for the appointment schedule. Paper-based appointment books can be purchased with various time intervals. A computerized appointment system can also be set to the specific time interval that has been decided on. A computerized system can be customized for different providers, so that one provider could have 10-minute time slots and another could have 15-minute time slots. If an appointment, such as a complete physical, needs longer than 15 minutes, multiple time slots are used to cover that appointment. Once the minimum time period has been set, then the appointment matrix can be established.

CREATING THE APPOINTMENT MATRIX

Setting up the appointment **matrix** (Procedure 10-1) involves blocking out the times when the provider is not available to see patients, such as lunch time, hospital rounds, conferences, and vacation (Figure 10-1). In a paper-based appointment book the matrix is usually established for 6 months at a time. In a computerized system the matrix can be set up indefinitely.

Establishing Guidelines for Appointment Scheduling

Before establishing the appointment matrix, decide the length of the shortest office visit type. This visit type would usually be for a **follow-up** or **recheck appointment** for an established patient. Other specific appointment types should now be determined. General categories for appointment types are: follow-up or recheck, wellness examination, complete physical examination, urgent visit, new patient visit, and comprehensive visit. Each category has a specific amount of time assigned to it; for example, a follow-up or recheck appointment could be 15 to 20 minutes and a comprehensive visit could be 30 to 40 minutes. The providers and scheduling team should work together to come up with these time periods to ensure that the office runs smoothly and efficiently.

If it is decided that a complete physical examination should be scheduled for 30 minutes, yet the provider routinely spends 45 minutes with the patient for a complete physical, then the scheduling guidelines need to be adjusted. Well-planned scheduling and adherence to that schedule allow the provider to do more than run in and out of examination rooms with little time for the patient to talk with the provider. There will be a bit of trial and error when developing the priorities for the appointment schedule.

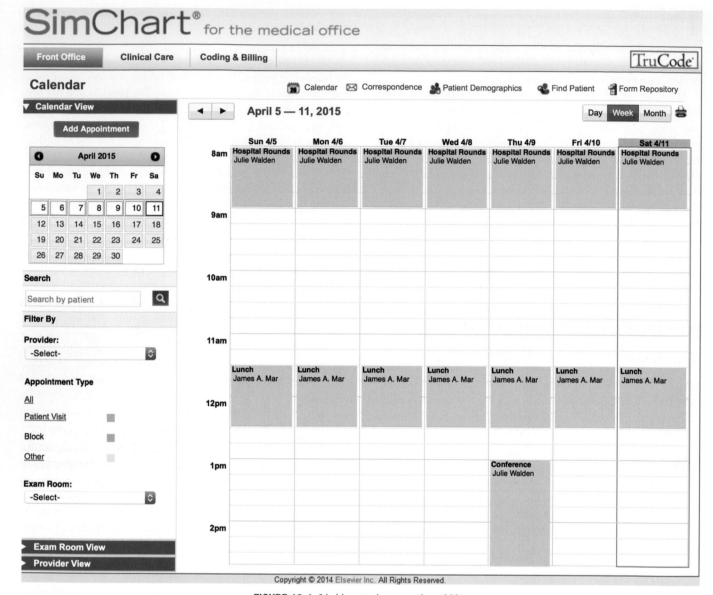

FIGURE 10-1 Schedule matrix showing provider availability.

Some providers need prompting to end the patient visit and move to the next patient. If there is a medical assistant in the examination room, he or she can help the provider remain on schedule by letting the provider know that the end of the appointment time is near. They may work out some type of signal, such as a hand gesture or phrase. A pager may be used when the medical assistant is not in room with the provider. When the provider's pager vibrates he or she will know that it is time to wind things up with that patient. The clinical medical assistant and the administrative medical assistant must work together to keep the healthcare facility running smoothly and efficiently.

CRITICAL THINKING APPLICATION   **10-1**

- Ramona has noticed that Dr. Brown is taking a little longer with patients than normal and that she is running consistently behind schedule by approximately 5 to 15 minutes. How can Ramona help rectify this situation?
- Discuss ways of approaching the provider when he or she is the cause of the delays in the schedule. What opening remarks can the medical assistant use to start the discussion in a positive way?

PROCEDURE 10-1	Manage Appointment Scheduling Using Established Priorities: Establish the Appointment Matrix

Goal: *To establish the matrix of the appointment schedule.*

EQUIPMENT and SUPPLIES

- Appointment book or computer with scheduling software
- Office procedure manual (optional)
- List of providers' availability and preferences
- Black pen, pencil, and highlighters
- Calendar

PROCEDURAL STEPS

1. Using the calendar, determine when the office is not open (e.g., holidays, weekends, evenings). If using the appointment book and a black pen, draw an *X* through the times the office is not open. If using the scheduling software, block the times the office is not open.
   PURPOSE: Blocking the closed times of the office helps prevent patients from being scheduled when the office is closed.

2. Identify the times each provider is not available. If using the appointment book, write in the providers' names on each column and then draw an *X* through their unavailable times. If using the scheduling software, select each provider and block the times the provider is unavailable.
   PURPOSE: Many providers do rounds in the hospital or long-term care facilities and cannot see patients in the clinic during those times. Providers also attend meetings and conferences during the workday. These events, along with vacations and lunch times, should be blocked on their schedules.

3. Using the office procedure manual or providers' preferences, determine when each provider performs certain types of examinations. In the appoint-

ment book, indicate these examinations either by writing the examination time or by highlighting the examination times. Follow the office's procedure on indicating these examination times in the appointment book. When using scheduling software, set up the times for the examinations or use the highlighting feature if available.
   PURPOSE: Some providers perform a variety of examinations. It can be more time efficient to have the same types of examinations on the same day. For instance, a provider in a women's health department may perform both gynecologic and prenatal examinations. The provider may prefer to set aside certain days to do prenatal examinations and other days to do gynecologic examinations.

4. Using the office procedure manual or the list of providers' preferences and availability, identify other times to block on the scheduling matrix. Some providers require catch-up times and these time slots are blocked. Some medical facilities save appointment times for same-day appointments. When saving time blocks for same-day appointments, make sure to use pencil so it can be erased and the patient's information entered on the day of the appointment. For the scheduling software, block those times when patients cannot be booked and indicate the times for the same-day appointments.
   PURPOSE: Allowing appointment times to be saved for same-day appointments provides the opportunity for the provider to see a patient who needs to get in immediately and prevents the patient from being turned away or double-booked.

Available Facilities

Another factor to keep in mind when scheduling appointments is the availability of facilities needed for the particular appointment type. Getting a patient into the office at a time when no facilities are available for the services needed is pointless. For example, suppose that a healthcare facility with two providers has only one room that can be used for minor surgery. Do not schedule two patients requiring minor surgery for the same time interval, even if both doctors could be available. If the healthcare facility has only one electrocardiograph, do not book two electrocardiograms (ECGs) at the same time. As the medical assistant gains **proficiency** in scheduling, it becomes easier to pair patient needs with the available facilities according to the provider's preference. Major equipment frequently used or a certain room with such equipment may need its own scheduling column in the appointment book or software system.

METHODS OF SCHEDULING APPOINTMENTS

The two most common methods of appointment scheduling are computerized scheduling and appointment book or paper-based

scheduling. Each has advantages and disadvantages, and the healthcare facility should weigh the benefits and choose the method that best suits the provider and the staff.

Computerized Scheduling

The computer has replaced the appointment book in many practices. Software for appointment scheduling, often referred to as **practice management software**, ranges from relatively simple programs that merely display available and scheduled times to more sophisticated systems that perform several other functions. Many programs can display such information as the length and type of appointment required and the patient's day or time preferences. The computer then can select the best appointment time based on the information entered into the computer.

Another advantage of a computerized scheduling system is the ability to search for future appointments. For example, when a patient calls and inquires about an appointment, the system can search by his or her name to find the time and date. With computerized scheduling, multiple users can access the appointment schedule at the same time, minimizing the wait time for patients. Another advantage of computerized schedules is the reports that can be generated. A hard copy of the provider's daily schedule can be created, showing the patients' names, telephone numbers, and the reason for the visit. Some healthcare facilities print these out, and others use them on screen. Healthcare facilities must have scheduling procedures to follow when the technology is down; some keep an appointment book as a backup to computer scheduling.

Appointment Book Scheduling

Office suppliers carry a variety of appointment book styles. Some appointment books show an entire week at a glance; many are color coded, with a special color used for each day of the week (Figure 10-2). This is very helpful when the provider asks the patient to return, for instance, in 2 weeks. If Wednesdays are colored yellow, the medical assistant can flip quickly to the correct day 2 weeks later and schedule the appointment. Multiple columns may be available to correspond with the number of doctors in a group practice, and the time can be divided according to their preferences.

Self-Scheduling

Allowing patients to schedule their own appointments using the Internet and the healthcare facility's Web site is becoming much more common. The patient is given limited access to the schedule, seeing only the available appointment times, not the other patients who are scheduled, thus protecting patient confidentiality. Other patients' names should never be visible on an online system.

Software is available that allows the patient to self-schedule through secure links to the provider's appointment book. The software or Internet site for the healthcare facility should give the patient guidelines as to the amount of time needed for certain appointments or should allow only a certain length of time to be self-scheduled, such as 15 minutes. These systems will reduce the number of calls and are available to the patient 24 hours a day. Some of these systems also send an automatic e-mail reminder to the patient the day before the appointment, requesting a reply to confirm. These systems are less frustrating to patients, who do not have to wait on hold to speak to the person who does scheduling for the healthcare facility. However, lengthy or complicated appointments should be scheduled through the staff.

Although this type of system for making appointments appeals to most technologically savvy people, some patients may not be comfortable using it. It does require minimal skills and Internet access. Others may object to online scheduling because they do not want their names anywhere on the Internet. This is a valid concern, and the facility should allow these patients to schedule over the telephone. If this system is used, some allowance must be made for patients who choose not to use it.

CRITICAL THINKING APPLICATION   **10-2**

The software used in Dr. Brown's office can allow patients to self-schedule. Ramona has heard about patient self-scheduling and would like to try this method in the office, but Dr. Brown is concerned that her patients will miss the personal contact and is not sold on the idea.

- What can Ramona say to convince Dr. Brown to try this new, time-saving method of scheduling?
- What challenges might the use of this system bring?

LEGALITY OF THE APPOINTMENT SCHEDULING SYSTEM

Because the paper-based appointment book can be used as a legal record, it must be accurate and maintained so that it provides correct information about the patients at the healthcare facility. Patients are expected to follow the provider's orders; this includes keeping appointments. If a patient does not show up for an appointment or cancels it and does not reschedule, a notation of this fact should be placed in the patient's health record. If a patient reschedules an appointment and subsequently keeps it, there is no need to document that it was rescheduled.

Pens are permanent, but the appointment book can become illegible if a number of patients change or cancel their appointments. Pencil is used in the appointment book so that making changes is easier. The information in the book includes the patient's name and a phone number where the patient can be reached. Some healthcare facilities list the reason for the appointment, but most note only the name and phone number. Listing the reason for the visit is not necessary if the medical assistant references the time needed for the appointment and blocks off that amount of time. Because the appointment book could be produced in litigation as a legal record, it should be kept for the number of years that constitute the statute of limitations in that individual state. If the appointment book is discarded, its contents should be shredded to protect patient privacy. Although the appointment book can be used as a legal record, actual medical records are more likely to be used in matters of litigation. Because **progress notes** are dated, a copy of the medical record shows all pertinent information about the patient's adherence to the provider's orders, including the appointments with the provider.

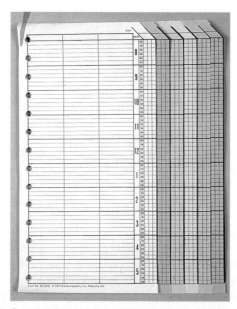

FIGURE 10-2 Color-coded appointment book pages help the medical assistant flip to the right day of the right week quickly. Appointments for multiple providers can be color-coded in the book.

Computerized scheduling systems can also be used to track patient appointments. Most computerized scheduling systems will allow the user to indicate if the patient has checked in, canceled, or missed the scheduled appointment. When a patient misses or cancels an appointment it should be documented in the electronic patient record for legal purposes.

TYPES OF APPOINTMENT SCHEDULING

Different types of appointment scheduling are used to meet the various needs of the medical facility, the providers, and the patients. Some offices use a combination of methods to create the right mix of activity during the day and to ensure that the day runs smoothly and efficiently. The medical assistant should become proficient at managing appointments. The following section presents several methods of appointment scheduling.

Time-Specified (Stream) Scheduling

When each patient is given a specific time for their appointment, this is referred to as time-specified or stream scheduling as it keeps a steady flow of patients moving through the office. This is the most common type of scheduling used in healthcare facilities. Studies have shown that providers can see more patients with less pressure when patient appointments are scheduled for a specific time slot. The medical assistant who is scheduling patients using this method should know the amount of time needed for each appointment type and keep time slots available for urgent visits.

Wave Scheduling

Wave scheduling is an attempt to create short-term flexibility within each hour. Wave scheduling assumes that the actual time needed for all the patients seen will average out over the course of the day. Instead of scheduling patients at each 15-minute interval, wave scheduling places three patients in the office at the same time, and they are seen in the order of their arrival. This way, one person's late arrival does not disrupt the entire schedule.

Modified Wave Scheduling

The wave schedule can be modified in several ways. For example, one method is to have two patients scheduled to come in at 10 AM and a third at 10:30 AM. This hourly cycle is repeated throughout the day. In another version, patients are scheduled to arrive at given intervals during the first half of the hour, and none are scheduled to arrive during the second half of the hour. This would allow time for urgent or walk-in patients to be seen.

Double-Booking

Booking two patients to come in at the same time is sometimes used to work in a patient with an acute illness or injury when there are no open appointments. This works out best if one of the patients needs laboratory work or another procedure done before seeing the provider. The provider can see one of the patients while the other one is being prepared.

Open Office Hours

With the open office hours method, the facility is open at given hours of the day or evening, and the patients are told that they can come in at any time. This type of system is often used in an urgent care setting. Patients are then seen in the order in which they arrive, although a patient with an urgent condition may be seen ahead of those who arrived before them.

The open office hours system can have many disadvantages. The office may already be crowded when the provider arrives, resulting in an extremely long wait for some patients. Patients may arrive in waves throughout the day, which causes parts of the day to be very busy and other parts to be slow. This makes accomplishing other office duties difficult. Without planning, the facilities and staff can be overburdened.

CRITICAL THINKING APPLICATION   **10-3**

Dr. Brown would like to implement evening appointments one night each week and open the office every other Saturday morning. She feels this will better serve her patients with children who have difficulty making daytime appointments. If this is her primary goal, should other types of patients be seen during these time slots? Why or why not?

Grouping Procedures

Grouping or categorizing of procedures is another method of scheduling that appeals to many practitioners. For instance, an internist might reserve all morning appointments for complete physical examinations, or a pediatrician might keep that time for well-baby visits. A surgeon might devote 1 day each week to seeing only referral patients. Obstetricians often schedule pregnant patients on different days from gynecology patients. The providers and staff can experiment with different groupings until the plan that works best for the practice eventually becomes evident. In applying a grouping system of appointments, the medical assistant may find it helpful to color-code the sections of the appointment book reserved for designated procedures.

Advance Booking

Often appointments are made months in advance. When any appointment is made, an appointment card should be completed and given to the patient. All appointment cards should mention that patients must give 24 hours' notice if they are unable to keep the time reserved. Most offices have some type of confirmation procedure by which patients are notified the day before to verify that they intend to keep the appointment. E-mail and text messages are becoming common methods of reminding patients of upcoming appointments. The medical assistant should be aware of the policies for his or her facility regarding patient reminders.

TIME PATTERNS

When booking appointments, the medical assistant should make it a policy to leave some open time during each day's schedule so that if a patient calls with a special problem that is not an immediate emergency, time will be available to book the patient for at least a brief visit. Mondays and Fridays generally are the most hectic days of the week. Keeping one time slot available in the morning and the afternoon specifically for emergencies also is a wise practice. A busy provider always fills these open slots, and having them in the schedule causes the least **disruption** during the day. If possible, set aside time in the morning and afternoon for a break. Even 15 minutes can give the provider time to return calls from patients, verify prescription calls, or answer questions.

TELEPHONE SCHEDULING

A pleasant manner and expressing a willingness to help are just as important on the telephone as when meeting patients face to face. This is especially true when making appointments, because the telephone contact may be the patient's first impression of the facility. Often the manner in which the booking is made makes more of an effect than the convenience of the appointment time.

Be especially considerate if the time requested for an appointment must be refused. Briefly explain why the time is not available and offer a substitute date and time. Comply with the patient's desires as much as possible, and do not show annoyance if the patient does not understand the scheduling process. Most people, however, understand the need for a well-managed office and are willing to cooperate.

Many offices offer the patient a choice when scheduling the appointment and let the patient decide which option is best for him or her. For example, the following dialog might take place during the scheduling call:

Medical assistant:	*"Mrs. Thomas, Dr. Stern is available to see you in the office next Tuesday or Wednesday, January 6 or 7. Which day is better for you?"*
Patient:	*"I will be working on Wednesday, so I would like to come in on Tuesday."*
Medical assistant:	*"Do you prefer a morning or afternoon appointment?"*
Patient:	*"The afternoon is best for me."*
Medical assistant:	*"Great. Would 1:30 or 3:30 be a better time?"*
Patient:	*"I can be there at 1:30."*
Medical assistant:	*"Then Dr. Stern will see you at 1:30 next Tuesday, January 6. Thank you for calling, Mrs. Thomas. We'll see you then!"*

These small courtesies give patients the feeling that they control their time. Always repeat the time to reinforce the appointment and do not hesitate to ask the patient if he or she has a pen ready to jot down the time and date. While repeating the information to the patient, check the appointment book or computer screen to ensure that it was posted correctly. When scheduling appointments over the telephone it is not possible to give the patient a reminder card for the appointment. Be sure to ask if they would like a telephone, e-mail, or text message reminder of the appointment.

Write legibly when using an appointment book. These records could be called into court, and the medical assistant must be able to read his or her own writing if asked to testify. Form the habit of entering the patient's daytime telephone number after every entry. The appointment may need to be canceled or the schedule rearranged in a hurry, and many precious minutes can be saved if the telephone number is handy. Cell phone numbers also are quite useful for tracking down a patient quickly.

SCHEDULING APPOINTMENTS FOR NEW PATIENTS

Arranging the first appointment for a new patient requires time and attention to detail (Procedures 10-2 and 10-3). This encounter provides the first impression of the healthcare facility and may set the tone for all subsequent visits. Tact, courtesy, and professionalism are extremely important. During the conversation with the new patient, request preliminary information to help determine how much time to allow for the visit on the appointment schedule. The provider may also expect the medical assistant to give general instructions to patients seeking care for specific complaints. For example, the patient may be required to be fasting for certain laboratory tests. Patient demographic information should be collected during the conversation, including the type of insurance the patient has. Some insurance carriers restrict which providers can be used.

After the necessary information has been collected, offer the patient the first available appointment. Whenever possible, offer a choice between two dates and times. Ask the patient to arrive 15 minutes before their scheduled appointment time to complete any paperwork necessary. Also ask whether he or she knows the directions to the healthcare facility or offer the physical address for those who use a GPS or want to obtain exact directions from one of the many Internet direction sites, such as MapQuest. Tell the patient whether any special parking conveniences are available and whether the healthcare facility provides a token or parking validation. The patient's options for the first payment should also be discussed. If payment is expected immediately, inform the patient. The staff should expect patient concerns about the amount of the first bill and should address this issue before the appointment so that there are no surprises or misunderstandings. Before ending the conversation, repeat the appointment date and time and then thank the patient for calling.

Some healthcare facilities mail an information packet/brochure to new patients, especially if the appointment is several days away. With the patient's permission and e-mail address, such information can also be sent via the Internet. An ideal tool to use to deliver this information is a new patient brochure (Procedure 10-3). This brochure can be printed with graphics and images to promote a professional impression of the healthcare facility. This brochure should include the following:

- Description of the practice
- Location or a map
- Telephone numbers
- E-mail and Web site addresses
- Staff names and credentials
- Services offered
- Hours of operation
- How appointments can be scheduled

In addition to the brochure, the packet could include a health history form, the **Notice of Privacy Practices (NPP),** and release of information form (to obtain records from their previous provider).

If another provider has referred the patient, the medical assistant may need to call the referring provider's office to obtain additional information before the patient's appointment. This information should be printed out and given to the attending provider before the patient arrives. Remember to send a thank you note to anyone who refers a patient to the facility.

Often, the medical assistant will need to conduct **preauthorization** or **precertification** to determine whether a patient is eligible for treatment or for certain procedures. The office manager must make certain that these procedures are being done and assign these duties to a specific person(s). More about preauthorization and precertification is included in the Basics of Health Insurance chapter.

PROCEDURE 10-2	Manage Appointment Scheduling Using Established Priorities: Schedule a New Patient

Goal: *To schedule a new patient for a first office visit and identify the urgency of the visit using established priorities.*

Role Play Scenario: Patricia Black, a new patient, calls. She just moved to the area and her asthma has flared up over the last 24 hours, but her albuterol inhaler is empty and she needs a new prescription for it. She states that she is doing okay, but without the albuterol she knows it will get worse within the next few days. According to your screening guidelines, she needs to be seen today and scheduling guidelines indicate she needs a 45-minute appointment.

EQUIPMENT and SUPPLIES

- Appointment book or computer with scheduling software
- Scheduling and screening guidelines
- Pencil

PROCEDURAL STEPS

1. Obtain the patient's demographic information (e.g., full name, birth date, address, and telephone number). Write this information down or enter it into the scheduling software. Verify the information.
   PURPOSE: It is important to verify the information. If you have difficulty hearing the patient, use a system to verify the spelling (e.g., "A" as in apple).
2. Determine whether the patient was referred by another provider.
   PURPOSE: You may need to request additional information from the referring provider and your provider will want to send a consultation report.
3. Determine the patient's chief complaint and when the first symptoms occurred. Utilize the scheduling and screening guidelines as needed.
   PURPOSE: You must know the amount of time that will be required for the visit and how quickly the patient needs to be seen based on the chief complaint.
4. Search the appointment book or scheduling software for the first suitable appointment time and an alternate time. Offer the patient a choice of these dates and time. Be open to alternative times if the patient cannot make the initial options you gave. Provide additional appointment options as needed.
   PURPOSE: Providing the patient with a choice of dates and times and additional options as needed helps to demonstrate sensitivity when managing appointments. It is an important customer service technique (Figure 1).
5. Enter the mutually agreeable time into the schedule. Enter the patient's name, telephone number, and add *NP* for new patient.
   PURPOSE: The *NP* in the appointment book indicates the patient is a new patient. Having the phone number available helps increase your efficiency if you need to contact the patient.
6. Obtain the patient's insurance information. If new patients are expected to pay at the time of the visit, explain this financial arrangement when the appointment is made.
   PURPOSE: Obtaining the patient's insurance information now ensures that the patient is seeing a provider covered by his or her insurance carrier. By explaining the payment policy before the appointment, the patient can come to the appointment prepared to pay.
7. Provide the patient with directions to the healthcare facility and parking instructions if needed.
   NOTE: Many facilities will e-mail or mail new-patient paperwork to the patient, who is instructed to complete the forms before the appointment and bring them to the appointment.
8. Before ending the call, ask if the patient has any questions. Reinforce the date and time of the appointment. Politely and professionally end the call, making sure to thank the patient for calling.
   PURPOSE: It is important to restate the appointment time and date to ensure the patient knows the correct information before ending the call.
   NOTE: For legal and safety reasons, many healthcare practices encourage patients with urgent same-day appointments to seek emergency care immediately if the condition worsens before the appointment time.

PROCEDURE 10-2   *—continued*

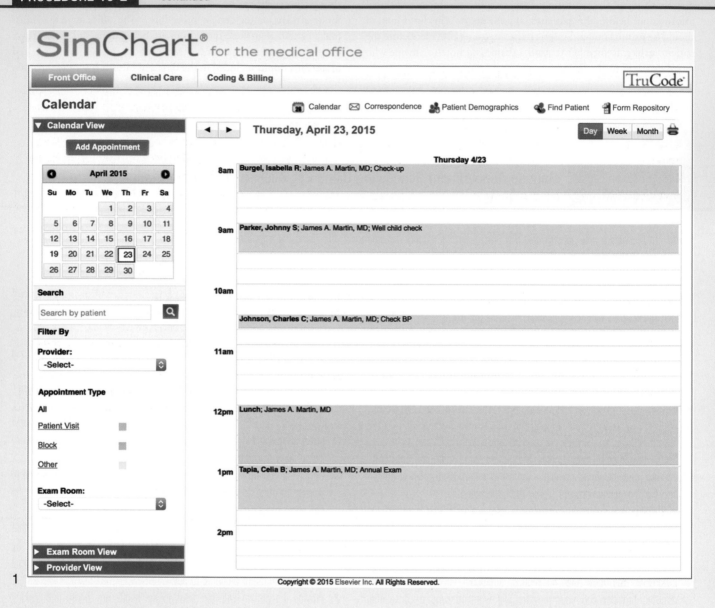

1

PROCEDURE 10-3   Coach Patients Regarding Office Policies: Create the New Patient Brochure

Goal: *Create a new patient brochure that provides an orientation to the practice and the office's policies and procedures.*

Role Play Scenario: Adam Burns stops by the office and he is interested in establishing a relationship with a provider. You need to coach him on the office's information, policies, and procedures.

EQUIPMENT and SUPPLIES

- Computer with word processing software
- Office procedure manual (optional)

PROCEDURAL STEPS

1. Using word processing software, design an informational brochure for patients that provides information about the practice and describes practice procedures. At a minimum, the information should include:

- Description of the practice (e.g., type of practice, mission statement)
- Location or a map of the practice
- Contact information (i.e., telephone numbers, e-mails, and Web site addresses)
- Staff names and credentials
- Services offered
- Hours of operation
- How appointments can be scheduled

- Practice policies and procedures (e.g., payment policies, appointment cancellations, medication refills, assistance after hours)

  <u>PURPOSE:</u> Providing patients with a written brochure listing the practice's information, policies, and procedures enables patients to use it as a reference.

2. Give a brief summary of the different parts of the brochure, including how appointments are scheduled and the practice's policies and procedures.

   <u>PURPOSE:</u> By discussing each part of the brochure with the potential patient, you can help explain what is stated. Summarize the information without reading the sections to the other person.

3. During the summary, use active listening skills by listening to what is said and how the message is said.

   <u>PURPOSE:</u> By actively listening to the other person's responses, you can understand more about what the person is unclear about or what the person wants. Actively listening helps to ensure you provide the necessary answers to the other person.

4. Ask if the person has any questions and listen to the person's questions and needs/wants. Address the questions and clarify any information that is required. Watch and listen for verification of the person's understanding.

   <u>PURPOSE:</u> Again, by using active listening skills, you can better understand what the person is unclear about and then address those areas.

SCHEDULING APPOINTMENTS FOR ESTABLISHED PATIENTS

In Person

Most return appointments for **established patients** are arranged when the patient is leaving the office. A good policy is to have all patients stop by the front desk to check out before leaving in case any information is needed from the patient or any outside scheduling must be done. The patient's health record can be reviewed to see whether the provider ordered any laboratory tests or procedures, and these can be scheduled and discussed with the patient. When making a return appointment, follow the same procedures as for scheduling any appointment by phone, offering the patient choices in the day and time slots (Procedure 10-4). If a certain time the patient specifically requests is not available, offer two alternatives. Always give the patient an appointment card and any necessary instructions at this time, along with a bright smile. Never forget to provide excellent customer service.

PROCEDURE 10-4   **Manage Appointment Scheduling Using Established Priorities: Schedule an Established Patient**

Goal: *To manage the provider's schedule by scheduling appointments for an established patient and handling rescheduling and a no-show appointment.*

Role Play Scenario: Celia Tapia has just completed seeing Dr. Martin and is checking out at your desk. You see that she needs to schedule a follow-up appointment in 2 weeks. The scheduling guidelines indicate a follow-up appointment is 15 minutes long.

EQUIPMENT and SUPPLIES

- Appointment book or computer with scheduling software
- Scheduling guidelines
- Pencil, red pen
- Reminder card
- Patient's health record

PROCEDURAL STEPS

1. Obtain the patient's name and information, purpose of the visit, the provider to be seen, and any scheduling preferences. If using the scheduling software, enter the patient's name and date of birth (DOB). Verify the correct patient is selected.

   <u>PURPOSE:</u> To schedule an appointment, the patient's information is required, along with the provider to be seen and the type of appointment required. Knowing any scheduling preferences or limitations will help you efficiently find an acceptable appointment time for the patient.

2. Identify the length of the appointment by using the scheduling guidelines.

   <u>PURPOSE:</u> Depending on the appointment type, each provider may require a different length of time for that appointment. Ensuring you schedule the appropriate amount of time will help facilitate the flow of patients on that day.

3. Search the appointment book or scheduling software for the first suitable appointment time and an alternate time. Offer the patient a choice of these dates and time. Be open to alternative times if the patient cannot make the initial options you gave. Provide additional appointment options as needed.

   <u>PURPOSE:</u> Providing the patient with a choice of dates and times and additional options as needed helps to demonstrate sensitivity when managing appointments. It is an important customer service technique (Figure 1).

PROCEDURE 10-4   —*continued*

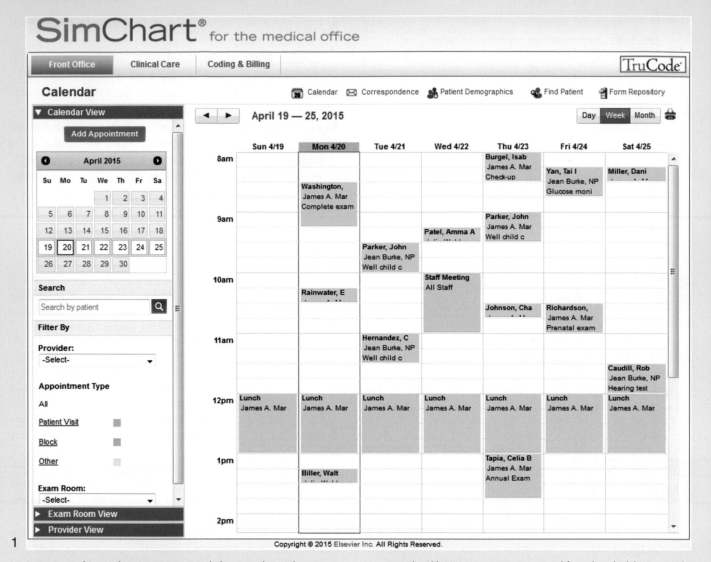

4. Using a pencil, write the patient's name and phone number in the appointment book and block out the correct amount of time. Add in any other relevant information per the facility's procedures. If using the scheduling software, create the appointment per the facility's guidelines.

   PURPOSE: By adding the patient's phone number to the appointment book, if the patient needs to be contacted, it saves time. Using pencil to write down the information in the book allows it to be erased if the patient cancels or reschedules for another time.

5. Complete the appointment reminder card and ensure the date and time on the card matches the appointment time. Give the card to the patient.

   PURPOSE: Using appointment reminder cards helps patients remember when their appointments are and helps decrease the number of no-show appointments.

Continuation of Scenario: Later that day, Mary Jones calls and needs to reschedule her appointment for the next day at the same time.

6. When a patient calls to reschedule an appointment, follow steps #1 through #4. When the new appointment is made, make sure to erase the old appointment from the appointment log. With the scheduling software, ensure the old appointment time is removed from the schedule. Repeat the appointment date and time to the patient.

   NOTE: It is important to erase the old appointment so the patient is not expected on two different days. By erasing or deleting the old appointment, it opens up that time for another patient.

Continuation of Scenario: Mary Jones no-shows for her follow-up appointment.

7. In the appointment book, using red pen, indicate the patient no-showed. Using the patient's health record, document that the patient failed to show for the follow-up examination with the provider. In an electronic system change the appointment status to no-show and ensure that it is documented in the health record.

   PURPOSE: For legal purposes, the healthcare facility must keep a record of patients who no-show for appointments. By indicating it in the appointment book and in the health record, the practice is covered if any issues should arise. Some medical practices have procedures that include contacting the patient regarding the no-show appointment and finding out the reason. This is then also charted in the health record.

By Telephone

Usually the medical assistant needs only to determine when the patient must return and to find a suitable time in the schedule. Established patients do not usually need directions and parking information unless the office has recently moved. The patient's address, telephone number, and insurance should always be verified and any changes documented in the health record. If an e-mail address and/or cell phone number is not on file, obtain one so as to have a quick, easy way to notify the patient of appointments and other events.

SCHEDULING OTHER TYPES OF APPOINTMENTS

The medical assistant may also schedule services other than appointments at the healthcare facility, and these will appear on the appointment schedule. This includes surgeries the provider will perform at a hospital or other facility, consultations, outside appointments and meetings, and even house calls if the provider makes them. The provider also must have time to get from one location to another, so driving time must be considered when arranging all appointments.

Some critical information is required when scheduling admission or treatments in other facilities. Always provide the facility with the patient's name, address, phone numbers (both home and cell), Social Security number, and insurance information and relay the procedures that are to be performed. Patient allergies should be mentioned if the patient is being admitted. Additionally, the facility may have forms that the patient needs to complete, so an e-mail address is helpful in such cases. Always provide the admitting diagnosis and orders to the healthcare facility before admission time. Some facilities require a history form before admission. The patient will be required to bring a form of picture identification, such as a state driver's license, and his or her insurance card.

Inpatient Surgeries

When scheduling a surgery, call the facility where the procedure will be performed as soon as the operation is planned. Provide all necessary information and state any special requests the provider may have, such as the amount of blood to have available for the patient. The facility may want the patient's insurance information and certainly will want a phone number so that the patient can be contacted before the surgery if necessary. Make sure all this information is available before placing the call.

Outpatient and Inpatient Procedure Appointments

A medical assistant often is asked to arrange laboratory or radiography appointments for patients. Before calling the facility to schedule the appointment, be sure all necessary information is available. Inform the patient of the time and place of the appointment, relay any special instructions, and then note these arrangements in the patient's health record. Some offices make a reminder call to the patient or send a reminder e-mail or text message.

Outpatient testing is common because most providers do not have extensive x-ray or laboratory equipment in their offices. Magnetic resonance imaging (MRI), computed tomography (CT) scans, numerous x-ray evaluations, ultrasonography, and simple blood tests all may need to be scheduled (Procedure 10-5). Provide the patient with the name, address, and phone number of the facility where the tests will be done.

Some patients may require a series of appointments (e.g., at weekly intervals). Try to set up these appointments on the same day each week at the same time of day. This considerably reduces the risk of the patient forgetting an appointment.

In some cases the medical assistant may be responsible for scheduling inpatient admissions or inpatient surgical procedures. This is similar to scheduling outpatient testing, but the medical assistant coordinates with a hospital rather than an outside facility and should also be documented in the patient's health record.

It is often the medical assistant's responsibility to provide the patient with any special instructions for the procedure or test that is going to be performed. The patient should be provided with written instructions as well. A patient undergoing general anesthesia will need to fast for approximately 12 hours before the procedure. If medications are to be taken the morning of the procedure the patient may take them with a small sip of water. The provider will instruct the patient about which medications to take. The patient should also be instructed to leave valuables at home. If it is an outpatient procedure and the patient will be sedated in any way, he or she should be instructed to have someone drive them home.

PROCEDURE 10-5 **Schedule a Patient Procedure**

Goal: *To schedule a patient for a procedure within the time frame needed by the provider, confirm with the patient, and issue all required instructions.*

Role Play Scenario: *Monique Jones has just completed seeing Dr. Walden and is checking out at your desk. She gives you an order from the provider that states she needs to have a magnetic resonance image (MRI) of her left ankle within a week. The radiology department in your facility performs MRIs.*

EQUIPMENT and SUPPLIES

- Provider's order detailing the procedure required
- Computer with order entry software (optional)
- Name, address, and telephone number of facility where procedure will take place

- Patient's demographic and insurance information
- Patient's health record
- Procedure preparation instructions
- Telephone
- Consent form (if required for procedure)

PROCEDURE 10-5   —continued

PROCEDURAL STEPS

1. Obtain an oral or written order from the provider for the exact procedure to be performed.
   PURPOSE: For you to schedule the procedure, you will need an order from the provider for the procedure to be performed.

2. Gather the patient's demographic and insurance information. If using an electronic health record, verify you have the correct patient.
   NOTE: For some procedures and diagnostic tests, precertifications or pre-authorizations need to be completed before scheduling the patient. This will be discussed in a later chapter.

3. Determine the patient's availability within the time frame provided by the provider for the procedure (Figure 1).
   PURPOSE: Make sure the patient will be able to comply with the arrangements for the test.

4. Contact the diagnostic facility and schedule the patient's procedure. If you are using a computerized provider order entry (CPOE) system and your facility performs the procedure, you also need to enter the order using the CPOE system.
   - Provide the patient's diagnosis and provider's exact order, including the name of procedure and time frame.
   - Establish the date and time for the procedure.
   - Give the patient's name, age, address, telephone number, and insurance information (i.e., insurance policy numbers, precertification information, and addresses for filing claims).
   - Determine any special instructions for the patient or special anesthesia requirements.
   - Notify the facility of any urgency for test results.
   PURPOSE: Schedule the procedure and provide needed information.

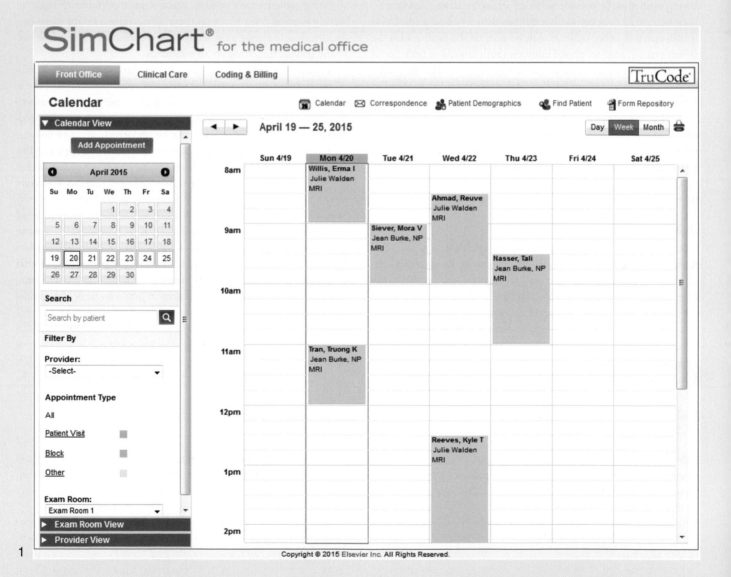

PROCEDURE 10-5   —*continued*

5. Notify the patient of the arrangements and provide the information in a written format.
   - Give the name, address, and telephone number of the diagnostic facility.
   - Specify the date and time to report for the procedure.
   - Give instructions on preparation for the test (e.g., eating restrictions, fluids, medications, enemas).
   - If using another facility, the patient will need to bring a form of picture identification and the insurance card.
   - If not using a CPOE system, explain whether the patient needs to pick up orders or whether the order will be sent to the facility in advance.
   - Ask if the patient has any questions and answer the questions.
   PURPOSE: Make sure the patient understands the necessary preparations and the importance of keeping the appointment. Providing written instructions to the patient will help reinforce what was discussed and give the patient a reference for the information.

6. If a consent form is required for the procedure, ensure the provider has reviewed the form with the patient and the patient has signed the consent form. A copy of the consent form may be required by the diagnostic facility before the procedure. The consent form should be scanned and uploaded into the electronic health record or placed in the paper record.
   PURPOSE: The consent form is used to make sure the patient understands the risks, benefits, and alternatives to the procedure.

7. Document the details of the scheduled procedure in the patient's health record. If applicable, create a reminder to check on the procedure results after the appointment date.
   PURPOSE: Document that the procedure was scheduled. It is legally important to show that what was ordered was scheduled. Creating a reminder for you to check up on the results of the procedure is also important in assisting the provider. 2/27/20XX Patient scheduled for colonoscopy on 3/10/20XX 8:00 am at Anytown Hospital. Patient preparations instructions given and patient verbalized understanding.

Outside Visits

If the provider regularly makes house calls or visits patients in skilled nursing facilities, a special block of time must be reserved in the appointment schedule. There has been an increase in the number of providers who are making house calls again, especially if they have an elderly patient base that are still living independently. The provider needs demographic information, such as addresses, room numbers, and the best route to each home or facility. Remember to allow for travel time.

There are a number of other situations that may have to be added to the schedule, sometimes without much advance warning. Handle all of these situations with care and courtesy.

Providers

Another provider dropping into the facility should be ushered in to see the provider as soon as possible, regardless of the appointment schedule. If the provider is seeing a patient, explain the situation and, if possible, take the visiting provider into a private room, such as the provider's office, to wait. Then notify the provider as soon as possible. Visits from other providers are usually brief and do not appreciably affect the schedule.

Pharmaceutical Representatives

Representatives from pharmaceutical companies are frequent visitors to healthcare facilities and generally are welcomed when the schedule permits. They are well trained and bring the provider valuable information on new drugs. The medical assistant often is expected to screen such visitors and turn away those whose products would not be used in that practice. If the representative or the pharmaceutical company is unknown to the office, ask for a business card and then check with the provider, who will decide whether to see the caller.

Pharmaceutical representatives will often bring samples of the medications that they are going to talk to the provider about. It is important for the medical assistant to understand the policies and procedures for the handling and dispensing of the samples. Most healthcare facilities will require that these samples be stored in a locked cabinet or closet and are given to patients only with provider approval.

Specialists usually limit their conferences with pharmaceutical representatives to their line of practice. The medical assistant, together with the provider, can prepare a list of the representatives with whom the provider is willing to spend time; the list is the determining factor in future conferences. The medical assistant can say whether the provider will be available that day and give an estimate of the waiting time or suggest a later time at which the representative may return. The representative then can decide whether to wait or return later. The pharmaceutical representative usually is quite understanding and cooperative and willing to wait patiently for a long time for just a brief visit with the provider. In turn, the medical assistant should treat the representative with courtesy, showing as much cooperation as possible.

Salespeople

Salespeople from medical, surgical, and office supply houses call regularly at healthcare facilities. Sometimes they want to see the provider, but the office manager or the medical assistant in charge of ordering supplies usually can handle these calls.

Unsolicited salespeople sometimes can present a problem in the professional office. If the provider does not want to see such callers, the medical assistant must firmly but tactfully send them away. Suggest that they leave their literature and cards for the provider to study and say that the provider will contact them if further information is desired.

SPECIAL CIRCUMSTANCES

Late Patients

Every medical practice has a few patients who are habitually late for appointments. This seems to be a problem for which no cure has been found. Emergencies and small delays can happen to anyone, but a patient who constantly arrives late can put a strain on the practice. Such patients can be booked as the last appointment of the day. Then, if closing time arrives before the patient does, the staff has no obligation to wait and other patients have not been inconvenienced. Some medical assistants tell the patient to come in 30 minutes before the appointment time actually scheduled. Make an attempt to work with patients who have occasional difficulties arriving on time, but do not allow the schedule to be constantly disrupted by late patients.

CRITICAL THINKING APPLICATION   **10-4**

Seth Jones is always late for his appointments. How might Ramona approach him about this? What can Ramona do to assist Mr. Jones in arriving for appointments on time?

Rescheduling Appointments

Changes sometimes must be made in the appointment schedule. Unexpected conflicts might arise that force a patient to change the appointment time. When rescheduling an appointment, make sure the first appointment is removed from the appointment book, and then set the new appointment. Otherwise, the patient will be expected in the office on 2 days, and time will be wasted with calls and follow-up, only to discover that the appointment was rescheduled. Most computerized scheduling systems will allow the medical assistant to open the appointment and change the date and time or to cut and paste the appointment into the new date and time.

Emergency Situations

Periodically, emergency or urgent calls come into the office, and an appointment needs to be scheduled. To some extent, all calls that come in go through a **screening** process to evaluate the urgency of the need to see the provider, and emergencies are prioritized. Screening is an extremely important function that requires experience, knowledge of signs and symptoms, and tact.

Emergencies may involve emotional crises in addition to the more obvious physical problems. Patients with emergencies and those who are acutely ill should be seen the same day. The urgency of the call initially can be determined by having a list of questions prepared for reference. The provider should help with this list; he or she should determine what is considered an emergency (life-threatening) or urgent (serious but not life-threatening). The patient may need to be referred directly to a hospital emergency department, or the provider may want to see the patient that day in the office. If patients are unable to get themselves to the hospital the medical assistant may need to contact the emergency medical services in your area. Remember to keep the patient on the phone until emergency medical technicians (EMTs) or other help arrives at the patient's location. Never place an emergency call on hold. Always obtain the name, phone number, and location at the start of the call so that the patient can be found if he or she loses consciousness or is disconnected.

Provider Referrals

If another provider telephones and requests that a patient be seen on the same day, most offices honor that request if at all possible. It is important to keep a schedule that is not intolerant of this type of request.

Patients Without Appointments

The provider and scheduling team should come up with a policy for patients without appointments, also referred to as walk-in patients. A patient who requires immediate attention most likely will be accommodated in the schedule somehow. If the patient does not need immediate care, a scheduled appointment at a later time may be the answer. Be sure to follow established office policy.

FAILED APPOINTMENTS

Why do patients fail to keep appointments? Some are simply forgetful. Once this tendency is detected in a patient, form the habit of telephoning or e-mailing a reminder the day before the appointment. **Automated call routing** offers the patient the option of canceling an appointment and can be programmed to keep calling until the patient responds and confirms or cancels the appointment.

A patient who has been pressed for payment may stay away because of an inability to pay for medical services. Do not make the mistake of classifying all such patients as "deadbeats." Many have every desire to pay, but they cannot afford to and feel embarrassed about their situation, so they avoid their appointments.

Patients also may fail to keep appointments because they are in a state of denial about their condition. For instance, if a patient recently tested positive for the human immunodeficiency virus (HIV), he or she may avoid appointments because going to see the provider forces the patient to face the reality of the disease. Take special care with such patients, and if denial is suspected, discuss this with the provider, who may want to refer the patient for counseling.

It is important to determine the reason for failed appointments and to do whatever is possible to remedy the situation. Telephone the patient to make sure no misunderstanding has occurred. If the patient's health is such that medical care must continue, the provider may write a letter explaining this to the patient. Send the letter by certified mail with return receipt requested. A copy of the letter needs to be added to the patient's medical record for legal protection.

Failed appointments need to be documented in the patient's health record and the appointment schedule for legal purposes. A patient may try to claim abandonment, when he or she has actually been the one to miss the appointments.

NO-SHOW POLICY

Some patients may not realize the importance of keeping their appointments. The patient who does not arrive for a scheduled appointment or reschedule it is called a **no-show**. A busy practice must have a very specific policy on appointment no-shows and must enforce it effectively. The first time a patient fails to show, note the fact on the health record and/or ledger card. The second time, warn the patient, and if a third no-show occurs, consider dropping the patient by using the customary methods that provide legal protection for the provider. Another option, instead of dropping a patient, is to only allow the patient to schedule for same day appointments.

The provider may wish to charge patients for not showing up for the appointment. Be understanding whenever possible, but do not let a patient take advantage of the provider's time. The office policy manual must state that patients may be charged for missed appointments and this should be explained to new patients when their first appointment is made. Because the time slot was scheduled and the provider was ready and available to treat the patient, it is ethical to charge the patient for missing an appointment, especially if he or she did not call to cancel or reschedule. Many providers do not press this issue, but it is an available tool if needed.

INCREASING APPOINTMENT SHOW RATES

Everyone benefits from a full schedule of kept appointments. Appointment show rates can be increased in several ways.

Automated Call Routing

As mentioned earlier, automated call reminders can contact patients scheduled for appointments. The patient is asked to press a certain key on the phone to confirm the appointment and a different key to cancel the appointment. This same tool can be used to send messages to patients (e.g., a reminder that it is the time of year to get a flu vaccination), to introduce a new provider at the office, or announce the availability of a new procedure. The provider can even record the call so that it sounds more personal. These systems can also be set up to send text messages to remind patients of their upcoming appointments.

Appointment Cards

Most healthcare facilities use appointment cards to remind patients of scheduled appointments and to eliminate misunderstandings about dates and times (Figure 10-3). Make a habit of reaching for an appointment card while writing an entry in the appointment book or scheduling it on the computer. After the date and time have been written on the card, double-check with the book/computer to make sure the entries agree.

Confirmation Calls

Patients who have made appointments in advance may appreciate a confirmation call to remind them they have a time set aside to see the provider. Always note the phone number the patient prefers the office to use for such calls. Many individuals have a home phone, cell phone, and work phone numbers; however, they may want calls from the provider to go only to their home phone. Highlight the preferred phone number in the medical record or indicate it on the computer. The office must use caution in making calls to patients because of the significance of privacy guidelines and standards. Some offices may want to prepare a release form in which the patient grants the office staff permission to contact the patient. Many providers

insist that messages left on voice mail not mention the term "doctor" or "doctor's office" for confidentiality reasons. The medical assistant might say, "This is Pam at Robert Welch's office confirming your appointment tomorrow at 2 PM. Please call us if you cannot make the appointment. Our number is 555-212-0909. Thank you!"

If the patient has signed the privacy policy and the policy states that messages from the provider's office may be left at certain numbers, the office certainly can leave messages at that number and mention that the call is from the healthcare facility. Still, it is a good idea to have an established policy on leaving messages that does not breach the patient's confidentiality.

E-Mail Reminders

Many computer scheduling programs can send an e-mail to patients the day before an appointment to remind them of it. This is a great timesaver for the office staff, because no time is taken to perform this duty other than the original scheduling of the appointment.

Mailed Reminders

The office staff may mail reminder letters to patients. This method is a bit time-consuming with a paper-based appointment system but worth the effort if the patients show up for their appointments. Computer scheduling systems can be set up to generate the reminder letters for scheduled appointments and also to remind patients that they are due for their annual physical or influenza vaccination.

HANDLING CANCELLATIONS AND DELAYS

When the Patient Cancels

Inevitably, cancellations occur. If a list is kept of patients with advance appointments who would like to come in sooner, the medical assistant can begin calling to try to get one of them in to fill the available opening. By keeping a list of patients willing to take the first canceled appointment, the medical assistant can readily identify which patients to call to fill the vacancy. Each cancellation should be noted in the medical record, along with a reason for the cancellation if that information is available. If the patient simply reschedules an appointment, a notation need not be made in the health record unless a pattern develops that might be significant to the patient's medical treatment.

When the Provider Is Delayed

Some days the provider will be delayed in reaching the office. If advance notice of the delay is received, start calling patients with early appointments and suggest that they come later. If some patients arrive before the office learns of the delay, explain that an emergency has detained the provider.

Show concern for the patient, but do not be overly apologetic, which might imply some degree of guilt. Most patients realize that a provider has certain priorities. The patient in the office may be inconvenienced, but it is not a "life or death" matter. If this kind of situation occurs frequently, however, consider devising a different scheduling system.

When the Provider Is Called to an Emergency

Providers are conscious of their responsibilities for responding to medical emergencies, and most patients understand if the medical

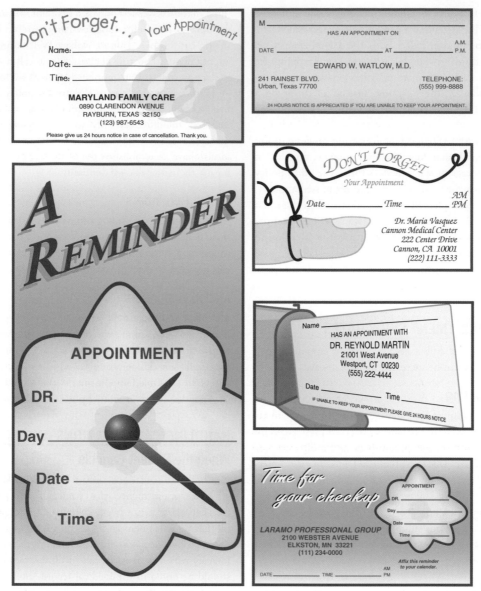

FIGURE 10-3 Examples of appointment cards.

assistant takes time to explain what has happened. The medical assistant may say, "Dr. Wright has been called away due to an emergency. She asked me to tell you she is very sorry to keep you waiting. There will be at least a 1-hour delay." The medical assistant should then ask the patient, "Would you like to wait? If that is inconvenient, I'll be glad to give you the first available appointment on another day. Or perhaps you'd like to have some coffee or do some shopping and return in an hour." It is also possible that another provider may be able to see the patient.

As quickly as possible, call the patients scheduled for a later hour. In many offices, especially those of obstetricians, surgeons, and general practitioners, a whole day's appointments must be canceled. For this reason, it is particularly important to have the daytime telephone number of each patient available so that the appointment can be rescheduled. If at all possible, cancel appointments before the patient arrives in the office to find that the provider is not available.

The **expediency** of the office staff in contacting patients who will be affected by an emergency is appreciated.

When the Provider Is Ill or Out of Town

Providers get ill, too, and patients scheduled to be seen during the course of the provider's recovery must be informed of this and their appointments rescheduled. They need not be told the nature of the illness.

When the provider is called out of town for personal or professional reasons, appointments must be canceled or rescheduled. Customarily, the patient is given the name of another provider, or possibly a choice of several, who will provide care during such absences. For security reasons, merely state that the doctor is unavailable. Stating over the telephone that the provider is out of town could lead to attempted burglary or other unauthorized intrusion on the premises.

PATIENT PROCESSING

The patient reception area should be an inviting place where patients feel comfortable. Visits to the provider can be times of great stress, and the staff must do everything possible to make the experience pleasant for patients. A patient usually has a choice of healthcare providers and should be given excellent customer service. Good patient relations result in referrals to the provider, and this helps the practice grow. When patients have a good experience with a provider, they are likely to tell others. When the staff is committed to making the patient feel welcome and the focus is on care of the patient, success of the practice is inevitable.

THE RECEPTION AREA

A first impression is a lasting one. Nowhere is this more important than in the healthcare facility, where the environment must appear orderly and faultlessly clean. The facility may be a provider's office, a hospital, a health maintenance organization, or one of the many other healthcare establishments. No matter the type of facility, the appearance of the reception room and the front desk, as well as a cordial greeting from the medical assistant, influence patients' **perception** of the entire facility and of the care they will receive.

The reception room is just that—a place to receive patients and visitors. The area should be planned for patients' comfort; it should be as attractive and cheerful as possible and kept clean and uncluttered. Some medical assistants have the opportunity to assist in the design and decoration of this very important area. Consider the traffic flow (i.e., the movement of patients from place to place) both in the reception room and through the rest of the facility so that it is unhindered and logical (Figure 10-4).

> **CRITICAL THINKING** APPLICATION   **10-5**
> Ramona believes that her patients enjoy a homey atmosphere, which is less intimidating than the sterile, clinical feel of some healthcare facilities. How might she give her facility this type of ambiance?

Fresh, **harmonious** colors and cleanliness are the foundation of an attractive room (Figure 10-5). Select comfortable furniture appropriate to the patients seen (e.g., higher chairs with arms for orthopedic patients, wider chairs for larger patients, small chairs for pediatric patients). Furniture should accommodate the peak load of patients seen each day; arrange it in conversational groups. Individual seating usually is the best choice for the provider's office. Provide good lighting, ventilation, and a regulated temperature. Reduce room clutter by providing a place to hang coats, rainwear, and umbrellas.

Most providers' offices are well supplied with recent magazines, and some have various books. Publications with short items of popular interest, such as *Reader's Digest,* are favorites. Any reading material placed in the reception room should be of interest to the general public; *Good Housekeeping, U.S. News and World Report, Real Simple, Oprah,* and *People* are examples of interesting magazines that most people enjoy reading. Some patients may donate magazines to the healthcare facility; if there is a name in the subscription area, be sure to mark through it so that the patient's name cannot be read.

The reception room is not the place for the provider's professional journals or pharmaceutical company's flyers.

A writing desk with writing paper in the reception area for the convenience of patients is a nice touch. A selection of tea and coffee is also appreciated by patients. Music from a concealed speaker is often used to make patients feel more comfortable while waiting and also provides white noise to help maintain patient confidentiality. A lighted aquarium or an educational display of some sort enhances the attractiveness and individuality of the reception area in the professional practice. Patients often are interested in health-related brochures. The provider also may have a DVD or healthcare book library that allows patients to check out items of interest to them. A telephone in the reception area is an asset and can be programmed by the telephone company not to allow long distance calls. A television or DVD player can help the time pass much faster, especially in pediatric practices. Children enjoy Disney movies and cartoon programs, and these hold their interest until it is time to see the provider. A children's corner equipped with small-scale furniture and some playthings works well. Youngsters who might otherwise get into mischief are kept pleasantly occupied. Toys should be easily cleanable; plastic washable items are especially good. Take extra care to ensure that no toy has sharp corners that could cause injury or small parts that could be swallowed. When selecting toys, make sure they will not stimulate the child toward noisy activity. Never place any type of ball in the reception area, because small children tend to throw them, and the balls can injure a patient or visitor.

> **CRITICAL THINKING** APPLICATION   **10-6**
> Ramona has a few patients who bring young children to their appointments. Sometimes the children are a bit disruptive and make other patients feel uncomfortable. How might Ramona handle this problem in the healthcare facility? Some children misbehave in public, and the parents do not respond or correct them. How might Ramona deal with this situation if it arises?

Many healthcare facilities offer a computer for patients to use while waiting to see the provider. This is a great **amenity**, because patients can make good use of their time in the reception area. Some patients may bring their personal laptop computers and use their wait time to complete projects. Providing Internet access for patients also is helpful; an amazing amount of work can be done just by checking e-mail. If patients are allowed to connect to the facilities network, the wise course is to provide one specific log-on name and password just for them so as to maintain control over access to private health information.

Periodically, take an objective look around the reception room. Could it use a little brightening or freshening up? Try to look at the room as if seeing it for the first time. The medical assistant is responsible for the appearance of the area by making sure the room remains neat and orderly throughout the day. Check the temperature and lighting for comfort. Scan the room at intervals during the day to ensure that it is in good order.

If the medical assistant's desk is in the reception area or in open view of patients, it should be free of clutter. In particular, patients' medical and financial records should not be in sight. To protect patient confidentiality, keep computer monitors turned so that those

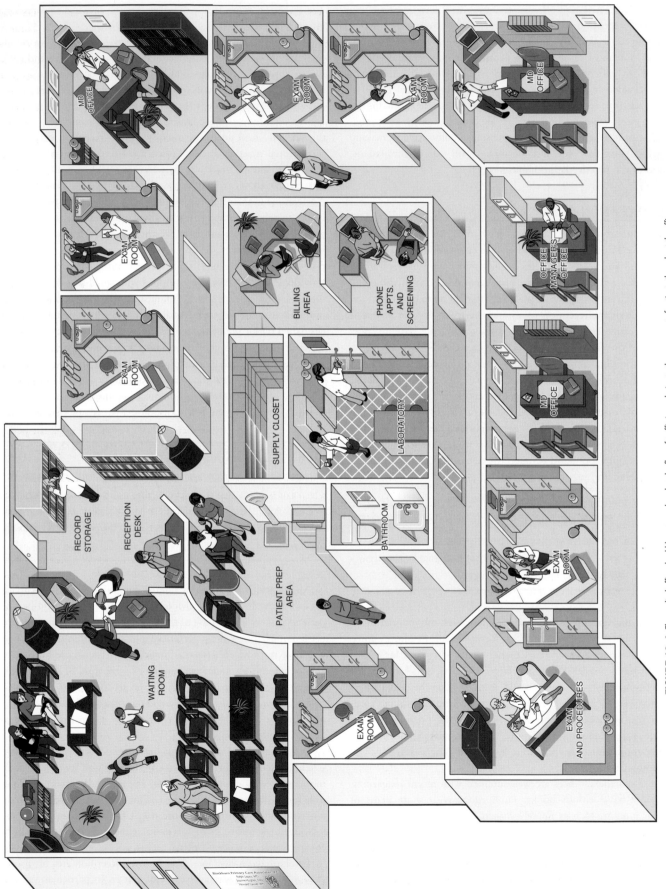

FIGURE 10–4 The medical office should be arranged so that the flow of traffic is conducive to the movement of patients throughout the office.

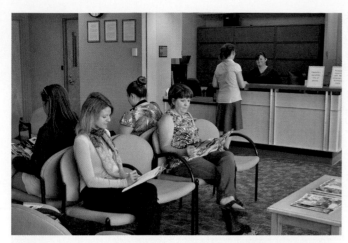

FIGURE 10-5 Patients appreciate cleanliness, restful colors, good ventilation, and light to read by when waiting in the reception area.

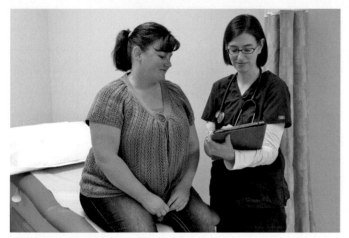

FIGURE 10-6 More providers and their staff members use electronic medical records to reduce paperwork and provide better, more efficient patient care.

waiting cannot view them. Some healthcare facilities use privacy screens that allow only the user to see the monitor, or they use a screen saver that activates after being idle for a few minutes. Medical assistants should not keep personal items on their desks.

PREPARING FOR PATIENT ARRIVAL

Advanced preparation helps make the day go smoothly and contributes to a more relaxed atmosphere for all. Some heatlhcare facilities prepare for the next day on the evening before, whereas others prepare each morning. The healthcare facility should be consistent, and the same routine should always be performed so that important preparations are not left undone.

Preparing Health Records

Review a list of patients who will visit the provider during the next appointment period. If an electronic health record system is used, this task could be as simple as pulling up and printing a report (Figure 10-6). If a paper-based appointment book system is used, pull the medical records for the day (or the next day if this is done in the evenings) and check off the patient's name on a copy of the appointment schedule; this helps ensure that all the records have

been located and are ready. Occasionally two or more patients may have the same or a similar name. Check the patient's Social Security number, date of birth, or other pertinent information to make sure the right medical record has been pulled. Review each record to verify that any recently received information (e.g., laboratory reports, radiograph readings) has been entered correctly and permanently attached to the record; if a document is missing, attempt to obtain it before the patient's arrival using a fax or other electronic means. Arrange the medical records **sequentially** in the order in which the patients are scheduled. The medical assistant may be expected to place the records of all the patients to be seen that day on the provider's desk, but the provider is more likely to prefer reviewing each record just before entering the examination room. Make sure enough space is available on the **progress notes** for the provider to write in the record. If not, place additional progress notes pages in the record.

Patient Check-in

The reception desk should be in clear view of all visitors who come into the office. If only one medical assistant is present, welcoming each new visitor personally sometimes is impossible. Develop an announcement system that alerts the staff when people enter the office. Patients who enter an empty reception room do not know whether to sit down, knock on the glass partition, or try to announce themselves in some other way. Glass partitions are used to maintain some privacy; however, some providers have eliminated them because they are so impersonal and they send the signal that the provider and staff are off limits to patients. If the partition is used, the policy and procedure manual should dictate when the glass should remain open and when it should be closed.

Make sure no patient medical records are on the reception desk and that the computer monitor is positioned so that it cannot be viewed by patients at the desk. This prevents violation of the regulations established by the Health Insurance Portability and Accountability Act (HIPAA).

The medical assistant should check the reception room each time he or she has been away from the desk to see whether more patients have arrived. Greet these patients by name; if you do not know the person who has entered the reception area, ask the individual's name. Use a sign-in register that promotes patients' privacy (Figure 10-7). Although patients can read the names of others who are in the healthcare facility to visit the provider, this is not considered a violation of HIPAA policy as long as the information disclosed is appropriately limited. This is one type of **incidental disclosure**. Pressure-sensitive labels printed with lines for the patient's name, the appointment time, and a "yes" or "no" question about changes in insurance coverage are a practical, inexpensive solution for confidential patient registers. Patients should not be expected to provide details of the reason for their visit in a public area.

During the patient check-in process it is vital that the medical assistant takes steps to protect the other patients in the reception area. One of the first questions that must be asked, according to the Centers for Disease Control and Prevention (CDC), is whether in the last 21 days, the patient has traveled to a country with widespread transmission or uncertain control for Ebola (e.g., Guinea, Liberia, or Sierra Leone) or had contact with someone with confirmed Ebola virus disease (EVD). If the patient answers yes, he or she should be isolated immediately. The medical assistant should

Patient Sign-In   Date: _____

Please sign-in and notify us if:

• **New patient**   • **Phone/address change**   • **Insurance change**

No.	Patient Name print	Appt. Time	Arrival Time	Appt. with	New patient (✓)	Phone/address change (✓)	Insurance change (✓)
1	P L E A S E						
2	2						
3	3						
4	4						
5	5						
6	6						
7	7						
8	8						
9	9						
10	10						
11	11						
12	12						
13	13						
14	14						
15	15						
16	16						
17	17						
18	18						
19	19						
20	20						
21	21						
22	22						
23	23						
24	24						
25	25						

FIGURE 10-7 Sign-in sheets contain very basic information about the patient and provide information for the medical assistant about changes that need to be edited on the patient's record.

follow the procedures of the facility for this process. During periods of increased respiratory infection activity (e.g., flu season) the health-care facility should make masks available for patients in the reception area. At check-in the medical assistant may need to ask patients to put on a mask while they are waiting if they are coughing. Tissues, along with waste containers and hand sanitizer, should be available for patients in the reception area.

GREETING THE PATIENT

Every patient has the right to expect courteous treatment in a pro-vider's office. Regardless of the patient's economic or social status, each person who enters the reception room should receive a cordial,

friendly greeting (Figure 10-8). A personal touch, such as greeting the patient by name, is an easy way to develop patient rapport. Use the patient's last name and title unless the patient insists on the use of his or her first name or prefers a nickname. For example, the medical assistant may say:

"How are you today, Mr. Roberts?"

"Ms. Nelson, the doctor will be in to see you shortly."

If the healthcare facility has a policy of obtaining a copy of all patients' photo identification cards, such as the driver's license, these can be used to identify patients and greet them by name, even if they do not visit the healthcare facility often. Some EHR systems allow for a patient's picture to be added so the medical assistant can be assured that they have the correct patient record opened during

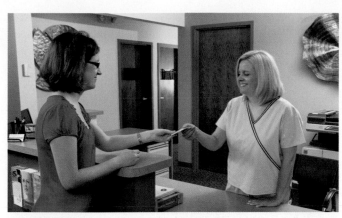

FIGURE 10-8 Greet all patients with a warm smile and assist them with forms they need to complete for the medical record.

check-in. Requesting a photo identification card or having the patient's picture on file also ensures that the person requesting benefits is actually the person covered by the insurance policy.

Patient Interaction

Although the healthcare facility can make patients feel uncomfortable, the medical assistant should try to make everyone feel at ease. Cultivate the habit of greeting each patient immediately in a friendly, self-assured manner. Establish eye contact and smile while introducing yourself to the patient. For example, "Good morning. I'm Elizabeth, Dr. Wade's medical assistant." Remember to ask about why the patient is here before asking about insurance coverage; no patient wants to feel that the provider's main interest is the collection of an insurance check.

Patients like to be acknowledged when they arrive. All staff members should review the day's schedule in the morning to be prepared to greet patients by name and to know whether the patient is new or established. Learn how to pronounce each patient's name correctly; incorrect pronunciations may offend or irritate some people. If the name is unusual, make a note of the **phonetic** spelling in the health record for reference. Note if the patient prefers a nickname. Documenting this information in the health record can help staff members remember names when talking to patients on the phone or in person. By using the patient's name often, the medical assistant also ensures that the correct patient is being treated.

Providers and staff members sometimes make brief notes in the health record about the current events in the patient's life. With this information, the medical assistant and the provider can read those notes before entering the examination room and share a short dialog with patients at the beginning of their visits. For example:

Medical assistant:	*"Hello, Mrs. Williams, how are you today?"*
Mrs. Williams:	*"I am doing very well, Ramona, how are you?"*
Medical assistant:	*"I'm fine. How was the cruise you took with your husband last month?"*
Mrs. Williams:	*"It was wonderful! The water was the bluest I have seen!"*
Medical assistant:	*"You went to Cozumel, didn't you?"*

Mrs. Williams:	*"Yes, we did! I'm surprised you remember, as many patients as you see each day!"*

This brief chat confirms that the staff members care about the individual patient, because they take an interest in their personal lives. Because the patient does not see the medical assistant or provider look at the notes before entering the patient room, the patient assumes that the information is recalled from memory. This is an impressive customer service technique. Most patients appreciate the provider and staff's interest in their families, hobbies, and work. Computer-based health records systems usually have a notes option where such information can be recorded.

Patients may feel somewhat anxious when visiting the provider's office, especially if they know they may be receiving bad news; perhaps a tumor has been discovered to be cancerous, or a family member may have been diagnosed with Alzheimer's disease. Watch the patient's body language. If a patient does not maintain good eye contact or seems otherwise uneasy, a gentle touch or a reassuring smile may be helpful as the office visit progresses. Remember to keep the patient's safety in mind and make certain that he or she has some type of support that will assure a safe arrival back home or at a family or friend's home after the office visit.

Some state regulations prohibit the placement of information other than health details in the health record; however, most health professionals agree that a patient's mental and emotional health are connected to the person's physical health. Details about what is happening in patients' lives provide clues to their physical problems. As a simple example, a patient going through a divorce may experience depression that needs to be treated with medication. Without knowledge of the divorce, the provider does not have all the information needed to make a sound medical decision. Providers can treat patients more effectively when such information is available in the health record.

REGISTRATION PROCEDURES

On a patient's first visit to the provider's office, the staff performs certain registration procedures. Most providers use a patient information or registration form to gather demographic information about the patient. The form may be attached to a clipboard and handed to the patient with instructions to complete sections. The medical assistant must be ready and willing to answer any questions

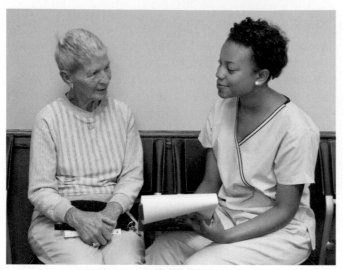

FIGURE 10-9 The medical assistant should take time to explain forms the patient does not understand and should always be willing to answer questions.

(Figure 10-9). The patient's name should appear prominently at the top of the form, followed by other pertinent facts in logical order. Most information sheets contain the following:

- Patient's full name and date of birth
- Responsible person's name and relationship to the patient
- Address and telephone number
- Name, address, and telephone number of contact person
- Occupation
- Place of employment
- Social Security number
- Driver's license number
- Nearest relative not living with the patient and his or her relationship
- Source of referral, if any

When the completed form is returned, check carefully to verify that all the necessary information has been provided. At this time the medical assistant should scan or obtain a copy of both sides of the patient's insurance card, verify the subscriber's date of birth, and collect any copayments. Ask the patient for payment, using phrases such as, "Your copay today is $15, Mrs. Williams. Will you be writing a check or would you like to charge this visit to your Visa?"

Some healthcare facilities insist that copays be collected before the office visit; this matter is handled according to the provider's discretion. Some patients do not believe they should have to pay before seeing the provider; they simply are not used to paying at the start of the visit. The medical assistant can say, "Mr. Thomas, would you like to go ahead and pay your copay now?" By giving the patient the option, it seems as if the medical assistant is helping the patient save time instead of insisting on collecting before seeing the provider. Follow the procedures outlined in the policy.

If this is a new patient, he or she will need to be given the healthcare facility's NPP document and sign an acknowledgment of receipt of the NPP that will need to be added to the patient's health record. In addition to scanning or copying the insurance card, many healthcare facilities also require the scanning or copying of patient's legal photo identification.

Some practices place their registration paperwork on their Web site, and the patient can download, complete, and print the paperwork before the first office visit. If a good length of time will pass between making the appointment and arriving for the office visit, the paperwork can be mailed to the patient with instructions to bring the completed documents to the office visit.

CRITICAL THINKING APPLICATION   **10-8**

Often some time is needed to complete forms when a new patient arrives in the healthcare facility. How might Ramona keep the healthcare facility on schedule when new patients arrive who require health record construction and form completion? What are some ways to trim time from these activities?

Obtaining a Patient's History

The patient's personal history, medical history, and family history may be obtained by asking him or her to complete a questionnaire. The questionnaire could be in a paper or electronic format. The paper form can be mailed to the patient to complete before they arrive for their appointment and the medical assistant may enter the information into the EHR. The electronic form can be completed at a private computer station once the patient has arrived at the healthcare facility, or the medical assistant may gather the information and enter it into the EHR. Another electronic option is for the patient to go to the healthcare facility's Web site and complete the form before the appointment. The provider can augment this information during the patient interview. Some experienced medical assistants conduct the interview to obtain the patient's personal and medical history, family history, and chief complaint.

SHOWING CONSIDERATION FOR PATIENTS' TIME

The patient expects to see the provider or practitioner at the appointed time. The medical assistant should bring the patient to the examination room for treatment or consultation as close to the appointment time as possible or explain delays. All patients want to be kept informed about how long they should expect to wait to see the provider. Any delay longer than 10 to 15 minutes should be explained (Figure 10-10). The medical assistant can also offer to reschedule the appointment for the patient. A crowded reception room is not always an indication of a provider's popularity. It may simply mean that the provider or assistant is inefficient at scheduling patients. Always consider the patient's time and make every effort to streamline the office visit.

A solo or small practice should seldom have more than three to five patients in the reception room. Patients complain that the wait time in medical facilities is one of the most frustrating aspects of the medical profession. The patient who complains about medical fees or the care received may first have become agitated during a long wait to see the provider. Many patients are fearful and tense; long wait times intensify these feelings. The medical assistant can often put patients in a better frame of mind with just a friendly smile and a show of concern.

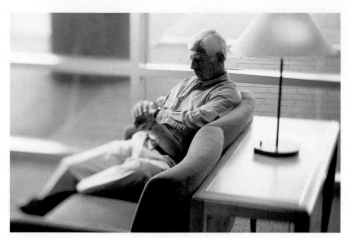

FIGURE 10-10 One of the most common patient complaints is the time spent in the reception area.

CRITICAL THINKING APPLICATION   **10-9**

Ramona offers to reschedule patient appointments if the schedule ever falls more than 15 minutes behind. If a patient becomes belligerent about the delays, how can Ramona handle the situation in a professional manner?

Patients With Special Needs

Some patients are physically challenged, some are very ill, and some are severely uncomfortable. Language or cultural barriers may exist. Observe the patient's appearance and behavior. Is the patient pale? Do the eyes or voice reflect pain or discomfort? Find out how the patient is feeling before suggesting that he or she be seated to wait for the provider. The patient may need to lie down in a cool room or perhaps be seen as an emergency case. Patients with disabilities, such as those who use a wheelchair, cane, walker, or crutches, may need extra attention. Some patients may need help disrobing even if a disability is not obvious. Always ask if the patient needs assistance and how you can actually help them. If there is a language barrier, having translation assistance available will help. This could be an actual person who does the translation or technology can be used do the translation. There are many online programs that can assist with translation in many different languages. In all special needs cases it is important to remain professional and treat everyone with respect.

ESCORTING AND INSTRUCTING THE PATIENT

While in the healthcare facility, most patients prefer to be escorted rather than simply told where to go. This usually is the clinical medical assistant's responsibility, but the task may be assigned to an administrative medical assistant. Pronounce the patient's name correctly when calling the person to the clinical area. If unsure of the pronunciation, ask the patient. Write the name phonetically on the health record for quick retrieval at the next appointment.

Some patients bring a family member or friend with them to the appointment. On occasion, several people want to accompany the patient when the person sees the provider. The healthcare facility policy and procedure manual should address the maximum number of patients allowed in. If the patient insists on more visitors, explain that the examination rooms are small and have only two chairs and suggest that the additional people may be uncomfortable standing in such a small room. If the patient still insists, make every attempt to satisfy the patient's needs.

Remember that, to an employee of the practice, the healthcare facility surroundings may become as familiar as home. A stranger to the practice's environment may be confused or disoriented by all the hallways, doors, and rooms. Uncertainty creates anxiety. Take the time to escort the patient personally to the appropriate examination or treatment room; do not point to the room and expect the patient to find the way. If a urine specimen is needed, direct the patient to the restroom and always explain how to collect the specimen and what to do with it. Having signs on the wall with room numbers and directions can be helpful to patients also.

HEALTH RECORD CARE

Health records should never be left in the examination room to be picked up and read by a patient. Doing so can cause misunderstandings, because patients rarely know medical terms and abbreviations. A number of methods are used to signal that a patient is ready to be seen. Often file holders are located on the doors of the examination rooms, and the health record can be placed in the holder horizontally when the patient is ready to be seen. The provider can signal the medical assistant that he or she is finished examining the patient by placing the health record in an upright position on leaving the examination room. Place the health record so that other patients in the hallway cannot see the patient's name. HIPAA considers names on health records to be incidental disclosures; however, protecting patient privacy by simply turning the record so that the name cannot be read is a good habit to cultivate.

With an EHR system, it is important to remember to log out of the computer when you are ready to leave the room. This will prevent any additions or deletions to the record and prevent the patient from viewing the record without a healthcare professional with them to explain any questions or concerns.

Some healthcare facilities have call light systems, by which a provider can press a button to call the medical assistant for help with the examination. Others have a flag system outside the door that signals what that particular patient needs next. Other healthcare facilities place patients in examination rooms in a certain order, and the provider knows, for instance, that when he or she has finished with the patient in room 1, the next patient will be waiting in room 2. The healthcare facility should develop a method that allows the most efficient use of time, provides high-quality care, and protects patient confidentiality.

CHALLENGING SITUATIONS
Talkative Patients

Any professional office has problem patients. Talkative patients, for example, take up far more of the provider's time than is justified. An alert medical assistant usually can spot this tendency during the initial interview. The patient's history can be flagged with a symbol to alert the provider. The medical assistant can buzz the provider's **intercom** and remind him or her that the next patient is ready. Once the medical assistant has learned which patients take extra time, they can be booked for the end of the day, or more time can be allowed for them.

CRITICAL THINKING APPLICATION   10-10
Ramona has one patient who insists on sitting close to her desk and attempting to chat the entire time she is waiting to see the provider. Even worse, she comes to her appointments at least an hour early. How might Ramona subtly deal with this patient?

Children

Children frequently present special management challenges, whether they are patients or they accompany a patient. Usually, the parent or guardian accompanies the child into the examination room, but some exceptions exist, such as cases of suspected child abuse. Older children certainly can see the doctor without a parent, especially for routine visits, such as a school sports physical. However, minors still need a parent to consent to treatment in most cases. The provider cannot force the parent to leave the examination room by any means. Although this practice of separating children from their parents to treat their needs is not always feasible, it sometimes can be applied with great success. By explaining to the parent that the child needs to develop a sense of independence and control of his or her own health care, they will often agree that they do not need to be in the exam room for the whole visit. Often there can be compromise by having the parent in the room before the examination to talk to the provider; the parent would then leave the room for the actual physical examination.

Parents are responsible for their children's behavior while at the healthcare facility. If children are doing something that could harm them or other patients, quietly speak to the parents and allow them to handle the situation. When children behave badly, the medical assistant can go to the child, kneel down to his or her level, and offer a book or toy, leading the child away from any objects that could be broken or from other patients. The medical assistant can say, "Let's come over here and play next to your mom!" The medical assistant should not discipline the child. If the child continues to behave badly, call the parent to the examination room early so that others in the reception area can relax and enjoy a pleasant office visit. Some patients may be anxious about receiving test results or have other issues, and an unruly child can make the situation even worse.

Angry Patients in the Reception Area

Every medical assistant eventually is confronted with an angry patient. The anger may simply reflect the patient's pain or fear of what the provider may discover during the examination. If possible, invite the patient into a room out of the reception area. Usually the best course is to let the patient talk out the anger. Present a calm attitude and speak in a low tone of voice. Under no circumstances should the medical assistant return the anger or become argumentative. Medical assistants must use good listening skills with angry people and must be empathetic.

There should be a policy in place for dealing with potentially dangerous individuals. Policies can include making sure that you can reach the exit if you take the patient to another room; having another employee close by; and knowing under what circumstances you should contact the police or building security for assistance.

Patient's Relatives and Friends

Patients are sometimes accompanied by a relative or well-meaning friend who may become restless waiting for the patient and attempt to discuss the patient's illness. The medical assistant should sidestep any discussion of a patient's medical care, except by direction of the provider. Avoid a "too casual" attitude, such as, "I'm sure there's nothing to worry about." A show of moderate concern and reassurance that "the patient is in good hands" usually takes care of the situation. Remember that health information cannot be released to anyone, including concerned friends and relatives, without the patient's consent.

THE FRIENDLY FAREWELL

The medical assistant can help convey a sense of caring by terminating the visit cordially. If the patient will return for another visit, the assistant can say something like, "We'll see you next week." If the patient will not be returning soon, a pleasant "I hope you'll be feeling better soon" is appropriate. Whatever words of goodbye are chosen, all patients should leave the facility feeling that they have received top-quality care and were treated with friendliness, respect, and courtesy.

PATIENT CHECKOUT

When the patient returns to the front office for checkout, greet him or her with a friendly smile and call the individual by name. Form the habit of asking patients whether they have any questions. Check the health record to determine when the provider wants the patient to return. Most providers note this information on the encounter form. Make the return appointment, remembering the technique of giving the patient choices for days, morning or afternoon, and specific times.

Be sure to thank the patient for coming and wish the person well as he or she leaves the facility.

PLANNING FOR THE NEXT DAY

As the day is winding down, look over the appointments scheduled for the next day. Review the health records for scheduled patients. If laboratory tests or other procedures were scheduled on the patient's last visit, determine whether the reports are available in the health record. If the patient is scheduled for specific procedures on this visit, make sure everything needed for the procedure is on hand and available. Planning can save many precious moments at the time of the patient visit.

CLOSING COMMENTS

The administrative medical assistant has a huge effect on the efficiency of the healthcare facility. A friendly, helpful attitude is a **prerequisite** for cordial **interaction** with patients, as is the ability to make compromises that benefit both the provider and patient. A personal touch is vital to projecting a sense of caring to the patients seen in the healthcare facility. Many healthcare facilities are not concerned enough about the customer service aspect of the business. Patients talk about their experiences with their friends and relatives and may be an excellent source of referrals if they are treated with dignity and courtesy. If they have a good experience, they tell several people. If they have a poor experience, they tend to tell everyone they know. Make sure to play a part in having each patient feel a sense of satisfaction as he or she leaves the office. All patients should feel that their time and money have been well spent. An office that runs smoothly and stays on schedule indicates professionalism and competence and is greatly appreciated by all who come in contact with it.

Patient Education

Providing patients with an information booklet about the healthcare facility can familiarize them with policies and procedures. Many providers compile an extensive booklet that even provides tips as to when the provider should be called immediately, listing symptoms and signs of emergencies.

Educating the patient about the healthcare facility's policies helps the facility run smoothly from day to day. All patients should be familiar with the policies about appointments. This leads to fewer misunderstandings and conflicts over bills that might include a charge for a missed appointment.

If the facility offers Internet-based appointment scheduling or forms completion, patients must be taught how to use the system. A printed pamphlet or information sheet is helpful for providing instructions to the patient. A wise option is to have a special phone number patients can call if they have problems with the system. For best results, choose a program that is simple to use, easy to understand, and does not breach patient confidentiality.

Legal and Ethical Issues

As mentioned earlier, the appointment schedule may be used as a legal record and could be brought by subpoena into a court of law. Make sure all handwriting in the book is completely legible and that information is routinely collected in a consistent manner for each entry. Do not fail to note a no-show both in the patient's health record and the appointment schedule. This often is helpful when a provider must prove that the patient did not follow medical advice or that the patient contributed to his or her poor condition by missing appointments. Old appointment schedules should be kept for a time equal to that of the statute of limitations in the state where the practice is located.

A medical assistant must never offer medical advice to a patient unless specifically instructed to do so by the provider. The patient sees the medical assistant as an extension of the provider and tends to weigh advice and comments by the medical assistant with the same validity as if they came from the provider. Provide only information the provider has approved or that is included in the healthcare facility's policy and procedure manual.

When a patient complains, listen carefully and try to resolve the problem or assure the patient that the issue will be discussed with the appropriate staff member to find a solution. If someone other than the patient asks for information about the patient, refrain from discussion unless the patient or provider has authorized the release of information.

Professional Behaviors

When working in scheduling and helping patients move through the healthcare facility, there are many opportunities to demonstrate professionalism. It is important to remember that we are often seeing patients when they are not at their best, so we must learn not to take all of the responses personally. When an angry patient approaches the reception desk you should smile politely, ask how you can help the person, and respond in a soothing tone of voice. When a patient calls for an appointment and demands a day and time when the provider is not available, you should remain calm and explain why that day and time is not an option. As a medical assistant in the front office you have the opportunity to make an amazing first impression on patients. Remember to always behave professionally.

SUMMARY OF SCENARIO

Ramona is an asset to the healthcare facility because her dedication and customer service skills help her interact with patients in a positive way. She genuinely cares about the patients and makes every effort to meet their needs while following Dr. Brown's preferences. She has found that her bright smile is a valuable aid when patients have been waiting and are growing restless.

Ramona cooperates with other staff members to get the patients seen as quickly as possible and to minimize wait time. She is flexible and can change the order of the patients seen, if needed, to maximize the use of time and facilities in the office. Because she is so cheerful and friendly, patients do not seem to mind when she asks for their cooperation. She keeps current phone numbers and cell phone information so that she can notify a patient quickly if Dr. Brown is running behind schedule. Ramona's proficiency on the computer also is an asset, and she makes frequent use of e-mail to take care of patient problems or rescheduling requests.

Because of the cooperation she receives from staff and patients alike, Ramona successfully runs an efficient office. She contributes to that efficiency by constantly refining her knowledge about her job. She pays attention to the times during the day that do not run as smoothly as others, evaluates the problems at those times, and then corrects them. Ramona also keeps the schedule moving by communicating with the clinical medical assistants, keeping them informed about arriving patients and those who have come early or are running late. She can quickly adjust and substitute a patient who already has arrived. Ramona has learned how to manipulate the schedule to accommodate an emergency. She knows that by making minor adjustments and keeping the waiting patients informed, the staff can handle any emergency.

All medical assistants need to develop skills in flexibility. Establishing a system that works and using it correctly makes patients and staff members more content with their experience in the healthcare facility.

SUMMARY OF LEARNING OBJECTIVES

1. **Define, spell, and pronounce the terms listed in the vocabulary.**
   Spelling and pronouncing medical terms correctly bolster the medical assistant's credibility. Knowing the definition of these terms promotes confidence in communication with patients and co-workers.

2. **Describe guidelines to establishing an appointment schedule and creating an appointment matrix.**
   When appointments are scheduled, a medical assistant must consider (1) the patients' needs, (2) the provider's preferences and habits, and (3) the available facilities. Make every attempt to schedule a patient at his or her most convenient time; this helps prevent no-shows. The provider will outline his or her preferences, which should be a high priority to the medical assistant. However, most providers are flexible and make adjustments according to the needs of the office. The availability of facilities in the office is perhaps the most inflexible factor. If a certain room or piece of equipment is being used for one patient, it usually cannot be used for another.
   Refer to Procedure 10-1 to create an appointment matrix.

3. **Discuss the advantages of computerized appointment scheduling.**
   Computerized scheduling programs are in demand because they are easy to operate and simplify both scheduling and changing of appointments. The computer can find the first available time much faster than a person scanning an appointment book. Most programs can prepare reports and even notify patients of the impending appointment automatically by e-mail, telephone, or text message. Web-based self-scheduling programs are becoming popular; these allow a patient to see the provider's available appointments and book his or her own date and time.

4. **Discuss appointment book scheduling and explain how self-scheduling can reduce the number of calls to the healthcare facility.**
   Office suppliers carry a variety of appointment book styles; many are color-guided.
   Self-scheduling can vastly reduce the number of calls to the office because a high number of everyday calls are requests to schedule appointments. With self-scheduling, patients can even make an appointment at midnight if they desire.

5. **Discuss the legality of the appointment scheduling system.**
   Because the paper-based appointment book can be used as a legal record, it must be accurate and maintained. Computerized scheduling systems can also be used to track appointments; missed or canceled appointments should be documented in the electronic system for legal purposes.

6. **Discuss pros and cons of various types of appointment management systems.**
   Scheduling of specific appointments is the most popular method of seeing patients. Wave and modified wave scheduling brings two or three patients to the office at the same time, and they are seen in the order of their arrival. This type of scheduling can be modified in many ways to suit the needs of the facility. Open office hours allow patients to come to the healthcare facility when it is convenient and wait their turn to see the provider. Other scheduling methods include double-booking and grouping of like procedures.

7. **Discuss telephone scheduling and identify critical information required for scheduling appointments for new patients.**
   Extend small courtesies to patients when on the phone with them to schedule an appointment. Write legibly when using an appointment book.
   Arranging the first appointment for a new patient requires time and attention to detail. Tact, courtesy, and professionalism are all extremely important. Collect patient demographic data and offer the patient the first available appointment. Some healthcare facilities mail an information packet/brochure to new patients; this can also be sent via e-mail. Often, the medical assistant will need to conduct preauthorization and precertification to determine whether a patient is eligible for treatment or for certain procedures.
   Refer to Procedure 10-2 to see how to schedule a new patient and to Procedure 10-3 to see how to coach patients regarding office policies and how to create a new patient brochure.

8. **Discuss scheduling appointments for established patients.**
   Most return appointments for established patients are arranged when the patient is leaving the healthcare facility. Refer to Procedure 10-4. Others are reserved by telephone, and the patient's address, telephone number, and insurance should always be verified and any changes documented in the health record.

9. **Discuss how the medical assistant should handle scheduling other types of appointments.**
   The medical assistant could be responsible for setting up other appointments such as inpatient surgeries, outpatient and inpatient procedure appointments, outside visits, providers, pharmaceutical representatives, and salespeople. Refer to Procedure 10-5 for specific procedures on how to schedule outpatient and inpatient procedure appointments.

10. **Do the following related to special circumstances in scheduling:**
    - Discuss several methods of dealing with patients who consistently arrive late.
      Patients who are habitually late for appointments might be told to arrive 15 minutes before the time written in the book. Some offices book these patients as the last appointment of the day, so that if they do not arrive promptly, they do not see the provider. Usually talking with the patient and gaining an understanding of why the patient arrives late improves the situation. The office can work with the patient to choose the best times that will result in a kept appointment.
    - Recognize office policies and protocols for rescheduling appointments.
      Changes sometimes must be made in the appointment schedule. When rescheduling an appointment, make sure the first appointment is removed from the appointment book, and then set the new appointment.
    - Discuss how to deal with emergencies, provider referrals, and patients without appointments.
      Periodically, emergency or urgent calls come into the office, and an appointment needs to be scheduled. Follow office procedures. Provider

referrals and patients without appointments should also be scheduled according to office policy.

11. **Discuss how to handle failed appointments and no-shows, as well as methods to increase appointment show rates.**

    It is important to determine the reason for failed appointments and to do whatever is possible to remedy the situation. Failed appointments need to be documented. A busy practice must have a very specific policy on appointment no-shows and must enforce it effectively. Methods to increase appointment show rates include automated call routing, appointment cards, confirmation calls, e-mail reminders, and mailed reminders.

12. **Discuss how to handle cancellations and delays.**

    Cancellations will occur because of a variety of reasons (e.g., when the patient cancels, when the provider is delayed, when the provider is called to an emergency, or when the provider is ill or out of town). All situations should be handled in accordance with office policy.

13. **Discuss patient processing, including the importance of the reception area.**

    The patient reception area should be an inviting place where patients feel comfortable. A first impression is a lasting one. Consider the traffic flow when designing the reception area, as well as fresh, harmonious colors and cleanliness. A writing desk with writing paper in the reception area for the convenience of patients is a nice touch. Some offices offer a computer for patients to use while waiting to see the provider.

14. **Describe how to prepare for patient arrival, including patient check-in procedures.**

    Advanced preparation helps make the day go smoothly and contributes to a more relaxed atmosphere for all. Health records should be prepared for the provider, arranged sequentially. The reception desk should be in clear view of all visitors who come to the office. Use a sign-in register that promotes patients' privacy. During the patient check-in process, it is vital that the medical assistant takes steps to protect the other patients in the reception area.

15. **Explain why using the patient's name as often as possible is important, as well as how the medical assistant can make patients feel at ease.**

    Using a patient's name as often as possible shows that the interaction is about the individual patient. By using the patient's name often, the medical assistant also ensures the correct patient is being treated. Providers and staff members make brief notes in the health record about the current events in the patient's life, which allows them to make friendly conversation.

16. **Describe registration procedures, including obtaining a patient history.**

    On a patient's first visit to the provider's office, the staff performs certain registration procedures. Most providers use a patient information or registration form to gather demographic information. The patient may also need the NPP document and to sign an acknowledgment of receipt

of the NPP. The patient's personal history, medical history, and family history may be obtained by asking him or her to complete a questionnaire, which could be paper or electronic.

17. **Do the following related to patient reception and processing:**

    - Show consideration for patients' time.
      The medical assistant should bring the patient to the examination room for treatment or consultation as close to the appointment time as possible or explain delays.
    - Properly treat patients with special needs.
      In all special needs cases, it is important to remain professional and treat everyone with respect.
    - Escort and instruct the patient.
      While in the provider's office, most patients prefer to be escorted rather than simply told where to go, and this is usually the medical assistant's responsibility.
    - Describe where health records should be placed.
      Health records should never be left in the examination room to be picked up and read by a patient. When using EHRs, it is important to remember to log out of the computer when you are ready to leave the room.

18. **Describe how the medical assistant should deal with challenging situations, such as talkative patients, children, angry patients, and patients' relatives and friends.**

    For talkative patients, the patient's history could be flagged with a symbol to alert the provider. Parents are responsible for their children's behavior while at the provider's office. The medical assistant should not discipline the child. Medical assistants should use empathy and good listening skills when dealing with angry patients, and there should be a policy in place for dealing with potentially dangerous individuals. Avoid a "too casual" attitude with patients' relatives and friends; show moderate concern and empathy.

19. **Discuss the friendly farewell, patient checkout, and planning for the next day.**

    The medical assistant can help convey a sense of caring by terminating the visit cordially. Be sure to thank the patient for coming and wish the person well as he or she leaves the office. As the day winds down, look over the appointments scheduled for the next day and plan ahead where possible.

20. **Discuss patient education, as well as legal and ethical issues, for scheduling appointments and patient processing.**

    The administrative medical assistant has a huge effect on the efficiency of the medical office. Educating the patient about office policies helps the facility run smoothly day to day. The appointment schedule may be used as a legal record and could be brought by subpoena into a court of law. When a patient complains, listen carefully and try to resolve the problem and assure the patient. If someone other than the patient asks for information about the patient, refrain from discussion unless the patient or provider has authorized the release of information.

CONNECTIONS

Study Guide Connection: Go to the Chapter 10 Study Guide. Read and complete the activities.

evolve   Evolve Connection: Go to the Chapter 10 link at *evolve.elsevier.com/kinn* to complete the Chapter Review Quiz. Check out the other resources listed for this chapter to make the most of what you have learned about scheduling appointments and patient processing.

DAILY OPERATIONS IN THE AMBULATORY CARE SETTING

SCENARIO

Marie Van Bakel, CMA (AAMA), is a new medical assistant in a small orthopedic clinic. She was hired by Dr. Carol Schmidt and Dr. Michael Michalski to be their clinical medical assistant. Marie just graduated from a medical assistant school and this is her first job. She is excited to work in orthopedics, which was the same specialty she worked in during her medical assistant practicum. In a small practice, Marie has a variety of different responsibilities compared with a medical assistant in a larger practice. She and the receptionist, Catherine, will be the only staff members in the office four out of five mornings a week because the doctors will be making hospital rounds and will be in surgery. Marie and

Catherine need to open the office and prepare for the patients. Marie is also responsible for the inventory of clinical supplies and equipment. During Marie's interview, Dr. Schmidt expressed her concern about the lack of procedures for ordering and maintaining inventory and would like Marie to develop those procedures. As part of her job, Marie is to manage ordering supplies and ensuring the proper quantities are in stock at all times. Not having much exposure to supplies and ordering during her practicum, Marie realizes she needs to learn about these procedures.

While studying this chapter, think about the following questions:

- What are the medical assistant's responsibilities when opening and closing the healthcare facility?
- What strategies are utilized to help keep the medical environment safe and secure?

- How do you perform a supply and equipment inventory?
- How does the healthcare facility utilize the United States Postal Service (USPS) and other delivery companies?
- How can a medical assistant practice proper body mechanics?

LEARNING OBJECTIVES

1. Define, spell, and pronounce the terms listed in the vocabulary.
2. Describe the administrative and clinical opening duties performed by the medical assistant.
3. Discuss the administrative and clinical closing responsibilities performed by the medical assistant, as well as daily and monthly duties.
4. Explain safety and security procedures important in the healthcare facility.
5. Do the following related to equipment in a medical practice:
   - Describe the elements of an equipment inventory list.
   - Explain the purpose of routine maintenance of administrative and clinical equipment.

- Explain the steps of creating a maintenance log, performing maintenance, and documenting the maintenance.
- Describe the medical assistant's role in ordering equipment.
6. Do the following related to supplies in the medical practice:
   - Discuss the elements on a supply inventory list.
   - List the steps involved in completing an inventory.
   - Perform an inventory with documentation.
   - Prepare a supply order.
7. Describe how the healthcare facility utilizes USPS and other delivery agencies.
8. Use proper body mechanics.

VOCABULARY

accounts payable Money owed by a company to other companies for services and goods; pertains to paying the bills of the facility.

answering service A business that receives and answers telephone calls for the healthcare facility when it is closed.

authorized agent A person who has written documentation that he or she can accept a shipment for another individual.

backordered An order placed for an item that is temporarily out of stock and will be sent at a later time.

billable service Assistance (i.e., service) that is provided by a healthcare provider that can be billed to the insurance company and/or patient.

bonded When an employer obtains a fidelity bond from an insurance company, which will cover losses from employee dishonest acts (e.g., embezzlement, theft).

buying cycle Refers to how often an item is purchased; depends on frequency of the use of the item and storage space available for the item.

VOCABULARY—*continued*

continuing medical education (CME) Activities (e.g., conferences, seminars) that promote further education for physicians and providers.

crash cart Emergency medications and equipment (e.g., oxygen, intravenous [IV], and airway supplies) stored in a cart, ready for an emergency.

depreciate To diminish in value (of an item) over a period of time; concept used for tax purposes.

discrepancies A lack of similarity between what is stated and what is found; for instance, when what is stated on the packing slip is different than what is found in the box.

disinfected The state of having destroyed or rendered pathogenic organisms inactive; does not include spores, tuberculosis bacilli, and certain viruses.

e-prescribing The ability of the provider to electronically send a prescription directly to the pharmacy.

girth The measurement around something; when referring to mail, it is the measurement around the middle of the package that is being shipped.

inventory The stored medical and administrative supplies that are used in the medical office. It is also the process of counting the supplies in stock.

invoices Billing statements that list the amount owed for goods or services purchased.

packing slip A document that accompanies purchased merchandise and shows what is in the box or package.

purchase order number Unique number assigned by the ordering facility that allows the facility to track or reference the order. Many vendors will add this number to the order documents (e.g., packing slip and statement).

quality control Manufactured samples with known values used to see if a test method is reliable by consistently producing accurate and precise results.

quantity to reorder The amount of supplies that need to be ordered.

restock Process of replacing the supplies that were used.

sanitized The state of having cleaned equipment and instruments with detergent and water, removing debris and reducing the number of microorganisms.

sterilized The state of having removed all microorganisms.

termination letters Documents sent to patients explaining that the provider is ending the physician-patient relationship and the patients need to see other providers.

vendor A company that sells supplies, equipment, or services to another company or individual.

white noise The sounds from a television or stereo that muffle or mute the conversation of others, thus helping to protect the confidentiality of patients.

zone A region or geographic area used for shipping.

MEDICAL OFFICE ENVIRONMENT

Opening the Healthcare Facility

In the healthcare facility, employees must arrive before patients to prepare for the patients. The preparation can differ based on the size of the facility and the practice's policies on preparation.

In smaller agencies, a few reliable employees are given keys to unlock the doors and the code to deactivate the alarm system. In larger facilities, employees must use the employee entrances, which are locked. Employees can unlock the doors by entering unique codes into a keypad or by using unique keycards (Figure 11-1, *A, B*). Both systems are developed to monitor who enters the building. Usually security, custodial, or supervisory personnel have the responsibility to deactivate the alarm system in larger facilities. The main patient doors are then opened by staff at a set time.

Regardless of the size of the agency, the medical assistant will be responsible for preparing the department or office for patients. For the administrative staff, voice mails need to be checked or messages from the **answering service** need to be obtained. The answering service may e-mail or fax the messages to the office, and these messages need to be addressed by staff and documented in the patients' health records. The phone voice mail message may need to be updated, and in some facilities the phones need to be "turned on" so patients can reach the healthcare facility and not get the answering service.

Computers, copy machines, and other equipment must be turned on. Some facilities require the medical assistant to print schedules of the day's appointments, keeping one for chart preparation and placing the other on the provider's desk. With the use of electronic health records (EHRs), providers and staff can utilize the software to see the appointments instead of having to rely on the paper schedule. Along with the list of appointments for the day, the medical assistant needs to pull the required paperwork for the patients. For practices without EHRs, the patients' medical records need to be pulled and prepared with any required documents. For practices with EHRs, required patient education literature (e.g., well-child visit documents) and preprinted paper screening forms may be prepared.

The administrative medical assistants need to prepare the reception area for patients. Magazines should be neatly displayed. Toys for children should be **disinfected** on a routine basis for infection control. Tissue boxes, hand sanitizer, and face masks should be well stocked and available for sick patients. Televisions and/or "**white noise**" music should be turned on. If the reception area includes beverages for patients, the medical assistant should prepare those and ensure they are adequately stocked.

CRITICAL THINKING APPLICATION   **11-1**

Catherine, the receptionist, utilizes low-volume music from a stereo as white noise in the reception area, which is near the reception desk. What are the benefits of the music?

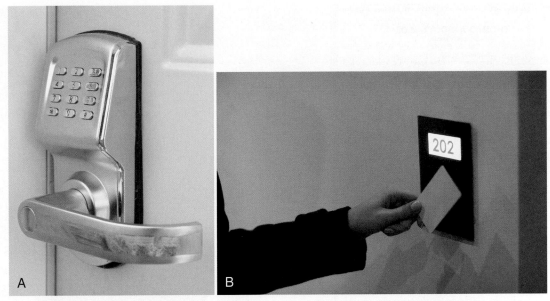

FIGURE 11-1 A, Keyless Access Locks allow employees to enter unique numbers that open the door and track who has keyed in. Once a person is no longer employed, the number is deleted. **B,** Employees can unlock doors using their unique key card. This system can track which keycard was used to open the door. (Photos copyright iStock.com.)

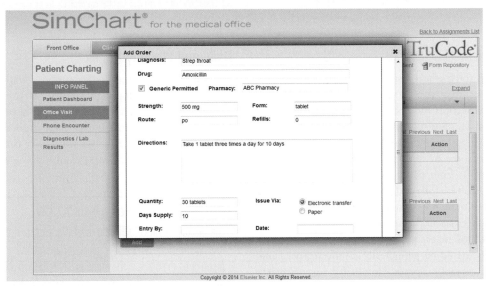

FIGURE 11-2 With e-prescribing, providers can enter the prescription information into the electronic health record (EHR) and send it to the pharmacy.

Medical assistants must also prepare the patient examination rooms by turning on the lights, checking that the supplies are stocked, and ensuring the rooms are cleaned appropriately. The medical assistant should scan the room, making sure it is neat, orderly, and safe for patients and children. For practices that do not use **e-prescribing**, prescription pads should not remain in examination rooms (Figure 11-2 and Figure 11-3). The provider should keep a pad in his or her pocket and the extra prescription pads should be stored in a locked cabinet. Prescription pads should never be accessible to patients because some might take the pads and try to forge a prescription, which is illegal.

Supply cabinets must be unlocked, except the narcotic cabinet. Narcotic medications should remain locked up at all times. The medical assistant must ensure restrooms have adequate supplies for patients (e.g., urine specimen containers, cleansing towelettes).

Quality control tests must be done on laboratory equipment. Outstanding patient issues from the prior day and any new reports on patients' diagnostic tests, including radiology tests and medical laboratory tests, need to be followed up. For facilities using paper records, the patient's record must be matched with the diagnostic report and then given to the provider to review. For facilities with EHRs, many times this process is completed electronically through the use of messaging systems in the software.

CRITICAL THINKING APPLICATION **11-2**

When opening the orthopedic office, what jobs does Marie, the clinical medical assistant, need to do? What jobs does Catherine, the receptionist, need to do to prepare for the day?

FIGURE 11-3 One prescription pad should be kept by the provider and extra pads should be locked up.

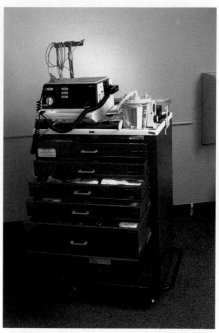

FIGURE 11-4 Crash carts must be inventoried monthly, ensuring medication and supplies have not expired and all the required supplies are available for an emergency.

Closing the Healthcare Facility

At the end of the day, the medical assistant needs to help with the closing duties. Some facilities have the administrative medical assistant prepare the patient records and documents for the next day. The administrative medical assistant must turn off the computers, copy machine, and other office equipment. The phones need to be switched to voice mail or the answering service. If the medical assistant handles co-payments from patients, the office procedures for handling the money must be followed. Any patient documents on the desk need to be put away for confidentiality purposes.

The medical assistant should clean up the reception area by gathering up the scattered magazines and returning them to their proper locations. Toys should be periodically disinfected per clinic protocol for infection control purposes. Unsolicited advertisements (e.g., pharmaceutical) and garbage need to be removed from the tables and chairs. The lights, television, stereo, and other devices should be turned off.

The clinical medical assistant must ensure that all the patients have left by checking the examination and treatment rooms. The medical assistant should **restock** the rooms and organize any reading materials in the room. The examination table, writing table, counters, computer keyboards, and chairs (i.e., those made of plastic, metal, or wood) should be disinfected. Patient-related documents should be put away. Computers and other devices should be shut down. Equipment and instruments should be **sanitized**, disinfected, or **sterilized**. Supply and medication cabinets need to be locked. If the department stocks narcotic medications, some facilities require the medications be counted by two staff members to verify the stock.

Depending on the facility, the medical assistant may be responsible for turning off the lights, activating the alarms, and locking the doors. In larger facilities, the custodial or security staff handles these responsibilities.

Daily and Monthly Duties

Medical facilities either employ custodial staff or hire cleaning services to clean. This cleaning takes place after hours each day. Larger facilities that employ custodial staff will have the staff clean high-traffic areas several times a day. These areas include the restrooms and the entrances. During wet weather, it is critical that the floors are kept dry to prevent people from slipping and falling.

CRITICAL THINKING APPLICATION   **11-3**

The orthopedic office utilizes a local cleaning service to clean the practice's rooms. The staff arrives after hours and are gone by the time Catherine and Marie open the office in the morning. Over the last month, Marie has noticed that the rooms do not look as clean as they should. Should she address this? If so, with whom should she discuss this?

The medical assistant also has responsibilities for cleaning and organizing the reception area and the examination rooms. During slow times, medical assistants are expected to do extra duties, including restocking medical and office supplies, forms, and patient literature. Just like at home, the cabinets and drawers in a medical office need to be straightened and reorganized. Medications and supplies that have expiration dates need to be checked monthly. **Crash carts** and other emergency supplies need to be inventoried monthly (Figure 11-4).

It is important that the medical practice be clean and organized. By taking the initiative to perform those tasks during quiet times, you will be considered a more valuable employee. Supervisors and providers value employees that look for additional activities to do during quiet times.

SECURITY IN THE HEALTHCARE FACILITY

Security and safety is important to the wellbeing of the medical practice staff, patients, and visitors. The healthcare facility can draw unwanted attention from those seeking drugs and money. Having plans in place that can be implemented when security is in question is critical for all.

Medical assistants need to stay alert for suspicious people. If a situation or a person makes you feel strange or on edge, listen to your instincts. Try to alert another staff person of the situation. Keep yourself at a distance from the person, including separating yourself from the person by a desk or piece of furniture if possible. If you are rooming a patient, position yourself so you are the closest to the door. If you feel uncomfortable rooming the patient, discuss the situation with the provider.

Medical facilities can be a target for those wanting to steal money, narcotic medications, and prescription pads. The staff should implement measures to limit the amount of money available in the building. Cash and checks from patients should be deposited daily to limit large quantities of money in the facility. Cash drawers should be stored out of sight of patients and visitors. Narcotic medications, if present in the agency, should always be in a double-locked cabinet with the keys hidden. Depending on the type of clinic, some will post signs stating there are no narcotic medications on site. As mentioned in a prior section, prescription pads are used in clinics that do not use e-prescribing. The prescription pads should remain out of view and reach of patients. They should not be stored in the patient examination rooms.

CRITICAL THINKING APPLICATION   11-4

Over the last 6 months, crime and break-ins have increased in the local area around the clinic. Many people believe the clinic has a supply of narcotic medication in stock, which is not true. What strategies can the staff implement to increase the security of the practice?

The healthcare facility should have procedures in place for dealing with suspicious people or potential robberies. Some clinics have code words that indicate specific situations. When these words are used by staff, they alert other staff members of the potential situation. Some clinics have installed alarm buttons under countertops and workstations. In a robbery situation or other security risk situation, the medical assistant can activate the alarm, which will trigger a notification to the clinic administration and the local police department. Remember it is always better to err on the side of caution and notify the police.

Many facilities have moved to locking employee entrance doors at all times during business hours and require either a key card or unique code to enter the building. In high crime areas, low-staffed clinics, or rural clinics, the doors to the patient care areas are also locked. This prevents unauthorized entry of people from the reception area to the patient care areas in the back, increasing the security.

After hours the facility should utilize alarms that are triggered when break-ins occur. When the alarm is triggered, an employee of the alarm company notifies the police department and the administrative personnel listed as emergency contacts. The police and the administrative personnel must determine what was the target and if anything was taken.

EQUIPMENT AND SUPPLIES

One of the most important responsibilities of the medical assistant is to manage the equipment and supplies in the medical office. In smaller facilities, the medical assistant may have more duties, including ordering and maintaining an inventory control system. In larger facilities, employees are hired for such roles in the purchasing department.

Equipment

In a medical practice, administrative and clinical equipment are used. The medical assistant needs to know how to operate, maintain, and handle issues with the equipment. For financial and tax purposes, the medical practice must know details about the equipment owned, including the purchase cost and age of each item. The process of gathering and creating a list of the equipment in the facility is called managing inventory.

Equipment Inventory

Each piece of equipment in the medical practice should be identified and records need to be maintained. The healthcare facility must be able to account for all of the equipment used and owned by the practice. In case of disaster or theft, the practice can provide these details to the insurance company to help facilitate the replacement of the equipment. In case of theft, equipment details can also be shared with the police to help identify equipment if it is found.

CRITICAL THINKING APPLICATION   11-5

Marie needs to learn more about managing inventory. She reviews her medical assistant textbook and reads articles online. She decides to start by creating an inventory list of the equipment in the medical office. What are some advantages of having an updated list of administrative and clinical equipment?

The practice's accountant utilizes the equipment inventory list while preparing the tax paperwork for the practice. Small equipment (e.g., thermometers, glucose monitors) is deducted as a practice expense for the year in which it is purchased. Computer hardware, calculators, and copiers are considered larger office equipment and **depreciate** over 5 years. Office furniture items (e.g., desks, files, safes, examination tables) depreciate over 7 years.

The equipment inventory list also helps the providers and supervisors identify equipment that needs to be replaced. Preplanning equipment purchases is a financial strategy for the practice. It allows the practice to be prepared and plan ahead for future investments.

To create an equipment inventory list, the medical assistant should create a spreadsheet and include all the administrative and clinical equipment (Figure 11-5). For each item, the medical assistant should document the following:
- Equipment name, manufacturer, and serial number
- Purchase date, cost, and supplier

Equipment Name	Manufacturer / Serial Number	Location / Facility Number	Purchase Date / Supplier	Cost	Warranty Information
Laser Printer	HP / HP3598XA	Medical Assistant Desk / LP59483	08/01/20XX / Best Office Supplies	$325	Parts and labor expires 07/31/20XX
AT2 Plus ECG / Spirometry	Schiller / WA4893X	Treatment Room / ES00012	05/02/20XX / Medical Equipment Supplies	$2987	Parts and Labor expires 05/01/20XX

FIGURE 11-5 An equipment inventory list can be created in a spreadsheet and provides useful information on the administrative and clinical equipment in the facility.

- Warranty information (e.g., start and end date, warranty coverage)

Larger facilities will also include the location of the equipment and the unique facility number of the equipment on the inventory list. For tracking purposes, larger facilities will place a sticker on the equipment and give each item a unique number. Procedure 11-1 explains how to create an equipment inventory.

The owner's or operation manual and warranty information for each item should be kept at a central location, available to users. Many manufacturers have the operation manuals available online as a convenience for users. The manuals are used to problem-solve performance issues, identify service schedules and routine maintenance, and identify parts or supplies needed for the operation of the machine.

PROCEDURE 11-1   Perform an Inventory with Documentation: Equipment Inventory

Goals: Perform an equipment inventory and document the inventory on the equipment inventory form.

EQUIPMENT and SUPPLIES

- Pen
- Administrative and/or clinical equipment
- Purchase information (e.g., date, cost, and supplier) and warranty information (e.g., start and end date, warranty coverage)
- Equipment inventory form

PROCEDURAL STEPS

1. For the equipment to be inventoried, gather the following information for each piece of equipment:
   - Name of equipment, manufacturer, and serial number
   - Location and facility number (if applicable)
   - Purchase date, cost, supplier, and warranty information

PURPOSE: To have the essential information required when creating the spreadsheet.

2. Complete an equipment inventory form by adding the gathered information for each item inventoried (see Figure 11-5).

PURPOSE: Creating an equipment inventory list on the computer will help you organize the information and also help you maintain the information easily.

3. Review the document created. Make any necessary revisions.

Equipment Safety and Maintenance

The medical assistant is responsible for monitoring equipment safety and proper functioning. Potential issues should not be overlooked and action should be taken to prevent injury to staff or patients and costly damage to the equipment. For administrative and clinical equipment, electrical cords should be checked for damage. Any suspected overheating issues should be immediately addressed. Any unusual noise or change in performance should be investigated. Equipment should be routinely cleaned and maintained in accordance with the operation manual, which will help promote the life of the machine.

CRITICAL THINKING APPLICATION   11-6

Marie realized that the practice did not have maintenance logs for the various pieces of equipment. She decided to start making logs, but realized there were a lot of logs she would have to make. How could she create logs in a very time-efficient manner? For a small office, describe options that she could use to organize all the logs so they are easy to locate and use.

Equipment operation manuals include information on cleaning, routine maintenance, service schedules, and how to troubleshoot common problems. The medical assistant should follow the cleaning procedures and the routine maintenance for the equipment utilized. Routine maintenance varies with the equipment. Copiers and printers may entail changing toner or cartridges. For clinical equipment, maintenance may include changing filters or batteries. Making a schedule as a reminder for routine maintenance can be helpful. Many facilities utilize logs to help track routine maintenance and service calls (Figure 11-6). The logs should include:

- Equipment name, serial number, location of machine, and facility's unique equipment number (if applicable)
- Manufacturer's name
- Date of purchase
- Warranty information (e.g., start and end date, warranty coverage)
- Service provider contact information
- Date and time maintenance activities performed
- Maintenance activities performed
- Signature of person performing maintenance

Procedure 11-2 explains the steps involved in creating a maintenance log, performing the maintenance, and then documenting the maintenance.

Maintenance Log

Equipment Name: **Laser Printer** Serial #: **HP3598XA** Location: **Medical Assistant Desk**

Facility #: **LP59483** Manufacturer: **HP** Purchased: **08/01/20XX**

Warranty Information: **Parts and labor expires 07/31/20XX**

Freqency of Inspections: **Every 6 months**

Service Provider: **Best Office Supplies**

Date	Time	Maintenance Activities	Signature
12/15/20XX	0956	**Replaced toner cartridge**	**Marie Van Bakel, CMA (AAMA)**
02/11/20XX	1235	**Service call: Office Repair Company – to fix stray ink marks on copies**	**Catherine Black, RMA**

Maintenance Log

Equipment Name: **AT2 Plus ECG/Spirometry** Serial #: **WA4893X** Location: **Treatment Room**

Facility #: **ES00012** Manufacturer: **Schiller** Purchased: **05/02/20XX**

Freqency of Inspections: **Every 12 months**

Warranty information: **Parts and Labor expires 05/01/20XX**

Service Provider: **Medical Equipment Suppliers**

Date	Time	Maintenance Activities	Signature
10/23/20XX	1123	**Replaced battery**	**Marie Van Bakel, CMA (AAMA)**
05/02/20XX	1445	**No tracing, cleaned stylus with alcohol**	**Marie Van Bakel, CMA (AAMA)**

FIGURE 11-6 Equipment maintenance logs are utilized to track maintenance activities by the staff and outside repair agencies.

PROCEDURE 11-2 Perform Routine Maintenance of Administrative or Clinical Equipment

Goals: *To perform routine maintenance of administrative or clinical equipment and document the maintenance on the log.*

EQUIPMENT and SUPPLIES

- Maintenance log(s)
- Administrative or clinical equipment (e.g., oral thermometers)
- Supplies for routine maintenance (e.g., battery)
- Operation manual if needed
- Pen
- Information regarding the equipment (i.e., name, serial number, location, facility number, manufacturer, purchase date, warranty information, frequency of inspections, and service provider)

PROCEDURE 11-2   —continued

PROCEDURAL STEPS

1. Gather information on the piece of equipment identified for routine mainte-nance, including: name, serial number, location, facility number, manufac-turer, purchase date, warranty information, frequency of inspections, and service provider.
   PURPOSE: To have the essential information required when completing the log.
2. Fill in the equipment details on the log (see Figure 11-6).
   PURPOSE: Adding the equipment details helps identify the machine and provides a quick reference to useful information that might be asked by the service provider. The form serves as a log for documenting the maintenance activities that are performed.
3. To perform the maintenance activities, gather the required supplies. If you are not familiar with the procedure or the required supplies, refer to the operation manual.

PURPOSE: You need to be familiar with the supplies and the procedure before you start the maintenance.
4. Perform the maintenance activities as directed in the operation manual. Take any required safety precautions necessary to protect yourself and others.
   PURPOSE: Following the outlined procedure in the operation manual will help you successfully complete the maintenance without injuring yourself and others or doing damage to the machine.
5. Clean up the work area.
6. Using a pen, document the date, time, the maintenance activity performed, and your signature on the log.
   PURPOSE: Completing the log indicating the activities performed will serve as a communication tool for future reference and services needed on that piece of equipment.

Service Calls and Warranties

When equipment is purchased, a warranty is given for a period of time. The warranty is the manufacturer's guarantee that if the piece of equipment needs to be repaired or has a defective part, the manu-facturer will pay for the cost of the repair and in some cases replace the item. Typically the warranty language includes details on what is covered and what is not covered. Some warranties are not honored if someone other than a "recognized" service person attempts to fix the machine. Extended warranties can be purchased for some machines, which lengthens the protection time.

Typically for complex and/or expensive equipment, the medical practice will contract with a service provider for repairs and routine service checks, which are explained in the operation manual. This assistance with equipment maintenance is necessary for some equip-ment and also helps to extend the lifetime of those machines. For repairs on other equipment, it might be necessary to ship or bring the machine to the repair service. Usually the cost for on-site repairs is more than if the machine is brought or shipped to the service provider for repairs. One of the main concerns when a piece of equipment breaks down is the effect on the medical practice. Some service providers will also loan equipment to healthcare facilities while the repairs take place. This service greatly lessens the burden on the practice.

Purchasing Equipment

Depending on the size of the medical organization, the process of purchasing equipment can vary. Large agencies typically have staff in purchasing departments who research the needs of the organiza-tion, identifying the best equipment to purchase. For smaller prac-tices, the medical assistant may be involved with the process.

If a provider or supervisor is considering replacing a piece of equipment, a number of factors are taken into consideration. The age of the machine and the availability of parts are considered. Sometimes repair parts are not available or are very expensive for older machines. The frequency and cost of repairs is a factor. Is the practice spending more on the repair costs compared with purchas-ing a new model? The utilization of the machine will be examined. If the machine is used often, it needs to be reliable. Does the new model have features that will enhance the practice or can the features provide extra **billable services** for the business? These factors are considered when a piece of equipment needs to be replaced.

CRITICAL THINKING APPLICATION   11-7

Currently, the providers are using an off-site radiology service. They are contemplating creating a small radiology room where they could take x-rays. How could Marie assist the providers with their plans for a potential purchase of x-ray equipment?

The provider and/or supervisor may also consider leasing a piece of equipment. With the frequency of technology changes in the medical field, leasing medical equipment is becoming a popular option for smaller facilities. Monitoring equipment, diagnostic testing equipment, examination tables, computer systems, and fur-niture are just some of the items that can be leased. The healthcare facility pays a fee to lease the machine or the furniture, which is less than what would be paid out if the item is purchased. The lease fees are tax deductible and allow the agency the ability to provide extra billable services.

The medical assistant may help the provider or supervisor identify potential new models. Using the Internet and contacting salespeople representing the models of interest are two ways to get additional information. Some salespeople will meet with the staff, demonstrat-ing the product and answering any questions they may have. In addition to research, the medical assistant may need to explain the usage of the machine and the frequency of repair checks. Usually the

Item Name	Size	Quantity	Item Number	Supplier's Name	Reorder Point	Quantity to Reorder	Cost	Stock Available	Order (✓)
Nonsterile gauze sponges, 8 ply	2"x 2"	100/pkg	NG0022	Midwest Medical	5	25	$2.31/pkg		
Sterile gauze sponges, 12 ply, 2/pkg	2"x 2"	25 pkg/box	NG0042	Midwest Medical	4	20	$3.99/box		

FIGURE 11-7 A supply inventory list shows details for items in inventory. For efficiency, use two extra columns ("Stock Available" and "Order") as shown. This list can be duplicated and utilized when performing inventory.

supervisor or provider has the final say on the new model and if the purchase should occur.

Supplies

There are many supplies required to run the medical office and treat patients. Supplies can include administrative items such as pens, paper, envelopes, and paperclips. Supplies can also include bandages, vaccines, medications, slings, and splints. The medical assistant needs to ensure the practice has enough supplies to treat patients. Running out of supplies can greatly affect the services provided to patients and can be more expensive for the healthcare facility because of last-minute ordering at higher prices. On the other hand, over-stocking supplies can be a financial waste to the practice. Many supplies have expiration dates and cannot be used beyond that date. Having adequate amounts of supplies in **inventory** is crucial.

Inventory Management

Inventory management involves ordering, tracking inventory, and identifying the quantity of product to purchase. The goal of inventory management is to have adequate supplies on hand to use in the healthcare facility, yet not have too much stock that will expire or take a long time to use.

The medical assistant in charge of ordering and managing supplies must keep a record on each item in inventory. The record can be a manual recording written in a notebook or on index cards, or it can be computerized in a spreadsheet or inventory control system software (Procedure 11-3 explains how to create the supply inventory list using a spreadsheet). For each inventory item, the medical assistant must record the following:

- Item details: Item name, size, quantity, item number, supplier's name, and cost (Figure 11-7).
- **Quantity to reorder**: Amount of product used during the **buying cycle**. For instance, the healthcare facility's buying cycle for 2x2 nonsterile gauze (100 per pack) is 1 month. The facility typically goes through 25 packs in 1 month. This would be the quantity used during the buying cycle and would be the quantity to reorder (see Figure 11-7).
- Reorder point: When the quantity of the item gets to a specific number, indicating that it needs to be reordered. For instance, when the inventory of 2x2 nonsterile gauze packs gets to 5 packs, the medical assistant must reorder (see Figure 11-7). Five is the reorder point or the quantity that triggers an order to be placed to replenish the inventory. The reorder point for

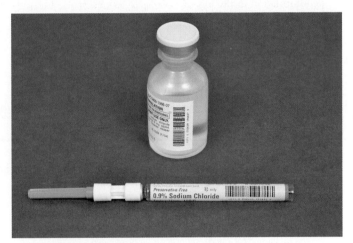

FIGURE 11-8 Using bar codes can make inventory control more efficient.

medical and administrative supplies can be different for each item because of the usage rate and the time it takes to receive the item after it is ordered. The reorder point for an item can be calculated based on the number used per day and the number of days it takes to order and receive the product. For instance, the practice uses half a pack of 2x2 nonsterile gauze per day. It takes 4 days to receive the order from the medical supply company. The medical practice may also want 6 extra days' worth of supplies on hand to prevent issues of running out of the item. Here is how you would figure out the reorder point:

Stock to cover order time: 0.5 pack per day × 4 days to receive order = 2 packs
Extra stock: 6 days × 0.5 pack per day = 3 packs
Reorder point: 2 packs (stock to cover order time) + 3 packs (6-day supply) = 5 packs

Inventory Control Systems

To make inventory management work well, an inventory control system should be in place. Large medical facilities may utilize computerized inventory control systems, which monitor usage and inventory in stock, and also identify items that need to be ordered. Smaller facilities may utilize simple computerized or manual systems.

To help create an efficient computerized system, many medical facilities utilize bar codes to track inventory and for billing for supplies (Figure 11-8). With this system, each item has a unique bar code. The bar code is scanned with a bar code reader when items are added or taken from inventory. Software can then help monitor the inventory quantity. For bar codes to work successfully, the staff must be diligent in scanning the bar codes when taking a product from stock. Bar code inventory control systems work successfully in large and small practices.

There are several manual systems utilized for identifying what supplies need to be ordered. The following are some of the more common methods utilized in medical facilities.

- When staff identify a product needs to be ordered, the item is written in a log. This process is similar to making a list of what you need at the grocery store. The person responsible for ordering supplies then prepares the order based on the information in the log.
- Another system includes using product identification slips, which contain the name of the product. The slips or cards are attached to the product or a box/package of items. When the

product is used, the slip is put in a special location like a box or plastic pocket. The slips in the box or pocket are then used by the medical assistant who prepares the supply order.

- The two-bin system consists of having a main bin for each item in inventory and then a backup bin for each. When the main bin is emptied, the backup bin is used and the product is reordered.
- The medical assistant responsible for ordering performs a hand count of the items in stock, identifying what needs to be ordered. This system is explained in the next section (see Procedure 11-3).

CRITICAL THINKING APPLICATION   **11-8**

Marie decided to implement a manual system for inventory. Of the manual systems discussed, which method might work best in the small orthopedic practice? Discuss your answer.

PROCEDURE 11-3   **Perform an Inventory with Documentation: Perform an Inventory of Supplies While Using Proper Body Mechanics**

Goals: *Perform a supply inventory using correct body mechanics. Document the inventory on the supply inventory form.*

EQUIPMENT and SUPPLIES

- Pen
- Administrative and/or clinical supplies to be inventoried
- Purchase information (e.g., item number, cost, and supplier) for supplies in inventory
- Reorder point and quantity to reorder for each item in inventory
- Supply inventory form

PROCEDURAL STEPS

1. For the supplies in inventory, gather the following information for each item:
   - Name, size, quantity (e.g., purchased individually, 100 per box)
   - Item number, supplier's name, cost
   - Reorder point and quantity to reorder
   PURPOSE: To have the essential information required when creating the spreadsheet.
2. Enter each supply's information on the inventory form, making sure the appropriate entry is in the right location (see Figure 11-7).
   Note: The "Stock Available" column will be empty for now.
   PURPOSE: Creating a supply inventory list on the computer will help you organize the information and also help you maintain the information easily.
3. Review the document. Make any necessary revisions.
   PURPOSE: Using a copy of the supply inventory list when counting the stock available will save time and help increase the accuracy of the information.

4. Using the supply inventory list, inventory the supplies in the department. Identify how the supply should be counted (e.g., individually, by the box) and count the number of items in stock.
   PURPOSE: By identifying the correct quantity that the item is inventoried by, you will increase the accuracy of the inventory. Counting an item by "each" when it comes as a package can cause confusion when identifying what needs to be ordered.
5. Add the number in the appropriate row under the "Stock Available" header.
6. Indicate which supplies need to be reordered by checking the appropriate columns.
7. After counting the item, place the stock neatly back, making sure the oldest stock is in the front.
   PURPOSE: It is important to clean up your workspace. The oldest stock must be moved to the front to ensure it is used first.
8. Continue steps 5 through 7 until all supplies are inventoried.
9. Use proper body mechanics when lifting and moving supplies by maintaining a wide, stable base with your feet. Your feet should be shoulder-width apart and you should have good footing. Bend at the knees, keeping your back straight. Lift smoothly with the major muscles in your arms and legs. Use the same technique when putting the item down.
   PURPOSE: Correct body mechanics will decrease your risk for injury when carrying or lifting heavy objects. See Figure 11-13 and 11-14 for proper body mechanics when lifting boxes.
10. Use proper body mechanics when reaching for an object. Clear away barriers and use a step stool if needed. Your feet should face the object. Avoid twisting or turning with a heavy load.
    PURPOSE: Straining when reaching or standing on tiptoes can increase your risk for injury.

Taking Inventory

No matter if a healthcare facility has an automated inventory control system or not, taking inventory at periodic times is critical. Many businesses that utilize automated inventory control systems hand count their inventory at least once a year, usually around the close of the business year. These companies compare their hand counts to the computer counts and identify discrepancies. The discrepancies are followed up on. The manual inventory procedure provides the company with information on the actual number of items in stock. With this information, the financial value of the inventory can be calculated and used for financial reports and taxes at the close of the business year.

For medical offices that do not implement inventory control systems, performing inventory or counting the items in stock is important before each buying cycle. See Procedure 11-3 for instructions on performing an inventory. One of the most frequent errors when performing inventory is to report a different quantity than what is on the supply inventory list, spreadsheet, or cards. For instance, if a medical assistant is counting nonsterile sponges, each package should be counted as 1 and not as 100 each. Looking at Figure 11-8, if there were 6 packages of sponges left in the supply cabinet, it should be noted as 6 packages, not 600 sponges or 600 each. Counting each item in a box or package when the product is inventoried by box or package creates conflict and confusion when looking at the reorder point.

To be most efficient when performing an inventory count, the medical assistant should utilize a supply inventory list (Figure 11-9). The supply inventory list shows all the items in stock. When using this document, the medical assistant can mark down the inventory counts for each item (see Procedure 11-3). If the supply inventory list is not available, then the medical assistant needs to write down the item number, size, quantity (e.g., 100/box), manufacturer, and any other identifying information. This process takes a lot more time.

When performing an inventory in the medical practice, the medical assistant should work in a systematic manner. The medical assistant starts with one supply cabinet, working from top to bottom, before moving onto another cabinet. All stock areas should be inventoried before preparing the supply order.

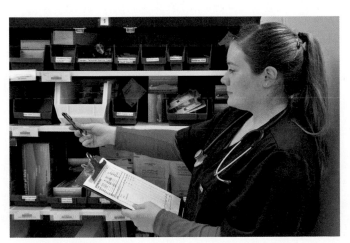

FIGURE 11-9 A medical assistant performing an inventory.

Price Consideration When Ordering Supplies

When ordering supplies, price comparison shopping is important, but it also takes time. The medical practice must balance the time it takes to the money saved. Some medical offices compare prices only on more expensive items or items that are used in vast quantities. They may compare prices every 6 to 12 months, instead of comparing prices with each order. When comparing prices, it is important to consider shipping and handling changes, as well as ensuring the products compared are the same quantity and quality.

Quantity discounts or price breaks are also a way to save money when ordering. The more of an item purchased, the cheaper the product becomes. For instance:

- Quantity 1 to 5, $1.50 per each item
- Quantity 6 to 15, $1.25 per each item

If the medical assistant purchased a quantity of 6, the price per each would be cheaper than if 4 were purchased. The medical assistant must consider storage space, how quickly the item will be used, and the shelf life (or expiration date) of the item. Buying too much just to get a price break may not be in the best interest of the medical practice if there is not adequate storage space or if the product will expire before it can all be used.

Some medical facilities join group purchasing organizations (GPOs), which combine orders from many different medical facilities and thus receive volume discounts from specific vendors. GPOs typically purchase both supplies and medications. Physician buying groups (PBGs) offer providers favorable pricing for vaccines, but the provider must only use the vaccines from the contracted manufacturers.

Ordering Supplies

If the medical practice does not join a GPO, then the medical assistant who orders typically identifies a couple of **vendors** from which to purchase administrative and medical supplies. The medical assistant can utilize the supplier's printed catalog, if available, or the company's online Web site store. Many medical and business supply companies only print the complete catalogs once or twice a year and they can become outdated between printings. The catalog provides a reference for supplies, but the Web site shows all the products available with the most updated prices and sale prices (Procedure 11-4).

Many suppliers require the medical assistant to create an account before ordering products. The account is set up using the practice's information. In some states, ordering sterile solutions (e.g., intravenous [IV] bags, normal saline vials), medications, and needles requires the provider's license number. The setup of the account will only be complete when a copy of the license is faxed to the company. If the medical assistant is ordering narcotics, the physician must authorize the order and provide a copy of his or her Drug Enforcement Administration (DEA) registration. Narcotics require special tracking documentation and thus a high level of authorization when purchasing them.

Some medical facilities utilize **purchase order numbers**, giving each order a unique reference number. This reference number should be included on the order sheets, added to the online information, or provided during the phone order. Vendors add the purchase order number to the order documentation and it can be used as a reference for both parties when discussing the order. The healthcare facility uses the purchase order number to track the order.

Payment terms may vary with suppliers, including credit cards, check, money order, or a line of credit. Typically, the line of credit is good for 30 to 60 days and **invoices** are sent to the ambulatory care clinic to be paid after the purchases have been received. Orders can typically be placed via fax, mail, or phone or online. If the medical assistant is faxing or mailing the order, the vendor usually requires the order to be placed on the vendor's order sheet. A copy of the phone, mailed, or fax order or a printout of the online order should be kept by the medical assistant to verify the order was correctly filled.

CRITICAL THINKING APPLICATION   **11-9**

Currently the practice has been ordering clinical supplies from two vendors. Marie would like to do some cost comparisons to get the best deals on supplies. She does not have a lot of time to spend on the research. How might she approach this situation? Where should she start first? What might be a long-term goal for her?

PROCEDURE 11-4   Prepare a Purchase Order

Goal: *Create an accurate purchase order for supplies.*

EQUIPMENT and SUPPLIES

- Pen
- Supply inventory list showing item name, size, quantity, item number, supplier's name, reorder point, quantity to reorder, cost, and current stock available
- Computer
- Internet
- Printer

PROCEDURAL STEPS

1. Review the supply inventory list with the current stock counts and determine what supplies need to be reordered.
   PURPOSE: By determining what needs to be reordered, you are preventing having too much or too little stock of a particular item.
2. Using the Internet, find the online store used for ordering the needed supplies.
3. Using the search box, type in the item number or description. Verify that the item from the search results is what you need to order.
   PURPOSE: It is important to verify you have the correct product before you add the product to your basket/cart.

4. Apply critical thinking skills as you identify the quantity to reorder for that item and order this amount.
   PURPOSE: The "Quantity to Reorder" column will indicate how much to reorder to prevent too many or too few of the product in inventory.
5. Repeat steps 3 and 4 until all items are ordered.
6. When you have finished, verify the contents in your basket/cart. Review the supply inventory list to ensure you have ordered everything that needs to be reordered and have ordered the correct quantity of each item.
   PURPOSE: Rechecking the order before finalizing the order will prevent costly mistakes.
7. Print a copy of the order.
   Note: For a real order, the payment information would be added and the order would be submitted at this time.
   PURPOSE: When ordering products, the copy of the order is then compared with the packing slips to ensure you have received the complete order. The copy and the packing slips are then stapled together and verified against the invoice when it is received. For prepaid orders, the packing slips and copy of the order are then filed once the entire order has been received.

Receiving the Order

Orders can arrive via the mail, a national delivery service (e.g., FedEx, United Parcel Service [UPS]), or a local delivery service. These services are discussed in a later section. The delivery person may require a signature from an employee. This signature is used to track who received the delivery.

The medical assistant must check the delivery as soon as possible to see if it needs immediate attention. Some medications are shipped on ice to maintain a constant cool temperature. These medications need to be immediately placed in the refrigerator or freezer upon arrival. If the temperature in the package warms up too much, the medication must be discarded. Storage information for medications can be found in the package insert or on the manufacturer's Web site.

For all orders, remove the **packing slip** from the box and compare the items in the package to the packing slip (Figure 11-10). Check off all items received. Some supply companies also indicate items that are **backordered** and will be arriving at a later time. Note any **discrepancies** or differences on the packing slip. Any items damaged should also be noted on the packing slip. The copy of the original order should be compared against the packing slip and any differences should be noted. Any discrepancies or damaged items should be addressed with the supply company as soon as possible.

Once the supplies have been reviewed, the packing slip should be attached to the copy of the order. When the complete order has been received, the copy of the order with the packing slips attached should be filed if the order was prepaid. If a line of credit was used, place the copy of the order with the attached packing slips in the

Vaccine Storage Guidelines

Frozen Vaccines

- Ideal temperature for frozen vaccines: −58° F to 5° F.
- Diluent storage directions are different from those for frozen vaccines.

Refrigerated Vaccines

- Each type of vaccine should be placed in its own container, which allows for air flow. Place newer vaccines behind older vaccines. Keep vaccine vials in their original boxes to prevent light exposure.
- Ideal temperature for refrigerated vaccines: 35° F to 46° F.
- Do not store vaccines next to the wall, top shelf, door, or floor of the refrigerator.
- Do not put food or beverages in the vaccine storage refrigerator.

Monitoring Guidelines

- To monitor temperatures, use a thermometer with a minimum and maximum reading. It will indicate the warmest and coldest temperatures since the thermometer was last reset.
- Read the thermometer when opening and closing the medical office.
- Document the readings and include the date, time, and your initials on the log.
- Leave a blank line if readings were not done.
- Report any out-of-range temperatures immediately.

Example of a Temperature Log

DATE	TIME	REFRIGERATOR TEMPERATURE			FREEZER TEMPERATURE			INITIALS
		MAX	MIN	CURRENT	MAX	MIN	CURRENT	
10/11/xx	0750	40° F	37° F	39° F	3° F	−13° F	−12° F	MVB
10/11/xx	1722	38° F	35° F	38° F	−8° F	−28° F	−19° F	BMN
10/12/xx	0752	42° F	36° F	39° F	−13° F	−23° F	−18° F	MVB
10/13/xx	0748	47° F	38° F	38° F	−8° F	−27° F	−22° F	MVB

Vaccine Storage and Handling, accessed 10/11/2015, http://www.cdc.gov/vaccines/recs/storage/default.htm.

CRITICAL THINKING APPLICATION   11-10

Using the Vaccine Storage Guidelines box, answer the following questions:

- Did all the refrigerator temperatures fall within the required range? Explain.
- Did all the freezer temperatures fall within the required range? Explain.
- If a temperature was outside the required range, what should be done?
- Why was a blank line left on the log?

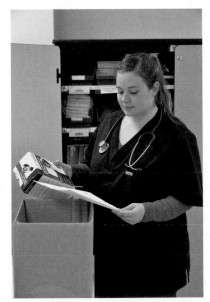

FIGURE 11-10 Comparing the packing slip to the contents in the box is an important step in receiving supplies.

accounts payable folder to wait for the invoice's arrival. The person responsible for paying the medical practice's bills will match the invoice with the copy of the order, ensuring everything is in order before paying the bill.

The items received should be put away as soon as possible and the boxes should be discarded. When putting supplies away, it is important to rotate stock. This means the new stock should go in the back and the older stock needs to be moved forward so it can be used first. Any items with expiration dates should be placed so the items expiring first are in front so they are used first. For stock without expiration dates, consider following the saying "First in, first out," which means when new stock comes in, it is placed behind the older stock. The older stock needs to be used first.

Common Inventory and Purchase Abbreviations	
BTL: Bottle	PO: Purchase Order
BX: Box	PPD: Pre-Paid
CS: Case	PYMT: Payment
EA: Each	QTY: Quantity
PKG: Package	

HANDLING MAIL

Depending on the size of the medical practice, medical assistants will have varying responsibilities with the mail. If the healthcare facility is large, there may be employees hired to prepare the mail for the United States Postal Service (USPS) and other shipping agencies. These employees also sort incoming mail and deliver the mail to the different departments in the facility. The medical assistant in the department is responsible for addressing the outgoing mail and sorting incoming mail. In smaller practices, the medical assistant is responsible for handling all the mail duties.

United States Postal Service

The USPS is an independent branch of the federal government that handles domestic and international mail services. Domestic mail includes items mailed and received within the United States, its territories and possessions, the military (i.e., Army Post Offices [APOs], Fleet Post Offices [FPOs], and Diplomatic Post Offices [DPOs]), and the United Nations in New York. International mail includes mail sent from a foreign country or to a foreign country. The majority of mail sent by a healthcare facility is domestic mail and the discussion will focus on these services.

To prepare mail to be sent, you will need to address the envelopes and packages following the USPS guidelines discussed in the Technology and Written Communication chapter. The postage is dependent on the:

- Weight and size of the item
- Urgency for arrival
- Delivery **zone**
- Services required

See Table 11-1 for domestic shipping sizes. Postage can be added to the item either by utilizing the USPS Web site or a local Post Office. The USPS Web site (www.usps.com) provides valuable resources for addressing and shipping mail. It allows you to buy stamps, schedule a pickup, calculate the shipping cost, look up ZIP codes, and track sent mail.

Domestic United States Postal Services

The medical assistant will utilize different types of mail services for the healthcare facility's business. It is crucial to understand the different services. For routine mail, the healthcare facility will use First-Class Mail, but for packages or urgent letters, other options are available (Table 11-2).

Priority Mail Express provides a 7-day-a-week delivery service. It guarantees overnight scheduled deliveries. This service is used for time-sensitive letters and packages up to 70 pounds (lb.) that need to get to the recipient quickly. The cost of this service is based on the item's weight and the delivery zone. Insurance is provided as part

TABLE 11-1   United States Postal Service Domestic Shipping Sizes

DOMESTIC SHIPPING	SIZE
Postcard	Height: 3.5"–4.25" Length: 5"–6" Maximum thickness: 0.016"
Letter	Height: 3.5"–6.125" (6⅛") Length: 5"–11.5" Maximum thickness: 0.25"
Large Envelopes	Height: 6.125"–12" Length: 11.5"–15" Maximum thickness: 0.75"
Packages	Maximum length plus girth: 108" (130" for Standard Post)

TABLE 11-2   Summary of the United States Postal Service's Domestic Services

Priority Mail Express	Very expensive; 7-days-a-week delivery service with guaranteed overnight scheduled delivery. Insurance is included.
Priority Mail	Expensive; delivery within 3 days. Insurance is included.
First-Class Mail	Most commonly used service. Cost based on size, shape, and weight. Add-on services are available for an extra fee.
Standard Post	Used for oversized packages, with delivery in 2–8 days.
Media Mail	Use for sending books and educational material, with delivery in 2–8 days.

of the service. Priority Mail Express envelopes and boxes are available at the Post Office and a flat rate fee is available.

Priority Mail provides delivery of letters and packages up to 70 lb. within 1 to 3 days. The cost of this service is based on the item's weight and the delivery zone. Priority Mail envelopes and boxes are available at the Post Office and a flat rate fee is available based on the size of the envelope or box for items up to 70 lbs. Priority Mail is cheaper than Priority Mail Express and insurance is part of the service.

First-Class Mail service provides delivery in 3 days or less. Envelopes and packages weighing up to 13 ounces (oz.) can be mailed using this service. This is the most common service used by the healthcare facility. The postage is based on the item's size, shape, and weight. Insurance and additional services can be added for an extra fee.

Standard Post service is an economical ground service for oversized, less urgent packages. This service can be used for larger packages weighing up to 70 lbs. and measuring up to 130 inches in combined **girth** and length. The cost is based on the item's weight and shape and the delivery zone. Insurance can be added with an extra fee.

Media Mail replaced the Book Rate and is used for sending books, electronic media, and educational materials. The cost is based on the weight of the item and insurance can be added for an additional fee.

Insurance and Additional Services

The USPS also has a host of optional services that can be added onto the standard services for an additional fee. In general, these services include insurance, shipping confirmation, delivery confirmation, and tracking. Some of these services, including Certified Mail and Return Receipt, are the options used more commonly by medical facilities.

The Standard Insurance option can be added to the postage to insure against loss or damage. The cost is based on the item's declared value. Priority Mail Express and Priority Mail insure the item to a point and additional coverage can be purchased.

Registered Mail can be added to First-Class and Priority Mail. This optional service can provide insurance for items valued up to $25,000. A mailing receipt is provided, and upon request, an electronic verification can be sent to the sender showing the item was delivered or an attempted delivery was made. If the healthcare facility was shipping an expensive machine to a repair service, Registered Mail may be used to help protect against loss or further damage.

Certified Mail is available for First-Class and Priority Mail. With Certified Mail, a mailing receipt showing the date when the item was mailed is included (Figure 11-11, *A*). It can be combined with Return Receipt to get additional information on when the delivery occurred and the recipient's signature (Figure 11-11, *B*). Many state laws mandate that **termination letters** be sent by Certified Mail with Return Receipt. The mailing receipt showing the letter was mailed and the Return Receipt along with a copy of the letter are uploaded into the EHR or filed in the paper medical record. These items provide proof the law was followed if there is ever a question.

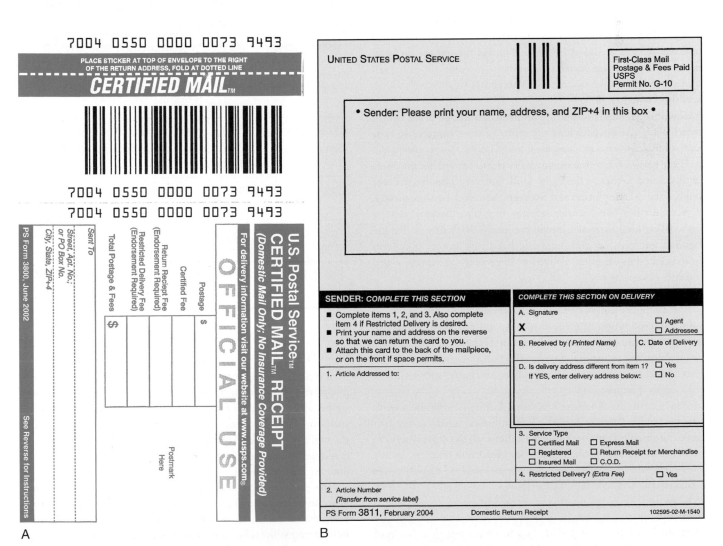

A   B

FIGURE 11-11 A, Receipt for Certified Mail. Attach the bottom portion of the receipt to the top of the package or envelope, just to the right of the return address. **B,** Return Receipt used to provide an automatic electronic or hardcopy record showing the recipient's signature.

Signature Confirmation is an optional service that can be added to First-Class, Priority Mail, and Media Mail. This service provides information about the date and time an item was delivered or a delivery attempt was made. The delivery record, which includes the recipient's signature, is kept by the USPS and is available electronically or by e-mail upon request.

The healthcare facility utilizes the Return Receipt more often than the Signature Confirmation (see Figure 11-11, *A*). The advantage of the Return Receipt service is that it provides an automatic e-mail or hardcopy mail delivery record showing the recipient's signature. The hardcopy is more expensive than the e-mail. Return Receipt can be added to the five domestic delivery services mentioned in the prior section.

With Restricted Delivery service and Adult Signature Restricted Delivery service, the mailed item can only be delivered to the addressee, an **authorized agent** of the addressee, or a parent/guardian. The receiver must verify his or her identity and must sign for the delivery. With the Adult Signature Restricted Delivery service, the person signing must also show proof that he or she is over 21.

The Certificate of Mailing provides evidence that the item was mailed. It shows the date and time the item was mailed. This service is limited because it doesn't show evidence of the delivery. It can be combined with other services for additional information. Additional optional services are listed in Table 11-3. For a complete list, refer to the USPS Web site (www.usps.com).

Private Delivery Services

The USPS only handles a portion of the mail delivered in the United States. Private companies have grown by offering competitive rates and additional services compared with USPS. Some companies provide national and international services, but others are more locally based. FedEx, UPS, and DHL are very popular national options for shipping letters and packages. Some offer on-site pickup.

Larger cities have courier services that have become popular options for local deliveries. Some companies have drivers that are **bonded**, professional, and trained to handle all aspects of delivery from medical to hazardous deliveries. Some of the services provided include:

- Pickup and delivery of medical specimens (e.g., take patient laboratory samples to a medical laboratory for testing).
- Transportation of medical records and documents from one location to another, complying with Health Insurance Portability and Accountability Act (HIPAA) requirements.
- Pickup and delivery of deposits to the bank, with return of cash if required.

The ultimate goal for the healthcare facility is to utilize a mail/courier service that provides the most efficient service at the best price. The medical assistant may have to research the delivery services available in the area to identify the best fit for the practice.

CRITICAL THINKING APPLICATION   **11-11**

The providers would like to utilize an off-site laboratory to process specimens. Marie would like to have a local courier service pick up specimens and deliver them to the off-site laboratory. When researching potential delivery couriers for this activity, what factors should Marie consider?

TABLE 11-3   Optional Services Provided by United States Postal Service

Standard Insurance	Protects against loss or damage. Cost is based on the item's declared value.
Registered Mail	Used to protect expensive items. A mailing receipt is given; upon request an electronic verification of delivery can be sent.
Certified Mail	Mailing receipt provides evidence the letter was mailed and the Return Receipt shows delivery information and the recipient's signature.
Signature Confirmation	Provides date and time of delivery, along with the recipient's signature. Copy of delivery record is available upon request.
Return Receipt	Provides an automatic electronic or mailed delivery record showing the recipient's signature.
Adult Signature Restricted Delivery	Addressee or authorized agent must verify identity and age (i.e., must be over 21); must sign for delivery.
Restricted Delivery	Addressee or authorized agent must verify identity and must sign for delivery.
Certificate of Mailing	Provides evidence (i.e., date and time) when an item was mailed.
United States Postal Service Tracking	Provides updates as an item is being shipped. Will include date and time of delivery or attempted delivery.
Special Handling	Used to get preferential handing when shipping very unusual items or items that need extra care.
Collect on Delivery (COD)	Recipient pays for merchandise and shipping when the package is received.
Hold for Pickup	Option to pick up item from a specified Post Office within 15 days, depending on service selected.

Incoming Mail

Mail can be collected at the post office or be delivered to the healthcare facility. If the facility is large, some employees have the responsibility to sort and deliver the mail to the different departments. In smaller practices, the medical assistant may be responsible for sorting the mail. Mail received by the healthcare facility greatly varies. The medical assistant must sort the mail following the practice's procedure for incoming mail.

The provider receives all mail marked *Personal* and correspondence from lawyers and accountants. Professional journals, pharmaceutical materials, and convention/**continuing medical education (CME)** events flyers are also given to the provider. Bills are given to the provider if he or she is responsible for paying them. If not, then the bills are given to the person responsible for the accounts payable

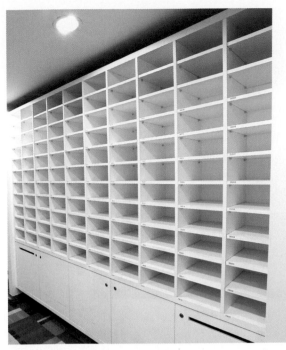

FIGURE 11-12 Mailboxes are efficient ways of sorting and storing mail for individuals in the department. (Photo copyright iStock.com.)

TABLE 11-4 Principles of Proper Body Mechanics

- To lift an object, maintain a wide, stable base with your feet. Your feet should be shoulder-width apart and you should have good footing. Bend at the knees, keeping your back straight. Lift smoothly, using the major muscles in your arms and legs. Use the same technique when putting the item down. Bending over to lift or to set down a heavy object will increase your risk of injury.
- When lifting and carrying heavy items, keep the item directly in front of you to avoid rotating your spine.
- Keep your movements smooth. Jerky or uncoordinated movements increase the risk for injury.
- When reaching for an object, your feet should face the object. Twisting or turning with a heavy load can cause injury.
- Prevent reaching and straining to get an object. Clear away barriers and utilize a firm and level surface (e.g., step stool) to get close to the object. Avoid standing on tiptoes.
- Get help if the item is too heavy to lift by yourself.
- Store heavy objects at waist-level or below.

activities. A provider may request the incoming mail be placed on his or her desk. In larger departments, mailboxes are utilized for each person in the department (Figure 11-12). The medical assistant can easily sort the mail and place it in the individual mailboxes.

CRITICAL THINKING APPLICATION 11-12

Catherine sorts the mail for the practice. Because the practice is small, they do not use the mailbox system. Mail has gotten lost when she has placed it on the providers' desks. What are some other options that Catherine can implement to prevent mail from getting lost or misplaced on providers' desks?

Mail related to patients, like diagnostic test and laboratory results and consultation letters, are opened and dated. If the practice uses paper medical records, the document should be clipped to the chart. If the ambulatory care facility uses an EHR, some practices have the medical assistant identify the patient in the system and write the patient's EHR number on the document. The provider can just type in this number, verify the patient's name, and proceed to reviewing the document and the EHR notes. This helps save time for the provider. Eventually the received document needs to be scanned and uploaded into the patient's EHR or filed in the paper record.

The medical assistant handles the magazines for the reception area, supply shipments, and correspondences from insurance companies. Payments from insurance companies and patients should be recorded immediately in the day's receipts.

The practice are procedures on handling mail that is not addressed to a specific person. Typically it is given to the department supervisor, office manager, or medical director. If a medical assistant has a question regarding who should get a specific piece of

mail, it is important to ask. If the medical assistant questions if a letter should be opened, it is better to not open it and ask the provider or office manager. When a provider is on vacation, the practice will have a procedure for handling the mail. If something is urgent or relates to a patient, procedures are in place to guide the medical assistant.

BODY MECHANICS

The Occupational Safety and Health Act (OSHA) of 1970 requires that employers provide a workplace that is free from serious recognized hazards and the employer must comply with OSHA standards. In the healthcare environment, the majority of injuries are sprains, strains, and tears. Back injuries are one of the most common injuries and can result from microtrauma related to repetitive activity over time or from one traumatic experience. Typically, improper lifting or lifting items too heavy for the back to support are the main reasons for acute back injuries. Other reasons for back injuries include:

- Reaching, twisting, or bending when lifting
- Bad body mechanics when lifting, pushing, pulling, or carrying items
- Poor footing or constrained posture

Medical assistants need to protect themselves from bodily harm while lifting, reaching, and carrying heavy boxes and equipment associated with supplies and equipment (Figure 11-13 and Figure 11-14). Using proper body mechanics is important to prevent injuries (Table 11-4). Proper body mechanics entails utilizing the appropriate muscles and body movements to maintain correct posture and body alignment. By utilizing proper body mechanics, coordination and endurance will be increased and the risk of strain and injury to the body will be decreased. See Procedure 11-3, which explains how to use correct body mechanics when performing a supply inventory.

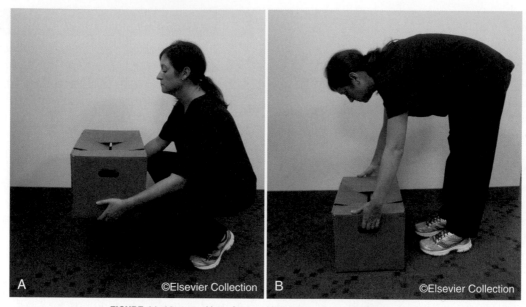

FIGURE 11-13 A, Bend knees for proper lifting technique. **B,** Improper lifting technique.

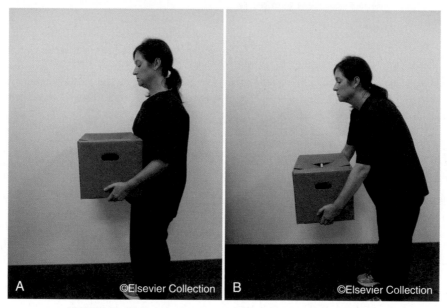

FIGURE 11-14 A, Carrying an item close to the body. **B,** Improper carrying technique.

CLOSING COMMENTS

Patient Education

The principles of body mechanics utilized by the medical assistant for tasks in the medical office can also be used in everyday life. The medical assistant may need to coach a patient on the correct techniques for lifting, reaching, and carrying heavy objects to prevent injury. With the frequency of back injuries, it is important to emphasize proper body alignment, proper posture, and good footing when moving heavy objects. Encourage patients to use a safe step stool when reaching high objects. The step stool should be sturdy and needs to accommodate the weight of the patient. Some step stools have a handle or grab bar, which can provide extra safety. Using proper body mechanics all the time is the key to preventing injuries that may last a lifetime.

Legal and Ethical Issues

The medical assistant must help to protect the medical practice from lawsuits. For any document sent to a patient, it is important for the medical assistant to file a copy in the medical record or to upload an electronic copy to the EHR. When using Certified Mail is required for what is being sent, the medical assistant needs to ensure that all the required paperwork is added to the health record, thus providing evidence that the laws were followed. Without evidence that a letter was sent and received, the medical practice could face a lawsuit.

Professional Behaviors

In the healthcare facility there is an abundance of administrative and clinical supplies. The medical assistant may be tempted to take some supplies for his or her personal use. This action could be looked upon as theft and is not professional.

Medical and administrative supplies cost the practice money. The medical assistant needs to appreciate the cost of supplies and help look for ways to decrease supply expenses. Being wasteful can cost the employer money. Making sure to rotate and use supplies before their expiration date will help prevent wasting money. Providers and supervisors appreciate staff that are cost conscientious.

SUMMARY OF SCENARIO

Marie has started to implement an inventory management process that is helping her identify when to reorder and how much to reorder. She initially started by hand counting the inventory, and then she identified how much was utilized each buying cycle. It took a few months for her to identify trends; even then, she found certain times of the year can affect the quantity of orthopedic products used. For instance, providers tend to use more casting products in the winter and summer months, which means Marie will need to increase her stock of those items during these times of the year. Marie knows that she can become more efficient with the inventory with the more she learns. She has already helped the practice save money by identifying cheaper vendors for commonly used expensive items. Marie loves her new job and the variety of responsibilities she has. She looks forward to continuing to learn in the future.

SUMMARY OF LEARNING OBJECTIVES

1. **Define, spell, and pronounce the terms listed in the vocabulary.**
   It is important to spell and pronounce terms commonly used in the healthcare setting. By using these terms correctly, the medical assistant will demonstrate professional traits and be credible when discussing the topics with others.

2. **Describe the administrative and clinical opening duties performed by the medical assistant.**
   The medical assistant has administrative and clinical duties that need to be performed to prepare the office for patients and the activities for the coming day. Some of the administrative responsibilities include preparing the reception area, turning on lights and equipment, and preparing the paperwork for patients' visits. In the clinical area, examination rooms need to be opened and stocked, supply cabinets need to be unlocked, quality control tests need to be completed, and outstanding patient issues need to be handled.

3. **Discuss the administrative and clinical closing responsibilities performed by the medical assistant, as well as daily and monthly duties.**
   At the end of the business day, the administrative duties include closing the office, cleaning and restocking the reception area as needed, turning off the equipment, switching the phones over to the answering service or voice mail, and following the facility's procedures for handling the money collected during the day. The medical assistant in the clinical area must clean and restock the examination rooms, turn off equipment, and lock cabinets. All patient information should be put away. During slow times, medical assistants need to do extra duties, including restocking medical and office supplies, forms, and patient literature. Crash carts need to be inventoried monthly.

4. **Explain safety and security procedures important in the healthcare facility.**
   The medical assistant must keep at a distance from a suspicious person. Being behind the desk or closest to the door in the examination room are a few ways to protect yourself. Healthcare facilities have implemented various strategies, including code words, alarms, and locked doors to help increase security.

5. **Do the following related to equipment in a medical practice:**
   - Describe the elements of an equipment inventory list.
     The equipment inventory list provides information about the administrative and clinical machines in the facility. This information is used by the provider, supervisor, and/or accountant for future planning and tax paperwork. Procedure 11-1 describes how to create an equipment inventory list and Figure 11-5 provides an example of an equipment inventory list.
   - Explain the purpose of routine maintenance of administrative and clinical equipment.
     Routine maintenance is crucial for the equipment to run correctly. The medical assistant should inspect equipment for unsafe issues. Equipment should be routinely cleaned as specified in the operation manual. The manual will also indicate routine maintenance and service schedules. Following these directions will help prevent problems with the equipment and will extend the machine's longevity.
   - Explain the steps of creating a maintenance log, performing maintenance, and documenting the maintenance.
     See Procedure 11-2 for the steps in creating a maintenance log. The procedure also provides directions for performing and documenting

Continued

maintenance. Figure 11-6 provides an example of an equipment maintenance log.

- Describe the medical assistant's role in ordering equipment.
  The medical assistant can help research potential equipment by utilizing the Internet and meeting with the salesperson. Leasing or buying the equipment are options to investigate, along with what additional billable services might be provided by using that machine. The provider or supervisor will make the final decision regarding the purchase or lease.

6. **Do the following related to supplies in the medical practice:**
- Discuss the elements on a supply inventory list.
  The supply inventory list can be created in a notebook, on index cards, or by using the computer and a spreadsheet or inventory control processing software. The elements on the list include the details about the item (i.e., name, size, quantity, item number, supplier's name, and cost), quantity to reorder, and reorder point. Procedure 11-3 describes how to create a supply inventory list and how to utilize it for inventory. See Figure 11-7 for an example of a supply inventory list.
- List the steps involved in completing an inventory.
  Procedure 11-3 describes how to perform an inventory by hand counting supplies.
- Perform an inventory with documentation.
  Procedure 11-3 discusses how to perform a supply inventory and document the inventory counts on the supply inventory list.
- Prepare a supply order.
  Procedure 11-4 describes how to identify which items need to be ordered. The steps on creating an online order using a supplier's Web site are described.

7. **Describe how the healthcare facility utilizes USPS and other delivery agencies.**
  The majority of the mail sent by the healthcare facility will be sent through the USPS. The USPS has a number of different types of mail services available to meet the needs of the healthcare facility. First-Class Mail is the most common service used in the healthcare facility to mail letters. Depending on the packages mailed or the urgency of the item, other services may be utilized. The USPS also offers insurance, shipping confirmation, delivery confirmation, and tracking services. These services can be added to other mail services for an additional fee. In some situations the medical office will need to use Certified Mail to send termination letters to patients.

  The facility may also use other national delivery agencies for urgent letters or large packages. Local delivery agencies' services can vary by location, but many assist healthcare facilities by transporting patients' medical records and laboratory samples to other agencies for processing or patient appointments. The medical assistant needs to be knowledgeable about the mail services available and the correct service to use to meet the needs of the healthcare facility.

8. **Use proper body mechanics.**
  The medical assistant must use proper body mechanics and posture to help decrease the risk of injury. See Table 11-4 for the principles of proper body mechanics when reaching, lifting, and carrying heavy items. Using proper body mechanics is important when performing inventory in the healthcare environment. Procedure 11-3 describes how to implement proper body mechanics when taking an inventory of supplies in the healthcare facility.

CONNECTIONS

Study Guide Connection: Go to the Chapter 11 Study Guide. Read and complete the activities.

evolve Evolve Connection: Go to the Chapter 11 link at *evolve.elsevier.com/kinn* to complete the Chapter Review Quiz. Check out the other resources listed for this chapter to make the most of what you have learned from Daily Operations in the Ambulatory Care Setting.

THE HEALTH RECORD

SCENARIO

Susan Beezler has just begun her career in the medical assisting profession. She is attending medical assisting school in the morning and works part-time for a family practitioner in the afternoons as a clerical record assistant. Susan is eager to learn about medicine and looks forward to taking on more responsibility at the office.

The practice is growing swiftly and recently added a new provider, Dr. Alex Thomas. Dr. Thomas has enjoyed working with Susan and feels that her energy will be just what his patients need. He has taken a professional interest in Susan and often lets her assist him with patients when her other duties allow.

Susan knows that although she is a beginner in the office, she will gain trust from her supervisors and patients as long as she projects a teachable attitude. The office has recently converted to an electronic records system but is still using paper records as well. Susan uses the information she learned in school about both types of health records. She cheerfully performs filing and even does some transcription for Dr. Thomas. The other staff members are pleased with her willingness to perform the most mundane tasks.

Susan enjoys sharing her experiences with her classmates. She is the only one currently working in the medical field, and the other students ask her lots of questions about the "real world" of medicine. She is very careful not to breach patient confidentiality; she discusses situations only in general terms, never mentioning any patients' names.

Susan feels a great sense of pride that she is already a member of the healthcare team and able to contribute to the lives of her patients.

While studying this chapter, think about the following questions:

- Why would some patients have concerns about the healthcare facility using electronic health records (EHRs)?
- How can the medical assistant earn the patient's trust so that the person is comfortable revealing the very private information required by a health history?
- Why is it so important to have a signed release of information form before sending patient information out?
- Why is it important that the health record be legible?
- Why is it important to know both administrative and clinical skills in the provider's office?

LEARNING OBJECTIVES

1. Define, spell, and pronounce the terms listed in the vocabulary.
2. Name and discuss the two types of patient records.
3. State several reasons that accurate health records are important.
4. Differentiate between subjective and objective information in creating a patient's health record.
5. Explain who owns the health record.
6. Distinguish between an electronic health record (EHR) and an electronic medical record (EMR).
7. Do the following related to healthcare legislation and EHRs:
   - Explain how the American Recovery and Reinvestment Act (ARRA) applies to the healthcare industry.
   - Define *meaningful use* and relate it to the healthcare industry.
   - List the three main components of meaningful use legislation.
8. Explore the advantages, disadvantages, and capabilities of an EHR system, and explain how to organize a patient's health record.
9. Discuss the importance of nonverbal communication with patients when an EHR system is used.
10. Discuss backup systems for the EHR, as well as the transfer, destruction, and retention of health records as related to the EHR.
11. Describe how and when to release health record information; discuss health information exchanges (HIEs).
12. Identify and discuss the two methods of organizing a patient's paper medical record.
13. Discuss how to document information in an EHR and a paper health record, and how to make corrections/alterations to health records.
14. Discuss dictation and transcription, and discuss transfer, destruction, and retention of medical records as related to paper records.
15. Identify filing equipment and filing supplies needed to create, store, and maintain medical records.
16. Describe indexing rules, and how to create and organize a patient's health record.
17. Discuss the pros and cons of various filing methods, as well as how to file patient health records.
18. Discuss organization of files, as well as health-related correspondence.
19. Discuss patient education, as well as legal and ethical issues, related to the health record.

VOCABULARY

age of majority The age at which a person is recognized by law to be an adult; can vary by state.

alleviate To partly remove or correct; to relieve or lessen.

alphabetic filing Any system that arranges names or topics according to the sequence of the letters in the alphabet.

alphanumeric Of or relating to systems made up of combinations of letters and numbers.

augment To increase in size or amount; to add to in order to improve or complete.

caption A heading, title, or subtitle under which records are filed.

computerized provider/physician order entry (CPOE) The process of entering medication orders or other provider instructions into the electronic health record (EHR).

continuity of care Continuation of care smoothly from one provider to another, so that the patient receives the most benefit and no interruption in care.

culpability Meriting condemnation, responsibility, or blame, especially as wrong or harmful.

dictation (dik-ta'-shun) The act or manner of uttering words to be transcribed.

direct filing system A filing system in which materials can be located without consulting an additional source of reference.

e-prescribing The use of electronic software to communicate with pharmacies and send prescribing information, taking the place of writing a prescription by hand and physically giving it to a patient; most new or refill prescriptions can be submitted electronically, cutting down on fraud and errors.

electronic health record (EHR) An electronic record of health-related information about a patient that conforms to nationally recognized interoperability standards and that can be created, managed, and consulted by authorized clinicians and staff from more than one healthcare organization.

electronic medical record (EMR) An electronic record of health-related information about an individual that can be created, gathered, managed, and consulted by authorized clinicians and staff within a single healthcare organization.

gleaned Gathered bit by bit (e.g., information or material); picked over in search of relevant material.

indirect filing system A filing system in which an intermediary source of reference (e.g., a card file) must be consulted to locate specific files.

interoperability The ability to work with other systems.

microfilm A film with a photographic record of printed or other graphic matter on a reduced scale.

numeric filing The filing of records, correspondence, or cards by number.

objective information Data obtained through physical examination, laboratory and diagnostic testing, and by measurable information.

obliteration (uh-blih-tuh-ra'-shun) The act of making undecipherable or imperceptible by obscuring or wearing away.

outguide A sturdy cardboard or plastic file-sized card used to replace a folder temporarily removed from the filing space.

parameters Any set of physical properties, the values of which determine characteristics or behavior.

patient portal A secure online Web site that gives patients 24-hour access to personal health information using a username and password.

personal health record (PHR) An electronic record of health-related information about an individual that conforms to nationally recognized interoperability standards and that can be drawn from multiple sources but that is managed, shared, and controlled by the individual.

pressboard A strong, highly glazed composition board resembling vulcanized fiber; heavy card stock.

provisional diagnosis A temporary diagnosis made before all test results have been received.

purging The process of moving active files to inactive status.

quality control An aggregate of activities designed to ensure adequate quality, especially in manufactured products or in the service industries.

reasonable cause Circumstances that would make it unreasonable for the covered entity, despite the exercise of ordinary business care and prudence, to comply with the administrative simplification provision (part of Health Information Technology for Economic and Clinical Health Act [HITECH]) that was violated.

reasonable diligence The business care and prudence expected from a person seeking to satisfy a legal requirement under similar circumstances.

requisites (reh'-kwuh-zihts) Entities considered essential or necessary.

retention schedule A method or plan for retaining or keeping health records and for their movement from active to inactive to closed filing.

reverse chronologic order Arranged in order so that the most recent item is on top and older items are filed further back.

subjective information Data or information elicited from the patient, including the patient's feelings, perceptions, and concerns; obtained through interview or questions.

subpoena duces tecum A court order to produce documents or records.

tickler file A chronologic file used as a reminder that something must be dealt with on a certain date.

transcription A written copy of something made either in longhand or by machine.

vested Granted or endowed with a particular authority, right, or property; to have a special interest in.

willful neglect Conscious, intentional failure or reckless indifference to the obligation to comply with the administrative simplification provision violated.

Health records can be found in basically two different formats, electronic and paper. Most healthcare facilities have switched to **electronic health records (EHRs)** for a number of reasons. The advantages of EHRs include easy storage of patient information, accessibility by multiple users at the same time, and making electronic claim submission a more efficient process, to name a few. The federal government has also offered financial incentives for providers to implement EHRs. Although most providers are using EHRs there are still some who are using paper records and others who are using a combination of both electronic and paper. When a provider is making a switch to an EHR he or she may decide to keep the patient's previous records in the paper format and just use the electronic format from now forward. Some providers may decide to scan in the last 3 to 5 years of the patient's record into the electronic record. Whatever the scenario the healthcare facility has chosen, it is important for the versatile medical assistant to be knowledgeable about both systems and able to perform well with either.

TYPES OF RECORDS

The two major types of patient records are the paper health record and the EHR. With the advances in computer technology, the paper health record has been shown to be much less efficient than the EHR. In most cases, only one person at a time can use the paper record. It is fairly common for information to be filed in the incorrect record, and the entire record also can be misfiled. Data cannot be accessed easily for research and **quality control,** and in facilities with multiple departments or locations, the information is difficult to share. The paper-based record is good evidence of patient care, but it is not nearly as useful in other capacities.

The EHR is much more efficient than the paper record. Multiple users can access the record at the same time. There are fewer errors because handwritten notes do not have to be interpreted. In addition, most EHRs also link the clinical information needed for billing purposes, and include practice management capabilities that allow for patient scheduling and generation of reports needed for research and quality control.

CRITICAL THINKING APPLICATION   **12-1**

Some of Dr. Thomas' patients are concerned that computer-based health records may not be completely private. They are worried that unauthorized individuals could access their information on the computer and do them harm. Should patients be allowed to decide whether their records are kept on computer or on paper?

THE IMPORTANCE OF ACCURATE HEALTH RECORDS

Health records are kept for five basic reasons. First, the health record helps the provider provide the best possible medical care for the patient. The provider examines the patient and enters the findings in the patient's health record. These findings are clues to the diagnosis. The provider may order many types of tests to confirm or **augment** the clinical findings. As the reports of these tests come in, the findings fall into place, much like the pieces of a jigsaw puzzle.

Then, with the confirmation data to support the diagnosis, the provider can prescribe treatment and form an opinion about the patient's chances of recovery, assured that every resource has been used to arrive at a correct judgment. The health record provides a complete history of all the care given to the patient.

Second, the health record also provides critical information for others. By reading through the record and discovering the methods used to treat the patient, healthcare professionals can provide **continuity of care.** Each person knows what the patient has experienced and can provide continuous care, even from one facility to another. For example, when a patient is transferred from a hospital to a skilled nursing facility, the information from the patient's hospital record helps the nursing facility staff to better care for the patient. When patients move from place to place or caregivers change, copies of the pertinent information should move with the patient to provide this continuity of care.

Third, health records are kept as legal protection for those who provided care to the patient. A documented health record is excellent proof that certain procedures were performed or that medical advice was given. An accurate record is the foundation for a legal defense in cases of medical professional liability. This is one reason that writing legibly in the paper record to document exactly what happened to the patient and the provider's response are critical. Remember: If it is not documented, it did not happen.

Fourth, health records provide statistical information that is helpful to researchers. The patient's record provides information about medications taken and the reactions to them. Health records may be used to evaluate the effectiveness of certain kinds of treatment or to determine the incidence of a given disease. Providers often take part in drug studies that track adverse reactions and side effects. The effects of various treatments and procedures also can be tracked and statistics **gleaned** from the information in patients' records. In tracking statistical information the information that would identify specific patients is removed. Correlation of such statistical information may result in a new outlook on some phases of medicine and can lead to revised techniques and treatments. The statistical data from health records also are valuable in the preparation of scientific papers, books, and lectures.

Fifth, health records are vital for financial reimbursement. The information in the health record supports claims for reimbursement and is required by most third-party payers.

CONTENTS OF THE HEALTH RECORD

The patient's health record is the most important record in a provider's practice. For completeness, each patient's record should contain **subjective information** provided by the patient and **objective information** obtained by the provider and staff of the healthcare facility. If all entries are completed, the health record will stand the test of time. No branch of medicine is exempt from the need to keep patient health records.

Subjective Information
Personal Demographics
The patient's health record begins with routine personal data, which the patient usually supplies on the first visit when the health record is established. Most patients are required to complete a patient

information form (Figure 12-1 and Procedure 12-1). The basic facts needed are:

- Patient's full name, spelled correctly
- Names of parents/guardians if the patient is a child
- Patient's gender
- Date of birth
- Marital status
- Name of spouse if married
- Home address, telephone number, and e-mail address
- Occupation
- Name of employer
- Business address and telephone number
- Employment information for spouse
- Healthcare insurance information
- Source of referral
- Social Security number

Past Health, Family, and Social History

The past health, family, and social history is often obtained by having the patient complete a questionnaire. The medical assistant may review the form for completeness and clarify any questions or missing information with the patient before the patient is seen by the provider. The provider will also augment this history with information provided during the patient interview. The responses provide information about any past illnesses (including injuries and/or physical defects, whether congenital or acquired), hospitalizations, or

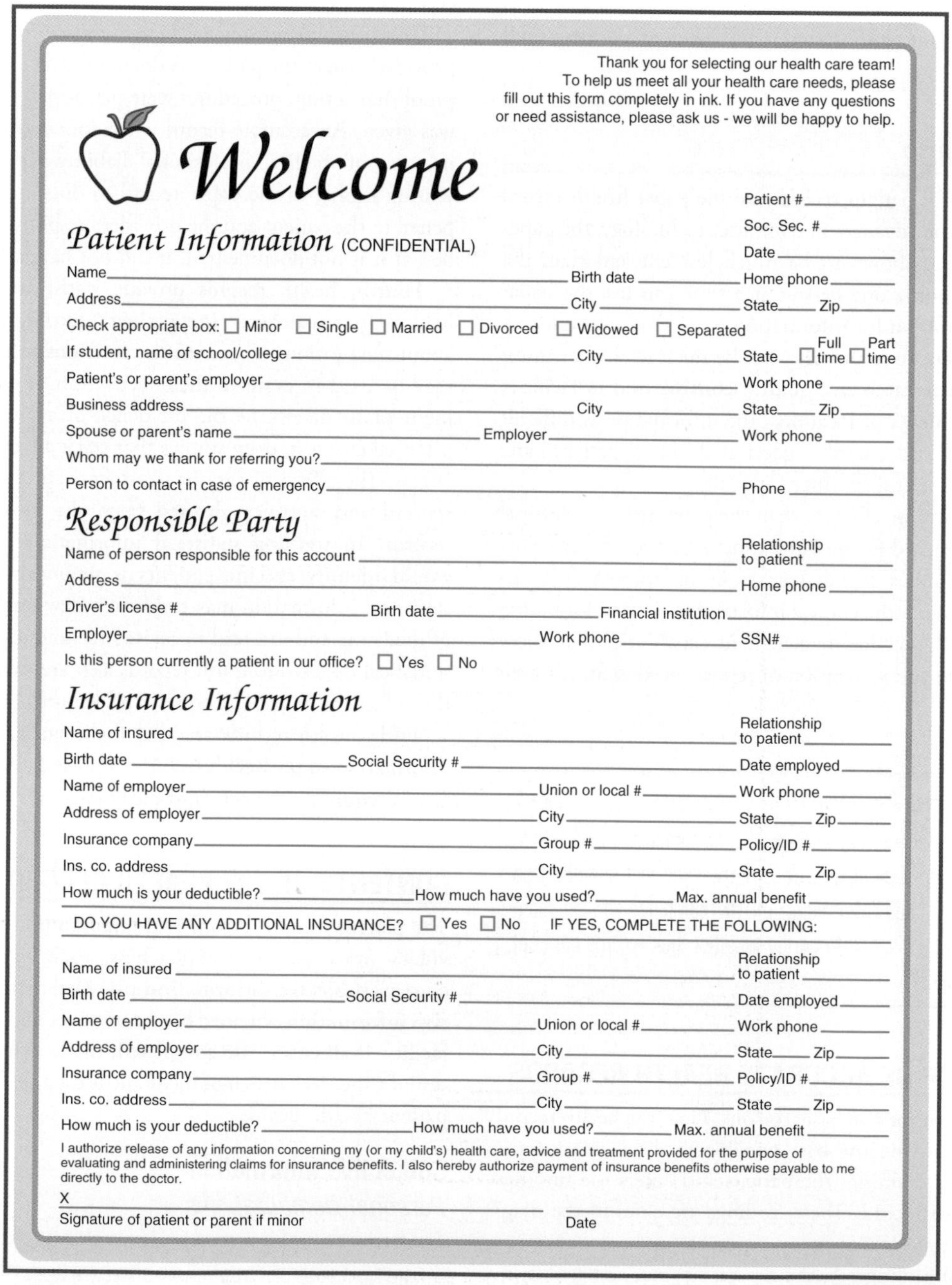
Thank you for selecting our health care team!
To help us meet all your health care needs, please fill out this form completely in ink. If you have any questions or need assistance, please ask us - we will be happy to help.

Welcome

Patient #
Soc. Sec. #
Date

Patient Information (CONFIDENTIAL)

Name ______ Birth date ______ Home phone ______
Address ______ City ______ State ______ Zip ______
Check appropriate box: ☐ Minor ☐ Single ☐ Married ☐ Divorced ☐ Widowed ☐ Separated
If student, name of school/college ______ City ______ State ______ ☐ Full time ☐ Part time
Patient's or parent's employer ______ Work phone ______
Business address ______ City ______ State ______ Zip ______
Spouse or parent's name ______ Employer ______ Work phone ______
Whom may we thank for referring you? ______
Person to contact in case of emergency ______ Phone ______

Responsible Party

Name of person responsible for this account ______ Relationship to patient ______
Address ______ Home phone ______
Driver's license # ______ Birth date ______ Financial institution ______
Employer ______ Work phone ______ SSN# ______
Is this person currently a patient in our office? ☐ Yes ☐ No

Insurance Information

Name of insured ______ Relationship to patient ______
Birth date ______ Social Security # ______ Date employed ______
Name of employer ______ Union or local # ______ Work phone ______
Address of employer ______ City ______ State ______ Zip ______
Insurance company ______ Group # ______ Policy/ID # ______
Ins. co. address ______ City ______ State ______ Zip ______
How much is your deductible? ______ How much have you used? ______ Max. annual benefit ______

DO YOU HAVE ANY ADDITIONAL INSURANCE? ☐ Yes ☐ No IF YES, COMPLETE THE FOLLOWING:

Name of insured ______ Relationship to patient ______
Birth date ______ Social Security # ______ Date employed ______
Name of employer ______ Union or local # ______ Work phone ______
Address of employer ______ City ______ State ______ Zip ______
Insurance company ______ Group # ______ Policy/ID # ______
Ins. co. address ______ City ______ State ______ Zip ______
How much is your deductible? ______ How much have you used? ______ Max. annual benefit ______

I authorize release of any information concerning my (or my child's) health care, advice and treatment provided for the purpose of evaluating and administering claims for insurance benefits. I also hereby authorize payment of insurance benefits otherwise payable to me directly to the doctor.

X ______
Signature of patient or parent if minor ______ Date

FIGURE 12-1 The patient information form provides all the information the medical assistant needs to construct the patient's record.

surgeries the patient has had (Figure 12-2). It also includes information about the patient's daily health habits. Stickers can be used on the front of paper health records to indicate allergies, advance directives, and other information (Figure 12-3). In an EHR there will be alerts that may appear as a pop-up window when the record is accessed that will indicate that the patient has allergies, that immunizations are due, or that there is no advance directive on file. These are useful for helping the health professional keep important facts about the patient in the forefront of the mind while treating the individual.

Past Health History. The past health history will include information about previous illnesses/injuries (including childhood illnesses such as chickenpox or measles), previous hospitalizations, and previous surgeries. The dates that these occurred will need to be documented, as well as any complications. The provider needs to be aware of this information because it could affect the patient's current condition.

Patient's Family History. The family history comprises the physical condition of the various members of the patient's family, any illnesses or diseases individual members may have had, and a record of the causes of death. This information is important because certain diseases may have a hereditary pattern. Most providers are interested in the immediate family: parents, grandparents, siblings, and children.

Patient's Social History. The social history includes information about the patient's lifestyle. If the patient drinks alcohol, how many drinks per day or per week are consumed? If the patient uses nicotine, how much is used in a day, and what type (i.e., cigarettes or smokeless tobacco)? Drug use, living situation, exercise, and nutrition information can be considered part of the social history.

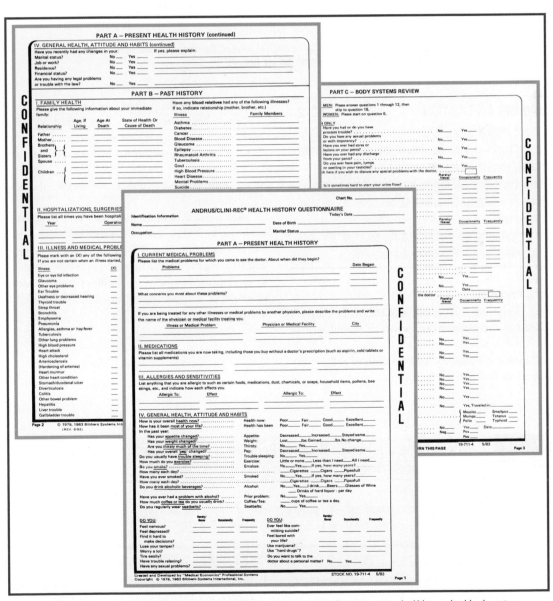

FIGURE 12-2 Database self-administered general health history questionnaire: Lengthy questionnaires should be completed by the patient before the individual is seen by the provider. Either mail the questionnaire to the patient in advance or ask the patient to come in early to complete the paperwork. (Courtesy Bibbero Systems, Petaluma, California.)

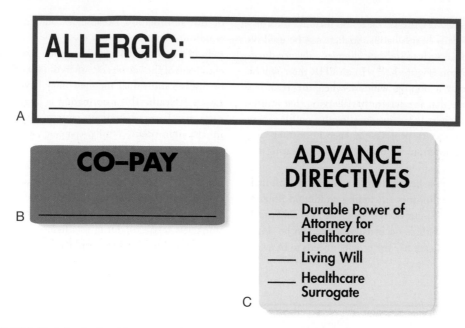

FIGURE 12-3 Record stickers: Information on stickers on the outside of the record allows the provider and medical staff to see important information about the patient quickly. (Courtesy Bibbero Systems, Petaluma, California.)

CRITICAL THINKING APPLICATION   **12-2**

While taking a patient's medical history, Susan asks about his social history. She asks whether he drinks alcohol. The patient immediately becomes defensive and accuses Susan of getting too personal about his affairs.

- How might Susan explain her reasons for asking these questions? What options are available if the patient refuses to discuss his social history with Susan?
- Could this opposition to questions about the social history raise suspicion in Susan's mind? What might she suspect?

Patient's Chief Complaint

The patient's chief complaint is a concise account of the patient's symptoms, explained in the patient's own words. It should include the following:

- The nature, location, frequency, and duration of pain, if any
- When the patient first noticed the symptoms

- Treatments the patient may have tried before seeing the provider and whether they have helped with the symptoms or not; when the last dose was taken
- Whether the patient has had the same or a similar condition in the past
- Other medical treatment received for the same condition in the past

Most medical facilities use a pain scale to determine the severity of the patient's discomfort. The medical assistant might ask, "How bad is your pain on a scale of 1 to 10, with 1 being almost no pain, and 10 being the worst pain you've ever experienced?" The pain scale or wording used in individual facilities should be documented in the office policy and procedures manual and followed by the medical assistant.

PROCEDURE 12-1	Create a Patient's Health Record: Register a New Patient in the Practice Management Software

Goal: *Register a new patient in the practice management software, prepare a Notice of Privacy Practices (NPP) form and a Disclosure Authorization form for the new patient, and document this in the electronic health record (EHR).*

EQUIPMENT and SUPPLIES

- Computer with SimChart for the Medical Office or practice management and EHR software
- Completed patient registration form
- Scanner

PROCEDURAL STEPS

1. Obtain the new patient's completed registration form. Log into the practice management software.
2. Using the patient's last and first names and date of birth, search the database for the patient.

PROCEDURE 12-1 — *continued*

PURPOSE: To help ensure the integrity of the practice management and EHR systems, a search for the new patient's name must always be done before registering that person. This prevents a double record from being created if the patient had been entered into the database at an earlier time.

3. If the database does not contain the patient's name, add a new patient and enter the patient's demographics from the completed registration form.

4. Verify that the information entered is correct and that all fields are completed before saving the data.

PURPOSE: Errors during the registration process can affect the communication with the patient (e.g., if a wrong address or e-mail is entered) or can affect billing (e.g., if the incorrect insurance information is added). Accuracy is extremely important when entering the patient's information.

NOTE: The software will generate a health record number for the patient.

5. Using the EHR software, prepare and print a copy of the NPP and a Disclosure Authorization form for the new patient. The Disclosure Authorization form should indicate the disclosure will be to the patient's insurance company.

PURPOSE: Before the medical office can release patient information to the insurance company, the patient has to give consent in writing.

SCENARIO UPDATE: The patient received both documents and signed the Disclosure Authorization form.

6. Using the EHR, document that the patient received a copy of the NPP and signed the Disclosure Authorization form. Scan the Disclosure Authorization form and upload it into the EHR.

PURPOSE: Documentation in the health record provides a legal record of what was done or communicated to the patient.

7. Log out of the software upon completion of the procedure.

PURPOSE: Logging into and out of the software helps to protect the integrity of the data saved in the software and prevents unauthorized people from viewing the information.

Objective Information

Objective findings, sometimes referred to as *signs,* are findings that can be observed and measured. They can include vital signs, measurements, and observations made by the medical assistant and findings from the provider's examination of the patient.

Vital Signs and Anthropometric Measurements

The medical assistant's responsibilities include taking the patient's vital signs (i.e., temperature, pulse, respirations, blood pressure, pulse oximetry) and height and weight. These measurements are documented in the patient's health record and are used by the provider in his or her assessment. If the medical assistant observes other signs such as a rash, this would also be documented in the patient's health record and brought to the provider's attention.

Findings and Laboratory and Radiology Reports

After the provider has examined the patient, the physical findings are documented in the health record. The results of other tests or requests for these tests are then documented or, if they appear on separate sheets, are attached to the health record. When an EHR is being used the separate sheet may be scanned so that it is in an electronic format and can be added to the patient's EHR.

Diagnosis

Based on all the evidence provided in the patient's past history, the provider's examination, and any supplementary tests, the provider notes his or her diagnosis of the patient's condition in the health record. If some doubt remains, this may be labeled a **provisional diagnosis**. A *differential diagnosis* is the process of weighing the probability of one disease causing the patient's illness against the probability that other diseases are causative. For example, the differential diagnosis of rhinitis, or a runny nose, could indicate allergic rhinitis (i.e., hay fever), the common cold, or even abuse of drugs or nasal decongestants.

Treatment Prescribed and Progress Notes

The provider's suggested treatment is listed after the diagnosis. Generally, instructions to the patient to return for follow-up treatment within a specific period also are noted here. If surgery or other treatment is going to be performed during the current visit, the patient must sign a consent form.

On each subsequent visit, when using a paper record, the date must be entered on the record; information about the patient's condition and the results of treatment, based on the provider's observations, must be added to the health record. Notations of all medications prescribed or instructions given, and the patient's own report of how they are doing, should be documented in the health record. If the patient is hospitalized, the name of the hospital, the reason for admission, and the dates of admission and discharge are documented. Much of this information can be obtained from the hospital discharge summary.

Condition at the Time of Termination of Treatment

When the treatment is terminated, the provider documents that information. For example: *August 18, 2016. Wound completely healed. Problem resolved.*

The Medical Assistant's Role

When the medical assistant is responsible for documenting the patient's history, care must be taken to ensure that the patient's answers are not heard by others. If privacy is not possible, the patient should be given a form to fill out, and the information should be transferred to the permanent record later. When privacy is available, the medical assistant may ask the patient questions and document the answers directly into the health record. This method offers an opportunity to become better acquainted with the patient while completing the necessary records and also ensures the patient understands what all the questions mean. If new patients must complete a lengthy questionnaire, the questionnaire may be mailed to the patient with a request that it be completed and returned to the provider before the appointment. If the record is electronic the patient may access his or her record through a **patient portal** and document the information directly into the EHR system. It would then be reviewed by the medical assistant and provider during the office visit. Another option with an EHR is for the patient to complete a paper form and the medical assistant to enter the information into the EHR while reviewing the form with the patient.

The medical assistant may document the patient's chief complaint, but the provider will question the patient in more detail. Many practitioners write their own entries on the record in longhand if a paper record is used. Some may document the findings directly into the computer if an electronic record is used. Others may dictate the material, either directly to the medical assistant or by using a recording device. If the material is dictated and transcribed, the provider should verify each entry and then initial the entry to verify its accuracy before it is entered into the patient's record. For a record to be admissible as evidence in court, the person dictating or writing the entries must be able to attest that they were true and correct at the time they were written. The best indication of this is the provider's signature or initials on the typed entry. In an EHR the provider's electronic signature is proof of the accuracy of the entries.

OWNERSHIP OF THE HEALTH RECORD

Who owns the health record? Patients often assume that because the information in the health record is about them, ownership of the record rightfully is theirs. However, the owner of the physical health record is the provider or medical facility, often called the "maker," that initiated and developed the record. The patient has the right of access to the information within the record but does not own the physical record or other documents pertaining to the record. The patient has a **vested** interest and therefore has the right to demand confidentiality of all information placed in the record.

The actual paper health record should never leave the medical facility where it originated. Even the provider should refrain from taking the record from the office to the hospital or nursing facility. If information from the record is needed, copies can be placed in a file, and progress notes can be written on site and inserted into the original record later. This is not an issue with an EHR because the record can be accessed by multiple users at the same time. Patients' paper records should be kept in a locked room or locked filing cabinets when the office is closed. EHRs must be protected from unauthorized access. Health Insurance Portability and Accountability Act (HIPAA) regulations state that each user must have a unique user name and password; individual access is determined by the system administrator.

Written health records must be legible. Each record should be written as if the provider and staff expect it to eventually be involved in a lawsuit; therefore every word must be legible to an average reader years after it is written. The record can help the provider prove that he or she treated a patient in a competent manner, or it can prove that the patient was not given competent care. Every person on staff at the provider's office is responsible for writing legibly in every health record.

EHRs eliminate the issue of legibility in the record, but it is just as important to be sure that all patient care is documented in the electronic record. If care is not documented, this will leave the healthcare facility open to potential lawsuits and can affect patient care. If services are not documented, they cannot be billed for either.

CRITICAL THINKING APPLICATION   **12-3**

On Susan's third day at work, a man comes into the office and demands to see his mother's health record. Susan accesses the record and sees that the mother has not granted permission for information to be given to her son. What should Susan do in this situation? Are there any viable reasons the son should have access to his mother's medical information?

TECHNOLOGIC TERMS IN HEALTH INFORMATION

Some confusion has arisen regarding the acronyms *EMR* and *EHR*. These acronyms have been used interchangeably for many years. To **alleviate** the confusion, the Office of the National Coordinator for Health Information Technology (ONC) has established definitions for EMR and EHR that are easy to understand. The EHR is an electronic record of health-related information about a patient that conforms to nationally recognized **interoperability** standards and that can be created, managed, and consulted by authorized clinicians and staff from *more than one healthcare organization*. The **electronic medical record (EMR)** is an electronic record of health-related information about an individual that can be created, gathered, managed, and consulted by authorized clinicians and staff *within a single healthcare organization*. An EMR is an electronic version of a paper record.

EMR is being used less and less as the federal regulations regarding electronic records have been established. There is a significant push toward having all electronic records meet the definition of an EHR. There are many advantages to having an electronic record system that can be accessed from more than one healthcare organization. The continuity of patient care is much more easily established when all providers have access to the same records regardless of what organization they are working for. There should be less running of duplicate tests and procedures, which will help reduce the cost of providing healthcare.

A **personal health record (PHR)** is defined by the ONC as an electronic record of health-related information about an individual that conforms to nationally recognized interoperability standards and that can be drawn from multiple sources, but that is managed, shared, and controlled by the individual. There are several ways that a PHR can be created. Some health insurance companies offer PHRs for those who they insure; some employers offer it as a service for their employees; and some healthcare facilities offer it to their patients. It is important to remember that the patient maintains a PHR. The information from an EHR does not automatically transfer to a PHR.

Another way for patients to access their healthcare information is through a patient portal. Patient portals allow patients to access their actual EHRs. At any time a patient can view progress notes, laboratory results, medications, or immunizations. Many patient portal systems also allow for communication between the patient and provider, completion of forms online, and ability to request prescription refills and schedule appointments. By establishing effective patient portals, healthcare facilities can meet some of the meaningful use requirements.

HIPAA uses the term *protected health information* (PHI), which is any information about health status, the provision of healthcare, or payment for healthcare that can be linked to an individual patient. HIPAA requires that all PHI be protected; this applies to EHRs, EMRs, PHRs, and patient portals.

AMERICAN RECOVERY AND REINVESTMENT ACT

The American Recovery and Reinvestment Act of 2009 (ARRA), commonly known as the Economic Stimulus Package, was passed to promote economic recovery. This legislation was signed into law by President Barack Obama on February 17, 2009. The health information technology aspects of the bill provide slightly more than $31 billion for healthcare infrastructure and EHR investment. The sections of the ARRA that pertain to healthcare are collectively known as the Health Information Technology for Economic and Clinical Health Act, or HITECH Act.

THE HEALTH INFORMATION TECHNOLOGY FOR ECONOMIC AND CLINICAL HEALTH ACT AND MEANINGFUL USE

The HITECH Act provides financial incentives for the meaningful use of certified EHR technology to achieve health and efficiency goals. It was incorporated into the ARRA to promote the adoption and meaningful use of health information technology. Remember, HIPAA was created in large part to simplify administrative processes using electronic devices. *Meaningful use,* defined simply, means that providers must show that they are using EHR technology in ways that can be measured significantly in quality and quantity. If providers meet the meaningful use requirements, they will qualify for incentive payments. Three main components of meaningful use can be identified, including:

- Use of certified EHR in a meaningful manner, such as **e-prescribing**
- Use of certified EHR technology for electronic exchange of health information to improve the quality of healthcare
- Use of certified EHR technology to submit clinical quality reports, procedure and diagnosis codes, surveys, and other measures

Criteria for meaningful use were designed to be implemented in three stages:

- Stage 1 (2011 and 2012): Electronic data capture and sharing
- Stage 2 (2014): Advanced clinical processes
- Stage 3 (expected to be implemented in 2016): Improved outcomes

In Subtitle D of the HITECH Act, privacy and security concerns related to the electronic submission of health information are addressed. Several provisions strengthen the civil and criminal penalties of the HIPAA rules, most of which became effective in February 2009. More of the provisions will become effective over the next few years, subject to future lawmaking.

Included in the February 2009 modifications of HIPAA were:

- Establishment of categories of violations that reflect increasing levels of **culpability**

TABLE 12-1 Categories of Health Insurance Portability and Accountability Act Violations and Associated Penalties		
CATEGORY: SECTION 1176(A)(1)	**EACH VIOLATION**	**ALL SUCH VIOLATIONS OF AN IDENTICAL PROVISION IN A CALENDAR YEAR**
(A) Did not know	$100 to $50,000	$1.5 million
(B) Reasonable cause	$1,000 to $50,000	$1.5 million
(C) (i) Willful neglect—corrected	$10,000 to $50,000	$1.5 million
(C) (ii) Willful neglect—not corrected	$50,000	$1.5 million

- Requirements that penalties be determined based on the nature and extent of the violation and the nature and extent of the harm resulting from the violation
- Establishment of tiers of increasing penalty amounts that determine the range of and authority to impose civil monetary penalties (Table 12-1)

As indicated in Table 12-1, minimum and maximum penalty amounts are established and can be assessed by the Department of Health and Human Services (HHS), depending on the nature of the violation. The HHS determines the penalties on a case-by-case basis and may provide or continue to provide a waiver for violations that arise from a **reasonable cause** and are not **willful neglect** incidents that are not corrected in a timely manner. The DHHS will also consider whether the covered entity has provided **reasonable diligence** in its attempts to bring the facility into compliance with the law. Providers can expect reductions in the amounts they are paid from Medicare and Medicaid if they are not in compliance. Remember, the computer system in the medical office must be more than a tool for data recall to be considered an EHR system; the provider must use the system for tasks, at a minimum, such as e-prescribing and **computerized provider/provider order entry (CPOE)**.

ADVANTAGES AND DISADVANTAGES OF THE EHR

According to a 2014 survey done by the National Ambulatory Medical Care Survey (NAMCS), 82.8% of providers in office-based practices use full or partial EMR systems. This is up from 18% in 2001.

The EHR has several advantages over a paper health record. Most experts agree that the EHR can reduce medical errors by keeping prescriptions, allergies, and other information organized; it also can reduce costs by preventing duplicate tests. Staffing needs also may be reduced, because fewer personnel are needed to manage an EHR system. Because a computer keyboard is used to enter information into the record, the record is not nearly as likely to be illegible as a written record. Typed copy certainly is easier to read than hand-writing, even if the record is several years old. EHR systems require individual user names and passwords, which secure the system from unauthorized users.

Compared with walls and file cabinets full of paper health records, the EHR requires less storage space. One or two external hard drives with a terabyte of disk space each conceivably could hold all the health records of all patients throughout the life of a provider's practice. This would eliminate the need to purge inactive files, and the resulting space requirement for the external hard drive may be no bigger than a large shoebox. The files may be duplicated regularly and placed off site as a backup. Using thumb drives as backup would meet HIPAA requirements as long as they were stored somewhere other than the healthcare facility. More facilities are using cloud storage to protect the EHR content.

Information can be accessed in a variety of locations, and more than one person can see the record at any given time. The patient database usually allows various types of statistical information to be recalled, which is a valuable tool. Patient information is available quickly in an emergency, even when the patient is not in his or her hometown. The provider and medical assistants can access progress notes, test results, and any other information about the patient, including patient education and appointment no-shows. The provider and medical assistants can access patient information using a smart phone or tablet.

Once the provider and staff become familiar with the system, they may find that they are able to see more patients in the course of a day than when paper records were used. All of these advantages lead to cost savings and more efficient patient care.

However, the EHR system is not without disadvantages. Studies show that lack of capital is the most significant obstacle to adoption of the system; another stumbling block is the reluctance of employees in providers' offices to make such substantial changes and to learn a new computer system. Employees who are not very familiar with computers may fear that they will not be able to learn the system or that an EHR may mean that they no longer will have a job. Providers may have the same fears of learning a new system and wonder about how much more time it will take them to do their job. Employees may not be the only individuals resistant to a changeover to electronic records; patients often are fearful that their private health information will be available to unauthorized individuals, and they often assume that their records will be posted on the Internet.

The startup costs of conversion to an EHR system usually are quite high, although most providers realize that the system eventually will be worth the cost. "The Financial and Nonfinancial Costs of Implementing Electronic Health Records in Primary Care Practices," an article in the online journal *Health Affairs,* suggests that the startup cost for a five-provider practice is approximately $162,000, with $85,500 going toward maintenance costs during the first year (Fleming et al., 2011). The study also suggested that the implementation team would need an average of 611 hours to prepare for the implementation, and end-users, such as the providers, medical assistants, and other staff members, would need about 134 hours of training to use the system. Both the provider and staff require extensive training in the EHR system and must be receptive to even more training to use the system to its full capacity. Training

is time-consuming and takes the provider and staff away from treating patients for certain periods. Because not all computer systems are user friendly, care must be taken to choose a system that has technologic support, both live and online, that is available during the hours the healthcare facility is operating. Space for the equipment can be an issue, although usually less space is required than for a paper record system. Finally, security and confidentiality are major concerns of both the healthcare professionals and the patients.

Reassuring Patients About the Security and Confidentiality of the Electronic Health Record

- Explain the conversion before the office changes and during the conversion.
- Never display a negative attitude about the change to an electronic health record (EHR) system; patients tend to reflect the attitude you show them.
- Prepare a pamphlet explaining the processes that will change in your particular office with use of the EHR.
- Take a moment to show the patient a little about the software once it has been implemented (using only their record). Most patients are interested in what the EHR can accomplish. Show the individual the log-in process (without revealing passwords) to reassure him or her that access to records is private and secure.
- Explain the records backup process to help alleviate patients' fears that their health information may be lost.
- Explain the office access policy regarding who can access and view patients' records.

Successful Conversion to an Electronic Health Record System

- Get the entire facility "on board" with the change.
- Provide leadership to the staff.
- Encourage and praise the staff's hard work in making the conversion successful.
- As a medical assistant, be loyal and promote loyalty to the facility during the change.
- Use good people management skills, especially with those who are against the conversion. Many people who were initially averse to conversions later say they do not know how they ever worked without the EHR.
- Always provide patients, visitors, and co-workers excellent customer service.
- Work as a team with other staff members.
- Use every employee's strengths where they are needed.
- Be willing to venture into a new system and keep a positive attitude.
- Remember that if healthcare is anything, it is constant change.

CRITICAL THINKING APPLICATION 12-4

Some of the patients who visit Dr. Adkins and Dr. Brooks have expressed concern that electronic health records (EHRs) may not be private enough and that their health information will be "floating around on the Internet." They are worried that unauthorized individuals could somehow access their information on the computer and do them harm.

- How might Susan alleviate the patients' fears about their records being available on the Internet?
- What disadvantages with regard to confidentiality are associated with the EHR?

Capabilities of Electronic Health Record Systems

The EHR system can perform a multitude of tasks, saving time and money in the provider's office (Figure 12-4). The following are some of the features of a typical EHR system.

- **Specialty software.** Patient data are captured and processed into a system that is specialty specific, so that the terminology and patient care treatments are compatible with the provider's specialty. However, additional features can allow the provider to include terminology from other specialties.
- **Appointment scheduler.** The appointment scheduler allows the staff to track and schedule appointments, matrix the schedule, and account for recurring time blocks (Figure 12-5). The appointments can be merged into specific types with default times so that lengthy procedures are not scheduled in short appointment blocks. The scheduler features also allow various search **parameters**; if a patient calls because he or she

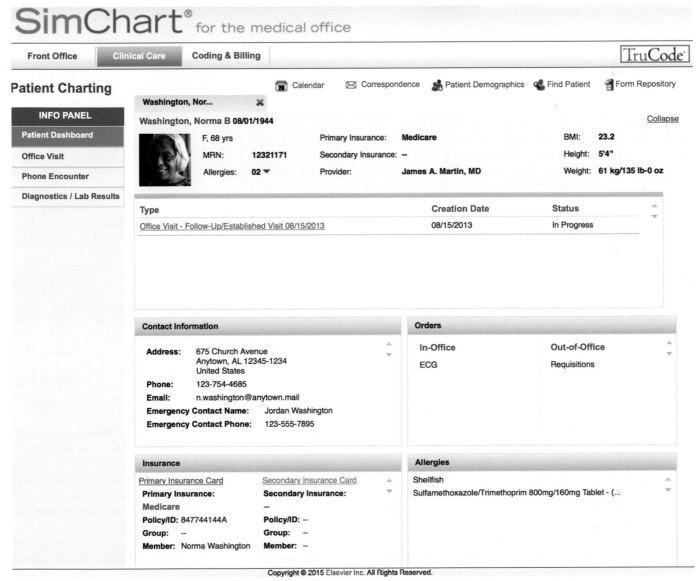

FIGURE 12-4 The electronic health record (EHR) can perform numerous tasks in addition to displaying personal information about the patient. This allows the provider and medical assistants to interact with patients and provide better service.

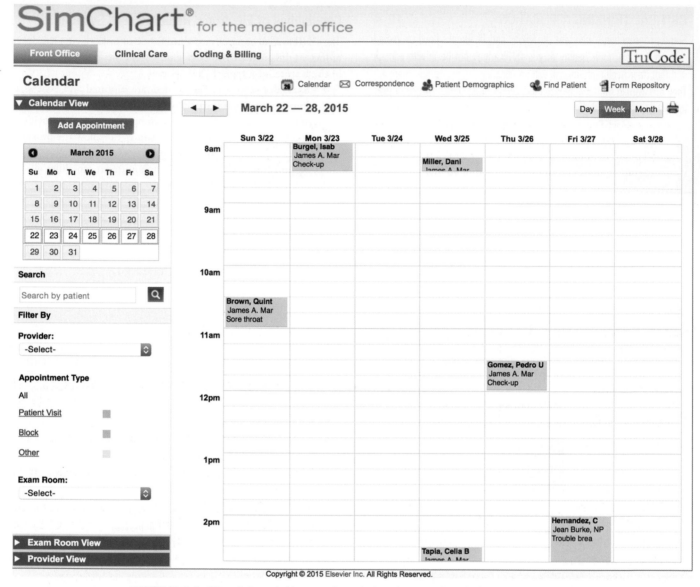

FIGURE 12-5 The EHR usually has a scheduling system that can be changed to manage the needs of the provider and office staff.

cannot remember the appointment time, a search can be initiated using the date, provider's name, patient's name, or other search keywords.

- **Appointment reminder and confirmation.** The system can be programmed to initiate automatic reminder or confirmation calls to patients. The staff can record the reminders, and patients are prompted to choose options, such as "Press one" to confirm or reschedule appointments.

- **Prescription writer.** The EHR system can produce electronic prescriptions, which can be printed and given to patients or automatically submitted to a pharmacy. Lists can be created with the provider's most common drug choices and dosages. A patient allergies function can block the prescription of drugs the patient cannot take, and the system can generate a patient information sheet on new prescriptions.

- **Medical billing system.** The EHR billing system can manage all of the practice's billing and accounting systems. The system also can interface with clearinghouses for electronic claims submission and tracking. Reports can be generated that

provide accurate details of the financial state of the practice at certain intervals or whenever requested.

- **Charge capture.** The charge capture functions can store lists of billing codes (e.g., International Classification of Diseases [ICD] and Current Procedural Terminology [CPT]) in addition to charges associated with procedures, supplies, and laboratory tests. Evaluation and Management (E/M) codes are used during office visits to obtain the highest possible reimbursement; these help the provider maximize profits while remaining in compliance with the law. Alerts can let the user know when a certain charge does not match a diagnosis code; for instance, a blood glucose done for a sore throat. In such cases, the software alerts the user and helps prevent errors that can lead to denial of insurance claims.

- **Eligibility verification.** EHR billing systems can perform online verification of insurance eligibility and can capture demographic data.

- **Referral management.** Current and referring providers can be coordinated and automated, allowing the provider to share patient information with another provider. This reduces the patient's physical effort of transporting copies of records back and forth to referring providers, eliminates the costs of such copies, and is faster and more efficient than copying and mailing patient records.

- **Laboratory order integration.** The laboratory order integration feature allows the user to interact with outside laboratories and to receive and post laboratory results to patients' records. Tests can be ordered from the provider's laptop, tablet, or smart phone. Results can be transmitted by fax, scan, or e-mail and uploaded directly into the patient's record (Procedure 12-2).

CRITICAL THINKING APPLICATION   **12-5**

Jennifer, the office manager, has noticed that Susan seems frustrated in the training classes for the EHR system used by the clinic. During a break, Jennifer asks Susan whether she is having any specific problems with the training classes. She also asks for Susan's input on the system. Susan says that she just prefers clinical work and that her typing skills are a little "rusty."

- How might Jennifer respond to Susan's comments?
- Why might this be a warning sign that Susan will not be a good match for the practice?

PROCEDURE 12-2	Organize a Patient's Health Record: Upload Documents to the Electronic Health Record

Goal: *Scan paper records and upload digital files to the EHR.*

Scenario: A new patient brings in a laboratory report and a radiology report that he would like to be added to his EHR. You need to scan in the original documents and upload them to the EHR.

EQUIPMENT and SUPPLIES

- Scanner
- Computer with SimChart for the Medical Office or EHR software
- Patient's laboratory and radiology reports

PROCEDURAL STEPS

1. Obtain the patient's name and date of birth if not on the reports.
   PURPOSE: You will need the patient's name and date of birth to find the patient's EHR.
2. Using a scanner that is connected to the computer, scan each document, creating an individual digital image for each.
   PURPOSE: The reports should be scanned separately and not combined to create one file. Each type of report must be uploaded separately to the correct location in the EHR.
3. Locate the file of the two scanned images in the computer drive. Open the files to ensure the images are clear.

PURPOSE: When scanning and uploading documents to the EHR, it is crucial that the image of the document is clear and can be easily read by the provider. If the image is blurred, rescan the document.

4. In the EHR, search for the patient, using the patient's last and first name. Verify the patient's date of birth.
   PURPOSE: Before uploading to or documenting in the EHR, it is critical to verify that the correct record is opened.
5. Locate the window to upload diagnostic/laboratory results and add a new result. Enter the date of the test. Select the correct type of result. Browse for the image file of the laboratory file and attach it. Save the information. Select the option to add a new result and repeat the steps to upload the second report. Verify that both documents were uploaded correctly.
   PURPOSE: Errors during the upload may affect the ability to see the files. Verifying at the time of the upload will help ensure providers can see the results in the future.

NONVERBAL COMMUNICATION WITH THE PATIENT WHEN USING THE ELECTRONIC HEALTH RECORD

Although many patients are covered under a type of insurance that requires them to choose a primary care provider (PCP) and to have a referral to a specialist, remember that the patient has the option of changing that PCP or specialist. The patient may decide to change providers simply because he or she does not feel comfortable with that particular provider.

Because the change process is relatively easy, the provider wants to keep his or her patients (in most cases), because losing patients means loss of income. If the care begins to seem impersonal, patients may feel a strong desire to change providers. Remember, patients are consumers of healthcare services, and they expect quality healthcare.

When using the EHR, the medical assistant must make sure his or her nonverbal communication sends the right message to the patient. Eye contact is absolutely essential (Figure 12-6). If the medical assistant constantly looks at the electronic device, the patient feels largely alienated from the information exchange process. Make eye contact with the patient while asking questions, looking at the screen only when needed to enter information. Do not insinuate by physical action that the EHR is a "hidden entity"; for example, do not necessarily shield the device from the patient's view when entering information. Although patients may not understand anything they see on the screen, they will feel more at ease if their information is not hidden from them. Also, modify your stance so that the patient feels like a part of the information process. Just as sitting in a chair

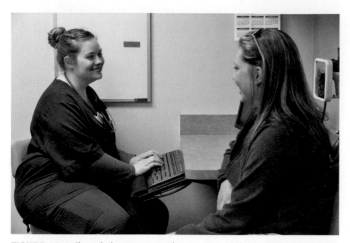

FIGURE 12-6 The medical assistant must make eye contact with the patient when using an EHR.

across from a supervisor's desk can be intimidating, the patient may feel the same emotions sitting across from a medical assistant entering information into the EHR. Take an open stance; sit next to or at an angle to the patient to support the impression that those in the healthcare facility and the patient are partners in the healthcare plan.

Remember that patients have the right to make decisions in most aspects of their healthcare plans; therefore offer choices wherever possible. Never expect patients to make quick decisions about their care. They may want to consult family members or give some thought to important medical decisions. The medical assistant needs to promote time to think unless the patient is faced with a critical, time-sensitive decision. Providers often assume that patients will automatically follow their instructions or orders; however, some patients prefer some time to think. Always follow up and make note of any wait time the patient requests, notify the provider, and enter that information into the EHR. Make sure timely communication is done with the patient and that any additional orders that need to be put in place are completed. The many features of the EHR allow the medical assistant to be efficient and highly competent if he or she is willing to make an extra effort to master the EHR system.

Also make sure patients understand all instructions given to them regarding test procedures or preparation for procedures. Most EHRs can print an instruction sheet, which the medical assistant can review with the patient. The customer service aspect of patient care is even more important when the facility uses an EHR system.

CRITICAL THINKING APPLICATION   12-6

Jennifer walks behind Susan's desk and notices that she is looking at the progress notes on a patient who was recently arrested and indicted for child abuse. The case has been in the newspaper and on television consistently for several weeks. Jennifer asks Susan why she has accessed that record. Susan hesitates and then says she must have entered the wrong patient ID number.

- Does Susan's explanation sound convincing?
- Why is Jennifer concerned about Susan looking at the patient's record?
- Just because the individual is a patient at the clinic, does that mean any employee has the right to look at the patient's EHR?

BACKUP SYSTEMS FOR THE ELECTRONIC HEALTH RECORD

Even the best or most expensive EHR system cannot function without power. If a natural disaster occurs and the provider's office is without electricity for several days or weeks, the provider must have a backup system for the EHR so that the office can function. HIPAA requires that the facility adopt a backup and recovery plan that includes daily off-site software backup for the EHR system. Several alternatives can be used for data preservation and backup.

- *External hard drive.* An external hard drive connects to the main computer, and with fairly simple programming can copy the information in the EHR daily. Seven electronic folders, one for each day of the week, can hold the information from the previous day; these folders are replaced with new, updated information at designated periods. CDs and DVDs can hold daily data, and some thumb drives have enough capacity to perform this task. Once a habit of a daily backup to the external hard drive has been established, the method is relatively simple and reliable.
- *Full server backup.* The provider may want to back up the EHR system on a dedicated server, which is a large-capacity computer set aside specifically for the EHR system. With these servers, a full backup should be performed monthly. Many large medical facilities and hospitals have one or more dedicated servers for the EHR system.
- *Online backup system.* An online backup system can be used, usually for a subscription fee. Although the cost may be higher than for some other methods, online systems are easy to use because there is no external drive to carry and no CD or thumb drive to put through the process of downloading data. However, a time investment is involved, because the process of contacting the company that offers the service and then downloading all the data takes several hours. Also, the initial download can take quite a while. Even so, an online system is very stable and reliable.

All these backup methods require an alternative power source in case of a disaster that interrupts electrical service. Remember that backup systems are not effective if the data are stored at the medical facility, and the disaster happens at or affects that physical address. Information technology professionals usually recommend using two of these three methods for the best protection. The system must be protected from theft and unauthorized use, just as is the on-site system.

Medical assistants should keep their paper health records skills sharp in case the EHR system is down for an extended period. Always have a supply of the most commonly used forms in a paper format available for alternative use in such instances. When the EHR system comes back up these paper forms can be scanned into the patients' EHRs.

Transfer, Destruction, and Retention of Electronic Health Records

In most medical offices, records are classified in three ways:

- *Active,* which are the records of patients currently receiving treatment.
- *Inactive,* which generally are the records of patients whom the provider has not seen for 6 months or longer.

- *Closed,* which are the records of patients who have died, moved away, or otherwise terminated their relationship with the provider.

The process of moving a file from active to inactive status is called **purging**. An EHR system can be set up to automatically move the inactive records to another server so that processing time will not be slowed down, but the records are still readily accessible if the patient returns to the healthcare facility. Closed EHRs are also separated from the active records and are typically stored elsewhere. They may be placed on CDs, computer hard drives, or maintained in inactive cloud space by the EHR vendor.

Retention and Destruction

Providers have an obligation to retain patient records, whether they are paper or electronic, that may reasonably be of value to a patient, according to the American Medical Association (AMA) Council on Ethical and Judicial Affairs. Currently, no nationwide standard rule exists for establishing a records **retention schedule**.

Medical considerations are the primary basis for deciding how long to retain health records. For example, operative notes and chemotherapy records should always be part of the patient's health record. The laws regarding the retention of health records vary from state to state, and many governmental programs have their own guidelines for specific records retention. When no rules specify the retention of health records, the best course is to keep the records for 10 years. However, for minors, the facility should keep the records until the minor reaches the **age of majority** plus the statute of limitations.

If a particular record no longer needs to be kept for medical reasons, the provider should check the state law for any requirement that records be kept for a minimum time (most states do not have such a provision). The time is measured from the last professional contact with the patient. In all cases, health records should be kept for at least the period of the statute of limitations for medical malpractice claims, which may be 3 years or longer, depending on state law. In the case of a minor, the statute of limitations may not apply until the patient reaches the age of majority. In summary, know the state requirements related to health records retention and follow those guidelines; the office policy manual should address records retention pertaining to the state where the practice exists.

The records of any patient covered by Medicare or Medicaid must be kept at least 10 years. The HIPAA privacy rule does not include requirements for the retention of health records. However, the privacy rule does require that appropriate administrative, technical, and physical safeguards be applied so that the privacy of health records is maintained.

Some providers refuse to destroy or discard old records. Storage is less of an issue with EHRs as they take up much less physical space. Always refer to state laws when discarding health records.

Before old records are discarded, patients should be given an opportunity to claim a copy of the records or have them sent to another provider. The medical facility should keep a master list of all records that have been destroyed. To legally destroy an EHR, the record, including the backup record, has to be overwritten using utility software.

RELEASING HEALTH RECORD INFORMATION

The healthcare facility must be extremely careful when releasing any type of medical information. The patient must sign a release for information to be given to any third party.

Requests for medical information should be made in writing (Figure 12-7). Electronic signatures may be accepted as long as they are obtained with proper process controls. HIPAA has designated that very specific information must be included on the Release of Information form, including specifically who the information is being released to, what specific information is to be released, and an expiration date for the release. Accepting a faxed request for medical information or a faxed release of information from a patient is unwise. Even requests from the patient's attorney or third-party payers must be cleared by the patient for them to obtain information.

If a provider is involved in a liability suit there will be a required exchange of information. As both parties to a lawsuit begin to prepare their cases, they enter the discovery process. Each side must disclose the pertinent facts of the case that may influence the final outcome of that case. On each occasion that information is needed from the provider, a separate request must be sent. Because this request form is signed by the patient, it serves as a release.

Most offices charge a fee to print or copy health records, whether it is a per-page charge or a per-record fee. If the records are sent electronically there is no fee charged. Follow the steps in the policy and procedures manual for the release of records. Some providers designate the office manager to handle requests for records releases.

Pay particular attention to records release requests involving a minor. In most cases, the parent or legal guardian is entitled to read through the patient's health records; however, according to the HHS, there are three situations in which the parent may not be legally entitled to review the records of his or her minor child:

- When the minor is the one who consents to care and the parent is not required to also consent to care under state law
- When the minor obtains medical care at the direction of a court or a person authorized by the court
- When the minor, parent, and provider all agree that the doctor and minor patient can have a private, confidential relationship

If the provider believes that the minor might be in an abuse situation or that the parent or legal guardian may be harming the patient, the provider is required, both legally and ethically, to report the abuse.

Sometimes patients want to look at their own records. They certainly have a right to see this information, but some patients may not understand the terminology used in the record. A staff member should always remain with a patient who is looking at his or her health record. Remember, the original health record should never leave the medical facility. Always follow office policy when releasing health records.

When a release is presented to the office, copy only the records requested in the release. Do not provide additional information that is not requested. The patient must specify that substance abuse, mental health, and/or human immunodeficiency virus (HIV) records are to be released. Remember that the patient ultimately decides

Central Texas Dermatology Clinic • 102 Westlake Drive • Austin, Texas 78746

AUTHORIZATION TO DISCLOSE HEALTH INFORMATION

I hereby authorize the use or disclosure of information from the medical record of:

Patient Name: _____   Date of Birth: _____

Social Security# _____   Daytime Phone: _____

I authorize the following individual or organization to disclose the above named individual's health information:

_____   Address: _____

This information may be disclosed TO and used by the following individual or organization:

_____   Address: _____

Please release the following:

____ Progress Notes   ____ Pathology Reports   ____ Lab Reports   ____ Any and all Records

____ Other Diagnostic reports (specify _____

____ Other (specify) _____

Including Information (if applicable) pertaining to:

____ Mental Health   ____ Drug/Alcohol   ____ HIV/AIDS   ____ Communicable Treatment

Purpose or Need for Disclosure:

____ Continued Patient Care   ____ Personal Use

____ Attorney/Legal   ____ Insurance Claim/Application

____ Disability Determination   ____ Other(specify) _____

I understand that the information in my health record may include information relating to sexually transmitted disease, acquired immunodeficiency syndrome (AIDS), or human immunodeficiency virus (HIV). It may also include information about behavioral or mental health services, and treatment for alcohol and drug abuse.

I understand that the information released is for the specific purpose stated above. Any other use of this information without the written consent of the patient is prohibited.

I understand that I have the right to revoke this authorization at any time. I understand that if I revoke this authorization I must do so in writing and present my written revocation to the individual or organization releasing information. I understand that the revocation will not apply to information already released in response to this authorization. I understand that the revocation will not apply to my insurance company when the law provides my insurer the right to contest a claim under my policy. Unless otherwise revoked, this authorization will expire on following date, event or condition: _____

If I fail to specify an expiration date, event or condition, this authorization will expire in six months.

I understand that authorizing the disclosure of this health information is voluntary. I can refuse to sign the authorization. I need not sign this form in order to ensure treatment. I understand that I may inspect or copy the information to be used or disclosed, as provided in CFR 164.524. I understand that any disclosure of information carries with it the potential for an unauthorized re-disclosure and the information may not be protected by federal confidentiality rules. If I have questions about disclosure of my health information, I can contact Theresa Farren at 512-327-7779.

_____   _____
Signature of Patient or Legal Representative   Date

_____   _____
Relationship to Patient (If Legal Representative)   Witness

COMPLETE ONLY IF INFORMATION IS TO BE RELEASED DIRECTLY TO PATIENT:

I understand that my medical record may contain reports, test results, and notes that only a physician can interpret. I understand and have been advised that I should contact my physician regarding the entries made in my medical record to prevent my misunderstanding of the information contained in these entries. I will not hold Central Texas Dermatology liable for any misinterpretation of the information in my medical record as a result of not contacting my physician for the correct interpretation.

_____   _____
Signature of Patient or Legal Representative   Date

_____   _____
Relationship to Patient (If Legal Representative)   Witness

Dr. review/signature/date _____

Date request completed _____   # of pages copied _____

Staff Signature _____

PHI Log completed _____

FIGURE 12-7 Authorization to release health records: All requests for health records should be made in writing, and the request should be kept in the patient's record.

whether a record can be released. If any question arises about what is to be released, consult the office manager or the provider.

Health Information Exchanges

The demand for electronic health information exchange (HIE) from one healthcare facility to another, together with nationwide efforts to improve the efficiency and quality of healthcare, is creating a demand for HIEs. As more and more providers move to EHRs it only makes sense to have a system in place that will facilitate the exchange of that information electronically to improve the timeliness of that exchange. Patient care can be improved because all providers will have access to the information needed to treat the patient.

The ONC states, "There are currently three forms of HIE:
- Directed Exchange—ability to send and receive secure information electronically between care providers to support coordinated care
- Query-Based Exchange—ability for providers to find and/or request information on a patient from other providers, often used for unplanned care
- Consumer-Mediated Exchange—ability for patient to aggregate and control the use of their health information among providers"

The implementation of HIE varies from state to state. There is some federal funding for the implementation of HIE that is being administered by the ONC.

CREATING AN EFFICIENT PAPER HEALTH RECORDS MANAGEMENT SYSTEM

The paper health records management system should provide an easy method of retrieving information. The files should be organized in an orderly fashion, the information must be documented accurately, and corrections should be made and documented properly. The wording in the record should be easily understood and grammatically correct. An efficient method of adding documents to the record must be established so that the provider always has the most up-to-date information.

Above all, the health records management system must work for the individual facility.

Organization of the Health Record

Source-Oriented Medical Records

The traditional patient record is a source-oriented medical record (SOMR); that is, observations and data are cataloged according to their source—provider (progress notes), laboratory, radiology, hospital, or consultant. Forms and progress notes are filed in **reverse chronologic order** (i.e., most recent on top) and in separate sections of the record according to the type of form or service rendered (e.g., all laboratory reports together, all x-ray reports together, and so on). Reverse chronologic order is used so that the provider and staff members do not have to search to the bottom of the record to find a recent laboratory report or a test.

Problem-Oriented Medical Records

The problem-oriented medical record (POMR) is a departure from the traditional system of keeping patient records. The POMR is a

record of clinical practice that divides medical action into four categories:
- The *database,* which includes the chief complaint, present illness, patient profile, review of systems, physical examination, and laboratory reports.
- The *problem list,* a numbered, titled list of every problem the patient has that requires management or workup. This may include social and demographic troubles in addition to strictly medical or surgical ones.
- The *treatment plan* includes management, additional workups needed, and therapy. Each plan is titled and numbered with respect to the problem.
- The *progress notes* include structured notes that are numbered to correspond with each problem number.

Several companies have developed file folders for organizing patient data according to the POMR. The problem list (Figure 12-8) is placed at the front of the record. Special sections are provided for current major and chronic diagnoses/health problems and for inactive major or chronic diagnosis/health problems. Progress notes usually follow the SOAP approach. SOAP is an acronym for the following:
- *S*ubjective impressions or patient reports
- *O*bjective clinical evidence or observations
- *A*ssessment or diagnosis
- *P*lans for further studies, treatment, or management

Some medical offices also use an *E* in the record to represent evaluation; others include *E* for education and *R* for response. The education notation shows that the patient was educated about his or her condition or given a patient information sheet. The response section is used to record an assessment of the patient's understanding of and possible compliance with the treatment plan.

The POMR has the advantage of imposing order and organization on the information added to a patient's health record. The records are more easily reviewed, and the likelihood of overlooking a problem is greatly reduced. The SOAP method forces a rational approach to the patient's problems and assists the formulation of a logical, orderly plan of patient care (Figure 12-9). The POMR is especially advantageous in clinics, group practices, and hospitals, where more than one person must be able to find essential information in the record.

DOCUMENTING IN AN ELECTRONIC HEALTH RECORD

Documentation in an EHR involves using radio buttons, drop-down menus, and free-text boxes. The radio buttons and drop-down menus allow for standardization of the content in the EHR and the free-text boxes allow for the documentation of the unique circumstance found with each patient (Figure 12-10). It is important to carefully review the choices made with the radio buttons and drop-down menus. Information documented using the free-text boxes should be proofread before submitting.

DOCUMENTING IN A PAPER HEALTH RECORD

When documenting in a paper health record the entry will always start with the date in the MM/DD/YYYY format. The date will be followed by the time. This may be written in standard or military

MASTER PROBLEM LIST

For use of this form, see AR 40-66; the proponent agency is the Office of The Surgeon General

MAJOR PROBLEMS

PROBLEM NUMBER	DATE ONSET	DATE ENTERED	PROBLEM	DATE RESOLVED
1.				
2.				
3.				
4.				
5.				
6.				
7.				
8.				
9.				
10.				
11.				
12.				

TEMPORARY (MINOR) PROBLEMS

PROBLEM LETTER	PROBLEM	DATES OF OCCURRENCES					
A.							
B.							
C.							
D.							
E.							
F.							
G.							
H.							

PATIENT'S IDENTIFICATION (Use mechanical imprint if available; for typed or written entries give: Name, SSN, Unit, Sex, Birthdate, and Duty Phone)

SUMMARY OF PROBLEMS, ALLERGIES, MEDICATIONS, SURGERIES AND TRAUMAS:

NOTE: DO NOT DISCARD FROM CHART

FIGURE 12-8 A problem list designed for a problem-oriented health record (POMR).

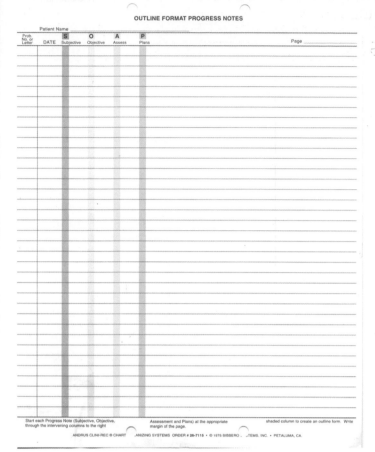

FIGURE 12-9 SOAP progress notes: The SOAP method keeps information organized and in a logical sequence. An actual progress note would include the provider's or medical assistant's signature or initials after this entry. (Courtesy Bibbero Systems, Petaluma, California.)

time. If standard time is used it must be followed by AM or PM (e.g., 2:00 PM). If military time is used it is in a four-digit format without a colon (e.g., 1400). All entries must be written in black or blue ink following the format designated by the healthcare facility. Documentation should be in the order in which the steps were completed. If temperature, pulse, and respiration (TPR) measurement is done it would be documented in the "O" or Objective section of the SOAP note starting with temperature, then pulse, and lastly respirations.

MAKING CORRECTIONS AND ALTERATIONS TO HEALTH RECORDS

Corrections sometimes must be made to health records. The first step is to verify the proper procedure for making corrections in the facility's policy and procedures manual. Some providers prefer a specific method for correcting errors in the health record. Erasing, using correction fluid, or any other type of **obliteration** is never acceptable. To correct a handwritten entry:

1. Draw a line through the error.
2. Insert the correction above or immediately after the error in a spot where it can be read clearly.
3. If indicated by the policy and procedures manual, write "Error" or "Err." in the margin.

4. The person making the correction should write his or her initials or signature below the correction and the date. Follow the format indicated in the policy and procedures manual (Figure 12-11).

Errors made while using the computer are corrected in the usual way. However, an error discovered in an entry at a later date is corrected in the same manner as for a handwritten entry. This is sometimes called an *addendum*. Never attempt to alter health records without using this specific correction procedure, because this alteration of records may indicate a fraudulent attempt to cover up a mistake made by a staff member or the provider. Do not hide errors. If the error could in any way affect the patient's health and well-being, it must be brought to the provider's attention immediately. An EHR system will track the changes made within the record.

DICTATION AND TRANSCRIPTION

With the increased use of EHRs and voice recognition software, there is decreased need for **transcription**. If **dictation** is still done in the healthcare facility the administrative medical assistant may find that transcribing the dictation is a job they perform periodically. Transcription can be done from handwritten notes, or more likely from machine dictation. Smooth operation of the facility may depend on the timely, accurate performance of assigned responsibilities, such as record documentation and preparation of special reports. Accuracy and speed are primary **requisites,** as is a strong grasp of medical terminology and principles, especially anatomy and physiology.

Dictation may be done using a machine transcription unit or a portable transcription unit. Many healthcare facilities now use a system that is accessed by telephone; the provider calls the system using passwords or access codes and records the information for the health record while speaking into the telephone. Later, employees transcribe the information into the health record. The provider must acknowledge and initial all transcription before it is placed in the health record.

Voice Recognition Software

Some healthcare facilities use voice recognition software for transcription. When first installed, the software requires the user to say several sentences into the unit so that it "learns" to recognize the user's voice. The system can be used to dictate progress notes, letters, e-mails, and virtually any document in the healthcare facility that needs to be created. These documents will need to be approved by the provider before they are permanently attached to the patient's record. Some systems have an authentication component that allows a type of electronic signature, such as those needed for hospital record dictation.

Transfer, Destruction, and Retention of Paper Health Records

As with EHRs, paper health records are also classified as active, inactive, and closed. A paper record system must have a system established for regular transfer of files from active to inactive status or possibly destruction. The expansion of records and the file space available can influence the transfer period. Records for patients currently hospitalized may be kept in a special section for quick

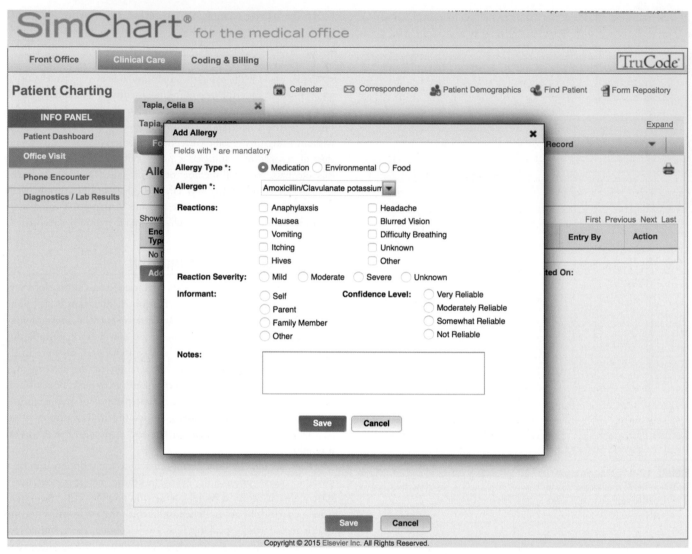

FIGURE 12-10 Documentation in an EHR is done using radio buttons, drop-down menus, and free-text boxes.

| 10/15/XXXX | 9:30 a.m. Tubersol Mantoux test: 0 mm induration. | 12   error 10/15/XXXX D. Bennett, CMA (AAMA) |
| | | D. Bennett, CMA (AAMA) |

FIGURE 12-11 Corrections to health records must be done in a legible manner and must be clearly understood. Always initial and date corrections to health records. (From Bonewit-West K: *Today's medical assistant,* ed 2, St. Louis, Saunders, 2013.)

reference and then placed in the regular active file when the patient is discharged from the hospital. In a surgical practice, the record frequently includes the specific date on which the patient is discharged from the provider's care, and the notation is made on the record, "Return prn" (from the Latin *pro re nata,* "as the occasion arises" or "when needed"). This record may safely be placed in the inactive file.

Most medical facilities use a year sticker on the file folder that indicates the last year the patient visited the clinic. If the file has a sticker showing that the patient's last visit was in 2014, and he or she presents to the clinic on January 5, 2016, a *2016* sticker should be placed over the one that indicates *2014.* These stickers often are

included with color-coded filing systems. The medical assistant can easily look at a group of files and see which ones need to be changed to inactive or closed status.

Retention and Destruction

Retention and destruction guidelines are the same for paper health records as for EHRs.

Long-Term Storage

Large healthcare facilities may find it advisable to convert their paper health records to **microfilm** for storage if the facility has not yet begun to scan documents into an EHR. If documents are stored electronically, they must be regularly backed up for storage. Another option is the transfer of paper records onto optical disks. Microfilm and optical disk technology are both expensive and probably are not practical for any but a very large group practice or health maintenance organization, so the facility should be moving toward some form of electronic storage. Using that method, health records can be kept indefinitely.

CRITICAL THINKING APPLICATION   **12-7**

Susan learned about SOAP documentation in school and is eager to use it in her new job. Dr. Thomas is seeing a patient that reports to Susan that she has had nausea and vomiting for the past 3 days. Susan obtains a weight of 132.5 pounds, temperature (T): 101.2° F tympanically, pulse (P): 94 beats/min, respiration (R): 14 breaths/min, and blood pressure (BP) 122/84 mm Hg in the right arm. What information would be documented in the Subjective field? What information would be documented in the Objective field? Who would document information in the Assessment field?

FILING EQUIPMENT

The vertical, four-drawer steel filing cabinet, used with manila folders with the patient's name on the tab, was the traditional system of choice for years. The most popular system today is color-coding on open horizontal shelves. Rotary, lateral, compactable, and automated files also are available. Some records are kept in card or tray files. Some factors that should be considered when selecting filing equipment are:

- Office space availability
- Structural considerations
- Cost of space and equipment
- Size, type, and volume of records
- Confidentiality requirements
- Retrieval speed
- Fire protection
- Cost

Drawer Files

Drawer files should be full suspension; they should roll easily, close securely, and be equipped with a locking device. The best cabinets have a center trough at the bottom of each drawer with a rod for holding divider guides. A drawback of the vertical four-drawer files is that only one person can use a file cabinet at a time. Filing also is slower, because the drawer must be opened and closed each time a file is pulled or filed.

File cabinets are heavy and can tip over, causing serious damage or injury unless reasonable care is taken. Open only one file drawer at a time, and close it when the filing has been completed. A drawer left even slightly open can injure a passerby.

Horizontal Shelf Files

Shelf files should have doors that lock to protect the contents. A popular type of shelf file has doors that slide back into the cabinet; the door from a lower shelf may be pulled out and used for work space. Open shelf units hold files sideways and can go higher on the

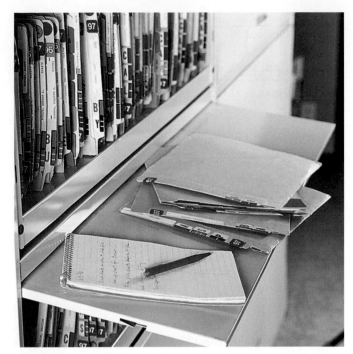

FIGURE 12-12 Open shelf filing is an efficient method, especially for color-coded filing systems. The shelf doors often can be used as workspace.

wall because no drawers need to be pulled out (Figure 12-12). File retrieval is faster, because several individuals can work simultaneously.

Rotary Circular Files

Rotary circular files can hold a large volume of records. They save space and clerical motion. The files revolve easily; some have push-button controls. Several people can work at one rotary file and use records at the same time. One disadvantage is that they afford less privacy and protection than files that can be closed and locked.

Compactable Files

An office with little space and a great volume of records might use compactable files, which are a variation of open shelf files. The files are mounted on tracks in the floor, and the units slide along the tracks so that access is gained to the needed records. One drawback is that not all records are available at the same time.

Automated Files

Automated files are very expensive initially and require more maintenance than other types of filing equipment. They are likely to be found only in very large facilities, such as clinics or hospitals. These files bring the record to the operator instead of the operator going to the record. When the operator presses a button indicating the appropriate shelf, the shelf automatically moves into position in front of the operator for record retrieval. The automated or power file is fast and can store large numbers of records in a small amount of space. However, only one person can use the unit at one time.

Card Files

Almost every office has some occasion to use a card file. This may be for patient ledgers, a patient index, a library index, an index of surgical tray setups, telephone numbers, or numerous other records. A good-quality steel box or tray is a sound investment.

FILING SUPPLIES

Divider Guides

Each file drawer or shelf should be equipped with plenty of dividers or guides. Some authorities recommend one guide for approximately each 1½″ of material, or every eight to 10 folders. Guides should be of good-quality **pressboard** or strong plastic. Less-well-constructed guides soon become bent and frayed and have to be replaced. Divider guides have a protruding tab, which may be an integral part of the card or may be made of metal or plastic. The guides reduce the area of search and serve as supports for the folders. They are available in single, third, or fifth cut (i.e., one, three, or five different positions).

Outguides

Outguides are made of heavyweight cardboard or plastic and are used to replace a folder that has been removed temporarily (Figure 12-13). They may also have a large pocket to hold any filing that may come in while the folder is out. They should be of a distinctive color for quick detection. This makes refiling simpler and alerts the file clerk that a file is missing. Several colors may be used, each color designating the temporary location of the file. The outguide may have lines for recording information, or it may have a plastic pocket for inserting an information card.

File Folders

Most records to be filed are placed in covers or tabbed folders. The most commonly used is a general purpose, third-cut manila folder that may be expanded to ¾″. These are available with a double-thickness, reinforced tab, which greatly extends the life of the folder. Folders kept in drawers have tabs at the top; those kept on shelves have tabs at the side. Many folder styles are available for special purposes.

The vertical pocket, which is of heavier weight than the general purpose folder, has a front that folds down for easy access to contents and is available with up to a 3½″ expansion. These are used for bulky histories or correspondence.

Hanging, or suspension, folders are made of heavy stock and hang on metal rods from side to side in a drawer. They can be used only with files equipped with suspension equipment.

Binder folders have fasteners that are used to bind papers in the folder. These offer some security for the papers, but filing the materials is time-consuming.

The number of papers that will fit in one folder depends on the thickness of the papers and the capacity of the folder. Near the bottom edge of most folders are one or more score marks, which should be used as the contents of the folders expand. Papers should never protrude from the folder edges, and they should always be inserted with their tops to the left. When papers start to ride up in any folder, the folder is overloaded.

Labels

The label is a necessary filing and finding device. Use labels to identify each shelf, drawer, divider guide, and folder. A label on the drawer or shelf identifies the nature of its contents. It should also indicate the range (i.e., alphabetic, numeric, or chronologic) of the material filed in that space.

The label on the divider guide identifies the range of folder headings following that divider guide up to the next divider (e.g., BaBo).

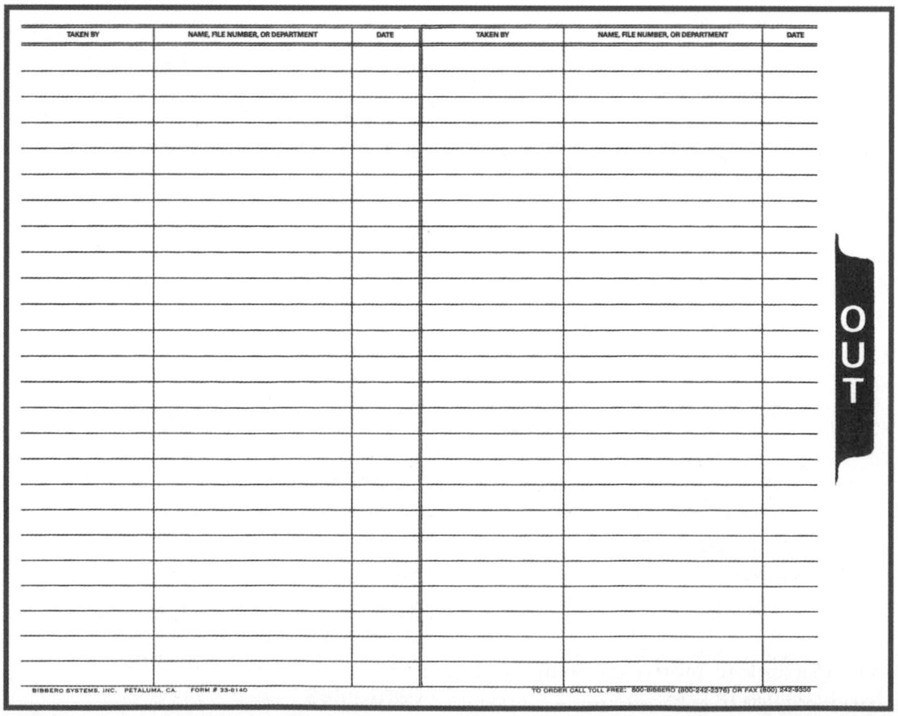

TAKEN BY	NAME, FILE NUMBER, OR DEPARTMENT	DATE	TAKEN BY	NAME, FILE NUMBER, OR DEPARTMENT	DATE

BIBBERO SYSTEMS, INC. PETALUMA, CA FORM # 33-8140

TO ORDER CALL TOLL FREE: 800-BIBBERO (800-242-2376) OR FAX (800) 242-9330

OUT

FIGURE 12-13 Outguides allow tracking of a file not in its proper location by providing information on the location of the file. (Courtesy Bibbero Systems, Petaluma, California.)

The label on the folder identifies the contents of that folder only. This may be the name of the patient, subject matter of correspondence, a business topic, or anything at all that needs to be filed. Label a folder when a new patient is seen, existing folders are full, or materials need to be transferred within the filing system.

Labels are available in almost any size, shape, or color to meet the individual needs of any facility. Visit an office supply Web site and review the catalogs to find the best product to meet the needs of the facility.

A narrow label applied to the front of the folder tab is the easiest to use and satisfactory for folders kept in a drawer file. Labels for shelf filing should be identifiable from both front and back. Always type the label before separating it from the roll or protective sheet. Type the **caption** on the label in indexing order (Procedure 12-3).

Indexing Rules

Indexing rules (Table 12-2) are standardized and based on current business practices. The Association of Records Managers and Administrators takes an active part in updating these rules. Some establishments adopt variations of these basic rules to accommodate their needs. In any case, the practices need to be consistent within the system.

1. Last names are considered first in filing; then the given name (first name), second; and the middle name or initial, third. Compare the names beginning with the first letter of the name. When a letter is different in the two names, that letter determines the order of filing.
2. Initials precede a name beginning with the same letter. This illustrates the librarian's rule, "Nothing comes before something."
3. With hyphenated personal names, the hyphenated elements, whether first name, middle name, or surname, are considered to be one unit.
4. The apostrophe is disregarded in filing.
5. When indexing a foreign name in which you cannot distinguish between the first and last names, index each part of the name in the order in which it is written. If you can make the distinction, use the last name as the first indexing unit.
6. Names with prefixes are filed in the usual alphabetic order, with the prefix considered part of the name.

TABLE 12-2   Applying Indexing Rules

INDEXING RULE	NAME	UNIT 1	UNIT 2	UNIT 3
1	Robert F. Grinch	Grinch	Robert	F.
	R. Frank Grumman	Grumman	R.	Frank
2	J. Orville Smith	Smith	J.	Orville
	Jason O. Smith	Smith	Jason	O.
3	M. L. Saint-Vickery	Saint-Vickery	M.	L.
	Marie-Louise Taylor	Taylor	Marielouise	
4	Charles S. Anderson	Anderson	Charles	S.
	Anderson's Surgical Supply	Andersons	Surgical	Supply
5	Ah Hop Akee	Akee	Ah	Hop
6	Alice Delaney	Delaney	Alice	
	Chester K. DeLong	Delong	Chester	K.
7	Michael St. John	Stjohn	Michael	
8	Helen M. Maag	Maag	Helen	M.
	Frederick Mabry	Mabry	Frederick	
	James E. MacDonald	Macdonald	James	E.
9	Mrs. John L. Doe (Mary Jones)	Doe	Mary	Jones (Mrs. John L.)
10	Prof. John J. Breck	Breck	John	J. (Prof.)
	Madame Sylvia	Madame	Sylvia	
	Sister Mary Catherine	Sister	Mary	Catherine
	Theodore Wilson, MD	Wilson	Theodore (MD)	
11	Lawrence W. Jones, Jr.	Jones	Lawrence	W. (Jr.)
	Lawrence W. Jones, Sr.	Jones	Lawrence	W. (Sr.)
12	The Moore Clinic	Moore	Clinic (The)	

7. Abbreviated parts of a name are indexed as written if that form generally is used by that person.
8. Mac and Mc are filed in their regular place in the alphabet. If the files have a great many names beginning with Mac or Mc, some offices file them as a separate letter of the alphabet for convenience.
9. The name of a married woman, who has taken her husband's last name, is indexed by her legal name (her husband's surname, her given name, and her middle name or maiden surname). There should be a cross-reference, such as an outguide placed where her maiden name falls directing you to her new name.
10. When followed by a complete name, titles may be used as the last filing unit if needed to distinguish the name from another, identical name. Titles without complete names are considered the first indexing unit.
11. Terms of seniority or professional or academic degrees are used only to distinguish the name from an identical name.
12. Articles (e.g., the, a) are disregarded in indexing.

PROCEDURE 12-3   Create and Organize a Patient's Paper Health Record

Goal: *Create a paper health record for a new patient. Organize health record documents in a paper health record.*

EQUIPMENT and SUPPLIES

- End tab file folder
- Completed patient registration form
- Divider sheets with different color labels (4)
- Progress note sheet (1)
- Name label
- Color-coding labels (first two letters of last name and first letter of first name)
- Year label
- Allergy label
- Black pen or computer with word processing software to process labels
- Health record documents (i.e., prior records, laboratory reports)
- Hole puncher

PROCEDURAL STEPS

1. Obtain the patient's first and last name.
   PURPOSE: To customize the record for the patient, the first and last name will be required.
2. Neatly write or word process the patient's name on the name label. Left-justify the last name, followed by a comma, the first name, middle initial and a period (e.g., Smith, Mary J.).
   PURPOSE: The label should be easy to read. The last name always comes before the first name.
3. Adhere the name label to the bottom left side of the record tab. When the record is held by the main fold in your left hand, the writing should be easy to read. (For directional purposes, assume the record main fold is on the left and the tab is at the bottom.)
4. Put the color-coding labels on the bottom right edge of the folder. Start by placing the first letter of the last name at the farthest right edge. Working left, place the second letter of the last name, then the first letter of the first name, and lastly the year label. The year label should be close to the name label.
   PURPOSE: When the folders are in the file cabinet, the folders are sorted by the colored labels, starting with the top label (first letter of the last name), followed by the second and remaining labels.

5. Place the allergy label on the front of the record. If allergies are known, clearly write the allergy on the label in red ink.
6. Place the divider labels on the record divider sheets, if they come separately. Ensure the labels on the divider sheets are staggered so they do not overlap. Print the name of the section on the front and back of the label. The print should be easy to read when the record is held by the main fold. (Suggested names for dividers: Progress Notes, Laboratory, Correspondence, and Miscellaneous.)
   PURPOSE: Placing divider labels on the divider sheets in a staggered pattern allows the provider to easily see all sections of the health record.
7. Using the prongs on the left-hand side of the record, secure the registration form.
   PURPOSE: The registration form should be in an easy-to-find location in the record.
8. Using the prongs on the right-hand side of the record, secure the index dividers with a progress note sheet under the progress note tab.
   PURPOSE: The provider will need the progress note sheet to document data regarding the visit.

Scenario: The patient authorized his/her prior provider to send health records to your agency. You need to organize these records within the paper health record.

9. Verify the name and the date of birth on the health records and ensure they match the information on the health record.
   PURPOSE: Before organizing and filing documents in a patient's health record, it is critical to ensure the health record is for the correct patient.
10. Open the prongs on the right side of the record and carefully remove the record to the point of where the documents need to be inserted. For the documents being inserted, punch holes in the proper location. Insert the papers into the record and then reassemble the remaining part of the record. Continue to do this until all the documents are filed within the health record.
    PURPOSE: Documents need to be placed in the correct location in the record so the provider can easily find information.

FILING METHODS

The three basic filing methods used in healthcare facilities are:
- Alphabetic by name
- Numeric
- Subject

Patients' records are filed either alphabetically by name or by one of several numeric methods. Subject filing is used for business records, correspondence, and topical materials.

Alphabetic Filing

Alphabetic filing by name is the oldest, simplest, and most commonly used system. It is the system of choice for filing patients' records in most small providers' offices.

The alphabetic system of filing is traditional and simple to set up, requiring only a file cabinet or shelf, folders, and some divider guides (Procedure 12-4). It is a **direct filing system** in that the person filing needs to know only the name to find the desired file. Alphabetic filing does have some drawbacks:
- The correct spelling of the name must be known.
- As the number of files increases, more space is needed for each section of the alphabet. This results in periodic shifting of folders to allow for expansion.
- As the files expand, more time is required for filing or retrieving each folder because of the greater number of folders involved in the search. The time can be greatly reduced by color-coding.

Numeric Filing

Some form of **numeric filing** combined with color and shelf filing is used by practically every large clinic or hospital. Management consultants differ in their recommendations; some recommend numeric filing only if more than 5,000 to 10,000 records are involved. Others recommend nothing but numeric filing. Numeric filing is an **indirect filing system**, or one that requires use of an alphabetic cross-reference to find a given file. Some object to this added step and overlook the advantages of numeric filing, which are:
- It allows unlimited expansion without periodic shifting of folders, and shelves usually are filled evenly.
- It provides additional confidentiality to the record.
- It saves time in retrieving and filing records quickly. One knows immediately that the number 978 falls between 977 and 979. By contrast, an alphabetic system, even with color-coding, requires a longer search for the exact spot.

Several types of numeric filing systems can be used. In the straight, or consecutive, numeric system, patients are given consecutive numbers as they first start using the practice. This is the simplest numeric system and works well for files of up to 10,000 records. It is time-consuming, and the chance for error is greater, when documents with five or more digits are filed. Filing activity is greatest at the end of the numeric series.

In the terminal digit system, patients also are assigned consecutive numbers, but the digits in the number usually are separated into groups of twos or threes and are read in groups from right to left instead of from left to right. The records are filed backward in groups. For example, all files ending in 00 are grouped together first, then those ending in 01, and so on. Next the files are grouped by their middle digits so that the 00 22s come before the 01 22s. Finally, the files are arranged by their first digits, so that 01 00 22 precedes 02 00 22.

Middle-digit filing begins with the middle digits, followed by the first digit, and finally by the terminal digits. Numeric filing requires more training, but once the system has been mastered, fewer errors occur than with alphabetic filing.

CRITICAL THINKING APPLICATION **12-8**

Susan is unsure whether alphabetic or numeric filing is best in the healthcare facility. What are some advantages and disadvantages of each method?

PROCEDURE 12-4 File Patient Health Records

Goal: *File patient health records using two different filing systems: the alphabetic system and the numeric system.*

Scenario: The agency utilizes the alphabetic system. You need to file health records in the correct location.

EQUIPMENT and SUPPLIES

- Paper health records using the alphabetic filing system
- Paper health records using the numeric filing system
- File box(es) or file cabinet

PROCEDURAL STEPS

1. Using alphabetic guidelines, place the records to be filed in alphabetic order.
   PURPOSE: Placing the records in alphabetic order before filing in the box or cabinet will make the filing process more efficient.

2. Using the file box or file cabinet, locate the correct spot for the first file.

3. Place the health record in the correct location. Continue these filing steps until all the health records are filed.

4. Using numeric guidelines, place the records to be filed in numeric order.
   PURPOSE: Placing the records in numeric order before filing in the box or cabinet will make the filing process more efficient.

5. Using the file box or file cabinet, locate the correct spot for the first file.

6. Place the health record in the correct location. Continue these filing steps until all the health records are filed.

Subject Filing

Subject filing can be either alphabetic or **alphanumeric** (e.g., A 1-3, B 1-1, B 1-2, and so on) and is used for general correspondence. The main difficulty with subject filing is indexing, or classifying; that is, deciding where to file a document. Many papers require cross-referencing. An example would be if you had a subject folder for Laboratory Supplies and the same organization provides you with your General Medical Supplies; there should be a notation in the Laboratory Supplies folder stating to See Also General Medical Supplies and vice versa. All correspondence dealing with a particular subject is filed together. The papers in the folders are filed chronologically with the most recent on top. The subject headings are placed on the tabs of the folders and filed alphabetically.

Color-Coding

When a color-coding system is used, both filing and finding files is easier, and misfiling of folders is kept to a minimum. The use of color visually restricts the area of search for a specific record. A misfiled record is easily spotted even from a distance of several feet. In color-coding, a specific color is selected to identify each letter of the alphabet. Any selection of colors may be used, and the division of the alphabet is determined by one's own needs. However, studies have shown that the frequency with which different letters occur varies widely.

Alphabetic Color-Coding

As medicine continues to consolidate into larger facilities with more patients in one system, the filing of patients' records becomes more complicated, and color-coding becomes more useful. Several color-coding systems use two sets of 13 colors: one set for letters A to M, and a second set of the same colors on a different background for letters N to Z.

Many ready-made systems are available for use. Self-adhesive, colored letter blocks with either two or three letters in the specific colors are supplied in rolls. The color blocks with the appropriate letter are placed on the index tab of the folder, along with the patient's full name. The letters are in pairs so that they can be seen from either side of the record. Strong, easily differentiated colors are used, creating a band of color in the files that makes spotting out-of-place folders easy (Figure 12-14).

Numeric Color-Coding

Color-coding is also used in numeric filing. Numbers 0 through 9 are each assigned a different color. In a terminal digit filing system, the colors for the last two numbers are affixed to the tab. If the number 1 is red and 5 is yellow, all files with numbers ending in 15 have a red and yellow band. Usually a predetermined section of the number is color-coded.

Other Color-Coding Applications

Color can work in many other ways for the efficient healthcare facility. Small tabs in a variety of colors can be used to identify certain types of insured patients and other specific information. For example, a red tab over the edge of the folder may identify a patient on Medicare; a blue tab may identify a Medicaid patient; a green tab may identify a workers' compensation patient; matching tabs may be attached to the insured's ledger card; research cases may be identified

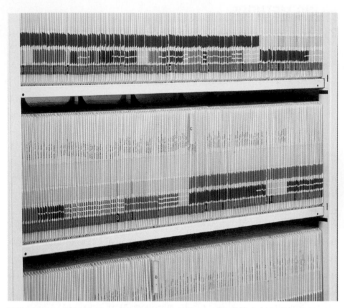

FIGURE 12-14 With color-coding of patients' records, a misplaced file is easily spotted. (Courtesy Bibbero Systems, Petaluma, California.)

by a special color tab; and brightly colored labels on the outside of a patient's record can indicate certain health conditions, such as drug allergies. In a partnership practice, a different color folder or label may identify each provider's patients. Color also can be used to differentiate dates: one color for each month or year.

The use of color in filing is limited only by the imagination. One word of caution: Every person in the facility who uses the files must know the key to the coding, and the key should also be written in the facility's policy and procedures manual.

ORGANIZATION OF FILES

Providers find studying a disorganized patient record very difficult. Some systematic method must be followed in placing items in the patient folder. From the filing standpoint, it should be emphasized that when a patient record is not in actual use, it should be in only one place—the filing cabinet or on the shelf. Many precious hours can be lost searching for misplaced or lost records carelessly left unfiled.

The patient's full name, in indexing order, should be typed on a label and the label attached to the folder tab. A strip of transparent tape can be placed on the label to prevent smudging. The patient's full name should also be typed on each sheet in the folder. Some of the types of records common to the healthcare setting, other than patient records, include health-related correspondence, general correspondence, practice management files, miscellaneous files, and tickler or follow-up files.

Health-Related Correspondence

Correspondence pertaining to patients' health should be filed in the patient's health record. Other medical correspondence should be filed in a subject file.

General Correspondence

The provider's office operates as both a business and a professional service. Correspondence of a general nature pertaining to the operation of the office is part of the business side of the practice. Usually, a special drawer or shelf is set aside for the general correspondence. The correspondence is indexed according to subject matter or the names of the correspondents. The guides in a subject file may appear in one, two, or three positions, depending on the number of headings, subheadings, and subdivisions.

Practice Management Files _Work book Ex. 5_

Of course, the most active financial record is the patient ledger. In facilities that still use a manual system, this is a card or vertical tray file, and the accounts are arranged alphabetically by name. At least two divisions are used: active accounts and paid accounts.

Miscellaneous Files

Papers that do not warrant an individual folder are placed in a miscellaneous folder. In that folder, all papers relating to one subject or with one correspondent are kept together in chronologic order, with the most recent on top, and then filed alphabetically with other miscellaneous material. Related materials may be stapled together. Never use paper clips for this purpose. When as many as five papers accumulate with one correspondent or subject, a separate folder should be prepared. Other business files include records of income and expenses, financial statements, income and payroll tax records, canceled checks, and insurance policies. These papers may be filed chronologically.

Tickler or Follow-Up Files

The most frequently used follow-up method is a **tickler file**, so called because it tickles the memory that something needs to be done or followed up on a particular date. The tickler file is always a chronologic arrangement. In its simplest form, it consists of notations on the daily calendar. If information, such as an x-ray report or laboratory report, is expected about a patient with an appointment to come in, the medical assistant might make a note on the calendar or tickler file a day ahead to check on whether the report has arrived.

The tickler file can be a part of a computerized health record system or could be as simple as an e-mail sent to oneself. Many people put reminders on their cell phones using an application (app) specially designed for memos and reminders. The tickler file could also be a card file; 12 guides, one for each month, are placed at the front of the cabinet, container, or other object used to hold the folders. Notations of actions to be taken are placed behind the guides for specific days of the current month. Notations for future months are placed behind the guide for that month. To be effective, the tickler file must be checked first thing each day.

The tickler file can be used in many ways. It is a useful reminder of recurring events, such as payments, meetings, and so forth. On the last day of each month, all the notations from behind the next month's guide are distributed among the daily numbered guides, and the guide for the month just completed is placed at the back of the file.

CRITICAL THINKING APPLICATION   **12-9**

Susan is responsible for checking the tickler file daily. What types of documents and duties might she find inside these files?

Transitory or Temporary File

Many papers are kept longer than necessary because no provision is made for segregating those with a limited usefulness. This situation can be prevented by having a transitory or temporary file. For example, if a medical assistant writes a letter requesting a reprint of the new patient brochure, the file copy is placed in the transitory folder until the reprint is received. When the reprint is received, the file copy is destroyed. The transitory file is used for materials with no permanent value. The paper may be marked with a T and destroyed when the action is completed.

CLOSING COMMENTS

Just as in every aspect of the medical profession, advances in health records management are occurring rapidly, allowing providers and other caregivers to perform their duties more efficiently and accurately. A medical assistant must constantly be willing to learn and to adapt to changes arising from legislation and technologic advances. Computers have become generally accepted as a means of recording health information.

A primary goal of all healthcare facilities is to provide efficient, high-quality patient care. The EHR system can help the staff reach that goal. In the future, every provider's office, hospital, pharmacy, and healthcare facility may be able to access information in minutes, which will improve patient care and save lives. Stay abreast of news and articles related to EHR systems. Remember, the healthcare industry is one of constant growth and learning, and today's information technology provides the medical assistant with endless opportunities to make that growth rewarding and applicable to your current position.

Patient Education

Patients worry about the security of their information, particularly about who can access it. Lawsuits often are filed when patients discover that an unauthorized person has accessed their PHI. The medical assistant should listen to a patient's concerns and explain the safety procedures that apply to the EHR in language the patient can understand. Some facilities prepare a brochure to explain the conversion process to the patient and the advantages of the EHR system.

The medical assistant should expect hesitation and even reluctance from patients who are concerned about the privacy of their health information. Patients are concerned about lack of control over who views their records. Be prepared to answer their questions about the safety of their records as related to the EHR. The medical assistant must know how the EHR is protected and what security measures are in place to be able to reassure the patients that their records are protected at all times.

Legal and Ethical Issues

The authority to release information from the health record lies solely with the patient unless such a release is required by law through a **subpoena duces tecum**. Ownership of the record often is a subject of controversy. The record belongs to the provider; the information belongs to the patient.

Remember that the EHR system contains information that is confidential at all times. The patient must authorize the release of health information in electronic form, just as if it were a piece of paper. EHR systems must:

- Maintain the security and confidentiality of data
- Be easily retrievable
- Have safeguards against the loss of information
- Protect patients' rights to confidentiality and privacy
- Require identification and authentication for access

By supporting these requirements, the medical facility remains in compliance with applicable laws and gains the trust of patients, who are reassured that their health information is secure and safe.

Professional Behaviors

Once the medical assistant has been trained on the EHR system and has had the opportunity to use it for a time, daily use should become second nature. In fact, it may be difficult to imagine a workday without the system! By being open to change and willing to learn, the medical assistant can set a good example for all employees and will be more receptive to the process of change. Be encouraging to other staff members while training on the system, and if technology comes easily to you, share your knowledge with others and assist wherever possible. Do not expect to master the system in a week; instead, realize that a new system has a learning curve and be patient with and receptive to the educational process. Keep technical support phone numbers handy and feel free to use them whenever a new or complicated issue arises. Work as a team, and if possible, help others who might find learning the system more of a struggle. Above all, while getting used to the new technology, make sure your attitude is one of enthusiasm, interest, and curiosity.

SUMMARY OF SCENARIO

Susan looks forward to attending her medical assisting classes each day and works diligently to perform to the best of her ability in the classroom. She strives to do well on each procedure check-off and each examination she completes. Her instructors provide excellent feedback and appreciate her contributions to the class.

Susan has the attitude that everything she is allowed to do in the healthcare facility is a learning tool. She regularly asks for additional responsibilities and is always ready to assist a co-worker. Dr. Thomas has recognized that she has the desire to learn, and he gives her many opportunities to glean more knowledge through the everyday activities in the office.

Although she is new to the medical profession, Susan learns quickly and thinks logically. She knows the rules and regulations on patient confidentiality and is always careful about the information she provides to those who request it. She is never hesitant about asking her office manager for guidance if she is unsure about any aspect of her duties. Susan is understanding and respectful when patients are concerned about their privacy. Her confidence and warm personality play a role in the trust she earns from the patients at the clinic.

Susan is willing to admit when she has made an error and has sought advice from Dr. Thomas and her office manager when an error needed correction. Although filing is not one of her favorite duties, she can be counted on to do her best while completing this important task. She realizes that filing is critical because the documents in the patient's health record direct the care provided to the patient. An abnormal laboratory report that is missing can make a crucial difference in the patient's care. She takes pride in her work and is efficient and accurate where health records are concerned. When she is faced with a task new to her, she considers it a learning experience and asks for help if she is not completely sure about the way to handle a situation.

Susan's co-workers are supportive and always willing to assist her as she learns to be the best medical assistant she can be. Her future as a professional medical assistant certainly holds opportunity and chances for advancement. Just as important, patients trust her. She has alleviated patients' concerns about EHRs by taking the time to explain privacy policies and exactly what information will be accessible to third parties. This trust also gives patients the confidence to reveal personal information and to know that it will be held in the strictest confidence, not just by Susan, but by each employee in the provider's office.

SUMMARY OF LEARNING OBJECTIVES

1. **Define, spell, and pronounce the terms listed in the vocabulary.**
   Spelling and pronouncing terms correctly bolster the medical assistant's credibility. Knowing the definition of these terms promotes confidence in communication with patients and co-workers.

2. **Name and discuss the two types of patient records.**
   The two major types of patient records are the paper health record and the electronic health record (EHR). The EHR is much more efficient than the paper record and most healthcare facilities have switched to EHRs for a number of reasons.

3. **State several reasons that accurate health records are important.**
   Health records must be accurate primarily so that the correct care can be given to the patient. The record also helps ensure continuity of care between providers so that no lapse in treatment occurs. The record serves as indication and proof in court that certain treatments and procedures were performed on the patient; therefore, it can be excellent legal support if it is well maintained and accurate. Health records also aid researchers with statistical information.

4. Differentiate between subjective and objective information in creating a patient's health record.

Subjective information is provided by the patient, whereas objective information is provided by the provider. Examples of subjective information include the patient's address, Social Security number, insurance information, and description of what he or she is experiencing. Objective information is obtained through the provider's questions and observations made during the examination.

Refer to Procedure 12-1 to see how to create a patient's health record and register a new patient in practice management software.

5. Explain who owns the health record.

The provider owns the physical health record, but the patient controls the information contained in it.

6. Distinguish between an electronic health record (EHR) and an electronic medical record (EMR).

The EHR is an electronic record of health-related information about an individual that conforms to nationally recognized interoperability standards and that can be created, managed, and consulted by authorized clinicians and staff from more than one healthcare organization. The EMR is an electronic record of health-related information about an individual that can be created, gathered, managed, and consulted by authorized clinicians and staff within one healthcare organization.

7. Do the following related to healthcare legislation and EHRs:

- Explain how the American Recovery and Reinvestment Act (ARRA) of 2009 applies to the healthcare industry.
  ARRA, commonly known as the Economic Stimulus Package, was meant to promote economic recovery. The health information technology aspects of the bill provide slightly more than $31 billion for healthcare infrastructure and EHR investment. The sections of the ARRA that pertain to healthcare are collectively known as the Health Information Technology for Economic and Clinical Health (HITECH) Act.
- Define meaningful use and relate it to the healthcare industry.
  Meaningful use, defined simply, means that providers must show that they are using EHR technology in ways that can be measured significantly in quality and quantity. If providers meet the meaningful use requirements, they will qualify for incentive payments.
- List the three main components of meaningful use legislation.
  The three main components of meaningful use are (1) use of certified EHR in a meaningful manner, such as e-prescribing; (2) use of certified EHR technology for electronic exchange of health information to improve quality of health care; and (3) use of certified EHR technology to submit clinical quality reports, procedure and diagnosis codes, surveys, and other measures.

8. Explore the advantages, disadvantages, and capabilities of an EHR system, and explain how to organize a patient's health record.

Advantages of the EHR include: reduction of errors, reduction of costs, reduction of staffing needs, legible documentation, easy accessibility, and less physical storage space than paper records. Disadvantages of the EHR

include: lack of capital, fear of something new, startup costs, and space for equipment. Some capabilities of an EHR system include specialty practice components, appointment scheduling features, prescription writers, medical billing systems, charge capture, eligibility verification, referral management, laboratory order integration, patient portals, and many other features that vary from system to system.

Refer to Procedure 12-2 for instructions on how to organize a patient's health record and upload documents to the EHR.

9. Discuss the importance of nonverbal communication with patients when an EHR system is used.

Eye contact is critical when an EHR system is used with patients. Body language must indicate that the medical assistant is open to and listening to the patient's concerns, not just concentrating on data entry. Providers and medical assistants alike may have to relearn how to interact with patients in a natural way while using the laptop or tablet in the examination room. Realize that during the implementation period, processing and serving patients may take longer because the staff is using new technology. Most patients are understanding about this if the medical assistant explains that a new system is in place and asks for patience. Because patients are not always technologically savvy, most will be supportive and interested in the EHR system.

10. Discuss backup systems for the EHR, as well as the transfer, destruction, and retention of health records as related to the EHR.

The provider must have a backup system for the EHR in case a medical office is without power for a significant amount of time. The EHR systems can be set to automatically back up the information at specified times during the day. This means that a minimum amount of data would be lost if the power went out. Options include external hard drive, full server backup, and online backup systems. In most medical offices, records are classified in three ways: active, inactive, and closed. The process of moving a file from active to inactive is called purging. Providers have an obligation to retain patient records. The records of any patient covered by Medicare or Medicaid must be kept at least 10 years.

11. Describe how and when to release health record information; discuss health information exchanges (HIEs).

The healthcare facility must be extremely careful when releasing any type of medical information; the patient must sign a release for information to be given to any third party. Requests for medical information should be made in writing. Pay particular attention to records release requests involving a minor.

There are currently three kinds of HIE—directed exchange, query-based exchange, and consumer-mediated exchange—and the implementation of HIE varies from state to state.

12. Identify and discuss the two methods of organizing a patient's paper medical record.

The source-oriented medical record (SOMR) categorizes the content by its source, such as provider, laboratory, radiology, hospital, and consultation. Within each source category the content is arranged in reverse chronologic order so that the most recent content is viewed first.

Continued

SUMMARY OF LEARNING OBJECTIVES—*continued*

The problem-oriented medical record (POMR) categorizes each of the patient's problems and elaborates on the findings and treatment plans for all concerns. Detailed progress notes are kept for each individual problem. This method addresses each of the patient's concerns separately, whereas a source-oriented record may address all problems and concerns at one time, usually covering one to three patient concerns per office visit. The POMR helps ensure that individual problems are all addressed.

13. **Discuss how to document information in an EHR and a paper health record, and how to make corrections/alterations to health records.**

Documenting information in an EHR involves using radio buttons, drop-down menus, and free-text boxes. When documenting in a paper health record, the entry will always start with the date in the MM/DD/YYYY format. All entries must be written in black or blue ink and follow the format designated by the healthcare facility.

To create a handwritten correction to a health record, a line should be drawn through the error, the correction inserted above or immediately after, and the person making the correction should write his or her initials or signature and the date below the correction. Errors made while using an EHR are corrected in the usual way; however, an error discovered in an entry at a later date is corrected in the same manner as for a handwritten entry.

14. **Discuss dictation and transcription, and discuss transfer, destruction, and retention of medical records as related to paper records.**

With the increased use of EHRs and voice recognition software, there is decreased need for transcription. Transcription can be done from handwritten notes, or more likely from machine dictation. Accuracy and speed are important. Some healthcare offices use voice recognition software for transcription.

As with EHRs, paper health records are also classified as active, inactive, and closed. Large healthcare facilities may find it advisable to convert their paper health records to microfilm.

15. **Identify filing equipment and filing supplies needed to create, store, and maintain medical records.**

Several types of equipment and supplies are needed to manage patients' records. Office space availability; structural considerations; cost of space and equipment; size, type, and volume of medical records; confidentiality requirements; retrieval speed; fire protection; and cost should all be considered when choosing filing equipment. Filing equipment includes: drawer files, horizontal shelf files, rotary circular files, compactable files, automated files, and card files. Filing supplies include divider guides, outguides, file folders, and labels.

16. **Describe indexing rules, and how to create and organize a patient's health record.**

Five basic steps are involved in document filing. (1) The papers are conditioned, which is the preparatory stage for filing. (2) The documents are released, which means they are ready to be filed because they have been reviewed or read and some type of mark has been placed on the document to indicate this. (3) The documents are indexed, which involves deciding where each document should be filed and coding it with some type of mark on the paper indicating that decision. (4) Sorting involves placing the files in filing sequence. (5) The actual filing and storing of the documents is the last step. Refer to Table 12-2 for indexing rules. Refer to Procedure 12-3 for information on creating and organizing a paper health record.

17. **Discuss the pros and cons of various filing methods, as well as how to file patient health records.**

Both the alphabetic and numeric filing systems have advantages and disadvantages. Perhaps most important is the staff's preference. Some find it easier to retrieve files that are in standard alphabetic order, whereas others prefer a numeric system. The numeric system is more confidential than an alphabetic system. Some staff members prefer a combination of the two, called the alphanumeric system. Both effectively keep health records in good order and allow the medical assistant to spot a misfiled record quickly.

Refer to Procedure 12-4 to see how to file patient health records.

18. **Discuss organization of files, as well as health-related correspondence.**

When a patient record is not in actual use, it should only be in the filing cabinet or on the shelf. Health-related correspondence, including general correspondence, should be filed appropriately. Practice management files are usually divided into active and paid accounts. Papers that do not warrant an individual folder are placed in the miscellaneous folder. Follow-up files are frequently called "tickler files." Transitory (i.e., temporary) files can be helpful for material with no permanent value.

19. **Discuss patient education, as well as legal and ethical issues, related to the health record.**

The primary goal of all healthcare facilities is to provide efficient, high-quality patient care. Patients worry about the security of their information and lawsuits can be filed when patients discover that an unauthorized person has accessed their protected health information (PHI). The authority to release information from the health record lies solely with the patient unless such a release is required by law through a *subpoena duces tecum.*

CONNECTIONS

Study Guide Connection: Go to the Chapter 12 Study Guide. Read and complete the activities.

evolve Evolve Connection: Go to the Chapter 12 link at *evolve.elsevier.com/ kinn* to complete the Chapter Review Quiz. Check out the other resources listed for this chapter to make the most of what you have learned from The Health Record.

13

PRINCIPLES OF PHARMACOLOGY

SCENARIO

Kathy Augustino, CMA (AAMA), was hired recently to work for a primary care practice in her hometown. Kathy is responsible for managing phone calls and answering patient questions about their medication and prescriptions. Part of her job description is to follow the provider's orders to administer medication to a wide range of patients. To be knowledgeable about the administrative side of medication management, and to give medications to patients accurately and safely, Kathy must understand the basic principles of pharmacology.

While studying this chapter, think about the following questions:

- What should Kathy know about the management of controlled substances in the ambulatory care setting?
- If Kathy is not familiar with a medication, how can she learn about the properties of the drug?
- Is it important that Kathy understand the clinical uses of prescribed drugs and over-the-counter (OTC) drugs?

- The practice uses an electronic prescription program as part of its electronic health record (EHR) package. How does Kathy transmit the provider's drug orders electronically?
- A primary care practice has patients of all ages. What factors related to age might affect the action of medications on Kathy's patients?
- What role does patient education play in drug safety?

LEARNING OBJECTIVES

1. Define, spell, and pronounce the terms listed in the vocabulary.
2. Do the following related to government regulation of medications in the United States:
   - Distinguish among the government agencies that regulate drugs in the United States.
   - Cite the areas covered in the regulations established by the Drug Enforcement Administration (DEA) for the management of controlled or regulated substances.
   - List the DEA regulations for prescription drugs for each of the five schedules of the Controlled Substances Act.
3. Explain the medical assistant's role in preventing drug abuse.
4. Differentiate a drug's chemical, generic, and trade names.
5. Describe the use of drug reference materials, and explain the five pregnancy risk categories for drugs.
6. Discuss tips for studying pharmacology, and define the five medical terms used to describe the clinical use of drugs.

7. Cite safety measures for the use of OTC drugs.
8. Do the following related to prescription drugs:
   - Diagram the parts of a prescription.
   - Demonstrate the ability to transcribe a prescription accurately.
   - Describe e-prescription methods.
9. Relate the principles of pharmacokinetics to drug use.
10. Describe factors that affect the action of a drug, including the physiologic changes associated with aging.
11. Identify the classifications of drug actions.
12. Differentiate among commonly used herbal remedies and alternative therapies.
13. Examine the role of the medical assistant in drug therapy education.
14. Identify the medical assistant's legal responsibilities in medication management in an ambulatory care setting.

VOCABULARY

angina pectoris (an-ji′-nuh/pek′-tuh-ruhs) A spasmlike pain in the chest caused by myocardial anoxia.

bronchodilator (brahn-ko-di′-la-tuhr) A drug that relaxes contractions of the smooth muscle of the bronchioles to improve lung ventilation.

cirrhosis (suh-ro′-suhs) A chronic, degenerative disease of the liver that interferes with normal liver function.

colloidal (kah-loid′-uhl) Pertaining to a gluelike substance.

enteric coated A term describing an oral medication that is coated to protect the drug against the stomach juices; this design is used to ensure that the medicine is absorbed in the small intestine.

formulary A list of drugs compiled by a health insurance company that identifies the drugs the insurance company will cover under benefits.

generic A medication that is not protected by copyright.

hypercholesterolemia (hi-per-kuh-les-tuh-ruh-le′-me-uh) Elevated blood levels of cholesterol.

identity proofing The process by which a credential service provider validates that a person is who he or she claims to be; the provider must complete this verification before being allowed to e-prescribe controlled substances.

lumen An open space, such as within a blood vessel or the intestine, or within a needle or an examining instrument.

metabolic alkalosis A condition characterized by significant loss of acid in the body or an increased amount of bicarbonate; severe metabolic alkalosis can lead to coma and death.

over-the-counter (OTC) drugs Medications sold without a prescription.

spermicide (spuhr′-muh-side) A chemical substance that kills sperm cells.

therapeutic range The blood concentration of a drug that produces the desired effect without toxicity.

tinnitus A noise sensation of ringing heard in one or both ears.

*P*harmacology is the broad science of the origin, nature, chemistry, effects, and uses of drugs. *Clinical pharmacology* is the study of the biologic effects of a drug used as a medical treatment and the actions of a drug in the body over time, including the rate at which it is absorbed by body tissues; where it is distributed or localized in the tissues; the route by which it is excreted; and its toxicity, or poisonous effect.

Medical assistants must have a general understanding of the types of drugs available and their uses. For every medication administered, a medical assistant must understand the drug's action, typical side effects, route of administration, and recommended dose, in addition to the individual patient factors that can alter the drug's effects and elimination. Drugs are constantly being developed and released for patient treatment; therefore, medical assistants must continually update their knowledge of specific drugs used in the ambulatory care setting. Correct management of drug administration and patient education are crucial factors in providing safe drug therapy for all patients.

GOVERNMENT REGULATION

Several federal agencies combine forces to regulate, safeguard, and manage the development and use of medications in the United States. The Food and Drug Administration (FDA), a division of the Department of Health and Human Services (HHS), regulates the development and sale of all prescription and **over-the-counter (OTC) drugs**. Pharmaceutical companies developing new medications must gain FDA approval before the drugs can be sold to consumers. The approval process begins with chemical testing in the laboratory and progresses to toxicity testing in laboratory animals, and finally to human clinical trials, which involve volunteers who participate in controlled drug studies. Only 1 of 10 new drugs ever reaches the clinical testing phase. If the drug is found to have an acceptable *benefit-to-risk* ratio (i.e., it is effective without causing an unacceptable degree of harm to the user), the FDA approves the medication for release.

The original manufacturer of the drug is awarded copyright protection on that particular chemical compound. Patents expire 20 years from the date of filing; this means that during the 20-year period, other pharmaceutical companies cannot produce **generic** copies of the drug. However, when patents on brand name drugs are near expiration, manufacturers can apply to the FDA to sell generic versions. Besides approving new drugs for the marketplace, the FDA establishes manufacturing standards for drug purity and strength and ensures that generic brands are effective and safe.

Standards for Generic Drug Manufacturers

On average, the cost of a generic drug is 80 to 85 percent lower than the brand name product. The U.S. Food and Drug Administration (FDA) has found no difference in the rates of reported side effects between brand name and generic drugs. Generic drugs must meet the following standards:

- The generic version must have the same active ingredients, labeled strength, route of administration, and dosage form (tablets, patches, and so on). However, generic drugs do not need to contain the same inactive ingredients or fillers as the brand name product. This difference may alter the absorption rate of a generic product. Because of this, some patients may require continued use of brand name drugs even after a generic becomes available.

- Generics do not have to replicate the human clinical trials of the brand name drugs, but applicants must prove that the product performs exactly as the brand name version does.

- Generic versions must act in the same period of time as the brand name version, delivering the same amount of active ingredient into the bloodstream in the same amount of time.

- The label of the generic drug must contain the same information as the brand name version for patient education.

- The generic manufacturing process must ensure comparable quality and production standards. The FDA continues to monitor the quality of the generic drug and periodically inspects manufacturing facilities to conduct quality control procedures.

www.fda.gov/Drugs/ResourcesForYou/Consumers/BuyingUsingMedicineSafely/. Accessed August 24, 2015.

Controlled Substances

The Drug Enforcement Administration (DEA) was established in 1973 as part of the Department of Justice to enforce federal laws regarding the use of illegal drugs. According to the Controlled Substances Act (CSA) of 1970, a drug or other substance that has the potential for illegal use and abuse must be placed on the controlled substance list. Any new medication with an action similar to a drug already on the controlled substance list also is considered to have the potential for abuse.

Most controlled drugs provide significant assistance to patients in need of their particular actions, such as pain relief or anesthesia for surgery. However, certain guidelines must be followed to comply with the storage of controlled substances, their record keeping, and security requirements. In addition, federal law mandates that all medical personnel, including medical assistants, share the responsibility for managing controlled substances on site. Precautions must be taken to monitor patients' drug use, protect prescription pads and e-prescription programs, maintain the records required by law, and report any known or suspected drug diversion or theft.

According to the guidelines set forth in the CSA, controlled substances are divided into five sections, or *schedules,* depending on their addictive abilities and likely degree of abuse. The classifications range from Schedule I drugs, which are illegal and cannot be prescribed, to Schedule V medications, which have the least potential for addiction and abuse (Table 13-1). A limited number of states also have a Schedule VI category for marijuana (cannabis) and synthetic cannabis products.

Every medical practice that stores and administers medications that fall into any of the schedule categories should have a copy of the controlled substances regulations. This list can be obtained from the regional DEA office or online. It is also important to ensure that the facility is included on the DEA's contact list so that the practice receives updates as drugs are added, deleted, or moved from one schedule to another.

Regulation of Controlled Substances

Specific CSA regulations govern the record keeping, physician registration, and inventory of controlled substances. Complete, accurate records on the purchase and management of scheduled drugs in the ambulatory care setting must be maintained. These records must be kept separate from the patient's medical record for 2 years and must be readily available for inspection by the DEA at all times. Each time

a controlled substance is dispensed and administered in the office, documentation of that process includes the number of doses of the drug on site both before and after the medication is dispensed. Medical practices that dispense and administer controlled substances on site use forms developed for this purpose. Any discrepancy in the count of the medication available must be documented and co-signed by two employees.

Every physician who prescribes or has controlled substances on site must register with the DEA for a Controlled Substance Registration Certificate. The physician receives a specific DEA registration number that must be included on all controlled substance prescriptions. The certificate is renewable every 3 years and is specific to a particular site of practice. Therefore, if the physician dispenses or prescribes scheduled drugs at more than one site, a DEA registration number must be obtained for each site.

All controlled substances must be stored in a safe or immovable double-locked cabinet, and the keys must be kept in a secure location. Prescription forms should be kept out of areas used by patients and preferably secured in an area that prohibits unauthorized or illegal use. All DEA forms used by the facility to order controlled substances also must be kept in a locked area.

Many ambulatory practices no longer keep controlled substances on site. However, if drugs are lost or stolen, the incident must be reported immediately to the regional DEA office and to local law enforcement authorities. If the facility needs to dispose of controlled substances a DEA-authorized collector should be contacted to safely and securely collect and dispose of controlled substances and other prescription drugs. Authorized collection sites may be retail pharmacies, hospital or clinic pharmacies, and law enforcement locations. If these disposal options are not available, the DEA recommends that some medicines, such as Demerol, Dilaudid, and OxyContin

TABLE 13-1   Schedule System of Classification of Controlled Substances

SCHEDULE	GUIDELINES	DRUG EXAMPLES
I	• No accepted medical use • Never prescribed for use • High potential for abuse • Possession of these drugs is illegal	Heroin, lysergic acid diethylamide (LSD), methaqualone (Quaalude), mescaline (peyote), amphetamine variations, phencyclidine (PCP), Ecstasy, gamma hydroxybutyrate (GHB), Acetylcodone, Dipipan. Marijuana is still considered a Schedule I drug by the DEA, even though some U.S. states have legalized marijuana for personal or medical use.
II	• Accepted for medical use but with severe restrictions • High potential for abuse • May cause severe psychological or physical dependence	Opium extracts, morphine, methadone, cocaine precursors, amphetamine, barbiturates, methylphenidate (Ritalin), lisdexamfetamine (Vyvanse); oxycodone (Percocet or OxyContin), hydromorphone HCl (Dilaudid), meperidine HCl (Demerol), codeine, alfentanil (Alfenta), alphaprodine (Nisentil), Burgodin, secobarbital (Seconal), pentobarbital (Nembutal), fentanyl, anileridine (Leritine)
III	• Accepted for medical use • Potential for abuse is less than for Schedule I or II drugs • May cause moderate to low physical dependence or high psychological dependence • Includes combination drugs that contain limited amounts of narcotics or stimulants	Acetaminophen and codeine (Tylenol with codeine), benzphetamine, suppositories with barbiturates, anabolic steroids, testosterone, butabarbital (Butisol), Fiorinal, Empirin, hydrocodone (Vicodin), buprenorphine, Boldione, paregoric, other opium combination products
IV	• Accepted for medical use • Low potential for abuse • May cause limited physical or psychological dependence compared with Schedule III drugs • Includes minor tranquilizers and hypnotics	Chlordiazepoxide (Librium), diazepam (Valium), flurazepam (Dalmane), chloral hydrate, Rohypnol ("date rape" drug), alprazolam (Xanax), triazolam (Halcion), temazepam (Restoril), chlorazepate dipotassium (Tranxene), lorazepam (Ativan), Klonopin, zolpidem tartrate (Ambien), barbital, clonazepam (Klonopin), diethylpropion (Tenuate), Motofen, midazolam (Versed), Donnatal Extentabs, Carisoprodol (Soma), eszopiclone (Lunesta), butorphanol (Stadol), Zaleplon (Sonata)
V	• Accepted for medical use • Low potential for abuse • May cause limited physical or psychological dependence compared with Schedule IV drugs • Includes drug mixtures containing limited amounts of narcotics	Cough medicines containing limited quantity of codeine (Robitussin A-C), alkaloids, kaolin and pectin belladonna (Donnagel), diphenoxylate with atropine (Lomotil), ezogabine (Potiga), lacosamide (Vimpat), pregabalin (Lyrica). May be sold by a pharmacist in some states; buyer must be 18 years old and must show identification

www.dea.gov/druginfo/ds.shtml. Accessed May 26, 2015.

oral doses, be flushed down the sink or toilet as soon as they are no longer needed. A list of medicines recommended for disposal by flushing can be found at http://www.fda.gov/Drugs/Resources ForYou/Consumers/BuyingUsingMedicineSafely/EnsuringSafeUse ofMedicine/SafeDisposalofMedicines/ucm186187.htm#Flush_List.

CRITICAL THINKING APPLICATION   **13-1**

Kathy is responsible for maintaining the inventory of controlled substances in the office. While checking the supply of meperidine, she notices that the expiration date on the medication is today. She must dispose of the remaining two pills. According to DEA regulations, how should she dispose of the medication?

Individual states also may regulate controlled substances; therefore, it is essential that medical assistants know their state's legal requirements. Specific federal guidelines apply to both written and e-prescriptions for controlled substances:

1. A written, oral, faxed, or DEA-compliant electronic prescription order must include the date the drug is prescribed; the name and address of the patient; and the name, address, and DEA number of the physician.
2. The amount prescribed must be written out ("ten" rather than "10"); the prescription usually is written for small amounts of the drug.
3. The provider must manually sign all paper prescriptions for controlled substances, although the medical assistant can prepare the prescriptions for the provider's signature.
4. Other specific rules may apply, depending on the schedule to which the prescribed controlled substance is assigned. The

symbols C-II, C-III, C-IV, and C-V are used to indicate the specific schedule.

- Schedule II (C-II) prescriptions
  - Must be either a written or an e-prescription; telephone or fax orders are not permitted
  - Cannot be refilled
  - May require specific types of order forms in some states
- Schedules III (C-III) and IV (C-IV) prescriptions
  - May be ordered orally, in writing, or transmitted electronically
  - May be refilled up to five times within 6 months of the original order
- Schedule V (C-V) prescriptions
  - May be ordered orally, in writing, or transmitted electronically
  - May be refilled up to five times within 6 months of the original order
  - Depending on the state, may be dispensed by the pharmacist without a prescription but typically require a photo ID

CRITICAL THINKING APPLICATION   13-2

Kathy is responsible for the orientation of a new medical assistant in the practice. Summarize the important points about government regulation of controlled substance prescriptions that she should include in the orientation.

DRUG ABUSE

Any drug, from aspirin to alcohol, can be misused or abused. The use of illegal and legal drugs has increased tremendously. Treatment programs for drug abuse are available throughout the United States for people from all walks of life. Programs include detoxification, rehabilitation, and long-term rehabilitation maintenance.

Medical assistants may encounter patients who are misusing or abusing drugs. It is important to be alert to the symptoms of drug dependence and to notify the provider when you suspect that a patient, or a co-worker, may have a problem with drug or alcohol dependency.

Drug *misuse* is the improper use of common drugs that can lead to dependence or toxicity. Examples of people with chronic dependencies include those who cannot have a bowel movement unless they take a laxative; those who have used nasal decongestants for so long that they cannot breathe without the use of nasal sprays; and those who take so many antacids that they suffer systemic **metabolic alkalosis**.

Drug *abuse* is the continuous or periodic self-administration of a drug that could result in addiction (physical dependence). Drug *dependency* is the inability to function unless under the influence of a substance; it may be psychological or physical. *Psychological dependency* is the compulsive craving for the effects of a substance. *Habituation* is a form of psychological dependency on a substance but without physiologic dependence, such as the need for tobacco. *Physical dependency*, or addiction, is a person's need to use a substance

continuously so that the body can function and also to prevent physical discomfort. This type of dependency occurs when abused substances produce biochemical changes in cells and tissues, most commonly in the nervous system. When a substance that causes physical dependency is discontinued, withdrawal symptoms occur. Withdrawal symptoms may be mild or serious, leading to convulsions and possibly death.

Regardless of the type of drug abused, it will have two effects on the person: acute and chronic. The acute effect is what the person feels when intoxicated, or directly under the influence of a particular substance. Chronic effects include the temporary or permanent physical and mental changes that result from long-term abuse.

Patients may question medical assistants about drug abuse. The medical assistant should read and keep up to date on drug-related issues. Booklets, websites, and agency referral names should be available for patients. In addition, patients' concerns and questions about drug abuse should be conveyed to the provider.

The Medical Assistant's Role in Preventing Drug Abuse

By following these guidelines, the medical assistant can help prevent drug abuse:

- Carefully monitor patients who repeatedly call for prescription refills of controlled substances.
- Request health records from other facilities for patients who report previous prescriptions for scheduled drugs.
- If the facility uses paper prescription pads, keep blank pads in a safe place, away from patient treatment areas, and minimize the number of prescription pads in use at any given time.
- Never use prescription pads for notepads, and never use preprinted or presigned forms.
- Secure computers used for electronic health record (EHR) documentation to prevent patient access to prescription generation.
- Keep only a limited supply of controlled substances on hand.
- Keep accurate, complete records of controlled substances dispensed on site and those prescribed; include specific documentation in the patient's record for all prescribed controlled substances.

DRUG NAMES

A single drug may have up to three names: a chemical name, a generic name, and a trade name. The chemical name represents the drug's exact formula. For example, the chemical name of the analgesic acetaminophen is *N*-(4-hydroxyphenyl); *acetaminophen* is the generic name, and the trade name is *Tylenol*. All drugs are assigned a generic, or nonproprietary (official), name. This name is much simpler than the chemical name, and it is not protected by copyright. The trade (brand) name is assigned by the manufacturer and is protected by copyright. To prevent confusion, the use of generic names rather than trade names is encouraged for medical professionals; however, patients may only recognize the trade names of drugs. Drugs also are classified by their use. For example, Advil is a brand name for the generic drug ibuprofen, which is classified as an analgesic and an antiinflammatory agent.

APPROACHES TO STUDYING PHARMACOLOGY

A pharmaceutical glossary could be a book in itself. Many terms are combinations of the condition to be treated plus the prefix *anti-* (e.g., antianginal, antianxiety, antiarrhythmic, anticoagulant, anticonvulsant, antidiarrheal). Notice how these names emphasize the drug's effect (use) rather than its action in the body. More recent classifications, such as parasympathomimetic and cholinesterase inhibitor, describe the pharmacologic action rather than the therapeutic use. Both viewpoints are necessary for a more complete understanding of drugs and their action in the human body. No one can remember all there is to know about clinical pharmacology. The number of new drugs introduced into use far exceeds the number of older drugs replaced or discontinued. The number of drugs available for clinical use grows beyond the ability to learn all there is to know about each medication. Therefore, it is essential that the medical assistant understand how to use pharmacology resources as references. Several drug index resources are available online that can be used to search for medication information. Examples of these are Rxlist at http://www.rxlist.com/script/main/hp.asp and Drugs.com at http://www.drugs.com/. If the facility promotes online drug research, preferred websites should be posted for staff use.

Drug Reference Materials

Reference books that are updated annually or periodically should be available for easy reference at all medical facilities. Most references list drug information in the following sequence:

1. *Action:* How the drug provides therapeutic results in the body, or the use of the drug.
2. *Indication:* The conditions for which the drug is used.
3. *Contraindications:* Conditions that make administration of the drug improper or undesirable. For example, aspirin is contraindicated in patients with GI bleeding.
4. *Precautions:* Necessary actions that must be taken because of special conditions of the patient, the drug, or the environment; these actions must be considered if the drug is to be successful or not harmful. The drug's pregnancy risk category is included in this section, as are precautions for nursing mothers (Table 13-2).
5. *Adverse reactions:* Commonly observed side effects on a tissue or organ system other than the one targeted by the medication. Adverse reactions include hypersensitivity, which causes an allergic reaction to the drug; idiosyncrasy, or an unexplained, unusual response to the drug; psychological dependence or habituation to the drug; and physical dependence on the compound, causing signs and symptoms of withdrawal in the patient if the medication is removed. For example, patients prescribed certain diuretics (e.g., Lasix) are at risk for potassium depletion, so they must take a potassium supplement or must eat a daily dietary source of potassium (bananas are a common source) to prevent complications.
6. *Dosage and administration:* Usual route, dosage, and timing for administering the drug.

TABLE 13-2	FDA's Pregnancy Risk Drug Categories
CATEGORY	**RISK LEVEL/DESCRIPTION**
A	Remote risk. Controlled studies in women have failed to demonstrate risk to fetus.
B	Slightly more risk than Category A. Animal studies show no risk, but controlled human studies have not been done; *or* animal studies show risk, but controlled studies in women have shown no risk.
C	Greater risk than Category B. Animal studies have shown risk, but no controlled human studies have been done; *or* no studies have been done in animals or women.
D	Proven risk of fetal harm. Human studies show proof of fetal damage, but the potential benefits of use during pregnancy may make its use acceptable.
X	Proven risk of fetal harm. Studies in women or animals show definite risk of fetal abnormality. Risks outweigh any possible benefit.

FDA, U.S. Food and Drug Administration.

7. *How supplied:* Description of how the medication is packaged and specifics on how it should be administered.

Package Inserts

Every drug package contains an insert describing all the significant aspects of using the drug, including information on the chemical formulation of the drug and clinical studies. The information in the insert is controlled by the FDA and serves as an excellent quick reference on new medications in the ambulatory setting.

Physicians' Desk Reference

The *Physicians' Desk Reference* (PDR) is published annually by Thomson Medical Economics (Oradell, New Jersey). It is supplied free to providers who subscribe to *Medical Economics* magazine. Copies can be purchased through the publisher or in local bookstores. Supplements are published quarterly throughout the year. The PDR contains information on approximately 3,000 drugs and includes product descriptions that are identical to the information provided in package inserts. The drug manufacturers pay for this space, so the PDR could be considered the Yellow Pages of the drug industry. The facility can also purchase an online version of the PDR and smart phone applications that can be used by staff and providers throughout the facility (*www.pdr.net/*).

The print version of the PDR contains color-coded sections, which allows for easy cross-reference. The various sections enable you to begin searching for information about a drug from any starting point. You can start with the usage, classification, generic name, manufacturer's name, or trade name of a drug, or what the drug looks like. A special photographic section allows visual identification of products. Once you know which drug you want to study, the product information section lists the actual package insert information alphabetically, first by the manufacturer, then by the brand name. (A separate PDR volume, the *Physicians' Desk Reference for Nonprescription Drugs,* is published annually for OTC drugs and dietary supplements.)

The six sections of the PDR are color coded as follows:

- *Manufacturer's index (white):* Alphabetical listing of pharmaceutical companies; it includes the drugs manufactured by each company and the contact information for each manufacturer
- *Brand and generic section (pink):* Alphabetical listing of all drugs in the PDR volume, with complete information for each
- *Product category index (blue):* Alphabetical listing compiled according to drug category; drugs with similar actions are listed alphabetically in each category
- *Product identification section (gray):* Illustrated section that shows actual-size photographs of the tablets and capsules listed in the PDR
- *General and diagnostic product information area (white):* Alphabetical listing of diagnostic product information and the uses of these products

United States Pharmacopeia/National Formulary

The *United States Pharmacopeia/National Formulary* (USP/NF) is the official source of drug standards for the United States. The *Pharmacopeia* was combined with the *National Formulary,* which lists the chemical formulas for all accepted drugs. This combined reference lists and describes all approved medications in the United States considered useful and therapeutic in the practice of medicine. Single drugs, rather than combined products (compound mixtures), are listed. If a drug name is the same as the official name in this volume, the drug is followed by the initials USP (e.g., digitoxin, USP).

Learning About Drugs

The study of pharmacology is difficult at best. However, the following steps can help make it easier:

1. Take advantage of opportunities to observe the use of drugs in patient care. Studying about atorvastatin calcium (Lipitor) becomes more meaningful when you see how its lipid-lowering action actually affects a patient's blood cholesterol level.
2. Concentrate on the most important drugs in each classification. As you expand your knowledge to other drugs in each category, you will easily understand new drugs by noting the similarities and differences between them and the basic, important drugs you studied first.
3. Learn about a drug's primary action and use, then expand your knowledge to its other actions and uses. Soon you will be able to name the drug that is usually indicated for a particular condition. Knowing a drug's secondary effects will help you understand the side effects that are likely to occur with use of the drug. More important, you will be aware of

contraindications to use of the drug. Knowledge of the drug's actions will enable you to predict what toxic reactions might occur from an overdose.

Terms Describing the Uses of Drugs	
Diagnostic	Helps to determine the cause of a particular health problem (e.g., injecting antigen serum for allergy testing).
Palliative	Indicates that the drug does not cure, but provides relief from pain or symptoms related to the disorder (e.g., the use of an antihistamine for allergy symptoms or narcotics for pain relief).
Prophylactic	Prevents the occurrence of a condition (e.g., vaccines prevent the occurrence of specific infectious diseases or contraceptives prevent pregnancy).
Replacement	Provides the patient with a substance needed to maintain health (e.g., insulin for patients with diabetes, levothyroxine sodium [Synthroid] for patients with hypothyroidism).
Therapeutic	Treats a disorder and cures it (e.g., antibiotics cure bacterial infections).

Dispensing Drugs

Drugs are dispensed in two ways: over the counter and by prescription. OTC drugs are available to the public for self-medication without a prescription. These drugs have been approved by the FDA for general consumer use, but patients taking prescription drugs should keep their healthcare providers informed about their OTC drug use.

A medical assistant directly involved in patient care should have an understanding of some basic facts about OTC drugs and herbal products. Today patients are better informed about their personal healthcare, and many want to be active participants in healthcare decisions. They need facts to make informed choices when using OTC preparations. Most OTC preparations are safe if used as directed on the package; however, patient education contributes greatly to the safe and correct use of OTCs. Patients should be encouraged to do the following when choosing or using an OTC:

- Carefully read the package label and insert for use guidelines.
- Take only the recommended dose.
- Monitor the expiration date and discard the medication when appropriate.
- Never combine an OTC with a prescription drug without the provider's knowledge.
- Recognize that many OTC drugs are contraindicated in pregnancy, for nursing mothers, and for young children, and if certain diseases are present.
- Check with the pharmacist if questions or concerns arise.

The number of prescription drugs that have been granted OTC status is constantly increasing, and as the list of OTC drugs increases, so does the need for consumer education. Many OTC medications influence the safety and effectiveness of prescription drugs; therefore,

TABLE 13-3   Commonly Used OTC Drugs and Possible Complications

DRUG NAME	CLASSIFICATION	INDICATIONS AND DESIRED EFFECTS	SIDE EFFECTS	DRUG INTERACTIONS
Acetylsalicylic acid (ASA), ibuprofen, naproxen	Nonsteroidal antiinflammatory drugs (NSAIDs); analgesics	Inflammation and pain relief	GI bleeding, compromised renal function, tinnitus, diarrhea, and nausea	ACE inhibitors, warfarin
Acetaminophen (Tylenol)	Analgesic, antipyretic	Relief of pain and fever	Liver damage	Warfarin
Pseudoephedrine (Sudafed)	Decongestant	Relief of common cold and allergy symptoms	Hypertension, vasospasm, arrhythmia, CVA	Beta blockers, digoxin
Diphenhydramine (Benadryl and other combination products)	Antihistamines	Cough, cold, allergy, and insomnia	Disrupted sleep, confusion, hallucinations, delirium	Oxybutynin (Ditropan)
Dextromethorphan (Dayquil Cough, Delsym, Robitussin)	Antitussive	Suppression of cough reflex	Dizziness, lethargy, nausea	
Tums, Gaviscon, Pepto-Bismol	Antacids	Treatment of heartburn, GERD symptoms	Diarrhea, constipation, kidney stones	Ibuprofen, tetracycline, isoniazid

ACE, Angiotensin-converting enzyme; *CVA,* cerebrovascular accident; *GERD,* gastroesophageal reflux disease; *GI,* gastrointestinal; *OTC,* over the counter.

gathering information for a complete and accurate pattern of the patient's use of OTC drugs should be part of every healthcare visit. Table 13-3 presents a list of commonly used OTC medications, their side effects, and possible prescription drug interactions.

Prescription Drugs

Federal law makes drugs that are dangerous, powerful, or habit-forming illegal to use except under a licensed provider's order. A prescription is an order written by the provider for the dispensing of a particular medication by the pharmacist and its administration to the patient. As electronic health records (EHRs) have come into use, electronic prescriptions have become commonplace, although some facilities continue to use paper prescription forms (Figure 13-1). The prescription must be signed by the provider, or the order cannot be carried out (Procedure 13-1). If the provider requests that the medical assistant phone or fax a prescription to the pharmacy, all pertinent information for the medication order must be written down and reviewed by the provider for accuracy before the call is made. A note is made in the patient's record that a medication order was phoned or faxed into the pharmacy, with all of the pertinent information about the order included.

Appropriate medical terminology and abbreviations must be used to complete the prescription. The more common terms and abbreviations are listed in Table 13-4. In an attempt to reduce the number of medication errors caused by incorrect use of medical terminology, The Joint Commission has developed a "Do Not Use" list of abbreviations, acronyms, and symbols that should not be used for documentation purposes in accredited institutions. In addition, the commission created an ancillary list of possible future inclusions. Both of these lists are presented in Table 13-5. Besides The Joint Commission lists, facilities have the option of creating their own list of problematic abbreviations that employees should avoid using.

Six Parts of a Prescription

- *Superscription:* Patient's name, address, and date need to be included at the top of the paper prescription; the symbol Rx (for the Latin word *recipe,* meaning "take")
- *Inscription:* Main part of the prescription; name of the drug, dosage form, and strength
- *Subscription:* Directions for the pharmacist; size of each dose, amount to be dispensed, and the form of the drug ordered (tablets, capsules, or some other form)
- *Signature:* Directions for the patient; usually preceded by the symbol Sig (for the Latin word *signa,* meaning "mark"); the place where the provider indicates the instructions to be put on the label to tell the patient how, when, and in what quantities to use the medication
- *Refill information:* May be regulated by federal law if the drug is a controlled substance; the provider must write on the script the number of times a refill is allowed
- *Provider's signature:* Must include the provider's signature (whether it is electronic or manual), in addition to his or her Drug Enforcement Agency (DEA) registration number when indicated

---

CRITICAL THINKING APPLICATION   13-3

Dr. Simon asks Kathy to prepare the following prescription for his signature: "Take one 20-mg tablet of Lipitor daily at bedtime. Dispense 4 weeks' worth, and the prescription may be refilled two times." How would Kathy write the prescription using the correct format, medical terminology, and abbreviations?

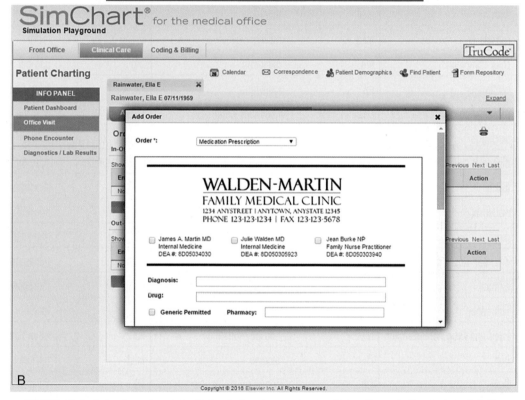

John Jones, M.D.   Tel: 724-544-8976
108 N. Main St.
City, State

Patient __Ms. Jean Smith__   DATE __10/7/XXXX__

ADDRESS __310 E. 70th St., Anytown, State__

Rx: Lipitor   40 mg tab

Disp: # 30

Sig: T̊ hs

Refill __3__ Times   _John Jones, M.D._
Please label ☑

A

B

FIGURE 13-1 A, Sample paper prescription. **B,** Sample electronic prescription entry. (**B** from Elsevier: *SimChart for the medical office,* St Louis, 2016, Elsevier.)

Electronic Prescriptions

Electronic health record (EHR) systems can create and send prescriptions directly to a pharmacy. EHR programs are designed to automatically check a prescribed drug against the patient's allergies, identify possible drug-drug interactions, access current databases for the patient's medication history, review the patient's insurance drug **formulary** for coverage, and electronically send the script to the patient's pharmacy to be filled. The Department of Health and Human Services (HHS) recognizes the importance of e-prescriptions in quality patient care because they reduce the chances of misinterpretation of a provider's handwriting and promote speed in filling prescriptions through the instant transfer of the script from the ambulatory care facility to the patient's pharmacy. The HHS recommends that an individual, such as a credentialed medical assistant, be designated the practice's expert for e-prescribing so that the process runs smoothly and all regulations for the delivery of prescriptions electronically are followed.

Details on Medicare incentive programs to encourage physicians to adopt e-prescribing programs can be found at the following website: *www.cms.gov/ Medicare/E-Health/Eprescribing/index.html?redirect=/Eprescribing.*

TABLE 13-4   Common Prescription Abbreviations

ABBREVIATION	MEANING	ABBREVIATION	MEANING	ABBREVIATION	MEANING
aa	of each	IM	intramuscular	pt	pint
ac	before meals	inj	injection	pulv	powder
ad lib	as desired	IV	intravenous	qh	every hour
agit	shake, stir	K	potassium	q2h	every 2 hours
am	morning	kg	kilogram	q3h	every 3 hours
amp	ampule	KVO	keep vein open	q4h	every 4 hours
ASA	aspirin	L	liter	qid	four times a day
aq	water	lb	pound	qm	every morning
bid	twice a day	LR	lactated Ringer's solution	qn	every night
C	cup, Celsius	mcg	microgram	qs	quantity sufficient
c̄	with	med	medicine	qt	quart
cap	capsule	mEq	milliequivalent	R	rectal
CC	chief complaint	mg	milligram	r/o	rule out
cm	centimeter	mL	milliliter	Rx	take, treatment
c/o	complaining of	MLD	minimum lethal dose	S, Sig	give the following directions
D/C	discharge	mn	midnight	s̄ or w/o	without
Dx	diagnosis	MO	mineral oil	SC, SQ, subQ	subcutaneous
dil	dilute	MOM	milk of magnesia	SOB	shortness of breath
disp	dispense	MTD	maximum tolerated dose	s̄s̄	one-half
dr	dram	NKA	no known allergies	stat	immediately
EENT	eye, ear, nose, throat	noct	at night	T, tbs	tablespoon
ext	extract	NPO	nothing by mouth	t, tsp	teaspoon
F	Fahrenheit	NS	normal saline	tab	tablet
FDA	Food and Drug Administration	N/V	nausea/vomiting	tid	three times a day
Fe	iron	O₂	oxygen	tinct	tincture
fl	fluid	OD	overdose	TO	telephone order
fx	fracture	OTC	over-the-counter (drugs)	tus	cough
gal	gallon	oz	ounce	ung	ointment
gm, g	gram	pc	after meals	vag	vagina
gr	grain	PL	placebo	ves	bladder
gtt	drops	pm	afternoon	VO	verbal order
h	hour	PMI	patient medication instruction	VS	vital signs
hs	at bedtime	po	by mouth	WNL	within normal limits
HTN	hypertension	pr	per rectum	W/O	water in oil
Hx	history	prn	as needed	x	times
ID	intradermal	pt	patient	y/o	years old

TABLE 13-5 The Joint Commission's Official "Do Not Use" List[1] and Possible Future Inclusions

DO NOT USE	POTENTIAL PROBLEM	USE INSTEAD
U (unit)	Mistaken for "0" (zero), the number "4" (four) or "cc"	Write "unit"
IU (international unit)	Mistaken for IV (intravenous) or the number 10 (ten)	Write "International Unit"
Q.D., QD, q.d., qd (daily) Q.O.D., QOD, q.o.d, qod (every other day)	Mistaken for each other Period after the Q mistaken for "I" and the "O" mistaken for "I"	Write "daily" Write "every other day"
Trailing zero (X.0 mg)* Lack of leading zero (.X mg)	Decimal point is missed	Write X mg Write 0.X mg
MS MSO4 and MgSO4	Can mean morphine sulfate or magnesium sulfate Confused for one another	Write "morphine sulfate" Write "magnesium sulfate"

[1]Applies to all orders and all medication-related documentation that is handwritten (including free-text)

*__Exception:__ A "trailing zero" may be used only where required to demonstrate the level of precision of the value being reported, such as for laboratory results, imaging studies that report size of lesions, or catheter/tube sizes. It may not be used in medication orders or other medication-related documentation.

Additional Abbreviations, Acronyms and Symbols (for possible future inclusion in the Official "Do Not Use" List)

> (greater than) < (less than)	Misinterpreted as the number "7" (seven) or the letter "L" Confused for one another	Write "greater than" Write "less than"
Abbreviations for drug names	Misinterpreted due to similar abbreviations for multiple drugs	Write drug names in full
Apothecary units	Unfamiliar to many practitioners Confused with metric units	Use metric units
@	Mistaken for the number "2" (two)	Write "at"
cc	Mistaken for U (units) when poorly written	Write "mL" or "ml" or "milliliters" ("mL" is preferred)
μg	Mistaken for mg (milligrams) resulting in one thousand-fold overdose	Write "mcg" or micrograms

www.jointcommission.org. Accessed November 16, 2015.

PROCEDURE 13-1 | **Prepare a Prescription for the Provider's Signature**

Goal: *To accurately prepare a prescription for the provider's signature using the appropriate abbreviations and prescription format.*

EQUIPMENT and SUPPLIES

- Patient's record
- Prescription pad
- Drug reference materials, if needed
- Black pen

PROCEDURAL STEPS

1. Refer to the provider's written order for the prescription. If the provider gives a verbal order to write a prescription, write down the order and review it with the provider for accuracy.
   PURPOSE: To ensure accuracy in writing the ordered medication.

2. If you are unfamiliar with the medication, look it up in a drug reference book (e.g., the *Physicians' Desk Reference* [PDR]).

PURPOSE: The medical assistant should be familiar with the details of the drug, including the correct spelling, form in which it is dispensed, strength, recommended dose, storage guidelines, drug-drug interactions, and possible side effects, to make sure the transcription is correct and to be prepared to answer the patient's questions about the medication.

3. Ask the patient about drug allergies.
   PURPOSE: The patient should be asked about drug allergies each time a medication is prescribed or dispensed because these can change over time.

4. Using a prescription pad that has the provider's name, address, and telephone number, begin to transcribe the provider's order. Add the provider's DEA number if the script is for a controlled substance (see Figure 13-1).

5. Record the patient's name and address and the date on which the prescription is being written.

6. Next to the Rx, write in legible handwriting the name of the drug (correctly spelled), the dosage form (e.g., tablet, capsule, or other, using correct abbreviations), and the strength ordered. This is the inscription. For example, if the provider orders Lipitor, 40-mg tablets, by mouth, one tablet at bedtime, the first line of the prescription should read: Lipitor 40 mg tabs.

7. On the next line, write *Disp.* This is the subscription, which includes directions to the pharmacist on the amount to be dispensed and the form of the drug. For the Lipitor order, the subscription would read: Disp: #30.

8. Next comes the signature. This includes directions for the patient, such as how and when to take the medicine; it usually is preceded by the abbreviation Sig: For the Lipitor order, the signature would read: Sig: Ť tab PO hs.

9. The provider has told you that the patient can get three refills of the prescription, so this information should be added at the bottom of the prescription on the designated line.

10. The provider must review and sign the prescription before it is given to the patient.

11. Document in the patient's health record the medication order and any pertinent details, including patient education and refill information.
    PURPOSE: All patient education should be documented for future reference. The details about the prescription, in addition to refill information, must be included for future prescriptions and/or refill orders.

Telephoning or Faxing a Prescription Into the Pharmacy or Transmitting an E-Prescription

Using the steps outlined previously, complete the prescription, making sure to include the following elements:

1. Patient's full name and address
2. Provider's full name and address
3. DEA number if the prescription is for a controlled substance (Schedule II drugs must be filled with a written prescription and/or an EHR program authorized to fill scheduled drugs)
4. For the prescribed drug:

- Name
- Strength
- Dosage form
- Quantity prescribed
- Directions for use
- Number of refills (if any) authorized

The provider must review the prescription for accuracy before the medical assistant telephones, faxes, or transmits the prescription to the pharmacy. Document the pharmacy order in the patient's health record as you would for any prescribed drug.

For an e-prescription, access the program for electronic transmission of prescriptions through the patient's record. Complete all the information required, and transmit the prescription to the patient's preferred pharmacy.

DRUG INTERACTIONS WITH THE BODY

Pharmacology is the study of drugs, their desired effects, and what happens to a drug while it is in the body. Different patients may react to the same dose of a drug in very different ways, and the same patient may react to the same dose of a drug differently at various times. Therefore, the management of medication therapy is concerned primarily with the effectiveness of a drug's action and the drug's potential side effects. *Pharmacokinetics* is the study of the movement of drugs throughout the body. Four basic actions occur when a drug is taken: absorption, distribution, metabolism, and excretion. If you know what happens to the drug in the body, you can know the *onset* of a drug's activity (when the drug action starts), when the effects of the drug are likely to peak, the minimum amount of the drug needed to bring about the desired effect (therapeutic dose), and the *duration* of a particular drug's activity. All these factors help the provider determine the appropriate form, amount, route, and frequency of administration of a medication for a particular patient.

Drug Absorption

The rate at which drugs are absorbed from the site of administration into the bloodstream depends on many factors, including the drug's ability to dissolve, the characteristics of the medication, the concentration of the dose, and the route of administration. Liquid oral medications dissolve more rapidly than solid forms because they do not have to be dissolved by GI fluids before they are absorbed. In addition, drugs soluble in fat pass more readily through the cell membrane because cell membranes have a fatty acid layer. More acidic drugs are absorbed well in the stomach, whereas others cannot be absorbed until they reach the small intestine. For some medications, such as antibiotics, the physician may order an initial *loading dose* of the drug, usually twice the typical amount, so that the patient's blood levels reach the **therapeutic range** more quickly.

Oral Route

Oral medications are convenient, safe, and relatively inexpensive. However, drugs that can be destroyed in any way by the digestive tract must be given by injection. Insulin and heparin are examples of drugs that are destroyed by the digestive process and therefore cannot be administered orally. Injection of medications leads to rapid absorption into the bloodstream, but this increases the danger of overdose or infection. Most oral medications are absorbed by the small intestine. After absorption into the bloodstream from the small intestine, drugs are carried to the liver. Much of the drug's potency is inactivated in this organ before the drug circulates to the tissues.

This inactivation by the liver often makes it necessary to administer higher doses orally than those given by injection.

Food slows the absorption of drugs; therefore, many medications are absorbed best when taken either 1 hour before or 2 hours after ingestion of food. Food also may bind with a medication or in some other way inactivate it. For example, tetracycline is destroyed by milk products and antacids containing calcium salts. Therefore, patients taking tetracycline should be advised not to eat dairy products or take liquid or solid forms of antacids. Stomach acid that naturally occurs during digestion may destroy certain drugs. Because some drugs are destroyed by the components of the digestive tract or irritate the empty lining of the stomach, oral drugs may be **enteric coated** to keep them intact for passage into the small intestine or to prevent gastric irritation or vomiting; therefore, enteric-coated medications should not be crushed or chewed.

Some drugs are not affected by digestive processes, but they cannot be absorbed through the intestinal walls into the bloodstream. For example, neomycin has no therapeutic effect when taken orally (unless it is used to sterilize the bowel before bowel surgery). Other drugs may be unable to cross the bowel mucosa because of their poor solubility in lipids (fats), or because they are inactivated by the pH of the GI tract.

It is important to remember these absorption factors when administering medication by the oral route. If a patient has previously responded to a drug but is no longer responding, it may be important to question the patient's food-medication cycle. It could be that the patient is no longer taking the medication on an empty stomach as directed.

Parenteral Route

Parenteral refers to the administration of drugs by injection. The parenteral route results in the fastest action because the medication is administered directly into the bloodstream or into tissues with a rich blood supply. However, several factors determine the effectiveness and rate of absorption of injected medications.

A drug in an aqueous (water) solution is absorbed more quickly in an area with more blood vessels. Therefore, drugs deposited in the muscle are absorbed faster than drugs given subcutaneously. The intramuscular (IM) route is chosen in an emergency for fast action or when larger amounts of the medication must be absorbed. The IM route is also used for oil-based medications (e.g., testosterone), which are typically prepared with oil to extend the absorption rate of the drug. The subcutaneous (SC) route is chosen when a slower, prolonged effect is desired.

Drug absorption also may be controlled physically. Absorption may be quickened by hand massage after injection, but massage should be done only if recommended. Absorption may be slowed by pharmaceutical preparation of the drug in a physical form that slows absorption. These methods include suspending the drug in a solution that prolongs absorption, such as **colloidal** substances, fatty substances (oil), or insoluble salts or esters. Drugs suspended in these substances slowly dissolve in the tissues over a long time, and the patient can be spared costly, frequent, and sometimes painful injections. Local anesthetics sometimes are mixed with epinephrine to keep the medication and its effects in an area longer because epinephrine (adrenalin) constricts blood vessels at the site, reducing circulation and the rate of absorption.

Another parenteral route is the *intravenous* (IV) route, in which the medication is injected directly into the vein. Because of the dangers of IV administration, only members of the medical team who are licensed to do so may inject medication intravenously. Other parenteral routes that are outside the medical assistant's scope of practice include:

- Intrathecal, or intraspinal, injections are used for spinal anesthesia and to administer certain medications into the spinal column.
- Intra-articular injections are used to administer corticosteroids into joints.
- Intralesional medications are injected directly into a lesion, such as an anticancer drug that is administered into a cancerous tumor.

Safety Alert

It is outside the medical assistant's scope of practice to perform IV administration of medications to patients. Because IV administration is so dangerous, medications given intravenously usually are administered in small doses through an IV infusion (IV drip) so that the effects in the body can be monitored.

Another form of parenteral route is an intradermal injection, which is injection of the drug within the dermal layer of the skin and superficial to the subcutaneous tissues. This route is used mostly for allergy testing and skin testing, such as testing for tuberculosis.

Mucous Membrane Absorption

Drugs may be absorbed by the mucous membranes of the mouth, throat, nose, eyes, rectum, vagina, and respiratory tracts. Some applications, such as nasal sprays, eye drops, and rectal suppositories for constipation, have a local effect. Others have a systemic effect, such as a rectal suppository given to control vomiting, or a nitroglycerin tablet dissolved under the tongue *(sublingual)* to dilate coronary arteries and relieve the pain of **angina pectoris**. *Inhalation* is used to concentrate drugs locally in the lower respiratory passages or to produce systemic effects, such as general anesthesia. For example, a **bronchodilator**, such as metaproterenol sulfate (Alupent), is inhaled during an asthma attack to relieve bronchospasms.

Topical Absorption

Topical routes include the application of medications to the skin, eyes, and ears. Drugs in ointments, creams, lotions, and aerosols can be applied for the treatment of skin itching, inflammation, or other discomforts, and for the treatment of skin infections with antibiotics. Nitroglycerin (for angina) can be absorbed through the skin from a dermal patch, which releases it systemically. Hormones such as testosterone and estrogen also can be administered via a dermal patch for systemic purposes.

Drug Distribution

Once a drug has been absorbed, it must be transported by the circulatory system to the area where it will have its effect. In the bloodstream, drugs can attach to plasma proteins and then are freed

Terms Related to Drug Interactions

Antagonism	The action of one drug diminishes the effect or shortens the duration of action of another drug. For example, Naloxone Injection and Evzio (a prefilled naloxone autoinjector) are used to reverse the life-threatening effects of a narcotic overdose.
Synergism	A drug enhances the intensity or prolongs the action of another drug. This can have a positive effect, as when two different antibiotics are used to treat an infection, or a negative effect, as when two drugs lower blood pressure to dangerous levels.
Potentiation	A form of synergism in which the effect of one drug is enhanced by the presence of another drug. In this case, the two drugs have different actions, but one increases the effect of the other. Promethazine, an antihistamine, when given with a painkilling narcotic such as Demerol, intensifies the narcotic's effect, thereby reducing the amount of the narcotic needed.

to pass from the blood into the site of action. Drugs are carried through the fluids into the cells of the tissues and organs. The blood supply to a part affects the speed with which drugs reach certain tissues.

The *blood-brain barrier* is a functional cellular barrier between the brain cells and the capillaries circulating blood through the brain. The barrier is poorly permeable to water-soluble materials, which makes it difficult for dissolved substances in the blood to pass through. For substances that do cross through, the barrier regulates the degree and rate of their absorption into the brain tissue. The general anesthetic thiopental is able to cross the blood-brain barrier immediately and produces sleep within seconds, whereas other sleep-producing drugs, such as the barbiturates, cross slowly and may take as long as 30 minutes to 1 hour to produce the same effect. The blood-brain barrier is a mixed blessing. It provides a physical barrier that protects the brain from potentially dangerous chemicals, but it also makes it very difficult to treat CNS disorders. In contrast, the placenta has no method for blocking substances, so whatever the mother consumes is readily passed through the placenta to the developing fetus. This means that childbearing women must be extremely careful of all chemicals they consume or inhale because they are quickly transferred to the baby's bloodstream.

Drug Action

Regardless of the route of administration, a drug can have one of two actions on the body: local (restricted to one spot or part; not general) or *systemic* (affecting the body as a whole). Most drugs are used for their systemic effects. Even when drugs are used for local purposes, no drug remains completely localized in the body. Any chemical that comes into contact with even the most superficial surface, such as the skin, has the potential to be absorbed into the bloodstream and circulate to other tissues and organs.

Multiple theories explain the actions of drugs. Drugs are believed to combine with body chemicals on the cell surface or within the

cell itself. Pharmaceutical developers create compounds that have an affinity for a specific target cell. The target cell recipient is called a *receptor*, and the drug that has the affinity for it and produces a functional change in the cell is called an *agonist*. Not all drugs that bind to specific cells cause a functional change in the cell. These drugs act as an *antagonist* to the natural process and work by blocking a sequence of biochemical events.

Some drugs are believed to act by affecting the enzyme functions of the body. Drugs attach to enzyme substances and rob the enzymes from cells. As a result, the enzyme products needed for normal cellular function are not supplied, and the cell fails to function properly.

Certain antiinfective drugs have a selected toxicity for pathogens or parasites that have invaded the body. Penicillin and sulfonamides work because they poison or interfere with the life processes of bacteria without affecting the life processes of normal human cells. Research scientists continue to look for differences between cancer cells and normal cells so that they can apply the principle of selected toxicity in cancer treatment. Both drugs that have a selective affinity for cells and those that bind with enzymes may be counteracted by administering large amounts of natural substances with which the drugs compete. This process is known as administering an *antidote* to a drug that may be acting as a poison. For example, an antidote such as naloxone hydrochloride can be administered if a patient receives too much anesthesia or has taken a drug overdose.

Some drugs alter the function of a cell by affecting the physical properties of the cell membrane rather than altering biochemical processes within the cell. This is especially true of drugs that affect nerve cells, such as anesthetics and alcohol. A change in the cell membrane alters the permeability of the membrane, which in turn changes the flow of ions into and out of the cells. This change in ion flow alters the *polarity* (opposite effects at two extremities, the two extremities being inside and outside the cell membrane) on which nerve pulses are conducted, resulting in general sleep or stupor.

Drug Metabolism

After the drug has been absorbed and distributed, it is metabolized for excretion. During metabolism, the drug is converted into harmless byproducts, which are more easily eliminated by the kidneys. Most drugs are broken down by the enzyme activity of the liver. For oral medications that are absorbed in the small intestine, this process begins in the liver before distribution.

The ability to break down the chemical components of a drug varies among individuals. Factors that determine this ability include age, the presence of other drugs, and liver disease. Infants and aging individuals have more difficulty effectively metabolizing medications. Patients taking multiple medications also may be at increased risk for liver-related problems with metabolism because of the sheer number of chemicals the liver is exposed to on a daily basis. Individuals with chronic liver disease, such as **cirrhosis**, may not be able to metabolize even normal doses of medications. A *cumulative effect*, meaning the total amount of the drug present in the body after multiple doses, may result in a toxic condition if the drug is absorbed faster than it is metabolized. Because of these factors, drug therapy must be monitored closely in very young and aging patients, those taking multiple medications, and patients with chronic liver disease.

In contrast, patients receiving long-term drug therapy may develop overstimulation of the enzyme activity of the liver. This results in rapid destruction of the drug, and the patient has to take larger and larger doses for the drug to be effective. This situation is called *tolerance*.

Drug Excretion

After the drug has been metabolized, its byproducts must be excreted from the body. The kidneys are the most important route for the elimination of drugs. Most chemicals are filtered out of the blood, circulated through the kidneys, and excreted in the urine. Because the kidneys are so important in the elimination of chemicals from the body, drug therapy must be carefully monitored in patients with kidney disease or malfunction. Drugs are also eliminated through the sweat glands, saliva, and feces. Exhalation, another mechanism for drug elimination, serves as the basis for measuring alcohol concentrations in the blood by the breathalyzer test. Drugs may be eliminated through the milk glands of a lactating mother, which means that a breastfeeding woman must be extremely careful about taking medications.

The combination of metabolism and excretion reduces the amount of drug in the body at any given time. The *therapeutic dose* of a medication depends on many factors, including the drug's half-life. The *half-life* is the amount of time it takes for half a dose of medication to be metabolized and excreted from the body. Some drugs have extremely short half-lives (only minutes), whereas others can take days to leave the body. The amount of drug lost during one half-life depends on how much drug is present. Providers use the half-life of a drug to determine the timing of medication administration, or the dose intervals. The shorter the half-life of the drug, the closer together are the times when it should be administered. If the next dose of the drug is not given within the half-life, blood levels drop and the patient does not receive adequate therapeutic effects from the treatment.

Pharmacokinetic Terms	
Absorption	The movement of a drug into the bloodstream. The rate of absorption depends on many factors, including the route of administration.
Distribution	The transport of a drug from the site of administration to the location in the body where it is meant to act (i.e., the target tissue).
Metabolism	The inactivation of a drug, including the time required for a drug to be detoxified and broken down into byproducts. The liver typically metabolizes medications.
Excretion	The elimination of a drug from the body, including the route of elimination and the time required for this process. The kidneys typically excrete drug metabolites.

FACTORS AFFECTING DRUG ACTION

As was stated earlier, different people react to the same dose of medication in different ways, and the same patient can react to the same dose of the same drug differently on various occasions. A

TABLE 13-6 Physiologic Changes of Age and Effects on Medication Usage	
CHANGES WITH AGING	**EFFECTS ON MEDICATION**
Stomach takes longer to empty, and gastric acidity is reduced.	Increases the risk of stomach irritation and ulceration.
Increased percentage of adipose (fat) tissue in the body.	Increases likelihood of drug storage in fat; may lead to drug toxicity.
Fewer protein-binding sites available in bloodstream.	Reduces drug passage through cell membranes; increases blood level of drug; may lead to toxicity.
Liver function declines.	Slows rate of drug metabolism; increases risk of toxicity.
Kidney function declines.	Slows rate of elimination of drug byproducts; increases risk of toxicity and complications.
Peripheral vascular disease present; venous tone diminished.	Reduces distribution of drug to the periphery.
Fat-soluble medications pass through blood-brain barrier more easily.	May affect central nervous system; increases risk of vertigo and confusion.

number of factors are important in determining the correct medication for a patient.

Body Weight

The effect of a medication is directly related to the person's weight. Basically, the same dose has a lesser effect on a patient who weighs more and a greater effect on a person who weighs less. Manufacturers of adult medications calculate dosages based on a normal adult weight (approximately 150 pounds). Sometimes the provider adjusts the dose to better suit the patient's body size. Pediatric medications are designed for the body weight of the child.

Age

The most significant effect of age on the body's response to a drug occurs in newborns and elderly individuals. This usually is related to immature or deteriorating body systems. In addition, both patient groups are particularly sensitive to drugs that affect the CNS and are at risk of developing toxic drug levels. Consequently, dosage amounts for these two groups must be carefully calculated. The provider may opt to start therapy with very small doses and increase the dose over time based on the presence or absence of side effects. Table 13-6 summarizes the altered effects of medications on aging individuals.

Gender

Drugs may affect men and women differently. As has been mentioned, a pregnant woman must be extremely cautious when taking medications to prevent possible damage to the developing fetus. In addition, the side effects of some drugs can stimulate uterine contractions, causing premature labor and delivery. Intramuscular medications are absorbed faster by men because they generally have higher levels of muscle mass, which is rich in blood vessels. Because women typically have a higher body fat content and less muscle (resulting in fewer blood vessels in peripheral tissues compared with men), intramuscular drugs remain in their tissues longer. In the past, most clinical trials were conducted only on men; therefore, until newer trial results are released that include women, the effect of gender on the action and safety of medications is impossible to predict accurately.

Time of Day

Diurnal refers to during the day or time of light. Diurnal body rhythms play an important part in the effects of some drugs. Sedatives given in the morning are not as effective as those administered before bedtime because the CNS is more alert in the morning, causing increased resistance to the effects of the drug. Corticosteroid administration is preferred in the morning because this best mimics the body's natural pattern of corticosteroid production and elimination.

Pathologic Factors

Patients may adversely respond to drugs if they have liver or kidney disease because the body is unable to metabolize and excrete chemicals properly. Drugs may also produce pathologic conditions of the liver or kidneys, and patients may need to be monitored for potentially serious drug complications. For example, patients taking statin medications (e.g., atorvastatin calcium [Lipitor]) for **hypercholesterolemia** should have liver function studies done routinely because these drugs are very hard on liver cells.

Patients with liver or kidney disease have an increased risk of drug toxicity, which may result in unconsciousness or death. Reactions in patients with other diseases or disorders may be quite different from the expected response. Therefore, a thorough medical history of the patient must always be taken before medications are prescribed and administered.

Immune Responses

The presence of a drug can stimulate a patient's immune response, causing the patient to develop antibodies to a particular chemical. If the same drug is administered again, the patient will have an allergic reaction to the drug, ranging from a mild reaction to anaphylaxis, a serious respiratory and circulatory emergency. Antibiotics are the group of drugs that most commonly cause allergic responses. A typical low-level allergic response to an antibiotic is *urticaria,* or the formation of hives.

Psychological Factors

People may respond differently to a medication because of the way they feel about the drug. If a patient believes in the therapy, even a placebo (a sugar pill or sterile water thought to be a drug) may help or bring about relief. In addition, a patient's personality can affect whether he or she will follow directions for a particular drug; also, a negative mindset or mental attitude can reduce an expected response to a drug.

Tolerance

Tolerance is the phenomenon of reduced responsiveness to a drug. *Acquired tolerance* occurs after a particular drug has been taken for a period of time. *Cross-tolerance* occurs when a patient acquires a tolerance to one drug and becomes resistant to other, similar drugs. *Physical dependence,* such as occurs with narcotic addictions, often accompanies tolerance. The body becomes so adapted to the presence of the drug that it cannot function properly without it. To withdraw the drug is to throw the body out of its equilibrium, causing withdrawal symptoms.

Accumulation

When a drug is taken too frequently to allow for proper elimination, it accumulates in the tissues. The result is a more intense effect and a longer duration. Accumulation can cause overdose and/or toxic effects. An example of a toxic accumulation of medication is *ototoxicity* (a toxic condition affecting the ears), which results in nausea, vomiting, **tinnitus**, and vertigo. Proper dosage and timing of administration are the best methods of preventing drug accumulation.

Idiosyncrasy

Occasionally a person reacts to a drug in a manner that is unexpected and peculiar to that individual. An idiosyncratic response may manifest in many different ways; for example, a hypnotic drug may keep a person awake, acting as a stimulant to this person rather than as a depressant. Usually these reactions cannot be explained.

Drug-Drug Interactions

Special care must be taken with patients who take more than one drug on a regular basis. One medication may increase or decrease the effects of another or may cause unexpected side effects. To safeguard patients from potentially negative drug interactions, it is important at each visit to record a complete list of all drugs the patient is taking, including OTC medications and herbal products. However, because many patients do not know or get confused about the names and dosages of their medications, the best way to maintain an accurate record is to ask that patients bring their medication containers with them to each office visit. This way, you can list information about the medications in the patient's EHR and at the same time ask whether the patient has any questions about his or her treatment. It is also a good idea to advise patients to fill prescriptions at the same pharmacy because the pharmacist can monitor medications for potential drug interactions. One of the positive aspects of EHRs is that the computer program reviews possible drug-drug interactions if a correct list of all a patient's medications is included in the person's electronic record.

An example of a drug interaction is the effect of some antibiotics on oral contraceptives. Certain antibiotics can interact with birth control pills, making the birth control pills less effective and pregnancy more likely. Patients should be told that spotting (midcycle bleeding) may be the first sign that an antibiotic is interfering with the effectiveness of birth control pills. Examples of antibiotics that interact with birth control pills include penicillin (Veetids), amoxicillin (Amoxil), ampicillin (Omnipen), sulfamethoxazole plus trimethoprim (Septra or Bactrim), tetracycline (Sumycin), minocycline (Minocin), metronidazole (Flagyl), and nitrofurantoin (Macrobid or

Macrodantin). If a woman wants to prevent pregnancy while taking an antibiotic, the provider may recommend that she use a condom and **spermicide** as a backup birth control method while taking the medication and for at least 1 week after the completion of treatment.

CRITICAL THINKING APPLICATION   **13-4**

Sylvia Kramer, a 72-year-old patient of Dr. Simon, calls today and asks Kathy how she should be taking her heart medicine, diltiazem HCl (Cardizem). Mrs. Kramer has diabetes, hypertension, and a history of heart disease. She is overweight, has the potential for kidney disease, and takes a number of other prescriptions. What factors may have an impact on the potential effect of Mrs. Kramer's medication?

CLASSIFICATIONS OF DRUG ACTIONS

Clinical pharmacology is a complex subject. To make it easier, drugs are classified into groups according to their actions in the body (e.g., diuretics, emetics); the symptoms they relieve (e.g., antihistamine); or the body system they affect (e.g., drugs that act on the cardiovascular system). The following examples of drug classifications serve as a glossary of terms that describe some basic drug actions. As you read some of the examples, remember that a drug classified as one type of agent may have other uses and actions in other body systems. For example, a drug classified as a diuretic may also be an antihypertensive drug, and a vasodilator may also be a respiratory antispasmodic. It takes time to understand not only the basic classification of a particular drug, but also the many secondary uses and effects the drug has on the human body.

Examples of Drug Classifications

Adrenergics
Desired effects: Cause vasoconstriction (i.e., narrowing of the **lumen** of a blood vessel); dilate pupils and bronchioles; relax muscles of the GI and urinary tracts.
Examples: *Adrenergics used to treat hypotension:* isoproterenol (Isuprel); norepinephrine (Levophed). *Adrenergics used for nasal and ophthalmic decongestion:* naphazoline (Naphcon); phenylephrine (Neo-Synephrine); pseudoephedrine (Sudafed); tetrahydrozoline (Visine).
Indications for use: Stop superficial bleeding; raise and sustain blood pressure; relieve nasal congestion and relieve redness, burning, irritation, and dryness of the eyes.
Side effects and adverse reactions: Chest pain, tachycardia, headache, increased blood glucose levels, nervousness, tremors.

Adrenergic Blockers
Desired effects: Cause vasodilation; reduce blood pressure; increase muscle tone of GI walls.
Examples: valsartan (Diovan); propranolol (Inderal); atenolol (Tenormin); carvedilol (Coreg); tamsulosin (Flomax); metoprolol (Lopressor).
Indications for use: Control hypertension and peripheral vascular disease; treat prostatic hyperplasia.

Side effects and adverse reactions: Confusion, lowering of blood pressure, lowering of blood glucose levels, fatigue, reduced heart rate.

Analgesics
Desired effects: Reduce the sensory function of the brain; block pain receptors.
Examples: *Nonnarcotic OTCs:* aspirin; acetaminophen (Tylenol); ibuprofen (Advil, Motrin). *Narcotic:* hydrocodone w/APAP (Tylenol with codeine); oxycodone (OxyContin); meperidine (Demerol); hydrocodone (Vicodin).
Indications for use: Relieve pain.
Side effects and adverse reactions: *Nonnarcotic:* GI disorders, liver and kidney disorders, tinnitus. *Narcotic:* Suppression of vital signs, agitation, blurred vision, confusion, constipation, oversedation, restlessness.

Anesthetics
Desired effects: Produce insensibility to pain or the sensation of pain; block nerve impulses to the brain, resulting in unconsciousness; dilate pupils; lower blood pressure; reduce respiratory and pulse rates.
Examples: *Local:* benzocaine (Dermoplast, Solarcaine); lidocaine (Xylocaine); bupivacaine (Marcaine); lidocaine topical (Lidoderm); procaine (Novocain). *General:* midazolam (Versed).
Indications for use: Produce local anesthesia (absence of sensation without loss of consciousness) or general anesthesia (loss of consciousness).
Side effects and adverse reactions: Hypotension, cardiopulmonary depression, sedation, nausea, vomiting, headaches.

Antacids/Proton-Pump Inhibitors
Desired effect: Reduce acidity in the stomach.
Examples: omeprazole (Prilosec); esomeprazole (Nexium); rabeprazole (Aciphex); lansoprazole (Prevacid); pantoprazole (Protonix). *OTCs:* magaldrate (Riopan); calcium carbonate (Maalox).
Indications for use: Treat gastric hyperacidity; treatment of gastroesophageal reflux disease (GERD).
Side effects and adverse reactions: Constipation, diarrhea, electrolyte imbalance, flatulence, kidney stones, osteoporosis.

Antianxiety Agents
Desired effects: Reduce anxiety and tension.
Examples: chlordiazepoxide (Librium); clonazepam (Klonopin); chlorazepate (Tranxene); diazepam (Valium); alprazolam (Xanax); temazepam (Restoril); triazolam (Halcion).
Indications for use: Produce calmness and release muscle tension; sedation.
Side effects and adverse reactions: Agitation, amnesia, bizarre behaviors, confusion, reduced white blood cell (WBC) count, depression, drowsiness, lethargy, oversedation, tremors, photosensitivity.

Antibiotics
Desired effects: Kill or inhibit growth of microorganisms.
Examples: azithromycin (Zithromax); levofloxacin (Levaquin); cefaclor (Ceclor); tetracycline (Sumycin); amoxicillin (Amoxil);

amoxicillin/clavulanic acid (Augmentin); cefadroxil (Duricef); ciprofloxacin (Cipro); cephalexin (Keflex); doxycycline (Vibramycin).

Indications for use: Treat bacterial invasions and infections.

Side effects and adverse reactions: Hypersensitivity reaction, nausea, diarrhea, GI distress, light sensitivity, urticaria.

Anticholinergics

Desired effects: Parasympathetic blocking agents; reduce spasms in smooth muscles.

Examples: scopolamine or atropine sulfate; tiotropium inhalation (Spiriva); dicyclomine (Bentyl); ipratropium (Atrovent).

Indications for use: Dry secretions before surgery; prevent bronchospasm.

Side effects and adverse reactions: Blurred vision, confusion, reduced GI and genitourinary motility, dilation of pupils, fever, flushing, headache, increased heart rate.

Anticoagulants

Desired effects: Delay or block clotting of blood.

Examples: rivaroxaban (Xarelto); heparin; enoxaparin sodium (Lovenox); warfarin sodium (Coumadin); tinzaparin (Innohep).

Primary uses: Treat blood clots, thrombophlebitis; prevent clot formation.

Side effects and adverse reactions: Increased bleeding; blood irregularities; GI, liver, and kidney disease.

Anticonvulsants

Desired effects: Prevent seizures; reduce excessive stimulation of the brain.

Examples: clonazepam (Klonopin); gabapentin (Neurontin); phenytoin (Dilantin); phenobarbital; carbamazepine (Tegretol); lamotrigine (Lamictal); pregabalin (Lyrica); topiramate (Topamax); valproic acid (Depakene).

Indications for use: Treat epilepsy and other neurologic disorders (e.g., peripheral neuropathy).

Side effects and adverse reactions: Sedation, vertigo, visual disturbances, GI disturbances, liver complications.

Antidepressants

Desired effect: Treat depression.

Examples: venlafaxine hydrochloride (Effexor); sertraline (Zoloft); escitalopram (Lexapro); duloxetine (Cymbalta); bupropion (Wellbutrin); trazodone HCl (Desyrel); fluoxetine (Prozac); imipramine pamoate (Tofranil); amitriptyline (Elavil); citalopram (Celexa).

Indications for use: Elevate mood; treat other neurologic disorders (e.g., migraines).

Side effects and adverse reactions: Anorexia, anxiety, sexual dysfunction, fatigue, drowsiness, vertigo, weight gain, confusion, blurred vision.

Antiemetics

Desired effect: Act on hypothalamic center in the brain to reduce or prevent nausea and vomiting.

Examples: prochlorperazine (Compazine); trimethobenzamide (Tigan); metoclopramide (Reglan); granisetron (Kytril); ondansetron (Zofran); promethazine (Phenergan).

Indications for use: Prevent and relieve nausea and vomiting; manage motion sickness.

Side effects and adverse reactions: Dry mouth, sedation, drowsiness, diarrhea, blurred vision.

Antifungals

Desired effects: Slow or retard multiplication of fungi.

Examples: miconazole (Monistat); nystatin (Mycostatin); fluconazole (Diflucan); ketoconazole (Nizoral); terbinafine (Lamisil).

Indications for use: Treat systemic or local fungal infections.

Side effects and adverse reactions: Anemia, chills, hypotension, vertigo, fever, kidney and liver damage, malaise, photophobia, muscle and joint pain.

Antihistamines

Desired effects: Counteract the effects of histamine by blocking action in tissues; may be used to inhibit gastric secretions.

Examples: cetirizine (Zyrtec); fexofenadine (Allegra); loratadine (Claritin, Alavert); chlorpheniramine (Chlor-Trimeton); diphenhydramine (Benadryl); promethazine (Phenergan); cimetidine (Tagamet); ranitidine (Zantac).

Indications for use: Relieve allergies; prevent gastric ulcers.

Side effects and adverse reactions: CNS depression, muscle weakness, epigastric distress, dry mouth.

Antihypertensive Agents

Desired effects: Block nerve impulses that cause arteries to constrict; slow the heart rate, reducing its contractility; restrict the hormone aldosterone in the blood.

Examples: amlodipine (Norvasc); atenolol (Tenormin); doxazosin mesylate (Cardura); metoprolol (Lopressor or Toprol); methyldopa (Aldomet); valsartan (Diovan); amlodipine plus benazepril (Lotrel); propranolol (Inderal); diltiazem (Cardizem); nifedipine (Procardia); benazepril (Lotensin); lisinopril (Prinivil, Zestril); losartan (Cozaar).

Indications for use: Reduce and control blood pressure.

Side effects and adverse reactions: Headache, vertigo, GI disturbances, rash, hypotension, nonproductive cough.

Antiinflammatory Agents

Desired effect: Reduce inflammation.

Examples: *Nonsteroidal antiinflammatory drugs (NSAIDs):* ibuprofen (Advil, Motrin); naproxen (Naprosyn); celecoxib (Celebrex); indomethacin (Indocin). *Steroidal antiinflammatory drugs (SAIDs):* dexamethasone (Decadron); prednisone (Cortisone); methylprednisolone (Medrol, Depo-Medrol); montelukast sodium (Singulair); fluticasone propionate (Flonase); mometasone (Nasonex). *Inhalers:* flunisolide (AeroBid); triamcinolone (Azmacort).

Indications for use: Treat arthritis and other inflammatory disorders, including asthma and allergic rhinitis.

Side effects and adverse reactions: GI upset, GI bleeding, hepatitis, drowsiness, tinnitus, irregular heart rate, kidney disorders.

Antimigraine Agents

Desired effect: Alter circulation to the brain.

Examples: topiramate (Topamax); sumatriptan (Imitrex); zolmitriptan (Zomig).

Indications for use: Treatment or prevention of migraine headaches.

Side effects and adverse reactions: Confusion, psychomotor slowing, difficulty concentrating, memory problems, rare but serious cardiac events.

Antineoplastics

Desired effects: Inhibit development of and destroy cancerous cells.

Examples: hydroxyurea (Hydrea); cyclophosphamide (Cytoxan); chlorambucil (Leukeran); raloxifene (Evista).

Indications for use: Cancer chemotherapy and/or prevention.

Side effects and adverse reactions: Nausea, vomiting, bone marrow depression, aplastic anemia, hair loss, GI ulcers.

Antipsychotics

Desired effect: Alter chemical actions in the brain.

Examples: quetiapine (Seroquel); risperidone (Risperdal); aripiprazole (Abilify); olanzapine (Zyprexa); chlorpromazine (Thorazine); haloperidol (Haldol).

Indications for use: Treat the symptoms of schizophrenia and bipolar disorder.

Side effects and adverse reactions: GI distress, hypotension, electrocardiographic (ECG) changes, vertigo, sedation, headache, photosensitivity.

Antipruritics

Desired effect: Relieve itching.

Examples: calamine lotion; hydrocortisone ointment; diphenhydramine (Benadryl).

Indications for use: Treat allergies or topical exposures that cause itching.

Side effects and adverse reactions: Topical agents have no side effects; Benadryl can cause vertigo, sedation, and nervousness.

Antipyretics

Desired effect: Lower body temperature.

Examples: aspirin; acetaminophen; ibuprofen.

Indications for use: Reduce fever.

Side effects and adverse reactions: GI disturbance, liver disease; with aspirin, possibility of Reye's syndrome if given during or after a viral disease.

Antispasmodics

Desired effects: Relieve or prevent spasms from musculoskeletal injury or inflammation.

Examples: methocarbamol (Robaxin); carisoprodol (Soma); cyclobenzaprine (Flexeril).

Indications for use: Treat sports injuries.

Side effects and adverse reactions: CNS suppression, drowsiness, vertigo.

Antitussives

Desired effect: Inhibit the cough center.

Examples: *Narcotic:* codeine sulfate. *Nonnarcotic:* dextromethorphan (Robitussin DM).

Indications for use: Temporarily suppress a nonproductive cough; reduce the thickness of secretions.

Side effects and adverse reactions: Codeine cough suppressants cause CNS depression and constipation.

Antiviral Agents

Desired effects: Inhibit the growth or reduce the spread of viral cells.

Examples: interferon beta-1a (Avonex); sofosbuvir (Sovaldi); dimethyl fumarate (Tecfidera); acyclovir (Zovirax); interferon; valacyclovir (Valtrex); oseltamivir (Tamiflu); famciclovir (Famvir); includes the human immunodeficiency virus (HIV) medications efavirenz, emtricitabine, and tenofovir (Atripla); emtricitabine and tenofovir (Truvada); darunavir (Prezista).

Indications for use: Treat viral infections, including oral and genital herpes, influenza, and HIV.

Side effects and adverse reactions: Confusion, diarrhea, headache, kidney disease, urticaria, vomiting.

Bronchodilators

Desired effect: Relax the smooth muscle of the bronchi.

Examples: theophylline (Theo-Dur); epinephrine (Adrenalin); albuterol (Ventolin HFA, Proventil, ProAir HFA); budesonide and formoterol (Symbicort); isoproterenol (Isuprel).

Indications for use: Treat asthma, bronchospasm; promote bronchodilation.

Side effects and adverse reactions: CNS stimulation, tremors, tachycardia, increased blood glucose level, elevated blood pressure.

Cathartics (Laxatives)

Desired effect: Increase peristaltic activity of the large intestine.

Examples: magnesium hydroxide (Milk of Magnesia); bisacodyl (Dulcolax); casanthranol (Peri-Colace).

Indications for use: Increase and hasten bowel evacuation (defecation).

Side effects and adverse reactions: Nausea, bloating, flatulence, cramping.

Central Nervous System Stimulants

Desired effects: Affect chemicals in the brain that contribute to hyperactivity and impulse control.

Examples: methylphenidate (Concerta, Ritalin); modafinil (Provigil); lisdexamfetamine (Vyvanse).

Indications for use: Treat attention deficit disorder (ADD) and attention deficit/hyperactivity disorder (ADHD).

Side effects and adverse reactions: Irregular heartbeat, rash, sore throat, aggression, hypertension, numbness, fainting.

Contraceptives

Desired effect: Inhibit conception.

Examples: medroxyprogesterone acetate (Depo-Provera); Ortho Evra; etonogestrel/ethinyl estradiol (NuvaRing).

Indications for use: Prevent pregnancy.

Side effects and adverse reactions: Breast enlargement and tenderness; cardiovascular risk; GI upset; headache; irregular menstrual bleeding; deep vein thrombosis; pulmonary embolus (PE).

Decongestants

Desired effect: Relieve local congestion in the tissues.

Examples: ephedrine or phenylephrine (Neo-Synephrine); pseudoephedrine (Sudafed); oxymetazoline (Afrin); mometasone (Nasonex).

Indications for use: Relieve nasal and sinus congestion caused by common cold, hay fever, or upper respiratory tract disorders.

Side effects and adverse reactions: Arrhythmias, hypertension, headache, nausea, dry mouth.

Diuretics

Desired effects: Inhibit reabsorption of sodium and chloride in the kidneys; promote excretion of excess fluid in the body.

Examples: hydrochlorothiazide (Dyazide, Esidrix, HydroDiuril); furosemide (Lasix); triamterene (Dyrenium).

Indications for use: Increase urinary output; lower blood pressure.

Side effects and adverse reactions: Dehydration, muscle weakness, fatigue, gout, hyperglycemia.

Erectile Dysfunction Agents

Desired effect: Facilitate an erection.

Examples: sildenafil (Viagra); tadalafil (Cialis).

Indications for use: Facilitates an erection in patients with erectile dysfunction (impotence) and symptoms of benign prostatic hypertrophy (enlarged prostate).

Side effects and adverse reactions: Headache, flushing, nasal congestion, myalgia, prolonged erections, vision and hearing problems, cerebrovascular accident (CVA), myocardial infarction (MI).

Expectorants

Desired effect: Liquefy secretions in the bronchial tubes so that they can be coughed out.

Examples: dextromethorphan (Benylin).

Indications for use: Relieve upper respiratory tract congestion.

Side effects and adverse reactions: Vomiting, diarrhea, abdominal pain.

Hematopoietic Agents

Desired effect: Promote red blood cell production.

Examples: epoetin alfa (Epogen, Procrit); pegfilgrastim (Neulasta).

Primary use: Treat anemia in patients undergoing chemotherapy.

Side effects and adverse reactions: Headache, arthralgia, nausea, hypertension, diarrhea.

Hemostatic Agents

Desired effects: Control bleeding; act as a blood coagulant.

Examples: phytonadione, vitamin K; absorbable hemostatic agents (e.g., Gelfoam, Surgicel) are applied directly to a wound.

Indications for use: Control acute or chronic blood-clotting disorder; promote formation of absorbable, artificial clot.

Side effects and adverse reactions: Hypersensitivity reactions, transient flushing, dizziness; newborn hyperbilirubinemia.

Hormone Replacement Agents

Desired effects: Replace hormones or compensate for hormone deficiency.

Examples: insulin (Levemir, NovoLog, Lantus Solostar, Humalog); levothyroxine sodium (Synthroid or Levoxyl); estrogen (Premarin); vasopressin (Pitressin).

Indications for use: Maintain adequate hormone levels.

Side effects and adverse reactions: *Estrogen replacement therapy:* Hot flashes, decreased sex drive, nausea, vomiting.

Hypnotics (Sedatives)

Desired effects: Induce sleep; lessen the activity of the brain.

Examples: zolpidem tartrate (Ambien); eszopiclone (Lunesta); secobarbital (Seconal); flurazepam (Dalmane); temazepam (Restoril); barbiturates.

Indications for use: Treat insomnia; obtain sedation (lower doses).

Side effects and adverse reactions: Daytime sedation, confusion, dry mouth, vertigo.

Lipid-Lowering Agents

Desired effects: Reduce blood cholesterol levels and/or increase high-density lipoprotein (HDL) level.

Examples: atorvastatin calcium (Lipitor); simvastatin (Zocor); ezetimibe (Vytorin or Zetia); rosuvastatin (Crestor); fenofibrate (Tricor).

Indications for use: Reduce low-density lipoprotein (LDL) and very low density lipoprotein (VLDL) levels and triglycerides; increase HDL.

Side effects and adverse reactions: GI discomfort, muscle pain and weakness, liver complications, hypersensitivity, cataracts, myopathy.

Miotics

Desired effect: Cause the pupil to contract.

Examples: carbachol (Isopto Carbachol); pilocarpine (Isopto Carpine).

Indications for use: Counteract pupil dilation.

Side effects and adverse reactions: Corneal edema, clouding, stinging, tearing, headache.

Monoclonal Antibodies

Desired effect: A class of highly specific antibodies that are produced in a laboratory and used to treat cancer and conditions that cause extreme inflammation, such as rheumatoid arthritis and psoriasis.

Examples: adalimumab (Humira); ustekinumab (Stelara); etanercept (Enbrel); trastuzumab (Herceptin); imatinib (Gleevec); fingolimod hydrochloride (Gilenya); infliximab (Remicade); rituximab (Rituxan); pemetrexed (Alimta); glatiramer (Copaxone); bevacizumab (Avastin).

Indications for use: Cancer treatment; treatment of rheumatoid arthritis, psoriasis, Crohn's disease, ulcerative colitis, multiple sclerosis.

Side effects and adverse reactions: Injection site reactions, headache, rash, sinusitis, hypersensitivity, neurologic complications, respiratory infections.

Mydriatic Agents (Anticholinergic)

Desired effect: Dilate the pupil.

Example: atropine sulfate (Isopto Atropine).

Indications for use: Ophthalmologic examinations.

Side effects and adverse reactions: Stinging, burning, photosensitivity.

Narcotics

Desired effects: Depress the CNS, causing insensibility or stupor.

Examples: *Natural narcotics:* opium group (codeine phosphate, morphine sulfate); buprenorphine and naloxone (Suboxone); oxycodone (OxyContin). *Synthetic narcotics:* meperidine (Demerol), methadone (Dolophine).

Indications for use: Relieve pain.

Side effects and adverse reactions: Suppression of vital signs; agitation, blurred vision, confusion, constipation, oversedation, restlessness.

Oral Hypoglycemic Agents

Desired effects: Reduce blood glucose level by increasing insulin production and/or reducing target cell resistance to insulin, or by delaying glucose absorption.

Examples: liraglutide (Victoza 3-Pak); rosiglitazone (Avandia); sitagliptin (Januvia); metformin HCl (Glucophage); acarbose (Precose); chlorpropamide (Diabinese); glimepiride (Amaryl); glipizide (Glucotrol); glyburide (Micronase).

Indications for use: Manage diabetes mellitus type 2.

Side effects and adverse reactions: GI irritation, fatigue, hypoglycemia, vertigo; possible hypersensitivity reactions.

Osteoporosis Agents

Desired effects: Inhibit bone reabsorption and/or promote use of calcium.

Examples: alendronate (Fosamax); risedronate (Actonel); calcitonin (Miacalcin nasal spray and Calcimar); ibandronate (Boniva); raloxifene hydrochloride (Evista); zoledronic acid (Reclast, Zometa).

Indications for use: Promote bone mineral density and reverse progression of osteoporosis.

Side effects and adverse reactions: GI disorders, esophageal irritation.

Respiratory Corticosteroid Agents

Desired effects: Reduce airway inflammation and bronchial resistance.

Examples: fluticasone and salmeterol (Advair Diskus); fluticasone propionate (Flovent HFA); budesonide and formoterol fumarate dehydrate (Symbicort); tiotropium bromide (Spiriva Handihaler); mometasone furoate monohydrate (Nasonex).

Indications for use: Long-term relief of asthma symptoms; decrease frequency of asthma attacks; manage chronic obstructive pulmonary disease (COPD) and seasonal allergies.

Side effects and adverse reactions: Headache, pharyngitis, myalgia, hypersensitivity, oral candidiasis. Advair Diskus is contraindicated in patients with a milk allergy.

Table 13-7 lists details about the top 50 prescribed drugs in 2014. Review this list to become familiar with some of the most commonly prescribed medications. These are just a few examples of the different classifications of medications. Remember to research and review all medications before administering them.

TABLE 13-7   Top 50 Prescribed Drugs in 2014

BRAND NAME	CLASSIFICATION	INDICATIONS AND DESIRED EFFECTS	SIDE EFFECTS	ADVERSE REACTIONS
Synthroid	Thyroid hormone	Increase BMR; enhance gluconeogenesis; stimulate protein synthesis	Reversible hair loss, dry skin, GI intolerance	Overdosage causes signs of hyperthyroidism, cardiac arrhythmias
Crestor	Cholesterol lowering (antihyperlipidemic)	Decrease LDL, VLDL, triglycerides; increase HDL	Pharyngitis, headache, epigastric distress, myalgia	Hypersensitivity, cataracts, myopathy
Nexium	Proton-pump inhibitor	Increase gastric pH; reduce gastric acid production; esophagitis; GERD; *Helicobacter pylori* ulcers	Headache, diarrhea, abdominal pain	Hepatitis, hypersensitivity, decreased WBC count
Ventolin HFA	Bronchodilator	Relieve bronchospasm, reduce airway resistance; can function as a rescue inhaler to relieve immediate symptoms of an asthma attack	Headache, nausea, restlessness, tremors, dizziness, throat irritation, hypertension	Palpitations, tachycardia, slight increase in BP, chest pain
Advair Diskus	Long-acting respiratory corticosteroid agent	Relieve symptoms of asthma; reduce airway resistance	Headache, pharyngitis, URI, myalgia, nausea	Hypersensitivity, palpitations, chest pain, oral candidiasis
Diovan	Antihypertensive	Cause vasodilation; decrease peripheral vessel resistance; decrease BP	Headache, dizziness, viral infection, fatigue, abdominal pain	Hypotension with overdosage, tachycardia, hypersensitivity
Lantus Solostar	Long-acting insulin	Control glucose levels	Localized reaction at injection site, hypokalemia, allergic reaction	Severe hypoglycemia with insulin overdose, diabetic ketoacidosis

Continued

TABLE 13-7   Top 50 Prescribed Drugs in 2014—*continued*

BRAND NAME	CLASSIFICATION	INDICATIONS AND DESIRED EFFECTS	SIDE EFFECTS	ADVERSE REACTIONS
Cymbalta	Antidepressant	Relieve depression	Nausea, dry mouth, diarrhea, insomnia, headache	Increased heart rate, orthostatic hypotension, skin rashes, GI disorders
Vyvanse	Stimulant	Improve attention span; decrease distractibility and impulsive behavior; treat ADHD	Abdominal discomfort and GI symptoms, decreased appetite, headaches, insomnia, dry mouth, dizziness	Cardiovascular complications in patients with heart problems, hypersensitivity; overdosage may cause arrhythmias, seizures, psychosis
Lyrica	Anticonvulsant	Seizure control; treat fibromyalgia; treat pain caused by nerve damage in diabetic neuropathy, herpes zoster (postherpetic neuralgia)	Muscle pain, weakness, or tenderness; vision problems; easy bruising or bleeding; swelling of hands or feet; rapid weight gain	Mood or behavior changes, anxiety, panic attacks, trouble sleeping, hyperactive, increased depression, suicidal thoughts
Humira	Monoclonal antibody	Reduce inflammation and joint destruction in rheumatoid arthritis	Injection site reactions, headache, rash, sinusitis, nausea	Hypersensitivity, neurologic events, respiratory infections and bronchitis
Enbrel	Antirheumatic, immunomodulator, monoclonal antibody	Relieve symptoms of rheumatoid arthritis, psoriasis, and other inflammatory conditions	Injection site reaction, abdominal pain, URI, headache	Infections, heart failure, hypertension, nervous system disorders
Remicade	Antirheumatic, immunomodulator, monoclonal antibodies	Decrease inflamed areas of intestine, synovitis, and joint erosion	Headache, nausea, fatigue, fever	Hypersensitivity, infusion reactions, lupuslike syndrome
Copaxone	Immunosuppressant	Slow progression of MS	Injection site reactions, arthralgia, vasodilation, anxiety	Infection, lymphadenopathy, hypertension, decreased WBC count
Neulasta	Hematopoietic agent	Increase phagocytosis and decrease incidence of infection during chemotherapy	Bone pain, nausea, fatigue, headache, arthralgia	Allergic reactions, spleen complications
Rituxan	Antineoplastic, monoclonal antibodies	Cytotoxicity, reduce tumor size; reduce joint destruction in RA	Fever, chills, headache, angioedema, nausea, rash	Arrhythmias, acute renal failure, hypersensitivity
Spiriva Handihaler	Bronchodilator	Relieve bronchospasm for patients with COPD	Dry mouth, sinusitis, pharyngitis, dyspepsia, UTI, rhinitis	Chest pain, angioedema, hypersensitivity
Januvia	Antidiabetic agent, oral hypoglycemic	Lower blood glucose and A_{1c} levels over time	Headache, nasopharyngitis, URI, hypoglycemia	Overdose causes severe hypoglycemia, pancreatitis, hypersensitivity
Atripla	HIV antiviral combination drug (three drugs)	Decrease viral load	Lactic acidosis, serious liver problems, serious psychiatric problems, kidney disorder, osteopenia, skin discoloration, diarrhea, dizziness, drowsiness	Serious complications from lactic acidosis and liver disorders
Avastin	Antiangiogenic agent, monoclonal antibody	Treatment of metastatic carcinoma of the colon; glioblastoma, and renal cell cancer	Fainting, anorexia, heartburn, diarrhea, weight loss, dry mouth, sores on the skin or in the mouth, voice changes	Gastric ulcers, bleeding, slow wound healing

TABLE 13-7   Top 50 Prescribed Drugs in 2014—*continued*

BRAND NAME	CLASSIFICATION	INDICATIONS AND DESIRED EFFECTS	SIDE EFFECTS	ADVERSE REACTIONS
OxyContin	Analgesic narcotic; contains codeine and acetaminophen	Relieve pain	Sleepiness, dizziness, hypotension, anorexia, constipation	Overdose causes respiratory failure, hepatotoxicity from overdose of acetaminophen; addiction
Epogen	Hematopoietic agent	Stimulate RBC production; raise H&H; treatment of anemia in chemotherapy patients	Fever, diarrhea, nausea, vomiting, edema	Encephalopathy, thrombosis, CVA, MI, seizures
Celebrex	NSAID, analgesic	Reduce inflammation and relieve pain; treatment of RA and other forms of arthritis	GI disorders, URI, back pain, peripheral edema, rash	Increased risk of CV events and GI bleeding
Truvada	HIV (combination of two antiviral drugs)	Prevent HIV cells from multiplying in the body; reduce risk of HIV infection	New infections, GI disorders, chest pain, dry cough, wheezing, cold sores, tachycardia	Hypersensitivity, lactic acidosis
Gleevec	Antineoplastic, monoclonal antibody	Suppress tumor growth	Nausea, diarrhea, vomiting, headache, fluid retention	Severe fluid retention, decreased WBC and platelet counts; pneumonia
Herceptin	Chemotherapeutic agent; adjunct therapy for cancers of the breast or stomach; monoclonal antibody	Interfere with growth and spread of cancer cells in the body	Nausea, diarrhea, weight loss, fever, headache, sleep problems, cough, trouble breathing, skin rash, bruising, cold symptoms	Cardiomyopathy, infusion reactions, embryo-fetal toxicity, pulmonary toxicity
Lucentis	Ophthalmic injection	Keep new blood vessels from forming under the retina; treat wet age-related macular degeneration and diabetic retinopathy	Itchy or watery eyes, dry eyes, swelling of the eyelids, blurred vision, sinus pain, sore throat, joint pain	Hypersensitivity, exophthalmos from increased intraocular pressure, detached retina, CVA, MI
Namenda	Alzheimer's disease	Reduce deterioration in moderate to severe Alzheimer's disease	Dizziness, headache, confusion, constipation, hypertension, cough	AV block, CNS reactions, hypersensitivity
Zetia	Cholesterol lowering (antihyperlipidemic)	Reduce total cholesterol, LDL, triglycerides; increase HDL	URI, headache, back pain, diarrhea, myalgia	None known
Levemir	Long-acting insulin	Control glucose levels	Localized reaction at injection site, hypokalemia, allergic reaction	Severe hypoglycemia with insulin overdose, diabetic ketoacidosis
Symbicort	Glucocorticoid inhaler, long-term treatment of asthma and COPD	Relieve symptoms of asthma and reduce airway resistance	Headache, URI, sore throat, sinusitis, oral candidiasis	Hypersensitivity, palpitations, ECG changes
Sovaldi	Antiviral	Prevent hepatitis C virus cells from multiplying	Headache, fatigue, mild itching, nausea, insomnia	Hypersensitivity, birth defects or death in unborn baby
Novolog	Combination insulin	Control glucose levels	Localized reaction at injection site, hypokalemia, allergic reaction	Severe hypoglycemia with insulin overdose, diabetic ketoacidosis
Tecfidera	Interferon	Treat relapsing multiple sclerosis	Nausea, diarrhea, stomach pain, flushing	Hypersensitivity, serious viral infection of the brain
Suboxone	Opioid narcotic	Treat narcotic addiction; not used as a pain medication	Tongue pain, redness or numbness inside mouth, constipation, headache, insomnia, swelling of arms or legs	Respiratory arrest, addictive, hypersensitivity

Continued

TABLE 13-7　Top 50 Prescribed Drugs in 2014—*continued*

BRAND NAME	CLASSIFICATION	INDICATIONS AND DESIRED EFFECTS	SIDE EFFECTS	ADVERSE REACTIONS
Humalog	Rapid acting or a combination insulin	Control glucose levels	Localized reaction at injection site, hypokalemia, allergic reaction	Severe hypoglycemia with insulin overdose, diabetic ketoacidosis
Xarelto	Anticoagulant	Prevent new clot formation	Bleeding, pruritus, pain in extremities, muscle spasms	Hemorrhage, hypersensitivity
Seroquel XR	Extended-release antipsychotic	Manage psychotic disorders and schizophrenia; adjunct antidepressant	Headache, sleepiness, dizziness, constipation, orthostatic hypotension	Heart block, hypokalemia, tachycardia
Viagra	Erectile dysfunction (ED) agent	Facilitate an erection	Headache, flushing, nasal congestion, UTI, diarrhea	Severe hypotension, prolonged erections, vision problems, CVA, MI
Alimta	Chemotherapeutic agent	Treatment of lung cancer; interfere with growth and spread of cancer cells in the body	Fatigue, anorexia, weight loss, N/V, diarrhea, rash, hair loss.	Hypersensitivity, kidney and liver damage
Victoza 3-Pak	Antidiabetic agent	Lower blood glucose and A_{1c}	Headache, nausea, diarrhea, GERD	Severe hypoglycemia, pancreatitis, hypersensitivity
Avonex	Interferon antiviral	Treatment of relapsing-remitting MS	Headache, flulike symptoms, myalgia, URI, generalized pain, sinusitis	Anemia, rare life-threatening reactions
Nasonex	Corticosteroid allergy agent	Decrease response to seasonal allergens; stabilize asthma	Nasal irritation, sore throat, headache	Hypersensitivity, stimulates wheezing in asthmatics
Cialis	ED agent	Facilitate erection in ED	Headache, myalgia, flushing, nasal congestion	Prolonged erections, vision and hearing problems, CVA, MI
Gilenya	Biologic response modifier, MS agent	Reduce progression of MS	Headache, flulike symptoms, diarrhea, back pain	Increased risk of infections, CVA, hypersensitivity, dyspnea
Stelara	Immunomodulator, antipsoriatic agent, monoclonal antibody	Reduce inflammation, scaling of psoriasis plaques	Headache, fatigue, nasopharyngitis, URI	Hypersensitivity, risk of skin cancer, neurologic complications
Flovent HFA	Corticosteroid inhaler	Prevent or control inflammation and asthma	Throat and nasal irritation, dry mouth, candidiasis	Anaphylaxis, glaucoma, nasal septal perforation
Prezista	Antiretroviral; protease inhibitor	Interrupt HIV replication; slow progression of HIV infection	Diarrhea, abdominal pain, headache, rash, N/V	Immune system reactions, pancreatitis, serious skin rashes, hepatitis
Procrit	Hematopoietic agent, erythropoiesis-stimulating agent (ESA)	Promote production of RBCs to raise H&H; treatment of anemia in chemotherapy patients	Fever, diarrhea, N/V, edema	Encephalopathy, thrombosis, CVA, MI, seizures
Isentress	Antiviral; integrase inhibitor	Prevents HIV cells from multiplying; treatment of HIV strains that are resistant to multiple antiretroviral drugs and for people with drug-sensitive HIV strains	Diarrhea, nausea, headache	Increase in total cholesterol, rash, increased liver enzymes, increased blood glucose, psychiatric disorders

www.medscape.com/viewarticle/825053; and www.webmd.com/news/20140805/top-10-drugs.
ADHD, Attention deficit/hyperactivity disorder; *AV*, atrioventricular; *BMR*, basal metabolic rate; *BP*, blood pressure; *CNS*, central nervous system; *COPD*, chronic obstructive pulmonary disease; *CV*, cardiovascular; *CVA*, cerebrovascular accident; *ECG*, electrocardiogram; *GERD*, gastroesophageal reflux disease; *GI*, gastrointestinal; *HCV*, hepatitis C virus; *HDL*, high-density lipoprotein; *H&H*, hemoglobin and hematocrit; *HIV*, human immunodeficiency virus; *LDL*, low-density lipoprotein; *MI*, myocardial infarction; *MS*, multiple sclerosis; *NSAID*, nonsteroidal antiinflammatory drug; *N/V*, nausea and vomiting; *RA*, rheumatoid arthritis; *RBC*, red blood cells; *URI*, upper respiratory infection; *UTI*, urinary tract infection; *VLDL*, very low density lipoprotein; *WBC*, white blood cells.

HERBAL AND ALTERNATIVE THERAPIES

The use of alternative therapies, often called *complementary* or *holistic medicine,* has become very popular in the United States. According to estimates, more than 42% of adult patients use some form of alternative therapy, such as herbal medicine, acupuncture, massage therapy, chiropractic care, or mind-body therapies. Even though only limited scientific studies prove the effectiveness of herbs, their use to relieve the symptoms of common patient complaints is definitely on the rise. It is estimated that 15 million adults take prescription drugs along with herbal and vitamin supplements. Patients typically are hesitant to discuss their use of herbal products with their provider, which makes it difficult for providers to assess potential drug-herb interactions. Therefore, it is important that medical assistants become familiar with common alternative therapies and that they include questions about the use of these therapies when gathering information about the patient's medication history.

Herbal Products

Regulation of Herbal Products

Herbal medicine uses plant-based products to promote health and treat the symptoms of a wide range of diseases. These remedies typically are marketed by manufacturers and are regulated by the federal government as dietary supplements. The FDA is responsible for regulating dietary supplements under the Dietary Supplement Health and Education Act of 1994 (DSHEA). Under DSHEA, manufacturers are responsible for performing tests and ensuring the safety of dietary supplements before they are sold. However, these products are not registered with the FDA and do not have to go through the rigorous process of FDA approval that new drugs face before they are produced and sold. In addition, there is no federal control over the standardization of herbal dietary supplements. Pharmaceutical companies must prove that each batch of a drug is standardized or consistent with previous batches. Because this is not the case with dietary supplements, there are no guarantees that the amounts of active ingredients in a herbal supplement remain the same over time or are similar to the amounts found in the same supplement produced by a different company.

The FDA has the authority to oversee the manufacture of domestically made and foreign-made supplements. Supplement manufacturers must provide evidence that their products actually contain what the labels claim and that the products are free of contaminants. According to FDA regulations, dietary supplement labels must list the following:

- Product name with the word "supplement" on the label
- Name and location of the manufacturer or distributor
- Structure/function claim: Claims of specific benefits may be made, but the following statement must be included: *This statement has not been evaluated by the Food and Drug Administration. This product is not intended to diagnose, treat, cure, or prevent any disease.*
- Directions for use
- For plant-based herbal preparations: the name of the plant or the part of the plant used
- For blended products created by the manufacturer: the components and the weight of each ingredient

- All nondietary ingredients (e.g., fillers, artificial colors, sweeteners, flavors), listed in descending order of weight
- The label may include warnings about use, but the lack of cautionary statements does not mean that no adverse effects are associated with the supplement.

Commonly Used Herbal Products

Table 13-8 summarizes the most commonly used herbal products. Information about herbal remedies is constantly changing, but the federal government has several websites that can be used as references. These include the National Center for Complementary and Alternative Medicine (*http://nccam.nih.gov/*) and the National Institutes of Health Office of Dietary Supplements (*http://ods.od.nih.gov/index.aspx*).

Alternative Therapies

Acupuncture

Acupuncture treatments are part of traditional Chinese medicine, which is based on the concept that disease is caused by a disruption in the flow of life force and an imbalance between yin and yang. In acupuncture treatments, thin metal needles are inserted through the skin to stimulate specific points in the body to restore and maintain health. Studies indicate that acupuncture may help reduce pain and relieve the nausea associated with chemotherapy treatments. Therapy involves a series of treatments, with the placement of as many as 12 needles in various locations on the body.

During the procedure, the patient is placed supine, prone, or in the Sims position, depending on the needle insertion site. Although the procedure is not painful, the patient may notice a sharp sensation when the needles initially are placed. After the needles have been in place for a time, they may be rotated gently, heated, or electrically stimulated to achieve the benefit sought by the treatment. The needles usually are left in place for 5 to 20 minutes, and after they have been removed, the provider typically discusses the results of treatment with the patient.

Chiropractic Care

Chiropractic providers apply techniques that focus on the body's physical structure (usually the spine) and perform manipulations or anatomic adjustments to correct alignment problems and help the body heal itself. Many patients combine chiropractic therapy with conventional medical treatment to obtain relief of chronic pain in the lower back and neck and to relieve persistent headaches. Chiropractors must earn a Doctor of Chiropractic degree at an accredited college and pass a state licensing examination before they can practice. Besides spinal adjustments, patient treatment plans may include a combination of hot and cold therapies; electrical stimulation; rest and rehabilitation exercises; dietary and lifestyle counseling; and the use of dietary supplements.

Mind-Body Therapy

Mind-body therapy uses biofeedback to teach patients to use their thoughts to control certain body reactions. It is based on the scientific principle that our thoughts can influence the body's involuntary functions. For example, a child experiencing the sudden onset of an asthma attack may become extremely anxious because he or she is having serious difficulty breathing. Panic and anxiety increase the

TABLE 13-8	Commonly Used Herbal Products	
NAME	USES	SIDE EFFECTS AND CAUTIONS
Acai	Weight loss and antiaging; antioxidant	Little scientific information about the safety of acai; no scientific evidence to support use for any health-related purpose; might affect magnetic resonance imaging (MRI) results.
Black cohosh	Relieve symptoms of menopause; treat menstrual irregularities and premenstrual syndrome; induce labor	Headaches, gastric complaints, heaviness in the legs, weight problems; safety unknown for pregnant women or those with breast cancer.
Echinacea	Treat or prevent colds, flu, and other infections; believed to stimulate the immune system	Most studies indicate echinacea does not appear to prevent colds or other infections; some people experience allergic reactions, including rashes, increased asthma, and anaphylaxis; gastrointestinal (GI) side effects.
Flaxseed	Laxative; treat hot flashes and breast pain; flaxseed oil used to treat arthritis; both flaxseed and flaxseed oil used to treat high cholesterol levels and prevent cancer	Few reported side effects; contains soluble fiber (such as that found in oat bran) and is an effective laxative; should be taken with plenty of water; may diminish body's ability to absorb medications taken by mouth; should not be taken at same time as oral medications.
Garlic	Treat high cholesterol, heart disease, hypertension; prevent certain types of cancer, including stomach and colon cancer	Some evidence indicates garlic can slightly lower blood cholesterol levels and may slow development of atherosclerosis; side effects include breath and body odor, heartburn, GI upset, and allergic reactions; acts as a mild anticoagulant (similar to aspirin); may be a problem during or after surgery—avoid dietary and supplemental garlic for at least 1 week before surgery; interferes with effectiveness of saquinavir, a drug used to treat human immunodeficiency virus (HIV) infection.
Ginger	Treat stomach aches, nausea, diarrhea; ginger extract is a component of many cold and flu dietary supplements; used to alleviate nausea associated with postoperative state, motion sickness, chemotherapy, and pregnancy; used for rheumatoid arthritis, osteoarthritis, and joint and muscle pain	Short-term use can safely relieve pregnancy-related nausea and vomiting; side effects most often reported are gas, bloating, heartburn, and nausea.
Asian ginseng	Support overall health and boost immune system; improve mental and physical performance; treat erectile dysfunction, hepatitis C, and menopause symptoms; lower blood glucose and control blood pressure	Some studies show ginseng may lower blood glucose and possibly boost immune function; when taken by mouth, it usually is well tolerated; most common side effects are headaches, sleep disorders, GI problems, and possible allergic reactions; patients with diabetes using medications for treatment should use ginseng with caution.
Ginkgo biloba	Treat a variety of conditions, including asthma, bronchitis, fatigue, and tinnitus (ringing or roaring sounds in the ears); typically used to improve memory; treat or help prevent Alzheimer's disease and other types of dementia; reduce intermittent claudication (leg pain caused by narrowing arteries); treat sexual dysfunction and multiple sclerosis	Research indicates that ginkgo is ineffective in treating Alzheimer's disease, dementia, and intermittent claudication; side effects may include headache, nausea, GI upset, diarrhea, dizziness, or allergic skin reactions; severe allergic reactions occasionally are reported; can increase bleeding risk, so people who take anticoagulant drugs, have bleeding disorders, or have scheduled surgery or dental procedures should use caution; uncooked ginkgo seeds contain a toxic chemical that can cause seizures.
Glucosamine plus chondroitin sulfate	Natural substances found in and around the cells of cartilage; used to treat arthritis and joint pain	Recent study shows participants with moderate to severe pain had significant relief with the combined supplement. Most common side effect is GI upset.
Green tea	Prevent and treat a variety of cancers and for mental alertness, weight loss, lowering cholesterol levels, and protecting skin from sun damage; laboratory studies suggest may help protect against or slow the growth of certain cancers	Safe in moderate amounts; possible complications include liver problems with concentrated green tea extracts but not when used as a beverage; contains caffeine; contains small amounts of vitamin K, which can make anticoagulant drugs less effective.

TABLE 13-8   Commonly Used Herbal Products—*continued*

NAME	USES	SIDE EFFECTS AND CAUTIONS
Melatonin	Treatment of sleep disorders	May help individuals with normal sleep patterns but has limited or no effect on those with sleep disorders. Most common side effects are nausea and drowsiness.
Milk thistle (silymarin)	Promote liver health, treat cirrhosis, chronic hepatitis, and gallbladder disorders; lower cholesterol; reduce insulin resistance	Studies suggest it may benefit the liver; associated with fewer and milder symptoms of liver disease in patients with hepatitis C; may lower blood glucose levels; can cause allergic reaction.
Saw palmetto	Primarily used to treat urinary symptoms associated with an enlarged prostate gland; also used for chronic pelvic pain, bladder disorders, reduced sex drive, hair loss, and hormone imbalance	Studies suggest it may be effective for treating prostate symptoms, but no evidence indicates that it reduces the size of an enlarged prostate; does not appear to affect readings of prostate-specific antigen (PSA) level, which is used as screening tool for cancer of the prostate; may cause mild GI upset, tender breasts, and decline in sexual desire in male patients.
St. John's wort	Traditionally used to treat mental disorders and nerve pain; may be used as a sedative; treatment for malaria; balm for wounds, burns, and insect bites; currently used for depression, anxiety, and/or sleep disorders	Some scientific evidence shows it helps treat mild to moderate depression; not effective in treating major depression. Side effects include photophobia (increased sensitivity to sunlight), anxiety, dry mouth, dizziness, GI symptoms, fatigue, headache, and sexual dysfunction. Affects the way the body processes or breaks down many drugs; may speed or slow a drug's metabolism. Combined with certain antidepressants, it may increase side effects such as nausea, anxiety, headache, and confusion. Drugs that can be affected include: • Antidepressants • Birth control pills • Cyclosporine (prevents rejection of transplants) • Digoxin (strengthens myocardial contractions) • Indinavir and possibly other drugs used for HIV • Irinotecan and possibly other drugs used to treat cancer • Warfarin and related anticoagulants St. John's wort is not a proven therapy for depression. If depression is not adequately treated, it can become severe.

Modified from the National Center for Complementary and Alternative Medicine. *https://nccih.nih.gov/health/herbsataglance.htm.* Accessed May 26, 2015.

urgency to breathe. If the child can be taught to relax and keep breathing at a normal rate, the asthma attack will not be influenced by the child's anxiety, and medications taken to relieve bronchospasm will be more effective.

Biofeedback specialists use special monitoring equipment to demonstrate the body's reaction to certain stimuli and to help teach patients how to control physical responses to stress. During a biofeedback session, the provider applies electrical sensors to various locations on the body. These sensors monitor and provide feedback about the body's physiologic responses to stress. For example, if a patient is experiencing chronic tension headaches, the sensors demonstrate that the headache is just part of overall muscular tension. Tension that is registering throughout the body may cause a beeping sound or lights flashing from the equipment as a cue for the patient to associate muscular tension with development of the headache. The goal is to help patients recognize that one body action results in another. Once this goal has been achieved, patients are taught

relaxation techniques designed to prevent the stressful response. Biofeedback methods are effective in managing multiple stress-related conditions, including muscle tension, headaches, chronic low back pain, altered heart rates, and hypertension.

Homeopathic Medicine

Homeopathy, or homeopathic medicine, is a medical approach that was developed in Germany over 200 years ago. The primary principle of homeopathic medicine is to administer very dilute substances that are designed to stimulate the body's ability to heal itself. Homeopaths work individually with clients to administer the lowest dose of medication possible, believing that the lower the dose, the more effective the treatment. Remedies are created from plants, minerals, or animals, and include red onion, arnica (mountain herb), and stinging nettle plant.

Homeopaths assess clients holistically and gather details on individual and family health histories, body type, and current physical, emotional, and mental symptoms. Treatments are specifically designed for each client; therefore, it is not unusual for people with the same condition to have different treatment protocols. People seek homeopathic assistance for a wide range of health problems, including allergies, asthma, chronic fatigue syndrome, depression, digestive disorders, ear infections, headaches, and skin rashes.

Homeopathic remedies are regulated in the same manner as OTC drugs. They do not have to comply with the strict testing guidelines required for prescription drugs. However, the FDA does require that homeopathic remedies meet strength, purity, and packaging standards. Labels must identify at least one health condition that the remedy can treat, provide an ingredient list, indicate the dilution of the ingredients, and explain safety instructions.

Homeopathic therapies are not known to interfere with prescription and OTC medications; however, it is important to gather information from patients about the use of homeopathic remedies and to document the details in the patient's record for the provider to review.

CLOSING COMMENTS

Patient Education

It is important for the patient to be aware of the effects a drug may have and should have on his or her system. The medical assistant plays an important role in helping patients understand their medications, promoting compliance with treatment, and preventing complications. Depending on the facility's policies, the administrative medical assistant may be expected to do many of the following tasks when gathering initial information from patients. These points should be considered when gathering a medication history and documenting in the patient's health record.

- Make a comprehensive list of all medications, including OTC agents and alternative therapies that the patient uses regularly.
- Ask female patients whether they are pregnant or breastfeeding.
- Preassess the patient for any adverse effects, such as drug allergies and drug-drug or drug-food interactions.
- Observe the patient for any adverse effects for a minimum of 20 minutes after administration of a medication in the office; also, inform the patient of possible adverse reactions to the medication that may occur at home.
- Discuss with the patient how and when the prescribed drug is to be taken, and whether any special storage precautions are required.
- Reassess that the patient is taking the medication properly.
- Provide comfort, encouragement, and guidance to patients to ensure their understanding, safety, and cooperation while using drug therapy.
- Answer any questions the patient may have. Remember: If you are not sure of the answer, consult the prescribing provider.

Therapeutic Communication with Patients from Diverse Cultures

Health beliefs can affect compliance with medication therapy. Patients from various cultures may be using home remedies or herbal treatments that could interfere with the effectiveness and safety of medications prescribed by the provider. Guidelines that the medical assistant may find helpful include the following:

- Investigate the healing practices of the primary cultures in your area so that you are better equipped to discuss these practices with your patients.
- Encourage cultural sensitivity in your co-workers.
- Provide patients with educational materials in their native language.
- Ask patients if they are using home remedies or are consulting a healer from their culture. If so, get as much detail as possible so that you can share this information with the provider.

Legal and Ethical Issues

The medical assistant plays a key role in the management of controlled substances in the ambulatory care setting. It is important that all rules for record keeping, inventory, prescribing, dispensing, and documenting scheduled drugs are followed according to state and federal regulations. The medical assistant may be responsible for requesting the provider's initial DEA registration and for continuing certification renewal. The area DEA office can provide instructions on this. Each DEA number is specific to a site, so multiple practice locations require a DEA number for each facility.

Accurate, complete documentation is essential for correct management of patient medications. Each time the patient is prescribed or administered a medication, complete details must be included in the patient's record using approved medical terminology and abbreviations. Failure to do this may result in a serious error that could harm the patient and result in litigation.

HIPAA Applications

According to the Health Insurance Portability and Accountability Act (HIPAA), patients have the right to request restrictions on the disclosure of protected health information (PHI) for treatment, payment, and healthcare operations (TPO). For example, if a patient has a history of substance abuse and this information is not pertinent to current TPO circumstances, the patient can request that this information not be disclosed. The facility does not have to agree to the patient's request; however, a process must be established within the practice to review the demand and explain the provider's decision to the patient. If the provider agrees not to release this information, the specific restriction must be documented in the patient's record, and staff members must review and comply with the restrictions each time material is sent out of the facility for TPO purposes.

Professional Behaviors

Participation in drug therapy requires absolute accuracy from the medical assistant. There is no room for error when gathering a medication history, documenting in the patient's health record, and understanding the purpose and effects of prescribed drugs. When a medical assistant performs his or her duties with accuracy, the message is sent that this is a professional who is dedicated to quality care and patient safety. Both the provider and patient rely on the medical assistant to possess accurate information about drug therapy and perform medication-related duties with meticulous care.

SUMMARY OF SCENARIO

Kathy has a great deal of responsibility in managing medications in the primary care practice where she works. She must be familiar with and follow DEA regulations governing the management of controlled substances. In addition, she must be able to use drug reference materials; identify the general clinical uses of prescribed drugs and OTC products; understand the parts of a prescription and use accepted medical terms and abbreviations; recognize the significance of patient education in the safe use of OTC drugs; and understand the factors that affect drug action.

SUMMARY OF LEARNING OBJECTIVES

1. **Define, spell, and pronounce the terms listed in the vocabulary.**
   Spelling and pronouncing medical terms correctly reinforce the medical assistant's credibility. Knowing the definitions of these terms promotes confidence in communication with patients and co-workers.

2. **Do the following related to government regulation of medications in the United States:**
   - *Distinguish among the government agencies that regulate drugs in the United States.*
     Several federal agencies combine forces to regulate drugs in the United States. The FDA regulates the development and sale of all prescription and OTC drugs; the DEA enforces laws designed to prevent drug abuse and educates the public about drug abuse prevention; and the FTC regulates OTC advertisement.
   - *Cite the areas covered in the regulations established by the DEA for the management of controlled or regulated substances.*
     DEA regulations for the management of controlled substances include specific record-keeping guidelines, in addition to information on physician registration and the inventory, storage, and disposal of controlled substances.
   - *List the DEA regulations for prescription drugs for each of the five schedules of the Controlled Substances Act.*
     Prescriptions written for controlled substances must comply with both state and federal regulations. The prescription must include details about the patient; information about the physician, including the DEA number; and the amount of the drug, written out ("ten" not "10"). The prescription must be manually or electronically signed by the physician. Orders for Schedule II drugs cannot be phoned in except in an absolute emergency, and these prescriptions cannot be refilled. Schedules III, IV, and V drugs may be prescribed by phone, faxed, or e-prescribed and refilled up to five times in a 6-month period. In some states, Schedule V drugs can be dispensed by the pharmacist without a physician's prescription. (See Table 13-1.)

3. **Explain the medical assistant's role in preventing drug abuse.**
   The medical assistant should keep track of patients who repeatedly call for prescription refills of controlled substances; secure computers so there is no access to e-prescription programs and keep prescription pads secure; and maintain a small supply of controlled substances in the office and accurately record their administration.

4. **Differentiate a drug's chemical, generic, and trade names.**
   The chemical name is the drug's formula. The generic (official) name is assigned to the drug and may reflect the chemical name. The trade (brand) name is given to the compound by the pharmaceutical company that developed it and is protected by law for 20 years.

5. **Describe the use of drug reference materials, and explain the five pregnancy risk categories for drugs.**
   The use of drug reference materials is crucial for the safe administration of medications. Most drug references include actions, indications, contraindications, precautions, adverse reactions, dosage, administration guidelines, and method of packaging. The most frequently used drug reference guide is the *Physicians' Desk Reference* (PDR), but package inserts also can be used. A number of websites provide FDA-approved information about medications such as Rxlist at *http://www.rxlist.com/script/main/hp.asp* and *Drugs.com* at *http://www.drugs.com/*. Table 13-2 presents the FDA's five pregnancy risk categories for drugs.

6. **Discuss tips for studying pharmacology, and define the five medical terms used to describe the clinical use of drugs.**
   Clinically, drugs are used as therapeutic medications (to cure a condition); palliative medications (to relieve symptoms); prophylactic medications (to prevent the occurrence of a condition); diagnostic medications (to help determine the cause of a disease); and replacement medications (to provide substances that normally occur in the body).

7. **Cite safety measures for the use of OTC drugs.**
   OTC drugs may interfere or interact with prescription drugs. Some safety measures for the use of OTC drugs include carefully reading directions, taking only the recommended dose, discarding the drug when it expires, informing the provider of OTC drug use, and being aware of contraindications to OTC drug use in certain conditions. (Refer to Table 13-3.)

8. **Do the following related to prescription drugs:**
   - *Diagram the parts of a prescription.*
     A prescription consists of the following six parts: (1) superscription, (2) inscription, (3) subscription, (4) signature, (5) refill information, and (6) provider's signature. A prescription also must provide the patient's name and address and the date the drug is prescribed.
   - *Demonstrate the ability to transcribe a prescription accurately.*
     Procedure 13-1 outlines the method for transcribing a prescription for the physician's signature. It is important that the medical assistant follow a written order; look up information about the medication in a drug reference text or online; ask the patient about drug allergies and record the patient's personal information on the prescription note; and correctly write the name of the drug, form, dosage, strength, route of administration, amount of the drug to be given to the patient, specifics about time of administration if appropriate, and the number

Continued

SUMMARY OF LEARNING OBJECTIVES—*continued*

of refills. The prescription should be reviewed and signed by the provider before it is given to the patient or before the medical assistant transmits an electronic prescription. (Refer to Tables 13-4 and 13-5 to review common prescription abbreviations and The Joint Commission's "Do Not Use" list.)

- *Describe e-prescription methods.*
  EHR systems can be used to create a prescription, print a paper copy of it, and/or send it directly to a pharmacy. EHR programs are designed to automatically check a prescribed drug against the patient's allergies, identify possible drug-drug interactions, access current databases for the patient's medication history, review the patient's insurance drug formulary for coverage, and either print out the prescription for the patient to take to the pharmacy or electronically send the script to the pharmacy.

9. **Relate the principles of pharmacokinetics to drug use.**
   Pharmacokinetics comprises the actions of absorption, which depends on the route of administration (oral, parenteral, mucous membrane, or topical); distribution through the bloodstream; metabolism in the liver; and excretion, primarily by the kidneys.

10. **Describe factors that affect the action of a drug, including the physiologic changes associated with aging.**
    Multiple factors affect a drug's action, including weight, age, gender, diurnal rhythms, pathologic factors, immune responses, psychological factors, tolerance, accumulation, idiosyncrasy, and drug-drug interactions. (Refer to Table 13-6 for the effects of aging on the body's processing of medications.)

11. **Identify the classifications of drug actions.**
    Drugs are classified into groups according to their actions in the body, by the symptoms they relieve, or according to the body system they affect. Drugs may have multiple actions and therefore multiple classifications.

(Refer to Table 13-7 for a summary of the top 50 prescribed drugs in 2014.)

12. **Differentiate among commonly used herbal remedies and alternative therapies.**
    Table 13-8 summarizes common herbal remedies, their uses, and possible side effects. Acupuncture treatments involve the use of thin metal needles inserted through the skin to stimulate specific points in the body to restore and maintain health. Chiropractic providers perform manipulations or anatomic adjustments to correct alignment problems and help the body heal itself. Mind-body therapy uses biofeedback to teach the patient to use his or her thoughts to control certain body reactions. The primary principle of homeopathic medicine is to administer very dilute substances that are designed to stimulate the body's ability to heal itself.

13. **Examine the role of the medical assistant in drug therapy education.**
    The medical assistant plays an important role in helping patients understand their medications, promoting compliance with treatment, and preventing complications. Conducting comprehensive interviews that ask detailed questions about patient use of drugs and documenting this information in the health record provides vital information for the provider. Culturally sensitive interviews with patients help the medical assistant gather details about home remedies and patient belief systems that may affect compliance with drug therapy.

14. **Identify the medical assistant's legal responsibilities in medication management in an ambulatory care setting.**
    The medical assistant's legal responsibilities in medication management include documenting compliance with DEA regulations for controlled substances; maintaining complete and accurate documentation on all medications administered and prescribed for each patient; and following HIPAA regulations on the release of confidential information.

CONNECTIONS

Study Guide Connection: Go to the Chapter 13 Study Guide. Read and complete the activities.

evolve Evolve Connection: Go to the Chapter 13 link at *evolve.elsevier.com/kinn* to complete the Chapter Review Quiz. Check out the other resources listed for this chapter to make the most of what you have learned from Principles of Pharmacology.

BASICS OF DIAGNOSTIC CODING

Mike Simeone, a recent medical assistant graduate, excelled in his diagnostic coding course. Recently he found an entry-level coding position in a gastroenterology practice managed by Dr. Marcia Buckner and Dr. Kevin Walker.

Mike is a little nervous but also excited about starting ICD-10-CM coding. He has studied the similarities and differences between the previous edition (ICD-9-CM) and the ICD-10-CM, and he knows that they share a similar foundation. Mike has used encoder software in some of his classes, which helped him determine the most specific and accurate code. Mike noticed that the new software update in the medical office has an ICD-10-CM module, which he is eager to try.

Mike has had some previous experience working in health records, which gives him a strong understanding of the importance of accurate, quality documentation. He knows where to look to find diagnostic statements in providers' orders, treatment plans, progress notes, surgical reports, and other medical reports.

While studying this chapter, think about the following questions:

- How do the format, layout, and conventions of the ICD-10-CM manual help the medical assistant search for the most accurate and specific diagnostic code?

- Why is the quality of health record documentation critical to diagnostic coding?
- Why does the medical assistant need to know the steps for performing diagnostic coding?

LEARNING OBJECTIVES

1. Define, spell, and pronounce the terms listed in the vocabulary.
2. Describe the historical use of the *International Classification of Disease* (ICD) in the United States.
3. Describe the transition from ICD-9-CM diagnostic coding to ICD-10-CM diagnostic coding.
4. Identify the structure and format of the ICD-10-CM.
5. Describe how to use the Alphabetic Index to select main terms, essential modifiers, and the appropriate code (or codes) and code ranges.
6. Do the following related to the Tabular List:
   - Explain how to use the Tabular List to select main terms, essential modifiers, and the appropriate code (or codes) and code ranges.
   - Summarize coding conventions as defined in the ICD-10-CM coding manual.

7. Review coding guidelines to assign the most accurate ICD-10-CM diagnostic code.
8. Explain how to abstract the diagnostic statement from a patient's health record.
9. Describe how to use the most current diagnostic codes and perform diagnostic coding.
10. Identify how encoder software can help the coder assign the most accurate diagnostic codes.
11. Explain the importance of coding guidelines for accuracy, and discuss special rules and considerations that apply to the code selection process.
12. Use tactful communication skills with medical providers to ensure accurate code selection.
13. Review medical coding ethical standards.

VOCABULARY

abstract A summary of the diagnostic statement and/or procedures and services performed.

acute The initial assessment and treatment of the disease, condition, or injury.

chronic A disease that manifests over a long period because medical treatment has not resolved it.

Coding Clinic An industry journal that provides insight into the coding of complex medical cases. The journal is sponsored by

the American Hospital Association (AHA), which also supports a website (*www.codingclinicadvisor.com*) that can accept questions from coders on specific cases.

diagnostic statement Information about a patient's diagnosis or diagnoses that has been extracted from the medical documentation, such as the history and physical finding, operative reports, and encounter form.

encounter Every meeting between a patient and a healthcare provider. The patient's history and chief complaint, in addition to the medical services provided, are documented in the patient's health record.

etiology The cause of a disorder; a claim may be classified according to the etiology.

histologic The microscopic composition of tissue.

impending A term used in the diagnosis of a condition that can be imminently threatening. For example, a patient showing signs of prediabetes may in the near future develop diabetes; therefore, in this case, diabetes is an impending condition.

manifestation An indication of the existence, reality, or presence of something, especially an illness; a secondary process.

neoplasm A growth of uncontrolled, abnormal tissue; a tumor. The ICD-10-CM assigns diagnostic codes for neoplasms based on six criteria, which can be found in a table that follows the Alphabetic Index.

notations Instructions or guides for assigning classifications, defining category content, or using subdivision codes. Notations are found in both the Alphabetic Index and the Tabular List.

reimbursement The process by which the medical office submits a claim to the insurance company, which then pays the provider for services rendered. All insurance claims must submit diagnoses and procedures as codes, not as descriptions.

THE HISTORY OF MEDICAL CODING

Medical coding began as medical classification in seventeenth century England. John Graunt, a statistician, wanted to study causes of mortality in children under age 6, so he developed a medical classification system. In the mid-1800s, William Farr, a medical statistician, established a more organized disease classification to widen the system to patients of all ages. The principles of Farr's classification method, and those of Jacques Bertillon, chief of statistics for the city of Paris, developed into the *International List of Causes of Death,* which was published in Chicago in 1893 by the International Statistics Institute. This list was revised every 10 years. After the League of Nations was established in 1920, its members saw the need for use of the classification system by a variety of stakeholders, including insurers, health administrators, hospitals, and military medical providers. The name of the list was changed to the *International List of Diseases.*

In 1946 the International Commission of the World Health Organization (WHO) established codes to define specific infectious diseases, parasites, symptoms, and causes of death. This code set was called the *Manual of the International Statistical Classification of Diseases, Injuries, and Causes of Death* (ICD).

(*Note:* It is important to understand the difference between the ICD and the *Clinical Modification* versions (i.e., ICD-9-CM and ICD-10-CM). The ICD is the international version, copyrighted and published by WHO. WHO authorized an adaptation for use in the United States, although all modifications had to conform to WHO conventions.* The adaptation currently used in the United States is the ICD-10-CM. [Other countries also may apply for adaptations.] The *Clinical Modification* version provides much more detail and sometimes has separate sections for procedures.)

The *Clinical Modification* version previously used in the United States (ICD-9-CM) was approved and put into use in 1975. This code set had 3-character categories, 4-character subcategories, and 5-character subdivisions.

In 1995 WHO approved the development of the *International Classification of Diseases, Tenth Revision, Clinical Modification* (ICD-10-CM) code set. This code set has a different format from that of the ICD-9-CM.

Medical Coding in the United States

As history dictates, the original purpose of medical coding was to collect statistical data. The United States is the only country in the world that uses coding for health insurance **reimbursement** purposes. Providers are responsible for billing the insurance company for any services rendered during the *encounter* (i.e., any meeting between a patient and a healthcare provider), and the provider must use approved medical codes for these procedures and services to obtain reimbursement. This means that the provider must supply diagnostic information that demonstrates the need for the rendered procedures and/or services. A *diagnosis* is the determination of the nature of a condition, illness, disease, injury, or congenital defect; the provider assigns a diagnosis through *assessment* of the patient.

All components of the encounter (i.e., diagnostic findings, procedures, and services) are used to determine the charges and to generate an insurance claim. This chapter focuses on the ways the medical assistant should gather diagnostic information and translate it into a diagnostic code. The ICD-10-CM coding manual is used for this purpose.

GETTING TO KNOW THE ICD-10-CM

What Is Diagnostic Coding?

Diagnostic coding is the translation of written descriptions of diseases, illnesses, or injuries into alphanumeric codes. The ICD-10-CM code set identifies the disease or injury for which a patient was treated as a code consisting of up to 7 characters, with a period after the 3rd character (Figure 14-1). Using the ICD-10-CM can help ensure accurate health record documentation and efficient claims processing.

The ICD-10-CM code set is available as online documents from the Centers for Medicare and Medicaid Services (*cms.gov*),

---

Conventions are abbreviations, punctuation, symbols, instructional notations, and related entities that help the coder select an accurate, specific code.

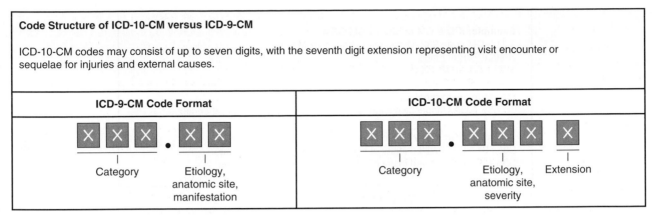

Code Structure of ICD-10-CM versus ICD-9-CM

ICD-10-CM codes may consist of up to seven digits, with the seventh digit extension representing visit encounter or sequelae for injuries and external causes.

ICD-9-CM Code Format	ICD-10-CM Code Format

FIGURE 14-1 Code structure and format in the ICD-9-CM and ICD-10-CM.

and as a manual, which is produced by several publishers. Different publishers may use different layouts, symbols, color coding, and some other features For the coding manual, however, the format, conventions, tables, appendixes, content, and basic structure are the same.

When you use the ICD-10-CM, you will choose a standardized alphanumeric code for the **diagnostic statement** assigned by the provider. Diagnostic statements are found in operative reports, discharge summaries, history and physical exam (H&P) reports, and reports on *ancillary diagnostic services* (e.g., radiology, pathology, and laboratory reports); all of these should support the patient's diagnosis or diagnoses. These reports are used by healthcare providers to code and report clinical information; this coding is required for participation in Medicare and Medicaid insurance programs and by most third-party payers and insurance carriers. The ICD-10-CM also keeps track of various healthcare statistics related to disease and injury. Practice management software, clearinghouses, and third-party payers recognize these codes, which simplifies the coding process and speeds reimbursement to healthcare providers.

Transitioning from ICD-9-CM to ICD-10-CM

As of the publication of this textbook, ICD-10-CM diagnostic coding will be a fairly new process, so it is important to be familiar with the differences between the ICD-9-CM and the ICD-10-CM.

The ICD-9-CM code set (see Figure 14-1) is made up of three volumes. Volumes 1 and 2 are used for diagnostic coding.

- Volume 1 contains the ICD-9-CM Tabular List of Diseases and Injuries (commonly called the *Tabular List*). It contains all the diagnostic codes for disease and injury, grouped into 17 chapters.
- Volume 2 contains the ICD-9-CM Index to Diseases and Injuries (also known as the *Alphabetic Index*). This is an alphabetic list of the *main terms* (discussed later) from the Tabular List and their associated codes. Volume 2 also contains *V codes* (Classification of Factors Influencing Health Status and Contact with Health Service) and *E codes* (Supplementation Classification of External Causes of Injury and Poisoning).

TABLE 14-1 Comparison of the ICD-9-CM and ICD-10-CM Code Sets

The ICD-10-CM differs from the ICD-9-CM in its organization and structure, code composition, and level of detail.

ICD-9-CM CODES	ICD-10-CM CODES
• Consist of 3 to 5 characters	• Consists of 3 to 7 characters
• Character 1: Numeric or alpha (E or V)	• Character 1: Alpha
• Characters 2, 3, 4, 5: Numeric	• Characters 2, 3: Numeric
• Always have at least 3 characters	• Characters 4, 5, 6, 7: May be alpha or numeric
• Decimal placed after character 3	• Decimal placed after character 3
	• Use all letters used except U

- Volume 3 is used by hospitals to code inpatient procedures and services performed in the hospital environment. Most medical offices do not use Volume 3 codes.

The ICD-10-CM follows the same hierarchal structure as the ICD-9-CM in that the first 3 characters represent the code category. Table 14-1 lists some of the significant differences between the ICD-9-CM and ICD-10-CM code sets.

General Equivalence Mappings

To assist with the changeover from the ICD-9-CM to the ICD-10-CM, the Centers for Medicare and Medicaid Services (CMS) has developed code maps, or general equivalence mappings (GEMs) (Figure 14-2). GEMs are used to accurately report ICD-10-CM codes that most closely match ICD-9-CM codes. The translation from ICD-9-CM codes to ICD-10-CM codes through GEMs is based on the description and meaning of the code. According to the CMS, "The purpose of GEMs is to create a useful, practical, code-to-code translation reference dictionary for both code sets, and to offer acceptable translation alternatives wherever possible."

As a medical assistant coder, you must still learn how to assign ICD-10-CM codes. However, GEMs can be helpful and can increase your efficiency in ICD-10-CM coding. A complete list of GEMs is available on the CMS website (*cms.gov*).

```
Example: ICD-9-CM to ICD-10-CM GEM
ICD-9-CM code 902.41 has the following GEM entry:
Source Target Flags
90241 S35403A 10000


902.41 Injury to renal artery
To S35.403A Unspecified injury of unspecified renal artery, initial encounter

Not included in ICD-9-CM to ICD-10-CM GEM
S35.401A Unspecified injury of right renal artery, initial encounter
S35.402A Unspecified injury of left renal artery, initial encounter
```

FIGURE 14-2 General equivalence mappings (GEMs).

CRITICAL THINKING APPLICATION   **14-1**

Mike is currently updating the electronic encounter form for the gastroenterology group. However, he is unsure of the accuracy of converting the ICD-9-CM codes to ICD-10-CM codes. What resource can he use to obtain accurate ICD-10-CM codes?

Structure and Format of the ICD-10-CM

The ICD-10-CM also has a Tabular List (officially, the ICD-10-CM Tabular List of Diseases and Injuries) and an Alphabetic Index (the ICD-10-CM Index to Diseases and Injuries). Every ICD-10-CM code begins with an alphabetic letter that indicates the chapter in the Tabular List from which the code originates (Table 14-2). (All the letters of the English alphabet are used except U, which WHO has reserved to assign to new diseases of uncertain **etiology**.) Some conditions use more than one alphabetic letter in their code ranges. For example, the codes in Chapter 1, Certain Infectious and Parasitic Diseases (A00–B99), begin with the letter A or B.

Every year the CMS reviews the ICD-10-CM coding manual, and the update is published on October 1. Additions, revisions, and deletions are made to many of the diagnostic codes, code descriptions, and guidelines. As mentioned previously, *you must always use the current year's coding manual to ensure accurate coding and to comply with regulatory guidelines.*

The CMS prepares Official Guidelines for Coding and Reporting to be used with the ICD-10-CM codes, in addition to instructions on how to report the codes on insurance claim forms. The guidelines are a set of rules that have been developed to accompany and complement the official conventions and instructions provided in the ICD-10-CM proper.

The Alphabetic Index

The Alphabetic Index consists of an alphabetic list of diagnostic terms and related codes. This index includes main terms, nonessential modifiers, essential modifiers, and subterms.

- **Main terms:** These terms appear in bold type.
- **Nonessential modifiers:** These terms follow the main term and are enclosed in parentheses. They are supplementary words or explanatory information; therefore, they do not affect the code assignment.

- **Essential modifiers:** These terms are indented one space to the right under the main term. They change the description of the diagnosis in bold type.
- **Subterms:** These terms are indented one space to the right under an essential modifier (two spaces to the right under the main term). These diagnoses are used when all conditions exist.

Figure 14-3 provides an example of the main term **Colitis**. Follow the list to the modifying term Ischemic, which is indented once. The subterm **acute** is indented once more, twice from the main term. The nonessential modifiers included with the subterm "acute" (i.e., catarrhal, chronic, noninfective, hemorrhagic) do not affect the code assignment.

```
Colitis (acute) (catarrhal) (chronic (noninfective)
     (hemorrhagic)—see also Enteritis K52.9
  allergic K52.2
  amebic (acute) (see also Amebiasis) A06.0
     nondysenteric A06.2
  anthrax A22.2
  bacillary—see Infection, Shigella
  balantidial A07.0
  Clostridium difficile A04.7
  coccidial A07.3
  collagenous K52.89
  cystica superficialis K52.89
  dietary counseling and surveillance (for) Z71.3
  dietetic K52.2
  due to radiation K52.0
  eosinophilic K52.82
  food hypersensitivity K52.2
  giardial A07.1
  granulomatous—see Enteritis, regional, large
     intestine
  infectious—see Enteritis, infectious
  ischemic K55.9
     acute (fulminant) (subacute) K55.0
     chronic K55.1
     due to mesenteric artery insufficiency K55.1
     fulminant (acute) K55.0
  left sided K51.50
     with
        complication K51.519
                                        continued
```

FIGURE 14-3 The main term **Colitis** in the Alphabetic Index.

TABLE 14-2   ICD-10-CM Tabular List of Diseases and Injuries

CHAPTER	TITLE	CODE RANGE	POSSIBLE DIAGNOSIS*	ICD-10-CM CODE
1	Certain Infectious and Parasitic Diseases	A00–B99	Measles	B05.9
2	Neoplasms	C00–D49	Colon cancer	C18.9
3	Diseases of the Blood and Blood-Forming Organs and Certain Disorders Involving the Immune Mechanism	D50–D89	Iron-deficiency anemia	D50.9
4	Endocrine, Nutritional, and Metabolic Diseases	E00–E89	Type I diabetes	E10
5	Mental, Behavioral, and Neurodevelopmental Disorders	F01–F99	Dementia	F03
6	Diseases of the Nervous System	G00–G99	Parkinson's disease	G20
7	Diseases of the Eye and Adnexa	H00–H59	Glaucoma	H40.9
8	Diseases of the Ear and Mastoid Process	H60–H95	Otitis media, left ear	H60.92
9	Diseases of the Circulatory System	I00–I99	Hypertensive heart disease	I11.9
10	Diseases of the Respiratory System	J00–J99	Acute sinusitis	J01.91
11	Diseases of the Digestive System	K00–K95	Inguinal hernia	K40
12	Diseases of the Skin and Subcutaneous Tissue	L00–L99	Pressure ulcer of right heel	L89.619
13	Diseases of the Musculoskeletal System and Connective Tissue	M00–M99	Rheumatoid arthritis	M05
14	Diseases of the Genitourinary System	N00–N99	Endometriosis	N80.9
15	Pregnancy, Childbirth, and the Puerperium	O00–O94	Ectopic pregnancy	O00.9
16	Certain Conditions Originating in the Perinatal Period	P00–P96	Neonatal jaundice	P59.9
17	Congenital Malformations, Deformations and Chromosomal Abnormalities	Q00–Q99	Cleft lip	Q37.9
18	Symptoms, Signs and Abnormal Clinical and Laboratory Findings, Not Elsewhere Classified	R00–R99	Abdominal pain	R10.9
19	Injury, Poisoning and Certain Other Consequences of External Causes	S00–T88	Left ankle fracture	S82.92xA
20	External Causes of Morbidity	V00–Y99	Snowboard accident Fall from cliff Exposure to excessive natural cold	V00.318A W15 X31
21	Factors Influencing Health Status and Contact With Health Services	Z00–Z99	Pregnancy state	Z33.1

*All diagnoses presented are NOS (not otherwise specified).

CRITICAL THINKING APPLICATION   14-2

Mike sometimes is confused as to which term is the main term and which are modifying terms. What documents or references can help him determine the main term? Whom can he consult in the practice to make sure he understands the main term? What can happen if he selects a modifier or subterm instead of a main term?

Supplementary Sections of the Alphabetic Index

The Alphabetic Index section includes two important tables.

- *Table of Neoplasms:* This table lists neoplasms by anatomic location. For coding purposes, neoplasms are further classified into six categories: Malignant Primary; Malignant Secondary; Ca [cancer] in situ; Benign; Uncertain Behavior; and Unspecified Behavior.
- *Table of Drugs and Chemicals:* This table presents a classification of drugs and other chemical substances; it is used to identify poisonings and external causes of adverse effects.

The six coding classifications are: Poisoning, Accidental (Unintentional); Poisoning, Intentional Self-Harm; Poisoning, Assault; Poisoning, Undetermined, Adverse Effect; and Underdosing.

The Tabular List

The Tabular List is divided into 21 chapters. Most chapter titles specify a particular group of diseases and injuries, and all titles are followed by a code range in parentheses; for example, Chapter 1, Certain Infectious and Parasitic Diseases (A00–B99) (see Table 14-2). Some chapters use a body part or an organ system to group the codes; for example: Chapter 8, Diseases of the Eye and Adnexa (H00–H59); and Chapter 10, Diseases of the Circulatory System (I00–I99). Other chapters group conditions by etiology or the nature of the disease process; for example, Chapter 2, Neoplasms (C00–D49). Chapter 17, Pregnancy, Childbirth, and the Puerperium (O00–O94) groups codes related to the prenatal and postnatal periods. Chapter 20, External Causes of Morbidity (V00–Y99), replaces the V and E codes used in the ICD-9-CM. Chapter 20 also groups codes related to external causes of injury and poisoning. Chapter 21 is Factors Influencing Health Status and Contact With Health Services (Z00–Z99).

Each chapter is subdivided into subchapters, or *blocks,* and each subchapter has a designated 3-character code; these subchapter codes and code ranges form the foundation of the ICD-1Ø-CM code set.

In each chapter, all the 3-character block codes begin with the alphabetic letter assigned to that chapter; for example, in Chapter 7, Diseases of the Nervous System (G00–G99), all the block codes (and their versions) begin with G. If a chapter's code range includes two letters [e.g., Chapter 1, Certain Infectious and Parasitic Diseases (A00–B99)] each 3-character block code begins with one of those two letters. The letter character is followed by a 2-character number.

A summary of the blocks (Figure 14-4) at the beginning of each chapter provides an overview of the chapter.

As mentioned, the ICD-1Ø-CM manual is produced by a variety of publishers, but many of the optional features are similar (remember, the important elements are always the same, regardless of the publisher). For instance, to enable the coder to better maneuver through the Alphabetic Index, each page has *guide words,* which are the first and last words on that page (this is the same arrangement used for the pages of a dictionary). Each chapter of the Tabular List has a different-colored border strip; in some manuals this strip shows the chapter title and the range of codes found on that specific page. In the chapters in the Tabular List, the codes for each category/block are arranged alphabetically (by the initial alpha character) and then numerically. Familiarizing yourself with these tools can help you improve your proficiency as you work through the manual to find the most accurate code.

It is important to note that some codes do not need to be extended beyond the 3-character code, and these are considered valid codes as is; for example, code I10 {**Essential (primary) hypertension**}. If a code has only three characters, do not add a decimal after the 3rd character. If a code has more than three characters, add a decimal point after the 3rd character; for example, **K11.7 {Disturbances of salivary secretion**}. Most ICD-1Ø-CM codes have 4 to 7 characters.

CRITICAL THINKING APPLICATION   **14-3**

Mike is reviewing the Tabular List of the ICD-1Ø-CM coding manual. He notices that each chapter begins with a list of diagnostic categories with a corresponding range of codes. What is this called? How can this feature be used as a tool for accurate ICD-1Ø-CM code assignment?

EXCLUDES 2	*certain conditions originating in the perinatal period (PØ4-P96)*
	certain infectious and parasitic diseases (AØØ-B99)
	complications of pregnancy, childbirth and the puerperium (OØØ-O99)
	congenital malformations, deformations and chromosomal abnormalities (ØØØ-Q99)
	endocrine, nutritional and metabolic diseases (EØØ-E9Ø)
	injury, poisoning and certain other consequences of external causes (SØØ-T98)
	neoplasms (CØØ-D49)
	symptoms, signs and abnormal clinical and laboratory findings, not elsewhere classified (RØØ-R94)

This chapter contains the following blocks:

NØØ-NØ8	Glomerular diseases
N1Ø-N16	Renal tubulo-interstitial diseases
N17-N19	Acute kidney failure and chronic kidney disease
N2Ø-N23	Urolithiasis
N25-N29	Other disorders of kidney and ureter
N3Ø-N39	Other disorders of the urinary system
N4Ø-N51	Diseases of male genital organs
N6Ø-N65	Disorders of male genital organs
N7Ø-N77	Inflammatory diseases of female pelvic organs
N8Ø-N98	Noninflammatory disorders of female genital tract
N99	Intraoperative and postprocedural complications and disorders of the genitourinary system, not elsewhere classified

FIGURE 14-4 Chapter blocks in the Tabular List.

Reporting NEC and NOS Codes

In some cases, because of limited documentation in the patient's health record, the medical assistant coder can find it difficult to assign an ICD-10-CM code with a higher specificity. The ICD-10-CM code set accommodates these coding circumstances by establishing "not elsewhere classified" (NEC) and "not otherwise specified" (NOS) guidelines.

- NEC means that the diagnostic statement contains specific wording, but no specific classification exists to match the wording. For example, an NEC code would be assigned if a patient seeks medical attention for **chronic** postoperative pain. The ICD-10-CM code would be **G89.28 {Other chronic postprocedural pain}**. For all NEC codes, the last character is always 8.
- NOS codes are used more often than NEC codes. For example, sinusitis with no documentation of the specific sinus site is assigned the NOS code **J32.9 {Chronic sinusitis, unspecified}**. The coder should keep in mind that the lack of documentation does not mean that all the patient's sinuses are inflamed; the provider must document the exact site of the sinusitis for a non-NOS code to be assigned. For all NOS codes, the last character is always 9.

Conventions Used in the Tabular List

As mentioned, *conventions* are abbreviations, punctuation, symbols, instructional **notations**, and related entities that help the coder select an accurate, specific code. Conventions are found in the Tabular List, but not in the Alphabetic Index. Understanding their meaning and using them as guides are crucial to accurate coding. The following are the most common conventions.

Placeholder Character. The ICD-10-CM uses the dummy placeholder X in two different ways. The dummy placeholder can be used as the 5th character in certain six-character codes; this allows for future expansion of the code set without interruption of the six-character structure.

Example 14-1—Using the Dummy Placeholder for the 5th Character. T43.4X1A Poisoning by butyrophenone and thiothixene neuroleptics, accidental, initial encounter (unintentional)

Specific categories have a 7th character, but may not use the 4th, 5th, or 6th characters. In these cases, the dummy placeholder X is used to fill the empty character spaces. Note that a dummy placeholder would not be needed for codes with less than 7 characters.

Example 14-2—Using the Dummy Placeholder in 7-Character Codes. S50.01XA Contusion of right elbow

In this case, the 7th character indicates "initial encounter" (see the following section).

> The appropriate 7th character is to be added to each code from category S03.
> A   initial encounter
> D   subsequent encounter
> S   sequela

FIGURE 14-5 A 7th character box below the main term.

Codes with 7 Characters. In the ICD-10-CM, the 7th character typically provides specificity about the coded condition. This extension may be a number or letter, and it is always assigned to the 7th character position. A list of possible 7th character codes can be found under the main term in the Tabular List (Figure 14-5).

When Additional Characters Are Required

Every ICD-10-CM code has at least 3 characters: an alphabetic letter followed by two digits. When additional characters are required for accurate coding, the ICD-10-CM coding manual includes symbols indicating how many characters are required. An additional symbol indicates that the 7th character code should follow placeholder X. These symbols are considered a coding convention and provide guidance to ensure coding accuracy.

CRITICAL THINKING APPLICATION   **14-4**

Mike is looking for the ICD-10-CM code for morbid obesity. From the Alphabetic Index, Mike looked up the code E66 in the Tabular List. The main term, **Overweight and obesity**, has a symbol that indicates a 4th character is needed. What is Mike's next step to assign the most accurate code? Can Mike just use E66? Why or why not?

Punctuation. Four basic forms of punctuation are used in the Tabular List: brackets, parentheses, colons, and braces (Figure 14-6). Each form serves a different purpose to help you read and understand the code descriptions.

Instructional Notations. Instructional notations, which are found in both the Alphabetic Index and the Tabular List, are critical to correct coding practices. They are located directly under the main term.

- **Includes** notes: The word "includes" is used in the Tabular List to clarify the conditions included within the particular chapter, section, category, subcategory, or code. Includes notes begin with the word "includes" when they appear at the beginning of a chapter, section, or category. At the code level, the word "includes" is not present; only a list of terms included in the code is

[ ]	Brackets enclose synonyms, alternative wording, or explanatory phrases.
( )	Parentheses are used to enclose supplementary words, which may be present or absent in the statement of a disease or procedure. These supplementary words do not usually affect the code number selected, but instead provide further definition or specificity to the code description.
:	Colons are used in the Tabular Index after an incomplete term that needs one or more of the modifiers or adjectives that follow to make it assignable to a given category.
{ }	Braces enclose a series of terms, each of which is modified by the statement appearing to the right of the brace.

FIGURE 14-6 Punctuation used in the ICD-10-CM.

provided. For example, to code the diagnostic statement "inflammation due to an infection" correctly, you must include the code for the infectious agent.

- **Excludes** notes: The ICD-10-CM uses two types of exclusion notes, Excludes1 and Excludes2. Either or both statements may be present under a category, subcategory, or code.
  - Excludes1: This is a clear "NOT CODED HERE!" message. It means that the excluded code should never be used with the code above the Excludes1 note. For example, code **G14** {**Postpolio syndrome**}, has this Excludes1 note: sequelae of poliomyelitis (B91). As another example, consider that a defect cannot be coded as both a congenital defect and an acquired defect.
  - Excludes2: This means "not included here." The excluded condition is not part of the condition represented by the code; however, a patient may have both conditions concurrently. Excludes2 notes have a corresponding code for the excluded condition. When an Excludes2 note is present, the coder may code both conditions if the patient presents with both. For example, code **F02** {**Dementia in other diseases classified elsewhere**} has the following Excludes2 note: vascular dementia (F01.5). This means that vascular dementia is not part of the condition coded as F02; therefore, you can code both dementia (F02) and vascular dementia (F01.5) if the patient has both.
- **Code first/Use additional code** notes: *Code first* notes (Figure 14-7) appear under *manifestation* codes. Manifestation codes specify the way in which an underlying condition appears, or manifests, as a result of an underlying etiology; the main terms of most manifestation codes include the words "in diseases classified elsewhere." A *Code first* note indicates that the underlying condition must be sequenced first, before that manifestation code. For these etiology/manifestation combination codes, a *Use additional code* note is found with the etiology code. The *Code first* and *Use additional code* notes indicate the order in which the codes are arranged: etiology code first, followed by the manifestation code.

  For example, when you code for pain, the code sequence depends on the reason for the encounter. If the reason is that the patient wants a pain management procedure, code for the site of the pain, such as lumbar region pain (**M54.5- Low back pain**) or shoulder pain (**M25.51- Pain in shoulder**). If the patient seeks treatment for an ailment such as an ankle fracture, but is also suffering from limb pain (**M79.6- Pain in limb, hand, foot, fingers and toes**), code the ankle fracture first and the limb pain second.

Cross Reference Notes. Cross reference notes in the Alphabetic Index instruct the coder to check elsewhere in the Index before assigning a code. The ICD-10-CM uses the following three types of cross reference notes:

- *See:* The *see* note (preceded by a long dash) follows a main term. It directs the coder to another main term. The correct code will be found with the main term indicated by the *see* note. For example, **Acidopenia**—*see* Agranulocytosis.
- *See also:* The *see also* note (preceded by a long dash) follows a main term. It indicates that another main term may be checked that may provide additional useful Index entries. For example, **Adiposis**—*see also* Obesity. However, if the original main term provides the necessary code, it is not necessary to follow the *see also* note.
- *See* category: The *see* category note directs the coder to a specific category (which is given as the category's 3-character code). For example: *[main term]* **Intoxication**, *[essential modifier]* meaning, *[subterm]* inebriation—*see* category F10. The *see* category instruction must *always* be followed.

Relational Terms. These terms are used in both the Alphabetic Index and the Tabular List to clarify the context of the disease or injury.

- *And:* In the Tabular List code titles, *and* should be interpreted as meaning "and/or."
- *With:* The term *with* should be interpreted as meaning "associated with" or "due to" when it appears in the Alphabetic Index, or in an instructional note or code title in the Tabular List. In the Alphabetic Index, the word *with* follows immediately after the main term, not in alphabetical order.
- *Due to:* In both the Tabular List and the Alphabetic Index, the term *due to* signifies relationship between two conditions. This assumption can be made when both conditions are present or when the diagnostic statement indicates this relationship.

Coding Guidelines

The coding manual begins with the ICD-10-CM Official Guidelines for Coding and Reporting every coding guideline for the entire ICD-10-CM code set is included in this section. The guidelines are a set of rules that have been developed to complement the official conventions and instructions provided in the ICD-10-CM proper. The guidelines are organized into four sections.

Section I. Conventions, General Coding Guidelines and Chapter Specific Guidelines: This section covers the structure and conventions of the ICD-10-CM classification system, in addition to the general guidelines that apply to the entire system. It also contains chapter-specific guidelines for each of the Tabular List's 21 chapters.

Section II. Selection of Principal Diagnosis: This section includes guidelines for selection of a principal diagnosis for non-outpatient settings.

G30	Alzheimer's disease
	Use additional code to identify:
	dementia with behavioral disturbance (F02.81)
	dementia with behavioral disturbance (F02.80)
F02	**Dementia in other diseases classified elsewhere**
	Code first the underlying physiological condition, such as:
	Alzheimer's (G30.-)
	F02.80 Dementia in other diseases classified elsewhere, without behavioral disturbance
	F02.81 Dementia in other diseases classified elsewhere, with behavioral disturbance

FIGURE 14-7 *Code first note.*

Section III. Reporting Additional Diagnoses: This section includes guidelines for reporting additional diagnoses in non-outpatient settings.

Section IV. Diagnostic Coding and Reporting Guidelines for Outpatient Services: As the title indicates, this section includes diagnostic coding and reporting guidelines for outpatient services.

The coding guidelines start with a table of contents for each of the four sections, including the related chapters of disease and injury. After the table of contents, the coding guidelines are presented in section order (i.e., Sections I through IV). For the purposes of outpatient medical office billing, you are most likely to need Sections I and IV.

PREPARING FOR MEDICAL CODING

Extracting Diagnostic Statements

To prepare for medical coding, you must analyze the patient's health record and **abstract** the diagnostic statement documented in the various reports. Sources of diagnostic statements include the encounter form, treatment notes, discharge summary, operative report, and radiology, pathology, and laboratory reports.

Encounter Form

The encounter form (also known as a *superbill*) can be viewed in the electronic health record (EHR). This form is most commonly used to obtain the list of medical services rendered and the treating diagnosis when the total charges are calculated. Although it is a convenient coding reference for the provider and medical staff, possible outdated codes can reduce or delay reimbursement. It is vital that the form used by the medical practice be reviewed annually to ensure that all codes on it have been updated, revised, or deleted according to the latest information from all current coding manuals. Medical practices should ensure that their current encounter form uses ICD-10-CM codes, not ICD-9-CM codes; otherwise, problems with reimbursement will result.

History and Physical Exam

The history and physical exam (H&P) are the starting point of the patient's narrative medical evaluation, which includes the reason the person sought medical attention. The H&P begins with a statement in the patient's own words that describes the reason for seeking medical attention. This statement, called the *chief complaint,* is often abbreviated in the history documentation in the health record. After the chief complaint, the provider documents any other pertinent history about medical, behavioral, and social factors, such as smoking, drinking, drug use, family history, previous surgeries, and hospitalizations.

After recording the patient's history, the provider performs a physical examination. This includes both objective and subjective assessments of the patient's physical status. The final sections of an H&P include an assessment and a plan. The assessment is the provider's evaluation of the findings from the H&P, and it includes a diagnostic statement. The plan is the treatment plan for the conditions noted in the assessment; it may include x-ray studies, laboratory tests, surgery, administration of medications, or other treatments.

Treatment or Progress Notes

Treatment notes are the second most common medical document from which diagnostic statements can be extracted. The format healthcare providers most commonly use for their notes is *SOAP notes,* a system of charting in which information is divided into subjective findings, objective findings, assessment, and plan for treatment. Just as in the H&P, the diagnostic statement can most often be found in the assessment section of the SOAP notes.

Discharge Summary

The discharge summary is used primarily for extracting diagnostic information for patients who were hospitalized, rather than those seen in a provider's office. The main elements of a discharge summary are the patient's admission date, date of discharge, H&P findings, clinical course during hospitalization, health condition on discharge, discharge diagnosis, and aftercare plan. Diagnostic statements are abstracted from the discharge diagnosis section. The medical office can use a discharge summary as an overview of the patient's condition, especially if the discharge was recent.

Operative Report

For patients who underwent surgery as an outpatient or inpatient, the operative report also is used to extract diagnostic statements. An operative report includes the preliminary diagnosis, the final diagnosis, and a detailed description of the operative procedure from start to finish. The medical assistant uses the final diagnosis when searching for and selecting a diagnosis code.

Radiology, Laboratory, and Pathology Reports

Radiology, laboratory, and pathology reports are used to support and/or establish the diagnostic statement. Any findings from these reports must be documented in the treatment notes in the health record so that they can be used for diagnostic coding, charge entry, or insurance billing purposes.

STEPS IN ICD-10-CM CODING

Accurate ICD-10-CM coding requires 8 basic steps (Table 14-3). The first step involves abstracting the diagnostic statement from the health record and determining the main and modifying terms from the various medical reports. The next steps are performed using the Alphabetic Index to search for the code, or code ranges that best fit the diagnostic statement. The remaining steps are performed using the Tabular List to verify and confirm that the code or codes located in the Alphabetic Index fully match the diagnostic statement and are the most specific and accurate diagnostic codes. Procedure 14-1 details the basic coding steps using the ICD-10-CM manual and also encoder software (i.e., TruCode).

CRITICAL THINKING APPLICATION **14-5**

In reviewing an encounter form, Mike noticed that the diagnostic statement indicated that the patient needed to be treated for a left inguinal hernia. However, Mike also noted that the surgical report indicated that the left inguinal hernia was obstructed. What should Mike use as the final diagnostic statement? Should he ask the provider which diagnostic statement to use?

TABLE 14-3 Diagnostic Coding Step-by-Step: Parkinson's Disease	
Step 1	• *Determine the correct diagnosis from the diagnostic statement.* Parkinson's Disease
Step 2	• *Use the main term to look up the diagnosis in the Alphabetic Index.* **Parkinson's disease, syndrome or tremor**—*see* Parkinsonism
Step 3	• *Look up the "see" term in the Alphabetic Index.* **Parkinsonism** (idiopathic) (primary) G20

Step 4	• *Review the essential modifiers under the main term.*
	Parkinsonism
	    with neurogenic orthostatic hypotension (symptomatic) G90.3
	    arteriosclerotic G21.4
	    dementia G31.83 *[F02.80]*
	        with behavioral disturbance G31.83 *[F02.81]*
	    due to
	        drugs NEC G21.19
	            neuroleptic G21.11
	    neuroleptic induced G21.11
	    postencephalitic G21.3
	    secondary G21.9
	        due to
	            arteriosclerosis G21.4
	            drugs NEC G21.19
	                neuroleptic G21.11
	            encephalitis G21.3
	            external agents NEC G21.2
	            syphilis A52.19
	        specified NEC G21.8
	    syphilitic A52.19
	    treatment-induced NEC G21.19
	    vascular G21.4

Step 5	• *Choose the correct essential modifier based on the diagnostic statement.* Because the diagnostic statement only indicates Parkinson's Disease, code G20 should be chosen.
Step 6	• *Look up code G20 in the Tabular List.* **G20 Parkinson's disease**

Step 7	• *Check for any coding guidelines, conventions, inclusion or exclusion notes, or an additional character symbol.*
	    Includes Hemiparkinson's
	                                 Idiopathic Parkinsonism or Parkinson's disease
	                                 Paralysis agitans
	                                 Parkinsonism or Parkinson's disease NOS
	                                 Primary Parkinsonism or Parkinson's disease dementia with
	    Excludes 1 Parkinsonism (G31.83)

Step 8	• Assign the final ICD-10-CM code. **G20 Parkinson's disease**

PROCEDURE 14-1 Perform Coding Using the Current ICD-10-CM Manual

Goal: *To perform accurate diagnosis coding using the ICD-10-CM manual.*

EQUIPMENT and SUPPLIES

- ICD-10-CM manual (current year)
- Encounter form and other relevant health records

PROCEDURAL STEPS

Preparation

1. Abstract the diagnostic statement from the patient's encounter form and/or other health records:
   (1) Determine the main terms in the diagnostic statement that describe the patient's condition.
   (2) Determine what essential modifiers describe the main term in the diagnostic statement.
   <u>PURPOSE</u>: To extract all diagnoses or diagnostic statements from the health record and to ensure that all parts of the diagnostic statement are included in the encounter form or health record, with nothing missing or added. Then, to identify the main term, essential modifiers, and subterms to be used to search the Alphabetic Index.

Alphabetic Index

1. Locate the main terms from the diagnostic statement in the Alphabetic Index.
   <u>PURPOSE</u>: To provide a starting point for searching the Alphabetic Index.
2. Locate the essential modifiers listed under the main term in the Alphabetic Index.
   <u>PURPOSE</u>: To ensure further specificity of the codes found in the Alphabetic Index.
3. Review the conventions, punctuation, and notes in the Alphabetic Index.
   <u>PURPOSE</u>: To ensure that no additional searches, exclusions, or similar terms are needed to complete the search in the Alphabetic Index.
4. Choose a tentative code, codes, or code range from the Alphabetic Index that matches the diagnostic statement as closely as possible.

<u>PURPOSE</u>: To prevent backtracking and repeated searches in the Alphabetic Index.

Tabular List

1. Look up the codes chosen from the Alphabetic Index in the Tabular List.
   <u>PURPOSE</u>: To begin the process of determining whether the codes selected from the Alphabetic Index are appropriate and accurate.
2. Review notes, conventions, and the Official Coding Guidelines associated with the code and code description in the Tabular List.
   1. Review conventions and punctuation.
   2. Review instructional notations:
      - *Includes* and *excludes* notes
      - *Code first, code also,* and *code additional* notes
      - *and, or,* and *with* statements
   <u>PURPOSE</u>: To ensure that the code or codes selected are appropriate for use and to determine whether they require additional codes or further specificity, or are excluded from use.
3. Verify the accuracy of the tentative code in the Tabular List.
   1. Make sure all elements of the diagnostic statement are included in the codes selected.
   2. Make sure the code description does not include anything not documented in the diagnostic statement.
   <u>PURPOSE</u>: To ensure that the most accurate and specific code is selected and that no contraindication exists to use of the code or codes selected.
4. Extend the codes to their highest level of specificity (up to the 7th character, if required). If a 7th character is required and no codes are present for the 4th, 5th, or 6th characters, it is appropriate to use the dummy placeholder X for these positions.
5. Assign the code (or codes) selected from the Tabular List as the appropriate code for the patient's condition by documenting it in the patient's health record.
   <u>PURPOSE</u>: To ensure that the health record and/or electronic encounter form contain documentation of the code or codes assigned.

PROCEDURE 14-1 —*continued*

Using the TruCode Encoder Software

1. Type in the diagnosis from the diagnostic statement in the search box as in Figure 1.

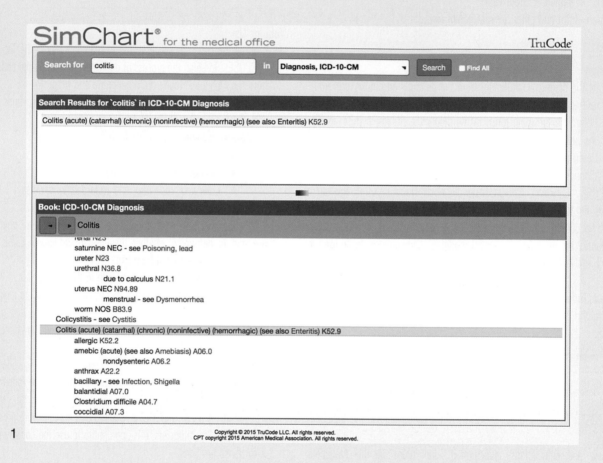

1

2. The software will provide a list of main terms that could be related to the diagnosis typed in the search box. The coder chooses the main term that represents the diagnostic statement.
3. Based on the main term chosen, a list of essential modifiers is presented (Figure 2). The coder must review the diagnostic statement to ensure that all documented modifying terms are identified. If the provider does not document a modifying term, the coder should not assume that a modifying term was implied.

PROCEDURE 14-1 *—continued*

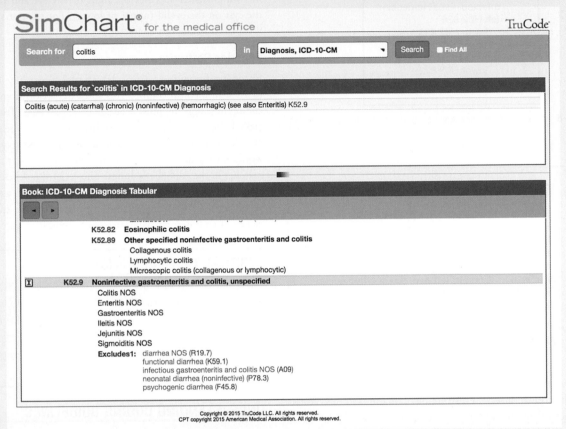

SimChart® for the medical office   TruCode®

Search for [colitis] in [Diagnosis, ICD-10-CM ▾] [Search] ☐ Find All

Search Results for `colitis` in ICD-10-CM Diagnosis

Colitis (acute) (catarrhal) (chronic) (noninfective) (hemorrhagic) (see also Enteritis) K52.9

Book: ICD-10-CM Diagnosis Tabular

[◄] [►]

K52.82 **Eosinophilic colitis**
K52.89 **Other specified noninfective gastroenteritis and colitis**
            Collagenous colitis
            Lymphocytic colitis
            Microscopic colitis (collagenous or lymphocytic)
[Ⅰ]   K52.9 **Noninfective gastroenteritis and colitis, unspecified**
            Colitis NOS
            Enteritis NOS
            Gastroenteritis NOS
            Ileitis NOS
            Jejunitis NOS
            Sigmoiditis NOS
            Excludes1: diarrhea NOS (R19.7)
                        functional diarrhea (K59.1)
                        infectious gastroenteritis and colitis NOS (A09)
                        neonatal diarrhea (noninfective) (P78.3)
                        psychogenic diarrhea (F45.8)

2

4. In the preceding figure, note the yellow on the left of the chosen diagnosis. In the TruCode program, click on the yellow area, and an instructional notes textbox, which includes coding guidelines, will appear as in Figure 3. To determine the most accurate code, follow these coding guidelines.

5. Once all the menus of essential modifiers and subterms have been presented, choose the most accurate and specific code based on the diagnostic statement.

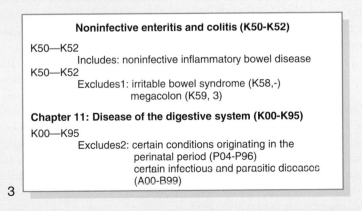

Noninfective enteritis and colitis (K50-K52)

K50—K52
            Includes: noninfective inflammatory bowel disease
K50—K52
            Excludes1: irritable bowel syndrome (K58,-)
                        megacolon (K59, 3)

Chapter 11: Disease of the digestive system (K00-K95)

K00—K95
            Excludes2: certain conditions originating in the
                        perinatal period (P04-P96)
                        certain infectious and parasitic diseases
                        (A00-B99)

3

Using the Alphabetic Index

After has been abstracted from the diagnostic statement from the health record have been identified the main terms, start searching for the best code, or code range, in the Alphabetic Index. It is important to note that the Alphabetic Index should be used only as a tool to locate the appropriate code or code range. The Tabular List, with its conventions, punctuation, notes, and guidelines, must always be used to confirm that the code or codes selected are accurate and specific and that no contraindications exist to the use of the code found in the Alphabetic Index. For this reason, never assign a code directly from the Alphabetic Index. Even if only one code is

> **Cyst**—*continued*
> eyelid (sebaceous) H02.829
>   infected—*see* Hordeolum
> left H02.826
>   lower H02.825
>   upper H02.824
> right H02.823
>   lower H02.822
>   upper H02.821

FIGURE 14-8 *Cross section of Cyst (main term); eyelid (essential modifier) in the Alphabetic Index.*

H02.82	**Cysts of eyelid**
	Sebaceous cyst of eyelid
H02.821	**Cysts of right upper eyelid**
H02.822	**Cysts of right lower eyelid**
H02.823	**Cysts of right eye, unspecified eyelid**
H02.824	**Cysts of left upper eyelid**
H02.825	**Cysts of left lower eyelid**
H02.826	**Cysts of left eye, unspecified eyelid**
H02.829	**Cysts of unspecified eye, unspecified eyelid**

FIGURE 14-9 *Tabular List main term:* **Cysts of eyelid**.

found in the Alphabetic Index, it may be used only if a thorough review of the conventions and instructional notations in the Tabular List does not contraindicate it.

Figure 14-8 presents an excerpt from the Alphabetic Index for the main term **Cyst.** The first essential modifier, which is indented one space under **Cyst,** is eyelid. Note the nonessential modifier—sebaceous—in parentheses after eyelid. (Remember, nonessential modifiers add detail, but they do not have to be present in the diagnostic statement for the code to be acceptable for use.) Directly below the essential modifier eyelid, and indented one space under it, are the subterms. Note that there are separate subterms for the left eye and for the right eye. In addition, the diagnostic codes for each eye are further modified by the location of the cyst (upper or lower).

Using the Tabular List

Once are identified at least the first three characters of the code in the Alphabetic Index, turn to the Tabular List. The chapters in the Tabular List are arranged alphabetically according to the initial letter of the 3-character code or codes assigned to each chapter. For example, Chapter 1 has code range A00–B99; Chapter 2 has code range C00–D49; Chapter 3 has code range D50–D89, and so on.

You've determined that the code you probably need is in the H02 code range, turn to the chapter that includes that range (Chapter 8). Figure 14-9, an excerpt from the Tabular List, shows **Cysts of eyelid** as a main term, with the code H02.82. (Note that the nonessential modifier, sebaceous, is not shown in parentheses; rather, it appears under the main term in the nonbold phrase "Sebaceous cyst of eyelid.")

In the coding manual, note the "additional character" symbol, which indicates that code H02.82 requires one more character. All

possible diagnoses with six-character codes are indented below the main term. A closer look at the disorders and their codes shows that the 6th character specifies the right or left eye and the location of the cyst on the eyelid (upper or lower). For the not specified code, 9 is placed in the 6th character position.

Encoder Software

Encoder software (e.g., TruCode) is a tool commonly used by coders to assist in medical coding. This software performs computer-aided coding to assign the most accurate code possible. (TruCode is especially helpful to students because it allows them to search the ICD-10-CM manual using a few key terms.) The coder types a few key words into a Search box, and the software finds the most likely matches in the Alphabetic Index. The coder then clicks on a specific code, and the software searches the Tabular List to assign the most accurate code. Encoder software can increase the speed and efficiency of coding for a wide variety of medical cases.

CRITICAL THINKING APPLICATION   **14-6**

Mike has determined a diagnostic statement to be "Perforation of the tympanic membrane in the left ear." What keyword should be used for the TruCode software search box? To what main term will the encoder go in the Alphabetic Index? What should Mike click to get to the Tabular List? At what point can Mike be sure that he has assigned the most accurate and specific code?

UNDERSTANDING CODING GUIDELINES

Remember that all ICD-10-CM coding manuals, regardless of the publisher, have comprehensive instructional notations and conventions to help the coder select the most accurate diagnostic code or codes. When any discrepancy occurs between reference sources (including this text), the current year's ICD-10-CM coding manual is the final authority; this fact cannot be overemphasized. When coding, you must always refer to and thoroughly review the conventions, instructional notations, code definitions, and other guidelines in the Alphabetic Index and Tabular List in the current year's version of the ICD-10-CM.

The following instructions are designed to provide some additional guidance in selecting diagnostic codes from various chapters in the ICD-10-CM; however, they are not to be considered a replacement for the ICD-10-CM manual, nor do they provide all the coding information, definitions, or explanations found in the manual. The steps for diagnostic coding (see Procedure 14-1) are the same for all chapters of the ICD-10-CM; however, special rules and considerations apply to some chapters that affect the code selection process.

Coding of Signs and Symptoms

Signs and symptoms are coded only if the provider has not yet reached a determination of the final diagnosis. For example, if the provider's notes contain terminology such as "rule out" or "suspected," the coder should use the patient's documented signs and symptoms, including subjective and objective findings. Subjective findings include the patient's chief complaint or statements about why the patient is seeking medical care. Objective findings

- Use only if there is no final or determining diagnosis
- Use if "rule out" or "suspected" are included in the assessment or diagnostic statement.
- Signs and symptoms can be subjective and/or objective findings
  - Subjective: Chief complaint or patient's verbal statements
  - Objective: Any measurable indicators found during the physical examination

FIGURE 14-10 Rules for coding signs and symptoms.

are any measurable indicators found during the physical examination.

In the Tabular List, ill-defined conditions, signs, and symptoms are found in Chapter 20, Symptoms, Signs, and Abnormal Clinical and Laboratory Findings, Not Elsewhere Classified (R00-R99). Figure 14-10 shows the signs and symptoms section of Chapter 20.

Conditions, signs, and symptoms included in Chapter 20 include the following:

- Not elsewhere classified (NEC) cases, even after all the facts of the medical case have been examined
- Signs or symptoms that existed on the first encounter but were temporary and for which causes could not be determined
- Conditional diagnosis for a patient who failed to return for further care and the cause of whose condition had not yet been determined
- Medical cases referred elsewhere for treatment before a diagnosis could be made
- Not otherwise specified (NOS) cases in which a more precise diagnosis was not available for any reason
- Certain symptoms, for which supplementary information is provided, that represent important problems in the medical care provided

Coding the Etiology and Manifestation

Etiology refers to the underlying cause or origin of a disease. *Manifestation* describes the signs and symptoms of the disease. In the Alphabetic Index, the etiology and manifestation codes are listed together. The etiology code is always listed first, and the manifestation code is listed beside it in italics and enclosed within brackets.

Multiple Coding

In addition to the signs and symptoms that require two codes to fully describe a single condition affecting multiple body systems, other single conditions may require more than one code. In the Tabular List, *Use additional code* notes appear with codes that are not part of an etiology/manifestation pair, but in which a secondary code is useful to fully describe a condition. The sequencing rule is the same as for the etiology/manifestation pair: *use additional code* indicates that a secondary code should be added after the condition code.

For example, consider a bacterial infection that is not included in Chapter 1, Certain Infectious and Parasitic Diseases (A00–B99). A secondary code may be required to identify the organism causing the infection. This secondary code may come from category **B95** {*Streptococcus, Staphylococcus,* and *Enterococcus* as the cause of diseases classified elsewhere} or from category **B96** {**Other**

bacterial agents as the cause of diseases classified elsewhere}. A *use additional code* note normally is found at the infectious disease code, indicating that the organism code must be added as a secondary code.

As mentioned, *code first* notes are used for certain conditions that involve both an underlying etiology and multiple body system manifestations caused by that etiology. In such cases, the underlying condition should be sequenced first, before the manifestations.

A *code, if applicable, any causal condition first* note indicates that this code may be assigned as a principal diagnosis when the causal condition is unknown or not applicable. If the causal condition is known, the code for that condition should be sequenced as the principal, or first-listed, diagnosis.

Multiple codes may be needed for sequelae, and complication codes and obstetric codes may be needed to more fully describe a condition. See the specific guidelines for these conditions.

Sequela (Late Effects) Codes

Sequelae are the lingering effects produced by a health condition after the acute phase of an illness or injury has ended. The acute phase is considered the first 30 days of a condition with no improvement. There is no time limit on when a sequela code can be used. The residual effect may be apparent early (e.g., another stroke), or it may occur months or years later (e.g., the consequences of a previous injury). Coding of sequelae generally requires two codes sequenced in the following order: the original condition or nature of the sequela is sequenced first; the sequela code is sequenced second.

An exception to the above guidelines are instances in which the code for the sequela is followed by a manifestation code identified in the Tabular List; or, the sequela code has been expanded (at the 4th, 5th, or 6th character) to include the manifestation or manifestations. The code for the acute phase of an illness or injury that led to the sequela is never used with a code for the late effect. The following box presents the rules for coding **impending**, or threatened, conditions.

Rules for Coding Impending or Threatened Conditions

Code any condition described at the time of discharge as "impending" or "threatened."

1. If it did occur, code as a confirmed diagnosis.
2. If it did not occur, consult the Alphabetic Index to determine whether the condition has a subterm for impending or threatened; also check main term entries for Impending and Threatened.
3. If the subterms are listed, assign the given code.
4. If the subterms are not found, code the existing underlying condition or conditions, signs, or symptoms and not the condition described as "threatened" or "impending."

Coding Complications of Care

A complication from medical care generally requires additional procedures or services for a patient, but often the complication is not mentioned as part of the diagnostic statement; this can result in reduced reimbursement. It is important to review the medical documentation to determine whether a complication exists and to code the complication in addition to the diagnostic statement. Keep in mind, not all conditions that occur during or after medical care or surgery are classified as complications. Two criteria must be met: a cause-and-effect relationship must be established between the care provided and the condition; and the documentation must indicate that the condition is a complication.

Coding Infectious and Parasitic Diseases

Multiple diagnostic codes are needed to code infectious or parasitic diseases. The first code identifies the disease or condition (e.g., throat infection), and the second code identifies the organism causing the disease (e.g., enterovirus). The second code can be found in the Tabular List in Chapter 1. The basic coding principles for the use of either combination or multiple codes apply throughout this section of the ICD-10-CM.

Coding Organism-Caused Diseases

The two-step process of coding organism-caused diseases begins with the affected anatomical site. In the case of a throat infection caused by enterovirus, you should first assign the diagnostic code for throat infection, or pharyngitis. In the Tabular List, code **J02.8 {Acute pharyngitis due to other specified organism}** is accompanied by the following *Use additional code* note: "Use additional code (B95–B97) to identify infectious agent." In the Tabular List, the B95–B97 category/block (found in Chapter 1) is titled Bacterial and Viral Infectious Agents. Starting with code B95, search for the code that specifies enterovirus; this happens to be code **B97.1 {Enterovirus as the cause of diseases classified elsewhere}.** Note that code B97.1 requires a 5th character; however, no other information is provided by the medical record. Therefore, you can assign code **B97.19 {Other enterovirus as the cause of diseases classified elsewhere}** as the final organism code.

Human Immunodeficiency Virus (HIV) Infection and Acquired Immunodeficiency Syndrome (AIDS)

To code HIV infection and AIDS correctly, it is essential first to understand the descriptions of the codes available. The key is whether the patient has symptoms.

- Human immunodeficiency virus (HIV): This indicates only that the virus is present.
- Acquired immunodeficiency syndrome (AIDS): AIDS is a syndrome; a syndrome is defined as a "group of symptoms occurring together." AIDS is the manifestation of signs and/or symptoms that can occur as a result of HIV infection.

Never code a patient as having HIV unless it is clearly documented as confirmed. Probable and suspected cases are never coded; instead, the signs and symptoms present should be coded. Remember that stringent restrictions are placed on the disclosure of medical information about patients with HIV infection and/or AIDS. Make sure the patient has signed the appropriate release of medical information form before any disclosures are made to third parties.

Selection and Sequencing of HIV Codes

(a) **Patient Admitted for HIV-Related Condition.** If a patient is admitted for an HIV-related condition, the principal diagnosis should be **B20 {Human immunodeficiency virus [HIV] disease},** followed by additional diagnostic codes for all reported HIV-related conditions.

(b) **Patient with HIV Disease Admitted for Unrelated Condition.** If a patient with HIV disease is admitted for an unrelated condition (e.g., a traumatic injury), the code for the unrelated condition (e.g., the nature of injury code) should be the principal diagnosis. Other diagnoses would be B20, followed by additional diagnostic codes for all reported HIV-related conditions.

(c) **HIV Infection in Pregnancy, Childbirth, and the Puerperium.** During pregnancy, childbirth, or the puerperium, a patient admitted (or presenting for a healthcare encounter) because of an HIV-related illness should receive a principal diagnostic code **O98.7- {Human immunodeficiency [HIV] disease complicating pregnancy, childbirth, and the puerperium},** followed by B20 and the code for the HIV-related illness. Codes from Chapter 17, Pregnancy, Childbirth, and the Puerperium (O00–O9A), always take sequencing priority.

Patients with asymptomatic HIV infection status who are admitted (or presenting for a healthcare encounter) during pregnancy, childbirth, or the puerperium should receive codes of O98.7- and **Z21 {Asymptomatic human immunodeficiency virus [HIV] infection status}.**

(d) **Encounters for Testing for HIV.** If a patient is being seen to determine his or her HIV status, use code **Z11.4 {Encounter for screening for human immunodeficiency virus [HIV]}.** Use additional codes for any associated high-risk behavior.

If a patient with signs or symptoms is being seen for HIV testing, code the signs and symptoms. An additional counseling code— **Z71.7 {Human immunodeficiency virus [HIV] counseling}** may be used if counseling is provided during the encounter for the test.

When a patient returns to be informed of his or her HIV test results and the test result is negative, use code Z71.7. If the results are positive, see previous guidelines and assign codes as appropriate.

Coding Neoplasms

A **neoplasm,** or new growth, is coded by the site or location of the neoplasm and its behavior. The Table of Neoplasms (Figure 14-11) is located just after the Alphabetic Index in the coding manual. This table lists the ICD-10-CM codes for neoplasms by anatomic site in alphabetic order. Six possible code numbers exist for each anatomic site, depending on whether the neoplasm is malignant or benign, exhibits uncertain behavior, or is of an unspecified nature. In the Table of Neoplasms, malignant neoplasms are categorized into three separate subclassifications: Malignant Primary, Malignant Secondary, and Ca in situ (carcinoma in situ).

Terms Defining Malignant Neoplasm Sites

- *Primary:* Identifies the originating anatomic site of the neoplasm. A primary malignancy is defined as the original site or sites of the cancer.
- *Secondary:* Identifies sites to which the primary neoplasm has metastasized (spread). A secondary malignancy is defined as a second location to which the cancer has spread from the primary location.
- *Ca in situ:* Carcinoma in situ is defined as the absence of invasion of surrounding tissues. Tumor cells are undergoing

	Malignant Primary	Malignant Secondary	Ca in situ	Benign	Uncertain Behavior	Unspecified Nature		Malignant Primary
bladder (urinary)	C67.9	C79.11	D09Ø	D30.3	D41.4	D49.4	marrow NEC	C96.9
dome	C67.1	C79.11	D09Ø	D30.3	D41.4	D49.4	unspecified side	C40.1Ø
neck	C67.5	C79.11	D09Ø	D30.3	D41.4	D49.4	marrow NEC	C96.9
orifice	C67.9	C79.11	D09Ø	D30.3	D41.4	D49.4	cartilage NEC	C41.9
ureteric	C67.6	C79.11	D09Ø	D30.3	D41.4	D49.4	clavicle	C41.3
urethral	C67.5	C79.11	D09Ø	D30.3	D41.4	D49.4	marrow NEC	C96.9
overlapping lesion	C67.8	—	—	—	—	—	clivus	C41.Ø
sphincter	C67.8	C79.11	D09Ø	D30.3	D41.4	D49.4	marrow NEC	C96.9
trigone	C67.Ø	C79.11	D09Ø	D30.3	D41.4	D49.4	coccygeal vertebra	C41.4
urachus	C67.7	—	D09Ø	D30.3	D41.4	D49.4	marrow NEC	C96.9
wall	C67.9	C79.11	D09Ø	D30.3	D41.4	D49.4	coccyx	C41.4
anterior	C67.3	C79.11	D09Ø	D30.3	D41.4	D49.4	marrow NEC	C96.9
lateral	C67.2	C79.11	D09Ø	D30.3	D41.4	D49.4	costal cartilage	C41.3
posterior	C67.4	C79.11	D09Ø	D30.3	D41.4	D49.4	costovertebral joint	C41.3
blood vessel—*see* Neoplasm,							marrow NEC	C96.9
connective tissue							cranial	C41.Ø

FIGURE 14-11 Table of neoplasms.

malignant changes but are still confined to the point of origin, without invasion of surrounding normal tissue. The *Ca in situ* column is used only if the provider documents that precise terminology.

Definitions of Benign, Uncertain Behavior, and Unspecified Nature Neoplasms

- *Benign:* The growth is noncancerous, nonmalignant, and has not invaded adjacent structures or spread to distant sites.
- *Uncertain Behavior:* The pathologist is unable to determine whether the neoplasm is benign or malignant.
- *Unspecified Nature:* Neither the behavior nor the **histologic** type of neoplasm is specified in the diagnostic statement.

The ICD-9-CM instructional notes state that the behavior of the neoplasm should be determined first for coding.

Most coding decisions on malignant neoplasms are between the primary and secondary classifications. Other terms are used in the following cases:

- *In situ* is used only when the diagnostic statement contains that exact phrase.
- *Unspecified* is used only when no pathologic study has been done, and the neoplasm is still described with a term such as "tumor" or "growth."
- *Uncertain* is used by the provider when it has not been determined whether malignant or benign.

Six Steps for Coding Neoplasms

The following steps can help determine the most specific and accurate diagnostic code for a neoplasm. These steps can be used in addition to the basic diagnostic steps.

1. Using the Table of Neoplasms, determine the site (anatomic location) of the neoplasm and select the row in the table in which it appears.
2. Determine whether the neoplasm is malignant or benign.

3. If the neoplasm is benign, select the column in the table by reviewing the diagnostic statement.
4. If the neoplasm is malignant, determine the table column that best fits its behavior: Malignant Primary, Malignant Secondary, or Ca in situ.
5. Link the appropriate column to the appropriate row.
6. Check the code in the Tabular List to make sure it complies with the guidelines, conventions, and instructional notations in the Tabular List.

The ICD-1Ø-CM manual always provides additional information, definitions, and guidelines for coding neoplasms in the tabular list, just as it does for all other diseases, illnesses, and injuries.

Coding for Diabetes Mellitus

Diabetes mellitus (DM) is classified as type 1 or type 2. Patients with DM type 1 develop the disease because the pancreas is unable to produce insulin. In individuals with DM type 2, the pancreas becomes unable to maintain the level of insulin the body needs to function, or the person has developed target cell resistance to insulin.

The diabetes mellitus codes are combination codes; they include the type of diabetes mellitus, the body system affected, and the complications affecting that body system. Use as many codes within a particular category/block as necessary to describe all the complications of the disease. These codes should be sequenced according to the reason for a particular encounter. Assign as many codes from category/block E08 to E13 (Diabetes Mellitus) as needed to identify all the patient's associated conditions.

Diabetes Mellitus and the Use of Insulin

In the ICD-1Ø-CM, the primary codes for diabetes mellitus (E08–E13) do not include whether the individual is using insulin. Therefore, if insulin use is documented in the health record, a second code is required: **Z79.4 {Long term (current) use of insulin}**. Code Z79.4 should not be assigned if insulin is given temporarily during an encounter to bring the blood glucose level under control in a patient with DM type 2.

Gestational Diabetes

Gestational, or pregnancy induced, diabetes can occur during the second and third trimesters of pregnancy in women who were not diabetic before pregnancy. Gestational diabetes can cause complications in the pregnancy similar to those of pre-existing diabetes mellitus. It also puts the woman at greater risk of developing diabetes after the pregnancy. Codes for gestational diabetes are in subcategory **O24.4 {Gestational diabetes mellitus}**. No other code from category O24 {**Diabetes mellitus in pregnancy, childbirth, and the puerperium**} should be used with a code from subcategory O24.4. The codes under subcategory O24.4 include diet controlled (O24.410) and insulin controlled (024.414). If a patient with gestational diabetes is treated with both diet and insulin, only the code for insulin controlled is required.

Code **Z79.4 {Long-term (current) use of insulin}** should also be assigned with codes from subcategory O24.4 if the patient is being treated with insulin.

An abnormal glucose tolerance level in pregnancy is assigned a code from subcategory **O99.81 {Abnormal glucose complicating pregnancy, childbirth, and the puerperium}**.

Coding for the Circulatory System

Providers use a wide variety of terms and phrases to identify components of the circulatory system. To code disorders of the circulatory system accurately, the coder must carefully review all inclusions, exclusions, conventions, guidelines, and instructional notations associated with each potential code selected.

Myocardial Infarction

A myocardial infarction (MI) is coded as follows:

* As *acute* if it is documented as such in the diagnostic statement or has a stated duration of 8 weeks or less.

* As *chronic* if it is so stated in the diagnostic statement or if symptoms persist after 8 weeks.

Other MI coding considerations include the following:

* If an MI is specified as "old" or "healed" without any current or presenting symptoms, it should be coded using category **I21 {ST elevation (STEMI) and non-ST elevation (NSTEMI) myocardial infarction}**.

* A history of an MI uses code **I25.2 {Old myocardial infarction}**. This code is used only if the patient has no symptoms and only if the old MI was diagnosed by means of an electrocardiogram.

* If the patient is symptomatic, code the underlying condition or symptoms only if the underlying condition is not known: **I21.3 {ST elevation (STEMI) myocardial infarction of unspecified site}**.

Hypertensive Disease

A distinction is made in the ICD-10-CM between "elevated" and "high" blood pressure. High blood pressure is defined as hypertension [**I10 Essential (primary) hypertension**]. If a diagnostic statement does not contain the word "hypertension" or the phrase "high blood pressure," the condition is coded as elevated blood pressure [**R03.0 Elevated blood-pressure reading, without diagnosis of hypertension**], not hypertension.

Hypertension frequently is the cause of various forms of heart and vascular disease; however, the mention of hypertension in the diagnostic statement does not mean that a combination code for hypertensive heart disease should be used. If a cause-and-effect relationship exists between the hypertension and the heart disease, it should be clearly documented in the clinical record or diagnostic statement.

The hypertension table in the ICD-9-CM was not included in the ICD-10-CM. Review Figure 14-12 for a comparison between ICD-9-CM and ICD-10-CM for hypertension coding.

Heart conditions classified to category **I50 {Heart failure}** or subcategories I51.4–I51.9 are assigned to a code from category **I11**

Hypertension	Malignant	Benign	Unspecified	Hypertension
Hypertension, hypertensive	401.0	401.1	401.9	I10 Essential (primary) hypertension
with CKD stage I-IV, or unspecified	403.00	403.10	403.90	I12.9 Hypertensive chronic kidney disease with stage 1-4 CKD, or unspecified chronic kidney disease
with CKD stage V, or ESRD	403.01	403.11	403.91	I12.0 Hypertensive chronic kidney disease with stage 5 CKD or end stage renal disease
Hypertensive heart	402.00	402.10	402.90	I11.9 Hypertensive heart disease without heart failure
Cardiorenal (disease)	404.00	404.10	404.90	I13.10 Hypertensive heart and chronic kidney disease without heart failure, with stage 1- 4 CKD, or unspecified CKD

FIGURE 14-12 Coding for hypertension in the ICD-9-CM and ICD-10-CM code sets. (Data from *www.ihs.gov/businessoffice/documents/2013pres/ICD-10CM-DiseasesOfTheCirculatorySystem.pdf.*)

{**Hypertensive heart disease**} when a causal relationship is stated in the health record ("as a result of hypertension") or implied ("hypertensive"). Use an additional code from category I50 to identify the *type* of heart failure in patients with heart failure.

The same heart conditions (category I50 or subcategories I51.4–I51.9) with hypertension, but without a stated causal relationship, are coded separately. The codes should sequence according to the circumstances of the admission or encounter.

Coding for Chronic Kidney Disease

Assign codes from category **I12** {**Hypertensive chronic kidney disease**} when both hypertension and a condition classifiable to category **N18** {**Chronic kidney disease (CKD)**} are present. Unlike for hypertension with heart disease, the ICD-10-CM presumes a cause-and-effect relationship and classifies chronic kidney disease with hypertension as hypertensive chronic kidney disease.

The appropriate code from category N18 should be used as a secondary code with a code from category I12 to identify the stage of chronic kidney disease.

If a patient has hypertensive chronic kidney disease and acute renal failure, an additional code for the acute renal failure is required.

Coding for Atherosclerotic Cardiovascular Disease

The ICD-10-CM has combination codes for atherosclerotic heart disease with angina pectoris. The subcategories for these codes are **I25.11** {**Atherosclerotic heart disease of native coronary artery with angina pectoris**} and **I25.7** {**Atherosclerosis of coronary artery bypass graft(s) and coronary artery of transplanted heart with angina pectoris**}.

When you use one of these combination codes, you do not need to use an additional code for angina pectoris. A causal relationship can be assumed in a patient with both atherosclerosis and angina pectoris, unless the documentation indicates that the angina is due to something other than the atherosclerosis.

If a patient with coronary artery disease is admitted because of an acute myocardial infarction (AMI), the AMI should be sequenced before the coronary artery disease.

Coding for Skin Ulcers

Codes from category **L89** {**Pressure ulcer**} are combination codes that identify the site of the pressure ulcer and the stage of the ulcer. The ICD-10-CM classifies pressure ulcer stages based on severity, which is designated by stages 1 to 4; unspecified stage; or unstageable. Unspecified and unstageable codes are used for pressure ulcers in which the stage cannot be clinically determined (e.g., the ulcer has been treated with a skin or muscle graft). These codes also are used for pressure ulcers documented as a deep tissue injury, but not documented as being due to trauma. The modifying term defines each stage, depending on the location of the ulcer (Figure 14-13).

Coding for Complications of Pregnancy, Childbirth, and the Puerperium

Coding for the obstetric patient is like using a specialty codebook within the ICD-10-CM coding manual. This is challenging for coders who do not code obstetrics often. Some important clinical terms regarding pregnancy are:

L89.21	**Pressure ulcer of right hip**
L89.210	**Pressure ulcer of right hip, unstageable**
L89.211	**Pressure ulcer of right hip, stage I**
	Healing pressure ulcer of right hip back, stage I
	Pressure pre-ulcer skin changes limited to persistent focal edema, right hip
L89.212	**Pressure ulcer of right hip, stage II**
	Healing pressure ulcer of right hip, stage II
	Pressure ulcer with abrasion, blister, partial thickness skin loss involving epidermis and/or dermis, right hip
L89.213	**Pressure ulcer of right hip, stage III**
	Healing pressure ulcer of right hip, stage III
	Pressure ulcer with full thickness skin loss involving damage or necrosis of subcutaneous tissue, right hip
L89.214	**Pressure ulcer of right hip, stage IV**
	Healing pressure ulcer of right hip, stage IV
	Pressure ulcer with necrosis of soft tissues through to underlying muscle, tendon, or bone, right hip
L89.219	**Pressure ulcer of right hip, unspecified stage**
	Healing pressure ulcer of right hip NOS
	Healing pressure ulcer of right hip, unspecified stage

FIGURE 14-13 Coding Example: Pressure Ulcer, Left hip.

- *Antepartum:* Meaning pregnancy (applies as soon as a pregnancy test result is positive)
- *Childbirth:* Meaning delivery
- *Postpartum:* The puerperium (the first 6 weeks after delivery)
- *Peripartum:* The period from the last month of pregnancy to 5 months' postpartum

Obstetrics cases use codes from Chapter 17, Pregnancy, Childbirth and the Puerperium (O00-O9A). These codes have sequencing priority over codes from other chapters.

Additional codes from other chapters may be used in conjunction with Chapter 17 codes to further specify conditions. If the provider documents that the pregnancy is incidental to the encounter, **Z33.1** {**Pregnant state, incidental**} should be used instead of any Chapter 17 codes. It is the provider's responsibility to state that the condition being treated is not affecting the pregnancy. Codes from Chapter 17 are documented only in the maternal health record; they are never used in the health record of the newborn.

Most of the codes in Chapter 17 have a sixth character indicating the trimester of pregnancy. Assignment of the final character for trimester should be based on the provider's documentation of the trimester (or number of weeks) for the current admission or encounter. This applies to the assignment of trimester for pre-existing conditions, in addition to those that develop during or are due to the pregnancy. The provider's documentation of the number of weeks may be used to assign the appropriate code identifying the trimester.

When a patient is admitted to a hospital for complications in pregnancy during a specific trimester and remains in the hospital into a subsequent trimester, the trimester character for the antepartum complication code should be assigned on the basis of the trimester when the complication developed, not the trimester of the discharge. If the condition developed before the current admission or encounter, or represents a pre-existing condition, the trimester character for the trimester at the time of the admission or encounter should be assigned.

7th Character for Fetus Identification

Where applicable, a 7th character is assigned for certain categories to identify the fetus for which the complication code applies. Assign the 7th character "0":

- For single gestations
- When the documentation in the record is insufficient to determine whether the fetus is affected and it is not possible to obtain clarification
- With more than one fetus, when it is not possible to determine clinically which fetus is affected

Outcome of Delivery and Liveborn Infant Codes

When a delivery occurs, the principal diagnosis should correspond to the main circumstances or complication of the delivery. In cases of cesarean delivery, the selection of the principal diagnosis should be the condition assigned after the encounter that was responsible for the patient's admission. If the patient was admitted with a condition that resulted in the performance of a cesarean procedure, that condition should be selected as the principal diagnosis. If the reason for the admission was unrelated to the condition resulting in the cesarean delivery, the condition related to the reason for the admission/encounter should be selected as the principal diagnosis.

For example, a maternity patient was admitted to the hospital for pneumonia, but because of complications, a cesarean section was performed. In this case, the pneumonia would be the primary diagnosis. A code from category **Z37** {**Outcome of delivery**} should always be included in the maternal health record when a delivery has occurred. Codes from category Z37 are not to be used in subsequent records or in the newborn's health record.

Code **O80** {**Encounter for full-term uncomplicated delivery**} should be assigned when a woman is admitted for a full-term vaginal delivery and delivers a single, healthy infant without any complications antepartum, during the delivery, or postpartum during the delivery episode. Code O80 is always a principal diagnosis.

Newborn Coding

Chapter 18, Certain Conditions Originating in the Perinatal Period (P00–P96), also is used for coding and reporting purposes. The perinatal period extends from just before the birth through day 28 after the birth. When you code the birth episode in a newborn's health record, assign a code from category **Z38** {**Liveborn infants according to place of birth and type of delivery**} as the principal diagnosis. A code from category Z38 is assigned only once, to a newborn at the time of birth. If a newborn is transferred to another institution, a code from category Z38 should not be used at the receiving hospital. When a newborn is admitted to another hospital, the newborn's admitting diagnosis is the health condition that required the hospital transfer.

Coding for Injuries

When you code injuries, assign separate codes for each injury unless a combination code is provided, in which case the combination code is assigned. Code **T07** {**Unspecified multiple injuries**} should not be assigned in the inpatient setting unless documentation for a more specific code is not available. Traumatic injury codes (**S00–T14.9**) are not to be used for normal, healing surgical wounds or to identify complications of surgical wounds.

The code for the most serious injury, as determined by the provider and the focus of treatment, is sequenced first.

Superficial Injuries

Superficial injuries, such as abrasions and contusions, are not coded when they are associated with more severe injuries at the same site.

Primary Injury With Damage to Nerves and/or Blood Vessels

When a primary injury results in minor damage to peripheral nerves or blood vessels, the primary injury is sequenced first. Any additional code or codes for injuries to nerves and the spinal cord and/or injury to vessels or nerves are coded as secondary.

Coding for Traumatic Fractures

The principles of multiple coding of injuries should be followed in the coding of fractures. Fractures of specified sites are coded individually by site in accordance with the level of detail furnished by the health record. The traumatic fracture categories include the following: A02, S12, S22, S32, S42, S49, S52, S59, S62, S72, S82, S89, and S92. A fracture not indicated as open or closed should be coded as closed. A fracture not indicated as displaced or not displaced should be coded as displaced.

Coding for Burns and Corrosions

The same principles for multiple coding apply to burns. Code each burn separately unless specific combination codes are given in the Tabular List. There are many combination codes. Most burn codes are found in Chapter 21 (Injury, Poisoning, and Certain Other Consequences of External Origin); the applicable codes are T20–T32. Because burns are coded by site and degree and by the extent of body surface involvement, all burn cases should have at least two codes and a third if the wound is infected. Other types of wounds, lacerations, punctures, and so on use a different 5th character to show that they are infected and therefore complicated. However, burn codes use the 5th character for other information; therefore, these diagnoses require an additional code to indicate infection.

The ICD-10-CM makes a distinction between burns and corrosions. The burn codes are used for the following: thermal burns (except sunburns) caused by a heat source, such as a fire or hot appliance; burns resulting from electricity; and burns resulting from radiation. Corrosions, on the other hand, are burns caused by chemicals. The guidelines are the same for burns and corrosions.

Current burns (T20–T25) are classified by depth, extent, and burn agent (X code). Depth is categorized as first degree (erythema), second degree (blistering), and third degree (full-thickness involvement). Burns of the eye and internal organs (T26–T28) are classified by site but not by degree.

Coding for Drug Toxicity

Chapter 21 also includes coding for the following drug toxicity classifications:

- *Poisoning* (T36–T50): A reaction to the improper use of a medication, which can be the result of an error made by the prescribing provider, intentional overdose, interaction with drugs or alcohol, or a reaction caused when a nonprescribed medication interacts with a prescribed and properly administered medication.
- *Adverse effect:* An unfavorable side effect that occurs even though a medication is correctly prescribed and properly administered.
- *Underdosing:* Patient takes less of a medication than is prescribed by the provider or by the manufacturer's instructions.
- *Toxic effect:* Patient ingests or comes in contact with a toxic substance.

Codes in categories T36–T65 are combination codes that include the substance taken and the intent. No additional external cause code is required for poisonings, toxic effects, adverse effects, and underdosing codes. When you are coding, do not code directly from the Table of Drugs and Chemicals. Always refer back to the Tabular List.

Coding for External Causes of Morbidity

In the ICD-9-CM, external causes of morbidity were coded with E codes (e.g., a fall from a ladder was coded E881.0). E codes were used to identify an accident or injury. However, E codes are not included in the ICD-10-CM code set.

Instead of using E codes, the ICD-10-CM has added Chapter 20, External Causes of Morbidity (V00-Y99). External cause codes are intended to provide data for research on injuries and for evaluation of injury prevention strategies. These codes capture how the injury or health condition happened (cause); the intent (unintentional or accidental; or intentional, such as suicide or assault), the place where the event occurred; the activity of the patient at the time of the event; and the person's status (e.g., civilian, military).

Place of Occurrence Guideline

Codes from category **Y92** {**Place of occurrence of the external cause**} are secondary codes; they are used after other external cause codes to identify the location of the patient at the time of the injury or other condition.

A place of occurrence code is used only once, at the initial encounter for treatment. No 7th character is used in Y92 codes. Only one code from category Y92 should be recorded on the patient's health record. Do not use place of occurrence code **Y92.9** {**Unspecified place or not applicable**} if the place is not stated or if it is not applicable.

Activity Codes

Activity codes **Y93** {**Activity codes**} are used to define the activity the patient was involved in at the time of injury or when the health condition developed. Only one code from category Y93 should be recorded in the patient's health record. An activity code should be used in conjunction with a place of occurrence code (Y92). The activity codes are not applicable to poisonings, adverse effects, misadventures. or sequelae.

Do not assign code **Y93.9** {**Unspecified activity**} if the activity is not stated.

A code from category Y93 can be used with external cause (Y99) and external cause codes if identifying the activity provides additional information about the event.

For example, you are coding a closed ankle fracture that occurred while the patient was playing soccer in a public park. First, you must identify what should be coded first. In this case, the ankle fracture is coded first: **S92.111A** {**Displaced fracture of neck of right talus**} (remember, "A" indicates initial encounter). The second code is the activity code; the patient was playing soccer, so the code for this activity is **Y93.66** {**Activity, soccer**}. Remember, if the report did not state an activity, do not add **Y93.9** {**Unspecified activity**}. Finally, when an activity code is used, a place of occurrence code should also be used. In this scenario, the patient was playing in a public park; therefore, the place of occurrence code is **Y92.830** {**Public park**}.

Coding for Health Status and Contact With Health Services

In the ICD-10-CM, Chapter 21, Factors Influencing Health Status and Contact with Health Services (Z00–Z99), replaces the V codes used in the ICD-9-CM to describe circumstances or encounters with a healthcare provider when no current illness or injury exists. The 16 categories of Z codes include contact/exposure, inoculations and vaccinations, health status, history of screening, observation, aftercare, follow-up, donor counseling, encounters for obstetric and reproductive services, newborns and infants, routine and administrative examinations, and other health encounters that do not fall into any one of the mentioned categories.

Maximizing Third-Party Reimbursement

The most important thing to remember in using the ICD-10-CM is to code the diagnosis to the highest level of specificity. Obtaining the correct reimbursement is important to the practice's cash flow, and it depends on proper coding and billing techniques. Some other crucial points to remember when submitting diagnostic codes for claims include:

- Use the current year ICD-10-CM manual and stay informed of all changes, revisions, and additions published for that year to both the codes and the official coding guidelines.
- Code accurately from documented information, making sure the appropriate code or codes are assigned for all parts of the diagnostic statement, with no additions or omissions.
- Be sure the diagnosis corresponds to the symptoms and treatment. Many codes are specific to age and gender.
- Review data entry to make sure no digits have been transposed.
- Know the insurance carrier's rules and requirements for completion and submission of claims.
- Incomplete or inaccurate codes may result in delay a possible or denial of reimbursement. An inaccurate diagnosis may have a lifelong negative effect on the patient.

Providers and Accurate Coding

Detailed documentation in the patient's health record can help coders to code to the highest specificity. Therefore, providers should be trained in how to document patient health records appropriately. Respectfully discuss with providers that diagnostic codes cannot be assigned unless clear documentation is found in the patient's health record. Some providers may feel that because they care for the same type of cases, specialized diagnostic statements should be implied. However, the medical assistant should stress to providers the high value of detailed documentation and how developing this practice not only improves ICD-10-CM code assignment, but also may result in higher health insurance reimbursements.

Staff meetings to review third-party requirements should be held regularly by the medical billing supervisor (Figure 14-14). Medical assistants should be respectful to the healthcare provider when third-party requirements compel more effort on their part. An understanding and patient attitude toward the healthcare provider goes a long way in building a trusting relationship.

---

if you know you need to query a provider about a health record that might yield a higher reimbursement, but that provider is on vacation for 7 days, enlist your office manager's help in flagging the health record until the provider returns to clarify it.

5. **Review notes from other health providers.** In most scenarios, coders are not allowed to code from documentation by anyone other than a provider; however, notes from ancillary staff members may encourage a coder to ask the provider whether the diagnosis does exist. For example, if a consultation with a dietitian suggests that a patient is malnourished, but the provider does not document this anywhere, you may be able to use the dietitian's clinical information as the basis for querying the provider. The diagnosis cannot be coded based solely on the dietitian's clinical information; the code can be assigned only after the provider confirms the diagnosis.

DeVault K. Know your ethical obligations regarding coding and documentation. www.hcpro .com/HOM-236942-5728/Know-your-ethical-obligations-regarding-coding-and-documentation .html. Accessed May 8, 2015.

Ethical Standards of Medical Coding

At times coders can feel pressured by decreasing insurance reimbursements and their employers to use fraudulent coding practices. However, if a medical practice is convicted of fraudulent billing, the coders may lose their coding license and face federal fines. A number of ethical standards have been established for medical coding, and most of these can help coders identify unethical coding behaviors. The following tips explain how to proceed in scenarios that may pose ethical dilemmas.

1. **Understand what ethical coding standards mean.** Coders face stress from all sides: financial issues, providers, and other coders. However, stress cannot be a compelling reason coders intentionally report diagnoses and/or higher specificity codes without sufficient documentation.

2. **Stand your ground.** When coding, be true to yourself, even though it can be hard in a stressful environment. When you know a chart needs additional documentation to justify reporting certain codes, don't be afraid to speak up to the provider. Conduct research ahead of time to strengthen your case. For example, search through and print out applicable issues of *Coding Clinic* from the American Hospital Association website: *ahacentraloffice.org*. The more backup documentation you have, the more likely it is that management will support your ethical coding decision.

3. **Say something.** Other coders may not follow the same ethical coding standards as you. If you observe unethical coding practices, bring it to the attention of the coder and allow him or her to make the needed adjustments. Broaching this issue with a colleague can be challenging, but encourage the other coder to reflect on the ethics of his or her actions. If the unethical coding practices continue, be sure to inform the next person in command.

4. **Keep in communication with the office manager.** Some coding situations require more management involvement than others. For example, if your conversation with a colleague does nothing to dissuade unethical behavior, bring your manager into the loop. Or,

---

CRITICAL THINKING APPLICATION   14-7

Mike used the GEMs to map the out-of-date ICD-9-CM codes to current ICD-10-CM codes, and then he updated the encounter form electronically. After a few days, Dr. Walker comes into Mike's office to ask that the old encounter form be printed out for him because he is not comfortable using the new electronic encounter form with the updated ICD-10-CM codes. What approach should Mike take in discussing Dr. Walker's concerns with him? How can Mike help Dr. Walker appreciate the need for the ICD-10-CM code updates?

CLOSING COMMENTS

Diagnostic coding using the ICD-10-CM, and its almost 70,000 codes, can seem overwhelming. Successful medical coders follow specific steps very closely to assign the most accurate ICD-10-CM code. Encoder software (e.g., TruCode) can search the ICD-10-CM electronically to facilitate faster coding. Detailed documentation in the patient's health record and accurate coding work hand in hand to maximize reimbursement for services rendered. The medical

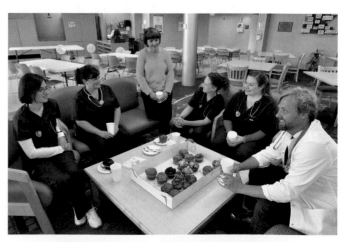

FIGURE 14-14 Regular staff meetings encourage accurate coding.

assistant can best communicate with healthcare professionals about accurate coding by showing them respect and patience. Medical assistants are expected to adhere to ethical standards, assigning and reporting only codes clearly supported by concise documentation in the patient's chart. When in doubt, a medical assistant should consult the attending healthcare provider for clarification. A coding professional is responsible for maintaining and continually enhancing his or her coding skills and for keeping informed of changes in the codes, guidelines, and regulations.

Patient Education

Most patients know very little about medical coding, so they may not understand how the codes on their encounter forms relate to their diagnosis. If the patient has questions, explain that the codes represent his or her diagnosis to the most specific and accurate level. Because the coding system is much like a foreign language to patients, be patient when explaining this process and answering questions, so that the patient is able to understand the insurance billing process.

Legal and Ethical Issues

Using the medical coding system allows providers to express the simplicity or complexity of a medical treatment or procedure. This specificity leads to the maximum reimbursement to the provider. The medical assistant must perform coding procedures accurately so that they reflect exactly what happened during the treatment. Codes must not be exaggerated to increase reimbursement to the provider.

Professional Behaviors

Although providers may be overly concerned about the need to maximize insurance reimbursements, coders should never feel coerced into fraudulent coding practices. Successful coders rely solely on medical documentation as the source of diagnostic statements. Coders should never assume that additional complications or conditions exist if they are not documented. In these cases, strong communication between the coder and the provider is necessary to clarify the appropriate diagnoses.

SUMMARY OF SCENARIO

Mike's experience using the ICD-1Ø-CM coding manual and encoder software on actual medical office cases has made him even more enthusiastic about his new responsibilities, and he enjoys the coding process more. He knows that as he gains experience in ICD-1Ø-CM coding, he will be able to set a positive example for the staff. As Mike progresses with diagnostic coding, he also will be able to help the providers and medical assistant staff be attentive to details when documenting in a health record.

Although the electronic encounter form for entering billing codes is an easy tool, Mike has learned that knowing how to use the ICD-1Ø-CM Alphabetic Index and Tabular List is a necessary asset to ensure accurate coding. He also knows

it is important when coding a diagnosis to make sure the medical documentation matches the encounter form and that all elements of the diagnostic statement are included. Furthermore, he must ensure that the diagnosis listed on the encounter form is fully documented in the patient's health record. Mike is feeling more comfortable about referring to coding guidelines to ensure the most accurate code and ensuring that every character for the ICD-1Ø-CM code is present. Every feature of the manual provides guidance in choosing and confirming a diagnostic code that matches the diagnostic statement on the encounter form and in the health record. Searching for codes in the encoder also has helped Mike develop his coding skills more quickly.

SUMMARY OF LEARNING OBJECTIVES

1. **Define, spell, and pronounce the terms listed in the vocabulary.**
   Spelling and pronouncing medical terms correctly reinforce the credibility of the medical assistant. Knowing the definition of these terms promotes confidence in communication with patients and co-workers. Also, understanding the medical terms found in the diagnostic statement is essential for identifying and selecting the most accurate and appropriate diagnostic code or codes.

2. **Describe the historical use of the *International Classification of Disease* (ICD) in the United States.**
   In 1946, the International Commission of the World Health Organization (WHO) established a code set called the *Manual of the International Statistical Classification of Diseases, Injuries, and Causes of Death* (ICD). Eventually, WHO approved an adaptation of this code set for use in the United States; the ninth edition, the *International Classification of*

Diseases, Ninth Revision, Clinical Modification (ICD-9-CM), was approved and put into use in 1975. The United States adopted ICD-1Ø-CM diagnostic coding on October 1, 2015.

3. **Describe the transition from ICD-9-CM diagnostic coding to ICD-1Ø-CM diagnostic coding.**
   As of the publication of this textbook, ICD-1Ø-CM diagnostic coding will be a somewhat new process, so it is important to familiarize yourself with the differences between the ICD-9-CM and the ICD-1Ø-CM. The ICD-1Ø-CM follows the same hierarchal structure as the ICD-9-CM, in which the first three characters represent the category of the code. (Review Table 14-1 to compare the differences in the ICD-9-CM and ICD-1Ø-CM code sets.) To aid the transition, the CMS has provided General Equivalence Mappings (GEMs), which help convert ICD-9-CM codes to the appropriate ICD-1Ø-CM codes.

Continued

SUMMARY OF LEARNING OBJECTIVES—*continued*

4. Identify the structure and format of the ICD-1Ø-CM.

Depending on the publisher, the ICD-1Ø-CM coding manual will vary somewhat in layout, symbols, color coding, and some other features. However, the format, conventions, tables, appendixes, content, and basic structure are always the same.

Every ICD-1Ø-CM code begins with an alphabetic letter that indicates the chapter of disease and injury in which the code is listed. (All the letters in the English alphabet are used except U, which WHO has reserved to assign to new diseases with uncertain etiologies.) Codes contain up to 7 alphanumeric characters; the first 3 characters are followed by a period. Codes that require a 7th character may use an X as a placeholder for the 4th, 5th, and 6th characters if no other code can be used for those characters.

5. Describe how to use the Alphabetic Index to select main terms, essential modifiers, and the appropriate code (or codes) or code ranges.

The ICD-1Ø-CM Index to Diseases and Injuries (commonly called the *Alphabetic Index*) consists of an alphabetic list of diagnostic terms and related codes. This index includes main terms, nonessential modifiers, essential modifiers, and subterms. Figure 14-3 provides an example of the *main term* **Colitis**; which is followed by the *nonessential modifiers* (acute), (catarrhal), (chronic), (noninfective), and (hemorrhagic). The second *essential modifier* listed under the main term is "amebic (acute)," and the *subterm* listed under amebic is "nondysenteric." The *main term* is bold face; the *nonessential modifiers* that follow it are enclosed in parentheses; the *essential modifier* is indented one space under the main term; and the *subterm* is indented one space under the essential modifier (two spaces under the main term). The nonessential modifiers (i.e., acute, catarrhal, chronic, noninfective, and hemorrhagic) do not affect the code assignment. The hyphen (-) at the end of the code indicates that additional characters are required to complete the code.

6. Do the following related to the Tabular List:

- *Explain how to use the Tabular List to select main terms, essential modifiers, and the appropriate code (or codes) or code ranges.*

  The ICD-1Ø-CM Tabular List of Diseases and Injuries (commonly called simply the *Tabular List*) is divided into 21 chapters. Each chapter is divided into categories, or *blocks,* that have been assigned 3-character codes. These codes form the foundation of the ICD-1Ø-CM code set.

  In most of the chapters, the title is composed of a group of diseases and injuries, followed by a code range in parentheses. For example, Chapter 1 is: Certain Infectious and Parasitic Diseases (AØØ—B99). However, some chapter titles use a part of the body or an organ system to group the codes; for example: Chapter 10, Diseases of the Circulatory System (IØØ—I99). Still other chapters group conditions together by etiology or the nature of the disease process, as in Chapter 2, Neoplasms (CØØ—D49). Chapter 17, Pregnancy, Childbirth, and the Puerperium (OØØ—O9A), groups codes related to the prenatal and postnatal periods. Chapter 20, External Causes of Morbidity (VØØ—Y99), replaces the V and E codes used in the ICD-9-CM. Chapter 20 also groups codes related to external causes of injury and poisoning. Chapter 21 is Factors Influencing Health Status and Contact with Health Services (ZØØ—Z99).

- *Summarize coding conventions as defined in the ICD-1Ø-CM coding manual.*

  Conventions are abbreviations, punctuation, symbols, instructional notations, and related elements that help the coder select an accurate, specific code. Conventions are found in the Tabular List, but not in the Alphabetic Index. Understanding their meaning and using them as guides are crucial to accurate coding.

7. Review the Official Coding Guidelines to assign the most accurate ICD-1Ø-CM diagnostic code.

An important section of the coding manual is the ICD-1Ø-CM Official Guidelines for Coding and Reporting. Every coding guideline for the entire ICD-1Ø-CM code set is included in this Coding Guidelines section at the beginning of the manual. These guidelines are a set of rules developed to accompany and complement the official conventions and instructions provided in the ICD-1Ø-CM proper.

8. Explain how to abstract the diagnostic statement from a patient's health record.

To prepare for medical coding, the medical assistant must analyze and abstract the diagnostic statements documented in the various reports in the patient's health record. Sources of diagnostic statements include the encounter form; treatment notes; discharge summary; operative report; and radiology, pathology, and laboratory reports.

9. Describe how to use the most current diagnostic codes and perform diagnostic coding.

Ten basic steps are required for accurate ICD-1Ø-CM coding (see Table 14-3). The first step involves abstracting the diagnostic statement from the health record and determining the main and essential modifiers from the various medical reports. The next steps are performed using the Alphabetic Index to search for the code, codes, or code ranges that best fit the diagnostic statement. The remaining steps are performed using the Tabular List to verify and confirm that the code or codes located in the Alphabetic Index fully match the diagnostic statement and are the most specific and accurate diagnostic codes.

The medical assistant's knowledge of accurate diagnostic coding contributes to the legal and financial health of the practice. In most cases, ICD-1Ø-CM codes are found on the encounter form. However, with literally thousands of current diagnostic codes, it may be necessary to code from the ICD-1Ø-CM manual. The process for diagnostic coding is outlined in Procedure 14-1.

10. Identify how encoder software can help the coder assign the most accurate diagnostic code.

Encoder software is computer-aided coding, which helps determine the most accurate code possible. The coder types a few key words into a Search box, and the software matches the entry with main terms in the Alphabetic Index. The coder then clicks on a specific code to hyperlink to the Tabular List.

SUMMARY OF LEARNING OBJECTIVES—*continued*

11. **Explain the importance of coding guidelines for accuracy, and discuss special rules and considerations that apply to the code selection process.**

    All ICD-10-CM coding manuals, regardless of the publisher, have comprehensive instructional notes and conventions to help the coder select the most accurate diagnostic code or codes. When a discrepancy occurs between reference sources, including this text, the current year's ICD-10-CM coding manual is the final authority. When coding, the medical assistant must always refer to and thoroughly review the conventions, instructional notations, code definitions, and other guidelines in the Alphabetic Index and Tabular List.

12. **Use tactful communication skills with medical providers to ensure accurate code selection.**

    The medical assistant coder must speak respectfully with providers about the importance of accurate health record documentation in maximizing reimbursements. Providers must understand that diagnostic codes cannot be assigned unless clear documentation is found in the patient's health record, even though some providers may feel that because they care for the same type of cases, specialized diagnostic statements should be implied.

13. **Review medical coding ethical standards.**

    At times medical coders can feel pressure from decreasing insurance reimbursements and their employers that they justify fraudulent coding practices. If a medical practice is convicted of fraudulent billing, it will lose its coding license, and it and the coder also may face federal fines. A number of standards have been established for ethical coding, and most of these can help coders recognize unethical coding behaviors.

CONNECTIONS

Study Guide Connection: Go to the Chapter 14 Study Guide. Read and complete the activities.

evolve Evolve Connection: Go to the Chapter 14 link at *evolve.elsevier.com/kinn* to complete the Chapter Review Quiz. Check out the other resources listed for this chapter to make the most of what you have learned from Basics of Diagnostic Coding.

15 BASICS OF PROCEDURAL CODING

SCENARIO

Sherald Vogt, a medical assisting student, works in an ambulatory surgery center run by Dr. John Caddell. Sherald really enjoyed learning about diagnostic coding in the *International Classification of Diseases, Tenth Revision, Clinical Modification* (ICD-10-CM), and now she looks forward to learning about procedural coding. Sherald recognized that a strong understanding of anatomy and pathophysiology was vital to correct diagnostic coding, and she believes the knowledge she has gained will help her in procedural coding. Sherald will be using the *Current Procedural Terminology* (CPT) coding system for most procedures and services provided in the medical office. In addition, she will use the *Healthcare Common Procedure Coding System* (HCPCS; pronounced "hic-pix") for auxiliary medical products and services.

As she did with the ICD-10-CM, Sherald will learn that accurate coding begins with the proper analysis of the clinical diagnosis (or diagnoses) and supporting documentation, from which she will abstract the correct data to assign an accurate procedure code. Just as does the ICD-10-CM, the CPT has coding guidelines, symbols, and formal steps specific to procedural coding, which Sherald will learn to use. However, unlike with ICD-10-CM diagnostic coding, in CPT and HCPCS coding, Sherald must determine how and when to use modifiers. Dr. Caddell wants to give Sherald some experience so he allows her to review some healthcare records so she can practice coding.

While studying this chapter, think about the following questions:

- What code set will be used for outpatient procedural coding?
- What will Sherald find similar to what she learned with the ICD-10-CM as she performs procedural coding?
- What will help Sherald select the most specific and accurate CPT code?
- What are the differences between CPT coding and HCPCS coding?
- How will Sherald use and apply modifiers in CPT and HCPCS coding?
- What will Sherald learn about the legal implications of inaccurate coding?

LEARNING OBJECTIVES

1. Define, spell, and pronounce the terms listed in the vocabulary.
2. Describe the organization of the *Current Procedural Terminology* (CPT) manual.
3. Report the history of procedural coding.
4. Distinguish between the Alphabetic Index and the Tabular List in the CPT code set.
5. Classify the six different sections of the CPT code set.
6. Discuss special reports, and explain the importance of modifiers in assigning CPT codes.
7. Review various conventions in the CPT code set.
8. Identify the required medical documentation for accurate procedural coding.
9. Describe how to use the most current procedural coding system and perform procedural coding for surgery.
10. Discuss how to use the Alphabetic Index.
11. Identify common CPT coding guidelines for evaluation and management (E/M) procedures.
12. Identify common CPT coding guidelines for anesthesia procedures.
13. Identify common CPT coding guidelines for surgical procedures.
14. Discuss coding factors for the integumentary system and muscular system, and for maternity care and delivery.
15. Identify common CPT coding guidelines for the Radiology, Pathology and Laboratory, and Medicine sections.
16. Do the following related to the HCPCS code set and manual:
    - Identify procedures and services that require HCPCS codes.
    - Describe how to use the most current HCPCS level II coding system.
17. Perform procedural coding of an office visit and an immunization.
18. Summarize common HCPCS coding guidelines.

VOCABULARY

Certified Registered Nurse Anesthetist (CRNA) A nursing healthcare professional who is certified to administer anesthesia.
CPT Assistant An online CPT coding journal, supported by the American Medical Association (AMA), that addresses subjects such as appealing insurance denials, validating coding to auditors, training staff members, and answering day-to-day coding questions.

debridement The surgical removal of dead, damaged, or infected tissue to improve the function of healthy tissue.

eponym In medical terms, a name of a medical diagnosis or procedure derived from the name of the person who discovered it.

global services For purposes of CPT coding, medical services and procedures performed for the patient before, during, and after a surgical procedure that is included with the assigned CPT code.

procedural statement The statement in the health record that specifically describes the procedures and services provided during the encounter.

special report Additional medical documentation required to confirm the need for the use of unlisted, unusual, or newly adopted medical procedures.

Procedural coding is the method of assigning a defined code for each specific medical procedure or service delivered by a qualified healthcare professional. Three types of procedure codes are used for medical coding for reimbursement: ICD-10-PCS, CPT, and HCPCS (Table 15-1). Because the medical assistant most likely will work in the outpatient setting, this chapter focuses on the CPT and HCPCS code sets. The medical biller is responsible for maintaining accurate medical recordkeeping and for processing insurance claims efficiently by using the CPT and HCPCS codes, which identify appropriate procedures and services common to the physician's office.

INTRODUCTION TO THE CPT MANUAL

The Current Procedural Terminology (CPT) system was developed and is maintained by the American Medical Association (AMA). It is updated each year and released on October 1. The CPT coding manual consists of descriptive terms and identifying codes for reporting professional and technical services. CPT codes convert free text procedural data into discrete data; that is, they establish a standard language that accurately describes medical and surgical services.

THE ORGANIZATION OF THE CPT MANUAL

Category I Codes

Category I codes are located in the Tabular List of the CPT manual and arranged by sections. For example, codes beginning with 7 (e.g., 70100—radiologic examination of the mandible, partial, with less

than four views) are located in the Radiology section of the manual. Each code has a description of the service or procedure performed. Some CPT codes (e.g., Category II and Category III codes, discussed later) are alphanumeric.

Category II Codes

Category II codes are a set of supplemental tracking codes that providers use for performance measurement. Category II codes are optional; they cannot be used as a substitute for Category I codes, and they are not reported as part of the insurance billing process. These codes describe clinical components that may be typically included in Evaluation and Management services or clinical services. In a Category II code, the 5th digit is the letter F.

Category II codes are described and listed in Appendix H of the CPT manual. They are listed in alphabetic order by condition. Category II codes are reviewed by the Performance Measures Advisory Group, which is composed of members from various medical organizations and government agencies. In some publishers' editions of the CPT manual, Category II codes are also listed in their own section, after the Medicine section and before the appendices.

Category III Codes

Category III codes are temporary codes assigned for emerging and new technology, services, and procedures that have not been officially added to the Tabular List of the CPT manual. Category III codes are intended to be used for data collection purposes, to substantiate widespread use, or as part of the approval process of the U.S. Food and Drug Administration (FDA). In a Category III code,

TABLE 15-1	Comparison of Procedural Code Sets					
CODE SET	**USED FOR**	**CODE FEATURES**	**EXAMPLE**	**DESCRIPTION**	**DEVELOPER**	**UPDATED**
ICD-10-PCS	Inpatient hospital procedures	7-digit alphanumeric code	0TTJ0ZZ	Appendectomy	National Center for Health Statistics	Annually, October 1
CPT	Outpatient procedures; professional and technical services	5-digit numeric code; a 2-digit modifier can be added	44970	Laparoscopic appendectomy	American Medical Association (AMA)	Annually, January 1
HCPCS	Auxiliary medical treatment, including vaccines, medical transport, drugs, durable medical equipment	5-digit alphanumeric code; a 2-digit modifier can be added	A0428	Ambulance service, basic life support, nonemergency transport	Centers for Medicare and Medicaid Services (CMS)	Annually, October 1

the 5th digit is the letter T. Category III codes may be used in billing and reporting if no code in the Tabular List accurately describes the technology, service, or procedure performed and no Category I code matches the medical documentation. Category III codes have no reimbursement value. In most publishers' editions of the CPT manual, Category III codes are also listed in their own section, after the Medicine section and before the appendices.

THE EVOLUTION OF CPT CODING

The AMA first published the CPT coding manual in 1966. The first edition contained only surgical codes, and the codes had only 4 digits.

The second edition of the CPT, published in 1970, presented an expanded system of five-digit codes to designate diagnostic and therapeutic procedures in surgery, medicine, radiology, laboratory, pathology, and medical specialties. At that time, the four-digit classification was replaced with the current five-digit coding system. The fourth edition, published in 1977, included significant updates in medical technology. At the same time, a system of periodic annual updating was introduced to keep pace with the rapidly changing environment.

Format of the CPT Coding Manual

- Comprehensive instructions for using the manual, including the steps for coding
- The Alphabetic Index
- Tabular List includes the following six sections:
  - Evaluation and Management
  - Anesthesia
  - Surgery
  - Radiology
  - Pathology and Laboratory
  - Medicine
- Coding Guidelines, Conventions, and Notes
- Appendices (15; A-O)

THE ALPHABETIC INDEX

The CPT coding manual is separated into the Alphabetic Index and the Tabular List. The Alphabetic Index is organized by main terms; these terms represent the type of surgery, the anatomic site, or **eponym** (Figure 15-1).

THE TABULAR LIST

The Tabular List is divided into six sections, with codes listed in numeric order in each section. As in the ICD-10-CM, the codes in the Tabular List include definitions, guidelines, and notes, which enable the coder to select the most specific code based on the procedural statement and service descriptions documented in the health record. The six sections of the Tabular List and their CPT code ranges are:

- Evaluation and Management (99201-99499)
- Anesthesia (00100-01999, 99100-99140)

Fracture	
Acetabulum	
Closed Treatment	27220-27222
Open Treatment	27226-27228
with Manipulation	27222
without Manipulation	27220
Alveolar Ridge	
Closed Treatment	21440
Open Treatment	21445
Ankle	
Bimalleolar	27808, 27810, 27814
Lateral	27786, 27788, 27792, 27808, 27810, 27814
Medial	27760, 27762, 27766, 27808, 27810, 27814
Posterior	27767-27769, 27808, 27810, 27814
Trimalleolar	27816, 27818, 27822-27823
Ankle Bone	
Medial	27760-27762
Bennett's	
See Thumb, Fracture	
Blow-Out Fracture	
Orbital Floor	21385-21387, 21390, 21395
Bronchi	
Reduction	31630
Calcaneus	
Closed Treatment	28400-28405
Open Treatment	28415-28420
Percutaneous Fixation	28406
with Manipulation	28405-28406
without Manipulation	28400

FIGURE 15-1 Alphabetic Index: Fractures.

- Surgery (10021-69990)
- Radiology, including nuclear medicine and diagnostic ultrasound (70010-79999)
- Pathology and Laboratory (80047-89398)
- Medicine (90281-99199, 99500-99607)

Sections are subdivided into *subsections*; *subsections* are subdivided into *categories*; and *categories* can be subdivided into *subcategories*. Each level of a section provides more specificity about the procedure or service performed and the anatomic site or organ system involved. Each section and subsection provides coding guidelines and, if needed, a reference to the **CPT Assistant**. In most instances, all four levels are found, although this is not a hard-and-fast rule.

In the CPT manual, the subsection is listed below the section and indented two spaces. The subsection usually describes an anatomic site or an organ system, as in the following examples:

- Anatomic site: heart, femur, or skull
- Organ system: digestive, integumentary, or cardiovascular

A category is listed below the subsection and indented two spaces. It generally refers to a specific procedure or service, but it can also indicate a more specific anatomic site:

- Procedures: esophagoscopy, incision and drainage, or cardiac catheterization
- Specific anatomic site: mitral valve, distal femur, or occipital bone

Subcategory is the lowest level of code description. The subcategory is listed below the category and indented two spaces. It provides even more specificity about an anatomic site or the procedure or service performed.

CRITICAL THINKING APPLICATION **15-1**

To practice her coding skills, Sherald is reviewing a surgical report for a gallbladder removal. Will she be able to find the main term "gallbladder" in the Alphabetic index? Why or why not? What main term should she be looking for? Once she finds the range of codes in the Alphabetic Index, what is her next step?

Evaluation and Management Section

The Evaluation and Management (E/M) section contains codes for the different types of encounters or patient visits. The code range in the E/M section is 99201 to 99499. The E/M section is further divided into subsections that include different types of services (e.g., office visits, hospital visits, consultations, skilled nursing facility, or nursing home visits). Each of these subsections is divided into codes that specify whether the patient is new or established. The subcategories of E/M services are further classified into levels of E/M services that are identified by specific codes. This classification is important because the nature of a provider's work varies by type of service, place of service, and the patient's status.

Anesthesia Section

The Anesthesia section includes CPT-4 codes for services by anesthesiologists and anesthetists. The code ranges in the Anesthesia section are 00100 to 01999 and 99100 to 99140. The CPT-4 codes include any type of anesthesia administered (e.g., general, local, and sedation anesthesia) for the surgery performed on the specified area of the body. Other support services, including the anesthesiologist's preoperative and postoperative encounters with the patient; evaluation of the patient's physical status; administration of anesthesia, fluids, and/or blood; and monitoring services, such as blood pressure, temperature, and electrocardiography, are also included in this code. Figure 15-2 presents examples of CPT-4 Anesthesia codes.

Forearm, Wrist, and Hand

01810	Anesthesia for all procedures on nerves, muscles, tendons, fascia, and bursae of forearm, wrist, and hand ➡ *CPT Assistant* Mar 06:15, Nov 07:8, Oct 11:3, Jul 12:13
01820	Anesthesia for all closed procedures on radius, ulna, wrist, or hand bones
01829	Anesthesia for diagnostic arthroscopic procedures on the wrist ➡ *CPT Changes: An Insider's View* 2003
01830	Anesthesia for open or surgical arthroscopic/endoscopic procedures on distal radius, distal ulna, wrist, or hand joints; not otherwise specified ➡ *CPT Changes: An Insider's View* 2003
01832	total wrist replacement
01840	Anesthesia for procedures on arteries of forearm, wrist, and hand; not otherwise specified
01842	embolectomy
01844	Anesthesia for vascular shunt, or shunt revision, any type (eg, dialysis)
01850	Anesthesia for procedures on veins of forearm, wrist, and hand; not otherwise specified
01852	phleborrhaphy
01860	Anesthesia for forearm, wrist, or hand cast application, removal, or repair ➡ *CPT Assistant* Nov 07:8, Jul 12:13

FIGURE 15-2 CPT-4 Anesthesia Codes.

Surgery Section

The Surgery section, the largest section of the CPT Tabular List, includes standardized codes for all *invasive surgical procedures* performed by providers or other qualified professionals. An invasive procedure is any medical procedure in which a body orifice or the skin must be penetrated by cutting or puncture (Figure 15-3 shows the Surgery section for procedures of the larynx). In most instances, each subsection is further divided into categories and subcategories, which describe procedures and services unique to that anatomic subsection. This section is divided into subsections that typically identify specific body systems, beginning with the integumentary system (skin) and ending with the ophthalmologic (eye) and otologic (ear) systems.

Larynx
Excision

31300	Laryngotomy (thyrotomy, laryngofissure); with removal of tumor or laryngocele, cordectomy
31320	diagnostic
31360	Laryngectomy; total, without radical neck dissection ➡ *CPT Assistant* Aug 10:4
31365	total, with radical neck dissection ➡ *CPT Assistant* Oct 01:10, Aug 10:4
31367	subtotal supraglottic, without radical neck dissection ➡ *CPT Assistant* Aug 10:4
31368	subtotal supraglottic, with radial neck dissection
31370	Partial laryngectomy (hemilaryngectomy); horizontal
31375	laterovertical
31380	anterovertical
31382	antero-latero-vertical
31390	Pharyngolaryngectomy, with radical neck dissection; without reconstruction
31395	with reconstruction
31400	Arytenoidectomy or arytenoidopexy, external approach (For endoscopic arytenoidectomy, use 31560)
31420	Epiglottidectomy

FIGURE 15-3 Surgery Section and Subsection: Larynx Excision.

Radiology Section

The Radiology section includes codes for diagnostic imaging, including x-ray studies, body scans, and for therapy used in the treatment of cancer. The code range in the Radiology section is 70000 to 79999. Radiology codes are designed for use by radiologists and other medical professionals by simply adding or changing a modifier. Radiology codes are differentiated by the number of views taken (Figure 15-4).

Pathology and Laboratory Section

Codes are included for all diagnostic tests performed on bodily fluids and tissues (including urine, blood, sputum, and feces); for those performed on excised or biopsied cells, tissue, or body organs; and for evaluation of those fluids and tissues to identify any pathology or disease present. The code ranges for the Pathology and Laboratory section are 80047 to 80076 for Organ or Disease-Oriented Panels and 80100 to 89999 for all other tests. Organ or Disease-Oriented Panel CPT codes are *bundled* into one specific code,

---

CRITICAL THINKING APPLICATION   15-2

Sherald reviewed a coded medical record for a Basic Metabolic Panel with total Calcium that had listed specific CPT codes for each panel test. Is this the correct way of coding for the organ panel? According to Figure 15-5, how should this organ panel be coded?

Spine and Pelvis

72010   Radiologic examination, spine, entire, survey study, anteroposterior and lateral
→ *CPT Assistant* May 02:18, Jan 07:29
→ *Clinical Examples in Radiology* Fall 09:10, Spring 13:9
72020   Radiologic examination, spine, single view, specify level
→ *CPT Assistant* Jul 13:10
→ *Clinical Examples in Radiology* Spring 13:8, 9
72040   Radiologic examination, spine, cervical; 2 or 3 views
→ *CPT Assistant* Sep 01:7, Jul 13:10; *CPT Changes: An Insider's View* 2001, 2013, 2014
→ *Clinical Examples in Radiology* Fall 09:10, Summer 11:8, Fall 11:9, Spring 13:8, 9
72050   4 or 5 views
→ *CPT Changes: An Insider's View* 2013
→ *Clinical Examples in Radiology* Summer 11:8, Fall 11:9, Spring 13:9
72052   6 or more views
→ *CPT Changes: An Insider's View* 2013
→ *Clinical Examples in Radiology* Summer 11:8, Fall 11:9, Spring 13:9

FIGURE 15-4 Radiology Section: Spine and Pelvis.

80047   Basic metabolic panel (Calcium, ionized)
This panel must include the following:
Calcium, ionized (82330)
Carbon dioxide (bicarbonate)(82374)
Chloride (82435)
Creatinine (82565)
Glucose (82947)
Potassium (84132)
Sodium (84295)
Urea Nitrogen (BUN)(84520)
→ *CPT Assistant* Apr 08:5, Apr 13:10; *CPT Changes: An Insider's View* 2008
80048   Basic metabolic panel (Calcium, total)
This panel must include the following:
Calcium, total (82310)
Carbon dioxide (bicarbonate)(82374)
Chloride (82435)
Creatinine (82565)
Glucose (82947)
Potassium (84132)
Sodium (84295)
Urea Nitrogen (BUN)(84520)
→ *CPT Assistant* Jan 98:6, Sep 99:11, Nov 99:44, Jan 00:7, Aug 05:9; *CPT Changes: An Insider's View* 2000, 2008, 2009

FIGURE 15-5 Laboratory Section: Organ Panel.

which lists the included tests, along with their specific CPT code (Figure 15-5).

Medicine Section

The codes for the Medicine section range from 90281 to 99199 and 99500 to 99607 (excluding the anesthesia code ranges described in

---

A View of the Outer Cochlear Implant
92601-92604

An example of the elements that are addressed in the diagnostic analysis and reprogramming of the cochlear implant.

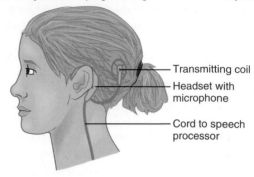

— Transmitting coil
— Headset with microphone
— Cord to speech processor

92601   Diagnostic analysis of cochlear implant, patient younger than 7 years of age; with programming
→ *CPT Assistant* Mar 03:1, Jan 06:7, Jul 11:17, Oct 13:7, Jul 14:4; *CPT Changes: An Insider's View* 2003
92602   subsequent reprogramming
→ *CPT Assistant* Mar 03:1, Jan 06:7, Oct 13:7; *CPT Changes: An Insider's View* 2003
(Do not report 92602 in addition to 92601)
(For aural rehabilitation services following cochlear implant, including evaluation of rehabilitation status, see 92626-92627, 92630-92633)
92603   Diagnostic analysis of cochlear implant, age 7 years or older; with programming
→ *CPT Assistant* Mar 03:2, 4, Jan 06:7, Jul 11:17, Oct 13:7; *CPT Changes: An Insider's View* 2003
92604   subsequent reprogramming
→ *CPT Assistant* Mar 03:2, 21, Jan 06:7, Jul 11:17, Oct 13:7, Jul 14:4; *CPT Changes: An Insider's View* 2003
(Do not report 92604 in addition to 92603)
92605   Evaluation for prescription of non-speech-generating augmentative and alternative communication device, face-to-face with the patient; first hour
→ *CPT Assistant* Mar 03:2, 4, Oct 13:7; *CPT Changes: An Insider's View* 2003, 2012
#✚ 92618   each additional 30 minutes (List separately in addition to code for primary procedure)
→ *CPT Changes: An Insider's View* 2012
(Use 92618 in conjunction with 92605)
92606   Therapeutic service(s) for the use of non-speech-generating device, including programming and modification
→ *CPT Assistant* Mar 03:2, 4; *CPT Changes: An Insider's View* 2003

FIGURE 15-6 Medicine Section: Analysis of Cochlear Implant.

the Anesthesia section). The Medicine section includes many and varied subsections, categories, and subcategories. This section can be considered a catchall section in that it includes codes for services and procedures that do not fit into any of the other sections of the CPT manual. Medical specialties, such as ophthalmology, otolaryngology, and allergy, which involve procedures and services that vary greatly from the traditional office encounter, are grouped in the Medicine section rather than the E/M section. Noninvasive diagnostic tests such as diagnostic analysis of cochlear implants, ECGs, and allergy testing, are included in the Medicine section rather than in the Surgery section (Figure 15-6).

UNLISTED PROCEDURE OR SERVICE CODE

Occasionally, even with the best, detailed documentation, an accurate, specific code to match the procedure or service performed cannot be found in the CPT manual. In each section (and sometimes in subsections, categories, and/or subcategories), nonspecific codes have been provided. These codes are known as Unlisted Procedures and Services. For example, code 29999 is found in the Surgery section, Musculoskeletal subsection. It describes an "unlisted procedure, arthroscopy." Unlisted codes can be used only when no Category I or Category III code exactly matches the medical documentation. When an unlisted code is used, a **Special Report** must be sent with the insurance claim that describes the procedure or service in detail.

CPT CODING GUIDELINES

Coding guidelines, which are found at the beginning of each section and some subsections of the Tabular List, add definitions and descriptions necessary to appropriately interpret and report the procedures and services in that section or subsection. Coding guidelines enhance the coder's understanding of when and under what circumstances specific codes may be used. Therefore, it is important to thoroughly read and apply the coding guidelines provided in the Tabular List. Because coding guidelines are updated every year on October 1, it is also important to reread the guidelines after every new edition is released. Selecting a code without reading the guidelines usually leads to selection of the wrong code. Not only will this result in possibly delayed or denied reimbursement, but also, continued inappropriate code selection can be considered fraud or abuse and can result in serious civil or criminal penalties.

Modifiers

Modifiers are two-digit, alphanumeric codes that report or indicate specific criteria, a specific condition, or a special circumstance. They are used with CPT codes to indicate that a service or procedure performed was altered by specific circumstances (Table 15-2). Modifiers are included with the five-digit CPT code to supply additional information or to describe extenuating circumstances that affected the rendered procedure or service. For instance, modifier -50 adds the detail that a procedure was performed bilaterally, or on both sides of the body. To describe a situation in which an assistant surgeon is needed for a surgical procedure, modifier -80 can be used to allow the assistant surgeon to submit charges for his or her time and services. Modifiers can also determine which side of the body a medical procedure was performed. The code 19100 RT indicates that the right breast was biopsied. A list of modifiers can be found in the CPT coding manual in Appendix A.

CPT CONVENTIONS

Conventions, or special symbols (Figure 15-7), are used to provide additional information about specific codes. For example, one of the codes in the Surgery section, Integumentary subsection, is +15401. Code 15401 describes "each additional 100 sq. cm ..." Just above code 15401 is code 15400, which describes a "xenograft of the skin ... the first 100 sq. cm. or less ..." If the medical documentation states that a "200 sq. cm. xenograft of the skin" was performed, the medical assistant would code the first 100 sq. cm. using code 15400, and the second 100 sq. cm. by using add-on code 15401 (+15401).

Another example of a symbol convention is a circle with a small round dot in the center. This symbol indicates that conscious sedation, rather than a general anesthetic, was used during a surgical procedure.

In the Tabular List in most CPT manuals, the legend explaining the meanings of the convention symbols is found at the bottom of each page of the Tabular List.

APPENDICES

The CPT coding manual uses appendices to organize changes to the original code set. There are 15 appendices. A list of appendices and the codes they contain can be found in Table 15-3.

TABLE 15-2   Commonly Used CPT Code Modifiers

MODIFIER	DESCRIPTION
-50	Bilateral procedure. If the procedure was performed on both sides of the body (e.g., both knees, both eyes) and the code description does not indicate that the procedure or service was performed bilaterally, modifier -50 is used.
-62	Two surgeons. When two surgeons work together as primary surgeons performing distinct parts of a procedure, each surgeon should report the procedure he or she performed to the insurance carrier using modifier -62. This prevents the insurance carrier from possibly rejecting a surgical charge as a duplicate.
-26	Professional component. This modifier is used when a technician performs the service to provide his professional opinion.
-RT, -LT	Indicates the side of the body on which the procedure took place. (e.g., 19100-LT — Breast biopsy, left side)

Symbols

▲   Revised code
●   New code
▶◀   New or revised text
⟳   Reference to *CPT Assistant*, *Clinical Examples in Radiology*, and *CPT Changes*
✚   Add-on code
⊘   Exemptions to modifier 51
⊙   Moderate sedation
✗   Product pending FDA approval
○   Reinstated or recycled code
\#   Out-of-numerical sequence code

FIGURE 15-7 CPT conventions.

TABLE 15-3   Appendices of the CPT Manual

APPENDIX	TITLE	DESCRIPTION
A	Modifiers	All modifiers applicable to CPT codes
B	Summary of Additions, Deletions, and Revisions	Shows the actual changes made to the annual CPT manual
C	Clinical Examples	Provides helpful narrative examples to aid selection of the correct and most specific level of Evaluation and Management (E/M) codes
D	Summary of CPT Add-on Codes	A list of CPT add-on codes
E	Summary of CPT Codes Exempt from Modifier 51	CPT codes that cannot use modifier 51, which indicates multiple procedures
F	Summary of CPT Codes Exempt from Modifier 63	CPT codes that cannot use modifier 51, which indicates procedures done on infants weighing < 4 kg
G	Summary of CPT Codes That Include Moderate (Conscious) Sedation	A list of CPT codes that do not use an additional code for conscious sedation
H	Alphabetic Listing of Performance Measures	Contains an alphabetic index of performance measures by clinical condition or topic
I	Genetic Testing Modifiers	Contains genetic testing modifiers
J	Electrodiagnostic Medicine Listing of Sensory, Motor, and Mixed Nerves	A list in which each sensory, motor, and mixed nerve is assigned its appropriate nerve conduction study code, to enhance accurate reporting of codes 95907 to 95913
K	Product Pending FDA Approval	Vaccine products that have been assigned a CPT code in anticipation of approval from the Food and Drug Administration (FDA)
L	Vascular Families	A diagram of veins to the first, second, and third order. assuming that the starting point is catheterization of the aorta
M	Renumbered CPT Codes— Citations Crosswalk	A summary of crosswalked, deleted, and renumbered codes, in addition to descriptors with the associated *CPT Assistant* references for the deleted codes
N	Summary of Resequenced CPT Codes	A list of CPT codes that do not appear in numeric sequence, which allows existing codes to be relocated to an appropriate location
O	Multianalyte Assays with Algorithmic Analysis	A list of CPT codes that includes a set of administrative codes for Multianalyte Assays with Algorithmic Analyses procedures; these typically are unique to a single clinical laboratory or manufacturer

CRITICAL THINKING APPLICATION   **15-3**

Sherald is trying to look up the CPT code for a left arm cyst biopsy. She has found the code, but how can she show that the procedure took place on the left side? Sherald also came across CPT code 32491 (removal of lung, pneumonectomy), but she needs to also code for the repair of a portion of the bronchus. The code has a (+) in front of it; what does this mean?

MEDICAL DOCUMENTATION FOR CPT CODING

Medical records used for procedural coding can include any or all of the following:

- Encounter form (Figure 15-8)
- History and physical report (H&P)
- Progress notes
- Discharge summary
- Operative report
- Pathology report
- Anesthesia record
- Radiology report

When comparing the medical documentation to the code, all of the elements of the description must match substantially, with nothing added or missing. For example, review CPT codes 21325 and 21320. Both codes describe the closed treatment of a nasal bone fracture. However, 21325 indicates that there is no stabilization and 21320 indicates that there is stabilization. The coder abstracts the procedural statement and then assigns the CPT code with the description that most closely resembles the medical document.

John Porter, MD Daniel Berg, MD
Roman Jagla, MD Katherine Olson, PNP
Ann Johnson, MD Emily Luther, FNP

YOUR NAME CLINIC
1234 College Avenue
Saint Paul, Minnesota 55316
Phone: (555) 555-2133   Fax: (555) 555-2134

TELEPHONE:
FAX:

PATIENT'S NAME		CHART #		DATE			

☐ MEDI-MEDI ☐ MEDICAL
☐ MEDICARE ☐ PRIVATE
☐ SELF PAY ☐ HMO _____

✔	CPT/Md	DESCRIPTION	FEE	✔	CPT/Md	DESCRIPTION	FEE	✔	CPT/Md	DESCRIPTION	FEE	✔	CPT/Md	DESCRIPTION	FEE
	OFFICE VISIT—NEW PATIENT					**LAB STUDIES**				**PROCEDURES (continued)**				**INJECTIONS**	
	99202	Focused Ex.			36415	Venipucture			93235	Holter, 24 Hour			90724	Influenza	
	99203	Detailed Ex.			81000	Urinalysis			10061	I & D Abscess Comp.			90732	Pneumococcal	
	99204	Comprehensive Ex.			81003	–w/o Micro			10060	I & D Abscess Simple			J0295	Ampicillin, 1 gr	
	99205	Complex Ex.			84703	HCG (Urine, Pregnancy)			94761	Oximetry w/Exercise			J0696	Rocephine	
	OFFICE VISIT—ESTABLISHED PATIENT				82948	Glucose			93720	Plethysmography			J1030	Depomedrol 40 mg	
	99212	Focused Ex.			82270	Hemoccult			94760	Pulse Oximetry			J2000	Lidocaine 50 cc	
	99213	Expanded Ex.			85023	CBC-diff.			10003	Rem. Sebaceous Cyst			J2175	Demerol	
	99214	Detailed Ex.			85024	CBC w/part diff			11100	Skin Bx			J3360	Valium 5 mg	
	99215	Complex Ex.			85018	Hemoglobin			94010	Spirometry			J1885	Toradol 30 mg IV	
	PREVENTATIVE MEDICINE—NEW PATIENT				88155	Pap Smear			92801	Visual Acuity			J1885	Toradol 60 mg IM	
	99381	< 1 year old			87210	KOH/Saline Wet Mount			17100	Wart Removal			90720	DTP–HIB	
	99382	1–4 year old			87430	Strep Antigen			17101	Wart Removal, 2nd			90746	HEP B—HIB	
	99383	5–11 year old			87060	Throat Culture			17102	Wart Removal, 3–15			90707	MMR	
	99384	12–17 year old			80009	Chem profile			11042	Wound Debrid.			86580	PPD	
	99385	18–39 year old			80061	Lipid profile			**X-RAY**				86580	PPD w/control	
	99386	40–64 year old			82465	Cholesterol			70210	Sinuses			90732	Pneumovax	
	99387	65+ year old			99000	Handling fee			70360	Neck Soft Tissue			90716	Varicella	
	PREVENTATIVE MEDICINE—ESTABLISHED PATIENT				**PROCEDURES**				71010	CXR (PA only)			82607	Vitamin B12 Inj.	
	99391	< 1 year old			92551	Audiometry			71020	Chest 2V			90712	Polio	
	99392	1–4 year old			29705	Cast Removal			72040	C-Spine 2V			90788	TD Adult	
	99393	5–11 year old			2900_	Casting (by location)			72100	Lumbrosacral			95115	Allergy inj., single	
	99394	12–17 year old			92567	Ear Check			73030	Shoulder 2V			95117	Allergry inj., multiple	
	99395	18–39 year old			69210	Ear Wax Rem. 1 2			73070	Elbow 2V					
	99396	40–64 year old			93000	EKG			73130	Hand 2V					
	99397	65+ year old			93005	EKG tracing only			73560	Knee 2V					
					93010	EKG. Int. and Rep			73620	Foot 2V					
					11750	Excision Nail			74000	KUB					
					94375	Flow Volume									

DESCRIPTION	ICD-10-CM
Abdominal pain/unspec	R10.9
Abscess	L02._
Allergic reaction	T78.40_
Alzheimer's disease	G30
Anemia/unspec	D64.9
Angina/unspec	I20.9
Anorexia	R63.0
Anxiety/unspec	F41.9
Apnea, sleep	G47.30
Arrhythmia, cardiac	I49.9
Arthritis, rheumatoid	M06.9
Asthma/unspec	J45.909
Atrial fibrillation	I48.0
B-12 deficiency	E53.8
Back pain, low	M54.5
BPH	N40
Bradycardia/unspec	R00.1
Broncitis, acute	J20._
Bronchitis, chronic	J42
Burritio/unopco	M71.0
CA, breast	C50._
CA, lung	C34._
CA, prostate	C61
Cellulitis	L03._
Chest pain/unspec	R07.9
Cirrhosis, liver/unspec	K74.60
Cold, common	J00
Colitis/unspec	K51.90
Confusion	R41.0
CHF	I50.9
Constipation	K59.00
COPD	J44.9
Cough	R05
Crohn's disease/unspec	K50.90
CVA	I63.9
Decubitus ulcer	L89._
Dehydration	E86.0
Dementia/unspec	F03
Depression, major/unsp	F32.9
Diab I, no complications	E10.0
Diab II, no complications	E11.9
w/kidney complic	E11.2_
w/ophthalmic compl	E11.3_
w/neurolog compl	E11.4_
w/circulartory compl	E11.5_
Insulin use	Z79.4
Diarrhea/unspec	R19.7
Diverticulitix	K57.92
Diverticulosis	K57.90
Dizziness	R42
Dysuria	R30.0
Edema/unspec	R60.9
Endocarditis	I38
Esophageal reflux	K21.0
Fatigue (lethargy)	R53.83
FUO	R50.9
Gaotritio	R20.70
Gastroenteritis (colitis)	K52.9
G.I. bleed	K92.2
Gout/unspec	M10.9
Headache	R51
Health exam	Z00._
Hematuria/unspec	R31.9
Herpes simplex	B00.9
Herpes zoster	B02.9
Hiatal hernia	K44.9
HTN (HBP)	I10
Hyperlipidemia/unspec	E78.5
Hypothyroidism/unspec	E03.9
Impotence	N52._
Influenza, respiratory	J10.1
Insomnia	G47.0
IBS, diarrhea	K58.
Lupus, systemic erythim	M32.9
MI, acute	I21._
MI, old	I25.2
Migraine	G43.9
Myalgia	M79.1
Neck pain	M54.2
Neuropathy	G62.9
Nausea	R11.1
Nausea/vomitting	R11.0
Obesity/unspec	E66.9
Osteoarthritis (site)	M19._
Otitis media	H66.9_
Parkinson's disease	G20
Pharyngitis, acute	J02.9
Pleurisy	R09.1
Pneumonia	J18.9
Pneumonia, viral	J12.9
Prostatitis/unspec	N41.9
PVD	I73.9
Radiculopathyp	M54.1_
Rectal bleeding	K62.5
Renal failure	N19
Sciatica	M54.3_
Shortness of breath	R03.02
Sinusitis, chr./unspec	J32.9
Syncope	R55
Tachycardia/unspec	R00.0
Tachy., supraventric	I47.1
Tedinitix/unspec	M77.9
TIA	G45.9
Ulcer, duodenal/unspec	K26.9
Ulcer, gastric/unspec	K25.9
Ulcer, peptic/unspec	K27.9
URI/unspec	J06.9
UTI	N39.0
Vertigo	R42
Weight gain	R63.5
Weight loss	R63.4

DIAGNOSIS: (IF NOT CHECKED ABOVE)

TODAY'S FEE

AMT. REC'D.

PROCEDURES: (IF NOT CHECKED ABOVE)

RETURN APPOINTMENT INFORMATION:

REC'D BY:
☐ CASH
☐ CR. CARD
☐ CHECK
_____

BALANCE

(DAYS)(WKS)(MOS)(PRN)

FIGURE 15-8 Encounter form.

Some providers have CPT and ICD-10-CM codes printed on their encounter forms; however, these codes should be treated only as a reference. Medical coders must also review the health record carefully and an abstract of all the procedures and services rendered during an encounter, regardless of all codes highlighted on the encounter form. For example, a provider may circle the procedure for a preventive health visit for a 4-year-old on the encounter form, but forgets to record the injections provided during the encounter. When the medical assistant reviews the patient's electronic health record (EHR), he or she discovers that the provider's notes state routine injections were indeed administered. If the medical assistant had not reviewed the EHR, the clinic would have lost reimbursement because the claim would not have included all the CPT codes applicable to the visit. Encounter forms should be updated annually to ensure that code additions, changes, and revisions are current.

STEPS FOR EFFICIENT CPT PROCEDURAL CODING

The CPT coding process, which includes use of the Alphabetic Index and the Tabular List, applies to all sections of the CPT manual, except for the E/M and Anesthesia sections.

To start the procedural coding process, you must first determine the procedures or services that were provided. This is accomplished with two basic steps:
1. Analyze and abstract the procedural statement documented in the health record.
2. Compare it with the encounter form, operative report, or other documentation to ensure that all services and procedures have been recorded.

For practice on CPT surgery coding, refer to Procedure 15-1.

Abstracting

The term *abstract*, used as a verb in this context, is the process of collecting pertinent medical information needed to assign the correct code.

Abstracting ensures that all medical procedures and services are identified and none are omitted. The abstracted data are then broken down into main terms and modifying terms. A main term is usually the primary procedure or service performed, and a modifying term further defines or adds information to the main term. Next, the main and modifying terms are used to find the code or code ranges in the Alphabetic Index. Last, the code selected is confirmed by reviewing the guidelines, notes, and conventions in the Tabular List to verify that the most accurate code has been chosen.

PROCEDURE 15-1   Perform Procedural Coding: Surgery

Goal: *To use the steps for CPT procedural coding to find the most accurate and specific CPT surgery code.*

EQUIPMENT and SUPPLIES

- CPT coding manual (current year)
- Surgery report (Figure 1)
- TruCode encoder software

PROCEDURAL STEPS

Using the CPT Coding Manual

1. Abstract the procedures and/or services from the procedural statement in the surgical report.
2. Select the most appropriate main term to begin the search in the Alphabetic Index.
3. Once the main term has been located in the Alphabetic Index, review and select the modifying term or terms if required.
   PURPOSE: For additional specificity and to narrow the search for the most accurate CPT code or code range in the Alphabetic Index.
4. If the main term cannot be found in the Alphabetic Index, repeat steps 2 and 3 using a different main term possibly based on the procedural statement.
5. Once the CPT code or code range is identified in the Alphabetic Index, disregard any code or code range containing additional descriptions or modifying terms not found in the health record.
6. Record the code or code ranges that best match the procedural statements in the surgical report.
   PURPOSE: To prevent repeated reference to the Alphabetic Index by recording all possible matches to the code or code range sought. This saves time and prevents redundant effort.

7. Turn to the Tabular List and find the first code or code range from your search of the Alphabetic Index.
   PURPOSE: To begin the process of finding the most specific and accurate code.
8. Compare the description of the code with the procedural statement in the surgical report. Verify that all or most of the health record documentation matches the code description and that there is no additional information in the code description that is not found in the documentation.
9. Review the coding guidelines and notes for the section, subsection, and code to ensure that there are no contraindications to use of the code. Review the coding conventions and add-on codes, if any.
   PURPOSE: To ensure there are no instructions that would prevent the use of the code selected.
10. Determine whether a modifier is needed.
    PURPOSE: To select any appropriate modifiers that provide additional information for the chosen code to explain certain circumstances or provide additional detail.
11. Determine whether a Special Report is required.
    PURPOSE: To clarify and add additional detail when an unusual or extenuating circumstance exists or if a Category III or unlisted procedure Category I code is used.
12. Record the CPT code selected in the health record documentation next to the procedure or service performed and in the appropriate block of the insurance claim form.
    PURPOSE: To complete the documentation and recording requirements.

PROCEDURE 15-1 —*continued*

Operative Report

PATIENT NAME: Sonia Sample
ROOM NUMBER: 222 West
MR NUMBER: 12-34-56

DATE OF PROCEDURE: 04/22/00
PREOPERATIVE DIAGNOSIS: Acute cholecystitis
POSTOPERATIVE DIAGNOSIS: Acute cholecystitis
NAME OF PROCEDURE: 1. Laparoscopic cholecystectomy
                                              2. Intraoperative cystic duct cholangiogram
SURGEON: Claude St. John, M.D.
ASSISTANT: Mark Weiss, D.O.
ANESTHESIOLOGIST: Angela Adams, M.D.
ANESTHESIA: General

DESCRIPTION OF THE OPERATION:
    The patient was placed in the supine position under general anesthesia. The oral gastric tube was placed. The Foley catheter was placed. The patient received appropriate antibiotics. The abdomen was prepped with iodine and draped in the usual fashion. Using a midline subumbilical incision, we entered the subcutaneous fat to find the aponeurosis of the rectus abdominis. Two stay sutures were placed 0.5 cm from the midline bilaterally and we left on these sutures, creating an opening in the linea alba.
    Under direct vision, the catheter was placed. The Hasson cannula was placed in the abdominal cavity and all was normal except an acute necrotizing and probably gangrenous gallbladder. There were multiple omental adhesions. Three other trocars were placed in the right subcostal plane in the midline, midclavicular line, and midaxillary line using a #10, #5, and #5 mm trocar, respectively. The gallbladder was punctured and emptied of clear white bile indicating a hydrops of the gallbladder. It was grasped at its fundus and at Hartmann's pouch retracted cephalad and to the right, respectively. We found the cystic duct and the cystic artery after circumferential dissection and isolated the cystic duct completely.
    When we were sure that this structure was a deep cystic duct, the clip was placed at the most distal aspect to make an opening immediately proximally and we placed a Reddick cholangiocatheter into it via #14 gauge percutaneous catheter. The cholangiogram showed normal arborization of the liver radicals. Normal bifurcation of the common hepatic duct. Normal common hepatic duct. Long large cystic duct. The common bile duct had numerous stones within it. They could not be emptied from the common bile duct. There was good flow into the duodenum.
    The impression was choledocholithiasis. This was corroborated by the radiologist. The decision was made to prepare the patient most probably for endoscopic retrograde cholangiopancreatography postoperatively, and no further intervention of the common bile duct was done in this setting.
    The cholangiocatheter was removed. An attempt was made to milk the bile out, but no stones came out. Three clips were placed on the proximal aspect of the cystic duct and the duct was then cut distally. The artery was isolated and double clipped proximally and single clipped distally and cut in the intervening section. We then peeled the gallbladder off the gallbladder bed with some difficulty because of the intense edema and inflammation. It was then removed from the liver bed completely. Cautery, suctioning and irrigation were used copiously to create a bloodless field. A last check was made and there was no bleeding and no bile leaking. A #15 Jackson-Pratt type drain was placed into Morrison's pouch and brought out through the lateral most port. We then removed, with great difficulty, the gallbladder from the umbilicus. Because of its enormous size and a 3 cm stone within it that was very difficult to macerate, the opening of the umbilicus had to be enlarged.
    As this was done, we removed the gallbladder completely and sent it for pathologic section. Two separate figure-of-eight 0 PDS were used to close the abdominal fascia. The Jackson-Pratt drain was then sutured in place with 2.0 nylon. The skin was closed throughout with subcuticular 3-0 PDS after copious irrigation of the subcutaneous plane. Mastisol and Steri-Strips were placed on the wound. The patient remained stable although she did have bigeminy during surgery and was on a Lidocaine drip. She will be going to the intensive care unit but as she left, she was extubated in the recovery room and was fully alert. She is moving all limbs.
    I will discuss with the gastroenterologist postoperative endoscopic retrograde cholangiopancreatography.
    SPECIMEN: Gallbladder.

Claude St. John, M.D.
CSJ/ld:
D: 04/22/00
T: 04/22/00 9:21 am
CC: Maria Acosta, M.D.

1

PROCEDURE 15-1   —continued

Using the TruCode Software

1. Abstract the procedures and/or services from the procedural statement in the surgical report.
2. Type the main term into the encoder Search box and select the CPT. Then click on Show All Results.
3. If the main term cannot be found through the search, repeat steps 2 and 3 using a different main term based on the procedural statement.
4. Choose the procedure description that is closest to the procedural statement in the surgical report as shown in Figure 2.

PURPOSE: To prevent upcoding or downcoding errors or other possible fraud and/or abuse circumstances.

5. Record the CPT code that best matches the procedural statements in the surgical report in the patient's health record.

PURPOSE: To prevent repeated reference to the Alphabetic Index by recording all possible matches to the code or code range being sought. This saves time and prevents redundant effort.

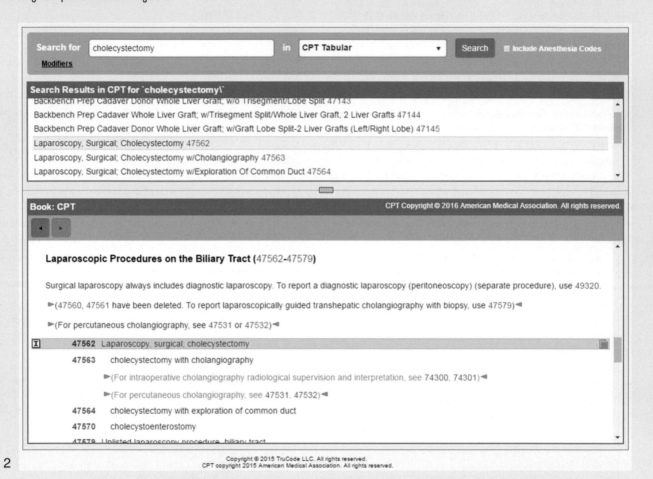

2

USING THE ALPHABETIC INDEX

Although the Alphabetic Index is a comprehensive, alphabetic listing of all main terms, there are no code descriptions. Therefore, it would not be effective to assign a CPT code simply by finding it through the Alphabetic Index. The Alphabetic Index is not a substitute for the Tabular List. Even if an individual is only looking for one code, the Tabular List must be used to ensure the code is accurate.

The Alphabetic Index is used as a guide to search for one or more codes or code ranges. The index is similar to that found in the back of any textbook; it is an alphabetic list of main and modifying terms found in the Tabular List of the coding manual. In a typical index,

the term or concept listed in the index is followed by a reference page or pages, where detailed information is presented in the body of the book. The Alphabetic Index in the CPT coding manual is used in the same way, except that it references codes or code ranges rather than pages. As discussed earlier, the Tabular List is divided into sections, and the procedures and services are listed in numeric order by the Category I code.

The Alphabetic Index is organized by main terms, and modifying terms are indented two spaces below the main term. Modifying terms further describe and add information needed to narrow the search for an appropriate procedure or service code. A main term can be a procedure, such as an excision, and each modifying term could provide further information about the anatomic location or the organ excised, the type of instrument used, a special technique, or whether other procedures were performed at the same time as the excision, such as obtaining biopsy tissue for examination. *Modifying terms affect the selection of appropriate codes; therefore, it is important to review the list of modifying terms when selecting a code or code range.*

Searching the Alphabetic Index

Begin the search of the Alphabetic Index by using one of the four primary classifications (or types) of main and modifying term entries:
- Procedure or service (e.g., examination, excision, scope, revision, repair, drainage)
- Organ or anatomic site (e.g., clavicle, mandible, humerus, liver, colon, uterus)
- Condition, illness, or injury (e.g., cholelithiasis, ulcer, fracture, pregnancy, fever)
- Eponym, synonym, abbreviation, or acronym (e.g., Naffziger operation, MRI [magnetic resonance imaging], TURP [transurethral resection of the prostate]).

When searching the Alphabetic Index, use the name of the performed procedure or service (anastomosis, splint, repair, stress test, therapy, vaccination); the organ or other anatomic site of the procedure (tibia, colon, salivary gland, aorta); the condition, illness, or injury (abscess, fracture, cholelithiasis, strabismus); or, if applicable, synonyms, eponyms, or abbreviations (ECG [electrocardiography], Stookey-Scarff procedure, Mohs' micrographic surgery).

Sometimes searching for a Main Term may not yield any results. When a Main Term cannot be found, search by another primary classification in the Alphabetic Index. Let's search the following procedural statement: Removal of Skin Tags on Neck. Begin by identifying the Main Terms that closely match the four primary classifications in the Alphabetic Index.
1. Procedure of Service: Removal
2. Organ or Anatomic Site: Neck Skin
3. Condition, Illness, or Injury: Skin Tag
4. Eponym: none in this case

Once all possible Main Terms have been abstracted, the coder can quickly search through the Alphabetic Index for the code or code range that matches the procedural statement.

Using *See* and *See Also* in the Alphabetic Index

The *see* statement in the Alphabetic Index points to another location in the Alphabetic Index to find the code or code range. The *see also* statement points to additional codes or code ranges in the Alphabetic Index that may be useful to the code found in the original search.

Use of the Semicolon

A semicolon (;) at the end of a main description indicates that modifying terms and descriptions follow. Every indented description below a stand-alone code is related to that stand-alone code. If a main term has no additional modifying terms, the next entry is a stand-alone description of a different procedure, which is positioned flush left, without indentation. As shown in Figure 15-9, the highlighted CPT code 61314 uses the semicolon and provides two locations.

| 61314 | Craniectomy or craniotomy for evacuation of hematoma, infratentorial; extradural or subdural |

FIGURE 15-9 Use of semicolon.

Stand-Alone Codes and Code Ranges

In the Alphabetic Index, a procedure or service may list a single code or a range of possible codes that may match the medical documentation. Remember that the Alphabetic Index is an index; it is designed as a guide to the most suitable codes that match the documentation. At this point, the search is only for the closest match or matches to the procedural statement.

Because some medical procedures and diagnostic tests can be quite complex, there may be a single (stand-alone) code or a code range that may include one main term but has several modifying terms from the Main Term. For example, the code for *Craterization, phalanges, toe* is 28124, a stand-alone code. However, using the same main term, *Craterization*, but adding *any of the phalanges* yields a range of codes: 26235-29236. The code range is shown with a hyphen to indicate that all codes within that range could be appropriate.

In some cases a stand-alone code and a range of codes are listed for the same service or procedure. For example, *Craterization, femur*, lists both the stand-alone code 27360 and the code range 27070-27071. Once a stand-alone code or code range has been found in the Alphabetic Index, the next step is to look up each of those in the Tabular List and select the code or codes that most closely match the medical documentation.

Steps for Using the CPT Alphabetic Index

1. Abstract the procedural statement from the medical documentation and determine the Main and/or Modifying Terms.
2. Select the most appropriate main term to begin searching in the Alphabetic Index.
3. Once the main term has been located, select one or more modifying terms, if needed, to narrow the search.
4. If no main or modifying term produces an appropriate code or code range, repeat steps 2 and 3 using a different main term.
5. Find the code or code ranges that include all or most of the description of the procedure or service found in the medical record.

CRITICAL THINKING APPLICATION   15-4

Sherald is having trouble finding a removal of a cataract procedure code in the Alphabetic Index. What are some options and/or alternative ways she can perform an Alphabetic Index search?

USING THE TABULAR LIST

Once the code or code ranges have been selected from the Alphabetic Index, the next stop is the Tabular List, where the procedural coding decision takes place. In the Tabular List, the conventions, symbols, guidelines, notes, and even the punctuation all play a part in choosing the most accurate code possible.

In the Tabular List, look up each code or code range found in the Alphabetic Index numerically. Read the description of each code thoroughly to ensure that the main terms abstracted from the procedural statement in the medical documentation are all included in the code description, with nothing substantial omitted or added. Read the section guidelines and notes to determine whether additional codes should be used, add-on codes or modifiers are required, or use of the code is contraindicated.

Steps for Using the CPT Tabular List

Except for the special considerations required for coding from the Evaluation and Management (E/M) and Anesthesia sections, the following steps apply to all sections of the CPT manual.

1. Look up the code or code range from the Alphabetic Index Search in the Tabular List numerically.
2. Compare the description of the code with the procedural statement from the medical documentation. Verify that all or most of the health record documentation matches the code description and that there is no additional element or information in the code description that is not found in the documentation.
3. Read the guidelines and notes for the section, subsection, and code to ensure that there are no contraindications to use of the code.
4. Evaluate the conventions, especially add-on codes (+) and exemption from modifier -51.

---

5. Determine whether any special circumstances require the use of a modifier or whether a Special Report is required.
6. Record the CPT code selected in the health record documentation next to the procedure or service performed and in the appropriate block of the insurance claim form.

SECTION-SPECIFIC CPT CODING GUIDELINES

Common CPT Coding Guidelines: Evaluation and Management Section

To properly code E/M services, the medical assistant must apply different code lookup techniques from the basic steps outlined earlier. Assigning the correct E/M code includes identifying the section, subsection, category, and subcategory of the procedure or service; reviewing the reporting instructions and guidelines for the code chosen; reviewing the level of E/M service; determining the extent of history obtained and examination performed; and determining the complexity of medical decision making.

The E/M section is divided into broad subsections, such as *office visit, emergency room visit, hospital visit,* and *consultation.* These subsections are further divided into subcategories, which include the place where the services were rendered (e.g., the provider's office, a hospital emergency department, a skilled nursing facility, or the patient's home) and the patient status (i.e., whether the patient is new or established). Procedure 15-2, part A, explains how to perform CPT coding for an office visit.

The first two steps in choosing an E/M code are:
1. Identify the place of service (POS)
2. Identify the patient status (new or established)

PROCEDURE 15-2   Perform Procedural Coding: Office Visit and Immunizations

Goal: *To use the steps for CPT Evaluation and Management coding and HCPCS coding to find the most accurate and specific CPT E/M and HCPCS codes using the coding manuals and the TruCode encoder.*

EQUIPMENT and SUPPLIES

- CPT coding manual (current year)
- HCPCS coding manual (current year)
- Progress Note (see Study Guide Chapter 15) (Figure 1)
- TruCode encoder software

Part A: CPT E/M Coding

1. Determine the place of service from the encounter form.
   PURPOSE: To determine the most accurate CPT E/M code, the place of service needs to be identified.
2. Determine the patient's status.
   PURPOSE: To determine the most accurate CPT E/M code, the patient should be identified as new or established.
3. Identify the subsection, category, or subcategory of service in the E/M section.

PURPOSE: To ensure that the correct place of service and patient status are used and the appropriate level of service is selected.

4. Determine the level of service:
   - Determine the extent of the history obtained.
   - Determine the extent of the examination performed.
   - Determine the complexity of medical decision making.
   PURPOSE: To ensure that the correct level is chosen for the history, examination, and medical decision making.

5. If necessary, compare the medical documentation against examples in Appendix C, Clinical Examples, of the CPT manual.
   PURPOSE: To help the coder select the appropriate level of service.

6. Select the appropriate level of E/M service code, and document it in the patient's health record.
   PURPOSE: To complete the documentation and reporting requirements.

PROCEDURE 15-2   *—continued*

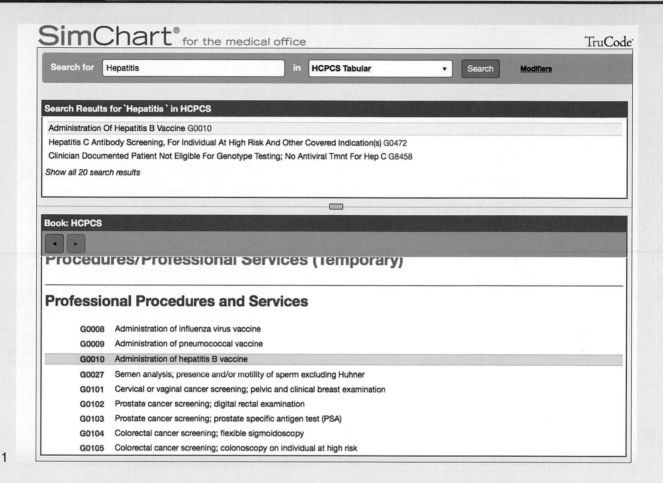

SimChart® for the medical office   TruCode®

| Search for | Hepatitis | in | HCPCS Tabular ▾ | Search | Modifiers |

Search Results for `Hepatitis` in HCPCS

Administration Of Hepatitis B Vaccine G0010

Hepatitis C Antibody Screening, For Individual At High Risk And Other Covered Indication(s) G0472

Clinician Documented Patient Not Eligible For Genotype Testing; No Antiviral Tmnt For Hep C G8458

Show all 20 search results

Book: HCPCS

◀ ▶

Procedures/Professional Services (Temporary)

Professional Procedures and Services

G0008	Administration of influenza virus vaccine
G0009	Administration of pneumococcal vaccine
G0010	Administration of hepatitis B vaccine
G0027	Semen analysis; presence and/or motility of sperm excluding Huhner
G0101	Cervical or vaginal cancer screening; pelvic and clinical breast examination
G0102	Prostate cancer screening; digital rectal examination
G0103	Prostate cancer screening; prostate specific antigen test (PSA)
G0104	Colorectal cancer screening; flexible sigmoidoscopy
G0105	Colorectal cancer screening; colonoscopy on individual at high risk

1

Part B: HCPCS Coding with TruCode Encoder Software

1. Review the provider documentation.
   PURPOSE: To ensure that all procedures and/or services are listed on the encounter form; that all procedures and services on the encounter form match the health record; and that nothing documented in the health record is missing from the encounter form.
2. Type the main term into the Search box of the encoder and choose the HCPCS Tabular code set for accurate coding.
3. If no modifying term produces an appropriate code or code range, repeat steps 2 and 3 using a different main term.

PURPOSE: To help find the most appropriate code or code range by using alternative methods of searching the Alphabetic Index.
4. Compare the description of the code with the medical documentation.
   PURPOSE: To avoid upcoding and downcoding errors and to ensure there are no contraindications to use of the code selected.
5. Select the appropriate HCPCS immunization code, and document it in the patient's health record.
   PURPOSE: To complete the documentation and reporting requirements.

Identifying the Place of Service

The place of service (POS) is the healthcare facility where the encounter between the patient and the provider occurred and where the medical service was delivered. The two most common places of service are "office" and "hospital." Table 15-4 presents a list of common POS locations and their two-digit identifying numbers, or POS codes.

Identifying the Patient Status

The patient status choices are "new" or "established" patient. A new patient (NP) is one who has not received any professional services from the provider, or from another provider of the exact same specialty and subspecialty who belongs to the same group practice, within the past 3 years. An established patient (EP) is one who has received professional services from the provider, or from another

TABLE 15-4   Commonly Used Codes for Place of Service

CODE	NAME
01	Pharmacy
11	Office
12	Home
13	Assisted Living Facility
14	Group Home
15	Mobile Unit
17	Walk-In Retail Health Clinic
20	Urgent Care Facility
21	Inpatient Hospital
22	Outpatient Hospital
23	Emergency Room—Hospital
24	Ambulatory Surgery Center
31	Skilled Nursing Facility
34	Hospice
51	Inpatient Psychiatric Facility
60	Mass Immunization Center
65	End-Stage Renal Disease Treatment Facility
71	Public Health Clinic
72	Rural Health Clinic
81	Independent Laboratory

Select the Appropriate Level of E/M Services Based on the Following

1. For the following categories/subcategories, **all of the key components**, ie, history, examination, and medical decision making, must meet or exceed the stated requirements to qualify for a particular level of E/M service: office, new patient; hospital observation services; initial hospital care; office consultations, initial inpatient consultations; emergency department services; initial nursing facility care; domiciliary care, new patient; and home, new patient.

2. For the following categories/subcategories, **two of the three key components** (ie, history, examination, and medical decision making) must meet or exceed the stated requirements to qualify for a particular level of E/M services: office, established patient; subsequent hospital care; subsequent nursing facility care; domiciliary care, established patient; and home, established patient.

3. When counseling and/or coordination of care dominates (more than 50%) the encounter with the patient and/or family (face-to-face time in the office or other outpatient setting or floor/unit time in the hospital or nursing facility), then **time** shall be considered the key or controlling factor to qualify for a particular level of E/M services. This includes time spent with parties who have assumed responsibility for the care of the patient or decision making whether or not they are family members (eg, foster parents, person acting in loco parentis, legal guardian). The extent of counseling and/or coordination of care must be documented in the medical record.

FIGURE 15-10 Appropriate assignment of E/M codes.

provider of the exact same specialty and subspecialty who belongs to the same group practice, within the past 3 years.

Once the POS and patient status have been established, the next step in selection of an E/M code is to determine the level of service provided.

Determining the Level of Service Provided

Key Components and Contributing Factors. The three key components for determining the level of service for E/M coding are the history, examination, and medical decision making. The four contributing factors are counseling, the nature of the presenting problem, coordination of care, and time. The history, examination, and medical decision-making components are considered primary key; that is, they are typically the three most important components for deciding the level of service. Counseling, the nature of the presenting problem, coordination of care, and time are secondary considerations. Figure 15-10 presents criteria for choosing the appropriate E/M code.

History. To understand the levels of the history, it is important to know the definition and components of the patient history. The history relates to the patient's clinical picture and depends on the patient for answers to specific questions.

Levels of History. The following are the four levels of history taking.

Problem-focused history: A problem-focused history concentrates on the chief complaint; it looks at the symptoms, severity, and duration of the problem. It usually does not include a review of systems (ROS) or the family and social histories.

Expanded problem-focused history: The provider proceeds as in the problem-focused history but includes a review of systems that relate to the chief complaint. Usually the past, family, and social histories are not included.

Detailed history: The detailed history consists of the chief complaint; extended history of present illness; problem-pertinent system review extended to include a review of a limited number of additional systems; and the pertinent past, family, and/or social histories directly related to the patient's problems.

Comprehensive history: A comprehensive history includes the chief complaint; extended history of present illness; an ROS that is directly related to the problem or problems identified in the history of the present illness plus a review of all additional body systems; and complete past, family, and social histories.

Examination. The examination is the objective part of the patient's visit. The provider examines the patient, obtains measurable findings, and makes notes referring to body areas and/or organ systems as follows:

- *Body areas:* Head, including face and neck; chest, including breasts and axillae; abdomen; genitalia, groin, and buttocks; and back, including spine and extremities
- *Organs and organ systems:* Constitution (e.g., vital signs, general appearance); eyes; ears, nose, throat, and mouth; cardiovascular; respiratory; gastrointestinal (GI); genitourinary; musculoskeletal; skin; neurologic; psychiatric; and hematologic, lymphatic, and immunologic

Levels of Examination. The examination is divided into the following levels:

- *Problem-focused examination:* The examination is limited to the single body area or single system mentioned in the chief complaint.
- *Expanded problem-focused examination:* In addition to the limited body area or system, related body areas or organ systems are examined.
- *Detailed examination:* An extended examination is performed on the related body areas or organ systems.
- *Comprehensive examination:* A complete multisystem examination is performed or a complete examination of a single organ system.

Medical Decision Making. When a provider makes medical decisions, the decisions are based on many years of education and experience. Three elements comprise the medical decision-making process:

1. The number of diagnoses and/or management options
2. The amount and/or complexity of data obtained, reviewed, and analyzed
3. The risk of significant complications and/or morbidity and/or mortality

Number of Diagnoses and Management Options. The provider's notes during the history and examination should help identify whether the patient's problem is minor, acute, stable, or worsening. The medical documentation should also identify whether a new problem exists or whether the provider plans to order any diagnostic tests to further investigate the patient's illness or injury.

Amount and Complexity of Data Reviewed. The medical documentation should also identify what laboratory tests, x-ray diagnostic procedures, and other tests have been ordered or reviewed.

Risk of Complications and Morbidity or Mortality. Risk is often involved in medical care, either from the treatment given to the patient or from the lack of treatment and professional care. *Morbidity,* the relative incidence of disease, and *mortality,* which relates to the number of deaths from a given disease, are integral parts of the provider's assessment of risks.

Complexity Levels in Medical Decision Making. The complexity of medical decision making is categorized into four levels: straightforward, low complexity, moderate complexity, and high complexity. Table 15-5 presents descriptions of the different levels of complexity of medical decision making.

Factors That Contribute to E/M Complexity

Counseling. Counseling is a discussion with a patient and/or family members about the diagnostic results, impressions, recommended diagnostic studies, prognosis, risks and benefits of management or treatment options, and instructions for management, treatment, and/or follow-up. Almost all E/M services involve a degree of counseling with the patient and/or family. This is factored into the E/M code, and as long as this factor does not exceed 50% of the time spent with the patient, it is included in the E/M code. It can be considered a contributing factor when the counseling exceeds 50% of the encounter.

Nature of the Presenting Problem. The presenting problem is usually explained in the chief complaint. It can range from something as simple as a cold in an otherwise healthy patient to a life-threatening problem. Unless dealing with the nature of the presenting problem exceeds half of the patient encounter, it is included in the E/M code description and is not a factor in selecting the level of service.

Coordination of Care. Some patients need assistance in arranging for care beyond the visit or hospitalization. Some will need care in a skilled nursing facility or home health care. Others will need hospice care. The primary provider usually coordinates this care. Coordination of care is also factored into the E/M code and is a consideration for determining the level of service only when it exceeds 50% of the patient encounter.

Time. Time is included in the E/M code descriptions only to assist providers in selecting the most appropriate level of E/M service. The times expressed in the code descriptions are averages, and time is not a determining factor in code selection unless counseling exceeds more than 50% of the encounter. Only then can time be used as a determining component to code level selection.

TABLE 15-5 Complexity of Medical Decision Making

NUMBER OF DIAGNOSES OR MANAGEMENT OPTIONS	AMOUNT AND/OR COMPLEXITY OF DATA TO BE REVIEWED	RISK OF COMPLICATIONS AND/OR MORBIDITY OR MORTALITY	TYPE OF MEDICAL DECISION MAKING
Minimal	Minimal or none	Minimal	Straightforward
Limited	Limited	Low	Low complexity
Multiple	Moderate	Moderate	Moderate complexity
Extensive	Extensive	High	High complexity

At first, E/M coding can be difficult to understand and put into practice. The E/M coding process provided here can serve as a guide to medical assistants in determining the place of service, patient status, and level of care provided, so that they can select the most accurate E/M code. Using the clinical examples in Appendix C of the CPT manual and comparing them to the medical documentation also can help medical assistants acquire a better understanding of E/M coding.

CRITICAL THINKING APPLICATION   **15-5**

Dr. Caddell performed a colonoscopy at the ambulatory surgery center on Cecil Matthews, who has been Dr. Caddell's patient for several years. Mr. Matthews came to the office with left lower quadrant pain and a history of colon cancer. What other factors or information would Sherald need to know to properly code Mr. Matthews' office visit? What medical documentation would Sherald need to properly code Mr. Matthews' colonoscopy?

Common CPT Coding Guidelines: Anesthesia

Anesthesiologists and **Certified Registered Nurse Anesthetists (CRNAs)** use codes in the Anesthesia section, which are also known as CPT-4 codes. These codes always start with a zero (0) and identify the anatomic location of the surgery performed. CPT-4 codes are used for unconscious sedation, or for putting patients to sleep during the medical procedure; codes for conscious sedation are found in the Medicine section.

Anesthesia coding differs from any other form of coding in the way anesthesia services are billed. These professionals are paid a standard amount per unit compared to surgeons, who are paid by the procedure. A standard formula has been established to determine the number of units they can bill for each procedure for which they provide anesthesia.

Basic unit values + Time units + Modifying units (B + T + M)

Anesthesia Formula

All healthcare providers who can administer anesthesia, including anesthesiologists and CRNAs, use CPT-4 codes for anesthesia services based on the anatomic region of the body where the surgery was performed.

Basic Unit Value (B)

The Anesthesia Society of America (ASA) publishes a Relative Value Guide (RVG) that lists the codes for anesthesia services. The RVG compares anesthesia services and assigns a numeric value to each service based on the level of complexity; this numeric value is called the *basic unit value.*

Time Units (T)

Anesthesia services are provided based on the time during which the anesthesia was administered, in hours and minutes. Typically 15 minutes equals 1 time unit, although this can vary because insurance carriers make that determination independently. The time starts when the anesthesiology provider begins preparing the patient to receive anesthesia, continues through the procedure, and ends when

the patient is no longer under the professional care of the anesthesiology provider. The hours and minutes during which anesthesia was administered are recorded in the patient's anesthesia record (Figure 15-11).

Modifying Units (M)

Modifying units reflect circumstances or conditions that change or modify the environment in which the anesthesia service was provided. The two modifying characteristics for anesthesia services are qualifying circumstances and physical status modifiers.

Qualifying Circumstances (QC). Sometimes anesthesia is provided in situations that make administration more difficult. These types of cases include provision of anesthesia in emergency situations, to patients of extreme age, during the use of controlled hypotension, and with hypothermia. There are four qualifying circumstances (QC) codes. Each of the five-digit codes is preceded by a plus sign symbol (+), indicating that it is an add-on code; these codes are used in addition to the Category I anesthesia code.

Physical Status Modifiers. Physical status modifiers are used to indicate the patient's physical condition at the time anesthesia was provided. There are five physical status modifiers, each composed of two characters: first the letter P, followed by a ranking of 1 to 6 (e.g., P1, P2, P3, and so on). P1 represents a normal, healthy patient, and P6 represents a brain-dead patient whose organs are being harvested. Table 15-6 presents a list of physical status modifiers and their

---

TABLE 15-6 Anesthesia Physical Status and Qualifying Circumstances Modifiers

MODIFIER	DESCRIPTION
Physical Status Modifiers*	
P1	A normal healthy patient
P2	A patient with mild systemic disease
P3	A patient with severe systemic disease
P4	A person with severe systemic disease that is a constant threat to life
P5	A moribund patient who is not expected to survive without the procedure
P6	A declared brain-dead patient whose organs are being removed for donor purposes
Qualifying Circumstances CPT Codes†	
99100	Anesthesia for a patient of extreme age (i.e., <1 yr or >70 yr)
99116	Anesthesia complicated by utilization of total body hypothermia
99135	Anesthesia complicated by utilization of controlled hypothermia

*A physical status modifier is required for performing anesthesia calculations.
†Use a qualifying circumstances modifier code, if appropriate, in addition to the primary CPT Category I Anesthesia code.

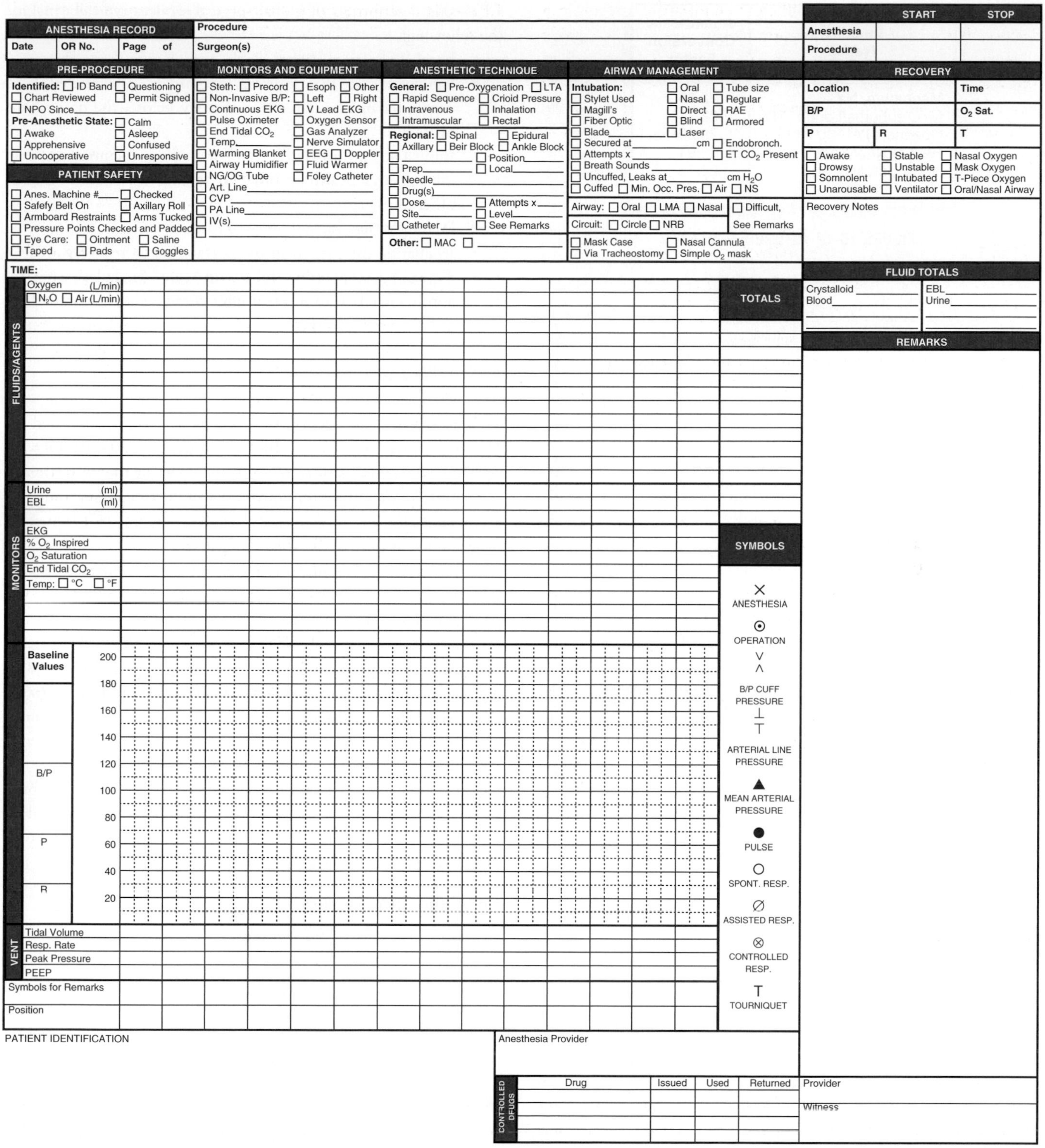

	START	STOP
Anesthesia		
Procedure		

ANESTHESIA RECORD

Date	OR No.	Page	of

Procedure _____
Surgeon(s) _____

PRE-PROCEDURE

Identified: ☐ ID Band ☐ Questioning
☐ Chart Reviewed ☐ Permit Signed
☐ NPO Since____
Pre-Anesthetic State: ☐ Calm
☐ Awake ☐ Asleep
☐ Apprehensive ☐ Confused
☐ Uncooperative ☐ Unresponsive

PATIENT SAFETY

☐ Anes. Machine #____ ☐ Checked
☐ Safely Belt On ☐ Axillary Roll
☐ Armboard Restraints ☐ Arms Tucked
☐ Pressure Points Checked and Padded
☐ Eye Care: ☐ Ointment ☐ Saline
☐ Taped ☐ Pads ☐ Goggles

MONITORS AND EQUIPMENT

☐ Steth: ☐ Precord ☐ Esoph ☐ Other
☐ Non-Invasive B/P: ☐ Left ☐ Right
☐ Continuous EKG ☐ V Lead EKG
☐ Pulse Oximeter ☐ Oxygen Sensor
☐ End Tidal CO_2 ☐ Gas Analyzer
☐ Temp____ ☐ Nerve Simulator
☐ Warming Blanket ☐ EEG ☐ Doppler
☐ Airway Humidifier ☐ Fluid Warmer
☐ NG/OG Tube ☐ Foley Catheter
☐ Art. Line____
☐ CVP____
☐ PA Line____
☐ IV(s)____

ANESTHETIC TECHNIQUE

General: ☐ Pre-Oxygenation ☐ LTA
☐ Rapid Sequence ☐ Crioid Pressure
☐ Intravenous ☐ Inhalation
☐ Intramuscular ☐ Rectal
Regional: ☐ Spinal ☐ Epidural
☐ Axillary ☐ Beir Block ☐ Ankle Block
☐ Prep____ ☐ Position____
☐ Needle____ ☐ Local____
☐ Drug(s)____
☐ Dose____ ☐ Attempts x____
☐ Site____ ☐ Level____
☐ Catheter____ ☐ See Remarks
Other: ☐ MAC ☐ ____

AIRWAY MANAGEMENT

Intubation: ☐ Oral ☐ Tube size
☐ Stylet Used ☐ Nasal ☐ Regular
☐ Magill's ☐ Direct ☐ RAE
☐ Fiber Optic ☐ Blind ☐ Armored
☐ Blade____ ☐ Laser
☐ Secured at____cm ☐ Endobronch.
☐ Attempts x____ ☐ ET CO_2 Present
☐ Breath Sounds
☐ Uncuffed, Leaks at____cm H_2O
☐ Cuffed ☐ Min. Occ. Pres. ☐ Air ☐ NS
Airway: ☐ Oral ☐ LMA ☐ Nasal ☐ Difficult,
Circuit: ☐ Circle ☐ NRB   See Remarks
☐ Mask Case ☐ Nasal Cannula
☐ Via Tracheostomy ☐ Simple O_2 mask

RECOVERY

Location	Time
B/P	O_2 Sat.
P	R	T

☐ Awake ☐ Stable ☐ Nasal Oxygen
☐ Drowsy ☐ Unstable ☐ Mask Oxygen
☐ Somnolent ☐ Intubated ☐ T-Piece Oxygen
☐ Unarousable ☐ Ventilator ☐ Oral/Nasal Airway

Recovery Notes

TIME:

FLUIDS/AGENTS

Oxygen (L/min)
☐ N_2O ☐ Air (L/min)

Urine (ml)
EBL (ml)

TOTALS

FLUID TOTALS

Crystalloid ____ EBL ____
Blood ____ Urine ____

REMARKS

MONITORS

EKG
% O_2 Inspired
O_2 Saturation
End Tidal CO_2
Temp: ☐ °C ☐ °F

SYMBOLS

Baseline Values
200
180
160
140
B/P 120
100
80
P 60
40
R 20

✕ ANESTHESIA
⊙ OPERATION
∨ ∧ B/P CUFF PRESSURE
⊥ ⊤ ARTERIAL LINE PRESSURE
▲ MEAN ARTERIAL PRESSURE
● PULSE
○ SPONT. RESP.
∅ ASSISTED RESP.
⊗ CONTROLLED RESP.
⊤ TOURNIQUET

VENT

Tidal Volume
Resp. Rate
Peak Pressure
PEEP

Symbols for Remarks

Position

PATIENT IDENTIFICATION

Anesthesia Provider

CONTROLLED DRUGS

Drug	Issued	Used	Returned	Provider
				Witness

FIGURE 15-11 Anesthesia record.

descriptions; a list also can be found in the Anesthesia section of the CPT manual.

Conversion Factors

A *conversion factor* is the dollar value of each basic unit value. Each third-party payer issues a list of conversion factors. The conversion factor for any given geographic location is multiplied by the number of basic unit values assigned to each procedure (Figure 15-12).

Calculating Anesthesia Services

Using the basic unit value (B), modifying unit (M), time unit (T), physical status (PS) modifier, if applicable, and the conversion factor

Locality Name	Anesthesia Conversion Factor
Manhattan, NY	22.65
NYC suburbs/Long I., NY	22.74
Queens, NY	22.28
Rest of New York	19.91
North Carolina	20.23
North Dakota	19.70

FIGURE 15-12 Anesthesia conversion factors.

Medical Narrative

A 25-year-old female patient in good physical condition has anesthesia services while undergoing laparoscopy (CPT-4 Code 00840). The time for the anesthesia administration was 2 hours. For the purposes of this example the RBV basic unit value will be 4.

Basic Unit Value	= 4
+ Modifying Units: PS	= 0
+ QC	= 0
+ Time Units	= 8
= 12 Total Units	

The total units value of 12 is then multiplied by the conversion factor for the geographic location of the anesthesiologist's office. For the purposes of this exercise, the conversion factor for Manhattan, NY, will be $20.48, and for North Carolina, $15.77. For the office located in Manhattan, NY, multiply $20.48 by 12. The fee for the anesthesia services would be $245.76. For the office located in North Carolina, multiply 12 times $15.77, for a fee of $189.24.

FIGURE 15-13 Anesthesia formula and calculation.

(Figure 15-13), the fee for anesthesia services is calculated according to the anesthesia billing formula:

$$(B + M + T + PS) \times Conversion\ factor$$

Common CPT Coding Guidelines: Surgical Section

Specific guidelines and notes related to surgery coding must be considered when a CPT code is assigned. Always review the current year's guidelines for the Surgery section for the most up-to-date information. The following sections discuss a few of the more common guidelines. When coding procedures and services, be sure to read the guidelines and notes thoroughly for accurate coding assignment.

Surgical Package Definition

The CPT code set is designed to include patient prep, surgical care, and postsurgical care in a single code; these are considered **global services** because they are already built into the surgical package cost of the assigned CPT code. Medical coders that include any of these global services as a separate CPT code are acting fraudulently. The

CPT code descriptions of global surgical services typically include the following:

- Local infiltration, digital block, and/or topical anesthesia
- Subsequent to the decision for surgery, one related E/M encounter on the day of, or the day before, the date of procedure
- Immediate postoperative care, including documentation in the patient's health record and talking with family and/or other physicians
- Writing orders for postsurgical care
- Evaluating the patient in the postanesthesia recovery area
- Typical postoperative follow-up care (includes care for approximately 6 to 8 weeks after surgery and is usually done at the provider's office)

NCCI Edits and Unbundled Codes

In 1996, in an effort to prevent fraudulent medical coding, the Centers for Medicare and Medicaid Services (CMS) established the National Corrective Coding Initiative (NCCI) edit list. This list contains two columns of codes, and the codes in the two columns are mutually exclusive. Submitted claims that contain mutually exclusive codes are automatically rejected. Figure 15-14 presents instructions on how to use the NCCI edits.

When a CPT procedure is billed, this code includes services related to prepping the patient for the procedure, performing the procedure, and suturing to complete the procedure; the single code for the procedure is called a *bundled code* because it represents all of the stages of surgery. When each step of the procedure is listed separately, these are called *unbundled codes*. Unbundled codes are used when the components of a major procedure are separated and reported separately. When these codes are separated and used individually, a special report should be used to describe the circumstances that made the unbundling necessary because unbundled CPT codes have higher reimbursements because each code is paid separately. Medical billers that regularly unbundle CPT codes may be cited for fraud and/or abuse.

Integumentary System

Excision of Lesions—Benign or Malignant

Excision of benign lesions includes a simple closure and anesthesia. If an incision, excision, or traumatic lesion requires intermediate or complex closure, the repair by intermediate or complex closure is coded and reported separately.

Levels of Closure (Repair)

- *Simple repair:* Performed when the wound is superficial (epidermis, dermis, or subcutaneous) without significant involvement of deeper structures. This includes local anesthesia and chemical or electrocauterization of wounds not closed.
- *Intermediate repair:* Includes simple repair with a need for a layered closure of one or more of the deeper layers of subcutaneous tissue and superficial fascia in addition to the skin closure. Single-layer closure of heavily contaminated wounds that required extensive cleaning or removal of particulate matter also constitutes intermediate repair.
- *Complex repair:* Includes wounds that require more than layered closure (e.g., scar revision, extensive undermining, or stents or retention sutures). Necessary preparation includes creation of a

A	B	C	D	E	F
Column 1/Column 2 Edits					
① Column 1	② Column 2	③ * = In existence prior to 1996	④ Effective Date	⑤ Deletion Date * = no data	Modifier ⑥ 0 = not allowed 1 = allowed 9 = not applicable
99215	G0101		19980401	19980401	9
99215	G0102		20000605	*	0
99215	G0104		19980401	19980401	9

① Column 1 indicates the payable code.
② Column 2 contains the code that is not payable with this particular Column 1 code, unless a modifier is permitted and submitted.
③ This third column indicates if the edit was in existence prior to 1996.
④ The fourth column indicates the effective date of the edit (year, month, date).
⑤ The fifth column indicates the deletion date of the edit (year, month, date).
⑥ The sixth column indicates if use of a modifier is permitted. This number is the modifier indicator for the edit. (The Modifier Indicator Table, shown on page 7 of this booklet, provides further explanation.)

FIGURE 15-14 Example of use of NCCI edits.

limited defect for repairs or **débridement** of complicated lacerations. Complex repair does not include excision of benign or malignant lesions, excisional preparation of a wound bed, or débridement, or the removal of damaged tissue or foreign objects from a wound, an open fracture, or an open dislocation.

Listing Services for Wound Repair
- The repaired wound or wounds should be measured and recorded in centimeters; it also should be indicated whether the wound was curved, angular, or in a starlike pattern.
- When multiple wounds are repaired, add together the lengths of those in the same classification (simple, intermediate, or complex) and from all anatomic sites that are grouped together into the same code descriptor. Do not add lengths of repairs from different groupings of anatomic sites (e.g., face and extremities) or from different classifications (intermediate and complex).
- When wounds of more than one classification are repaired, list the more complicated repair as the primary procedure and the less complicated repair as the secondary procedure, using modifier -59.
- Débridement is considered a separate procedure only when gross contamination requires prolonged cleansing, when large amounts of dead or contaminated tissue must be removed, or when débridement is carried out separately without immediate primary closure.
- Wound repair that involves nerves, blood vessels, and/or tendons should be reported under the appropriate system for repair of those structures. The repair of these associated wounds is included in the primary procedure unless it qualifies as a complex repair, in which case modifier -59 applies.

Musculoskeletal System
Fractures
- *Closed fracture:* The fractured bone does not protrude through the dermis or epidermis.
- *Open fracture:* The fractured bone cuts through the skin layers and can be directly visualized.

- *Closed treatment:* The fracture site is not surgically opened (exposed to the external environment and directly visualized). The three methods of closed treatment of fractures are (1) without manipulation, (2) with manipulation, and (3) with or without traction.
- *Manipulation:* Attempted reduction or restoration of a fracture or dislocated joint into its normal anatomic alignment by manually applied forces.
- *Open treatment:* Used when (1) the fractured bone is surgically opened or (2) an opening is made remote from the fracture site to insert an intramedullary nail across the fracture site.
- *Percutaneous skeletal fixation:* Fracture treatment that is neither open nor closed. The fracture fragments are not visualized, but a fixation device (e.g., pins) is placed across the fracture site, usually under x-ray imaging.

Maternity Care and Delivery
The services normally provided in uncomplicated maternity cases include antepartum care, delivery, and postpartum care.
- *Antepartum* care includes the initial and subsequent history; physical examinations; recording of weight, blood pressure, and fetal heart tones; routine chemical urinalysis; monthly visits up to 28 weeks' gestation; biweekly visits to 36 weeks' gestation; and weekly visits until delivery. Any other visits or services provided within this period should be coded separately, including any routine tests (e.g., sonography, routine laboratory tests).
- *Delivery* includes admission to the hospital, the admission history and physical examination, management of uncomplicated labor, vaginal delivery (with or without forceps or episiotomy), or cesarean delivery. Medical problems complicating labor and delivery should be identified by using the codes in the Medicine and E/M sections in addition to codes for maternity care.
- *Postpartum care* includes hospital and office visits after vaginal or cesarean section delivery.

Common CPT Coding Guidelines: Radiology Section

Assigning CPT codes for the Radiology section is the same procedure as the Surgery section. The Radiology section contains all diagnostic imaging codes, including x-ray studies, ultrasound, MRI, and nuclear medicine procedures, in addition to radiation oncology and several other types of diagnostic imaging procedures, services, and therapies. The Radiology section is divided into subsections: head and neck; chest, spine, and pelvis; upper and lower extremities; abdomen, gastrointestinal and urinary tracts; and gynecologic, obstetric, heart, and vascular procedures. The next subdivision, categories, defines the types or functions of various procedures (e.g., diagnostic ultrasound, radiation oncology, and so on) unique to the anatomic site subsection. In addition to the radiology procedure codes, codes are included for physician supervision and interpretation of diagnostic imaging data and for clinical and radiation treatment planning and administration of contrast materials during radiologic procedures.

Common CPT Coding Guidelines: Pathology and Laboratory Section

Assigning CPT codes for the Pathology section is the same procedure as the Surgery section. The subcategories for the Pathology and Laboratory section include organ panels and disease panels, drug testing, therapeutic drug assays, evocative or suppression testing, consultations, urinalysis, chemistry, molecular diagnostics, infectious agents, microbiology, anatomic pathology, cytopathology, cytogenetic studies, and surgical pathology.

For purposes of coding from the Laboratory section, organ or disease panels are groupings of numerous tests performed to diagnose the health or disease status of specific organ systems. A panel code can be used only if all the tests listed under the code selected were performed. Otherwise, the individual tests should be billed using a separate code for each. There are two types of drug testing, qualitative and quantitative. The codes for drug testing are *qualitative*; that is, they are based on the type of drug found. *Quantitative* assays, on the other hand, are performed to determine the amount of drug present.

Common CPT Coding Guidelines: Medicine Section

The Medicine section of the CPT contains codes for a variety of therapeutic procedures and diagnostic testing. This section also contains codes for dialysis, ophthalmology, acupuncture, chiropractic manipulation, and conscious sedation. The steps for determining Medicine codes are similar to those for choosing Surgery codes.

Immune Globulins

When you code administration of **immune globulins**, identify the immune globulin product administered and the method of administration using the codes in the hydration, therapeutic, prophylactic, and diagnostic injections and infusions subsection.

Hydration codes are intended to report a hydration intravenous (IV) infusion consisting of prepackaged fluid and electrolytes; they are not used to report the infusion of drugs or other substances. When multiple drugs are administered, report the service or services and the specific materials or drugs for each (Figure 15-15).

Medicine
Immune Globulins

▶Codes 90281-90399 identify the immune globulin product only and must be reported in addition to the administration codes 90765-90768, 90772, 90774, 90775 as appropriate. Immune globulin products listed here include broad-spectrum and anti-infective immune globulins, antitoxins, and various isoantibodies.◀

⊘ 90281 Immune globulin (Ig), human, for intramuscular use
⊘ 90283 Immune globulin (IgIV), human, for intravenous use
⊘ 90287 Botulinum antitoxin, equine, any route
⊘ 90288 Botulism immuno globulin, human, for intravenous use
⊘ 90291 Cytomegalovirus immune globulin (CMV-IgIV), human, for intravenous use
⊘ 90296 Diphtheria antitoxin, equine, any route
⊘ 90371 Hepatitis B immune globulin (HBIg), human, for intramuscular use
⊘ 90375 Rabies immune globulin (RIg), human, for intramuscular and/or subcutaneous use
⊘ 90376 Rabies immune globulin, heat-treated (RIg-HT), human, for intramuscular and/or subcutaneous use

FIGURE 15-15 Relationship of immune globulins and infusions in CPT.

Immunization Administration for Vaccines/Toxoids

Codes 90465-90474 must be reported in addition to the vaccine and toxoid code(s) 90476-90749.
Report codes 90465-90468 only when the physician provides face-to-face counseling of the patient and family, during the administration of the vaccine. For immunization administration of any vaccine that is not accompanied by face-to-face physician counseling to the patient/family, report codes 90471-90474.
In a significant separately identifiable Evaluation and Management service (e.g., office or other outpatient services, preventive medicine services) is performed, the appropriate E/M service code should be reported in addition to the vaccine and toxoid administration codes.
(For allergy testing, see 95004 et seq)
(For skin testing of bacterial, viral, fungal extracts, see 86485-86586)
▶(For therapeutic or diagnostic injections, see 90772-90779)◀
90465 Immunization administration under 8 years of age (includes percutaneous, intradermal, subcutaneous, or intramuscular injections) when the physician counsels the patient/family; first injection (single or combination vaccine/toxoid), per day
(Do not report 90465 in conjunction with 90467)
+90466 each additional injection (single or combination vaccine/toxoid), per day (List separately in addition to code for primary procedure)
(Use 90466 in conjunction with 90465 or 90467)

FIGURE 15-16 Relationship of immune vaccines/toxoids and administration codes in CPT.

Immunization for Vaccines or Toxoids

The immunization for vaccines or toxoids codes are for the administration of vaccines and toxoids only and should be reported in conjunction with the appropriate codes in the immunization administration for vaccine/toxoids subsection (Figure 15-16).
Vaccines/Toxoids Codes. These codes identify the vaccine product only. Codes in the immunization administration for vaccines/toxoids subsection must be used in addition to the vaccine or toxoid product codes. To meet the reporting requirements of immunization registries, vaccine distribution programs, and reporting systems, the exact

vaccine product administered must be reported on the insurance claim.

Home Health Procedures and Services

The home health procedures and services codes are used by non-physician healthcare professionals only. They are used to report services provided in a patient's residence, including assisted-living apartments, group homes, nontraditional private homes, custodial care facilities, and schools.

HCPCS CODE SET AND MANUAL

Healthcare Common Procedure Coding System (Level II) codes have five alphanumeric digits, beginning with one letter followed by four numerals. HCPCS uses five coding conventions for special instructions relating to specific codes (Figure 15-17). The modifiers for HCPCS are codes composed of two alphanumeric characters. Like the modifiers for CPT Category I codes, the HCPCS modifiers do not change the description of the code, but rather provide additional information or describe extenuating circumstances. Like the CPT manual, the HCPCS manual is divided into two parts: the Alphabetic Index and the Tabular List. As with the CPT, procedures and services can be looked up in the Alphabetic Index and then confirmed as the most accurate and appropriate code by using the Tabular List. The HCPCS manual has no subsections, categories, or subcategories; it has only sections. An appendix contains all the HCPCS modifiers and their descriptions.

The coding steps for HCPCS are almost identical to those for CPT Category I codes. Clinical documentation is the starting point for HCPCS coding, and the final code selected should add nothing to or omit anything from the description in the medical documentation. The final step is determining whether the code selected can stand alone or requires a modifier to further define or add needed information.

Sometimes HCPCS codes are used along with CPT codes, especially in the medical office setting. For example, a well-baby visit would include the E/M code for the patient visit and also HCPCS codes for the administration of immunizations. Procedure 15-2, part B, explains how to code an office visit involving immunizations.

Healthcare Common Procedure Coding System (HCPCS)

HCPCS is a collection of codes and descriptions for procedures, supplies, products, and services not covered by or included in the CPT coding system (Figure 15-18). As are CPT codes, HCPCS codes are updated annually by the Centers for Medicare and Medicaid Services (CMS). These codes are designed to promote standardized reporting and collection of statistical data on medical supplies, products, services, and procedures.

COMMON HCPCS CODING GUIDELINES

Ambulance Transport

HCPCS codes for ambulance transport range from A0021 to A0999. These codes require specific modifiers (Table 15-7) to be added to ensure code specificity. This section provides codes for a variety of medical transport, including ambulance services, nonemergency transportation, and medical supplies used during the transport. A waiting time calculation table also is available, if needed.

Medical and Surgical Supplies

HCPCS codes for medical and surgical supplies range from A4000 to A8999. The HCPCS manual provides some figures that offer guidance as to what the medical and surgical supplies look like, so they can be billed properly. Medical assistants can code only for surgical supplies purchased by the medical office. For example, pharmaceutical and medical equipment representatives can provide the medical office with some supplies that can be used for patient care. However, it is unethical to bill the patient's insurance company for supplies that were provided to the provider for free. All medical and

---

☼	**Special coverage instructions.** Indicates that there are instructions provided regarding circumstances in which the code might be included for reimbursment.
◆	**Not covered by or valid for Medicare.** These codes might result in reimbursement by private health insurance payors but not by Medicare. Their value may be only for statistical data collection but not for reimbursement.
✳	**Carrier discretion.** These codes may or may not be paid by health insurance carrier including Medicare.
▶	**New.**
⇒	**Revised.** The revised symbol is placed in front of codes with any data, payment, or miscellaneous change from the prior year.

FIGURE 15-17 HCPCS conventions.

	Humidifiers/Compressors/Nebulizers for Use with Oxygen IPPB Equipment
E0550	Humidifier, durable for extensive supplemental humidification during IPPB treatments or oxygen delivery
E0555	Humidifier, durable, glass or autoclavable plastic bottle type, for use with regulator or flowmeter
E0560	Humidifier, durable for supplemental humidification during IPPB treatment or oxygen delivery
E0561	Humidifier, nonheated, used with positive airway pressure device
E0562	Humidifier, heated, used with positive airway pressure device
E0565	Compressor, air power source for equipment which is not self-contained or cylinder driven
E0570	Nebulizer, with compressor
E0571	Aerosol compressor, battery powered, for use with small volume nebulizer
E0572	Aerosol compressor, adjustable pressure, light duty for intermittent use
E0574	Ultrasonic/electronic aerosol generator with small volume nebulizer
E0575	Nebulizer, ultrasonic, large volume
E0580	Nebulizer, durable, glass or autoclavable plastic, bottle type, for use with regulator or flowmeter
E0585	Nebulizer, with compressor and heater

FIGURE 15-18 *Healthcare Common Procedure Coding System (HCPCS) Tabular List.*

TABLE 15-7   Modifiers Used for HCPCS Ambulance Transport Codes

TRANSPORTATION SERVICES MODIFIERS*	DESCRIPTION
D	Diagnostic or therapeutic site other than P or H when those are used as origin codes
E	Residential, domiciliary, custodial facility
G	Hospital-based end-stage renal disease (ESRD) facility
H	Site of transfer (e.g., airport or helicopter pad) between modes of ambulance transport
I	Free-standing ESRD facility
J	Skilled nursing facility
N	Physician's office
P	Residence
R	Scene of accident or acute event
S	Intermediate stop at physician's office on the way to hospital

*Includes ambulance HCPCS origin modifiers.

surgical supplies used during patient care should be documented on the encounter form in the patient's EHR.

Durable Medical Equipment

HCPCS codes for durable medical equipment range from E0100 to E9999. Examples of durable medical equipment include crutches, wheelchairs, walkers, and other products that assist patients with mobility. Some equipment is kept in the medical office inventory. If the practice purchases the medical equipment wholesale, it is allowed to bill patients and/or their insurance company for the retail value of the equipment. Just as with medical and surgical supplies, it is important for the provider to document the dispensing of the durable medical equipment on the encounter form or medical record.

CLOSING COMMENTS

The CPT and HCPCS coding manuals are updated and published every year, so the updated manuals should be ordered in the early fall so that they arrive in enough time for the medical assistant to review them. Always use the current year's manuals so that the codes are accurate. The Introduction in each manual discusses and highlights changes and/or new coding guidelines. Annual updates should be uploaded to reflect any coding changes in the encoder to ensure that all codes are up to date for the current year.

Legal and Ethical Issues

Medical assistants are responsible for keeping up to date on CPT coding to ensure that no fraud takes place in the coding and claims submission process. Medical assistants should also ensure that proper precautions are taken to avoid incorrect coding, data entry errors, and false claims submissions because these activities can be considered fraud.

Medical coders should be familiar with the NCCI edits, which are published every year by the Centers for Medicare and Medicaid Services (CMS). Medicare can cite a healthcare facility for fraud or abuse (or both) if claims submitted by the facility regularly show unbundled codes. Not only is unbundling an unethical practice, it incurs very stiff monetary penalties. According to the Civil Monetary Penalties Law, medical practices can be cited for penalties of up to $50,000 per violation, and assessments of up to three times the amount claimed for each item or service, or up to three times the amount of remuneration offered, paid, solicited, or received.

Professional Behaviors

Two rules should be followed when you code any procedure or service:
1. Be as specific as possible in code selection, and use all pertinent words in the description given in your documentation.
2. Never add or delete any words, modifying terms, or descriptors to the procedure or service code description that change the definition of the procedure or service or that are not documented.

SUMMARY OF SCENARIO

Sherald has learned that procedural coding using the CPT is similar in many ways to ICD-10-CM diagnostic coding. The two coding manuals have unique but also similar steps, conventions, and guidelines. She also has learned that proper abstraction of procedural data from the health record is equally important for ICD-10-CM and the CPT coding. Sherald also has learned that HCPCS codes are used to describe procedures and services not found in the CPT, such as vaccinations, ambulance services, and durable medical equipment.

Sherald uses documentation by the provider in the encounter form, in a patient's electronic health record, to identify the procedures performed. However, she realizes that she also must know how to use the CPT manual because some notes must be coded from procedures or services delivered. As with diagnostic coding, Sherald reviews the patient's EHR for research and documentation if any questions arise about a claim. She knows that coding to the highest level of specificity helps to ensure accuracy and also enables the practice to obtain the maximum reimbursement allowed. Sherald also uses the Internet to network and research. She realizes the importance of keeping up to date with the CPT and HCPCS codes, so she plans to order the updated CPT manual every year. As Sherald continues to learn procedural coding, she envisions herself becoming well rounded in her knowledge of the practice's administrative operations.

SUMMARY OF LEARNING OBJECTIVES

1. **Define, spell, and pronounce the terms listed in the vocabulary.**
   Spelling and pronouncing medical terms correctly reinforce the medical assistant's credibility. Knowing the definitions of these terms promotes confidence in communication with patients and co-workers.

2. **Describe the organization of the *Current Procedural Terminology* (CPT) manual.**
   The CPT manual comprises three category codes: Category I, Category II, and Category III codes. Category I codes are 5-digit codes that are listed in the Tabular List. Category II codes are used for performance measurement, and their use is optional. Category III codes are temporary codes for emerging medical technologies.

3. **Report the history of procedural coding.**
   The second edition of the CPT, published in 1970, presented an expanded system of codes to designate diagnostic and therapeutic procedures in surgery, medicine, radiology, laboratory, pathology, and medical specialties. At that time, the 4-digit classification was replaced with the current 5-digit coding system. The fourth edition was published in 1977 and included significant updates in medical technology. At the same time, a system of periodic annual updating was introduced to keep pace with the rapidly changing environment.

4. **Distinguish between the Alphabetic Index and the Tabular List in the CPT code set.**
   The CPT has two primary divisions, the Alphabetic Index and the Tabular List. The Alphabetic Index is like any other index in a textbook; it is simply a guide to finding data in the body of the textbook. The Tabular List is divided into six sections, and codes are listed in numeric order in each section.

5. **Classify the six different sections in the Tabular List of the CPT code set.**
   The six sections of the Tabular List are Evaluation and Management, Anesthesia, Surgery, Radiology, Pathology and Laboratory, and Medicine. Sections are divided into subsections; subsections are further divided into categories; and categories can be subdivided into subcategories.

6. **Discuss special reports, and explain the importance of modifiers in assigning CPT codes.**
   When a bill is submitted for a service that is unlisted, unusual, or newly adopted, the third-party carrier requires a special consultation report. Modifiers are used in CPT codes to indicate that a service or procedure performed was altered by specific circumstances. Two-digit alphanumeric modifiers, included with the 5-digit CPT code, can be used to supply additional information or to describe extenuating circumstances that affected the rendered procedure or service.

7. **Review various conventions in the CPT code set.**
   Conventions are used to provide additional information about certain codes. Examples of conventions include triangular and round symbols, which indicate that a code or description was revised, removed, or added.

8. **Identify the required medical documentation for accurate procedural coding.**
   Medical records used for procedural coding can include any or all of the following: encounter form, history and physical report (H&P), progress notes, discharge summary, operative report, pathology report, anesthesia record, and/or radiology report. When the medical documentation is compared against any code description, all the elements of that code must substantially match, with nothing added or missing.

9. **Describe how to use the most current procedural coding system and perform procedural coding for surgery.**
   The basic steps in procedural coding are: (1) read, analyze, and abstract the procedure or service documented in the health record and (2) compare it with the encounter form, operative report, or other documentation to ensure that all services and procedures have been recorded. After searching the Alphabetic Index, the medical assistant should turn to the appropriate codes in the Tabular List to perform the final coding steps. Read the section thoroughly to determine the most accurate code to assign to the procedure or service, and then code the procedure or service. The process for procedural coding for surgery with the CPT code set is detailed in Procedure 15-1.

10. **Discuss how to use the Alphabetic Index.**
    The Alphabetic Index is a comprehensive, alphabetic listing of all main terms used in procedural coding. However, it is not a substitute for the Tabular List. It is organized by main terms, and modifying terms are indented two spaces below that term. Begin the search of the Alphabetic Index by using one of the four primary classifications of main and modifying term entries. In the Tabular List, look up each code or code range found in the Alphabetic Index.

11. **Identify common CPT coding guidelines for Evaluation and Management (E/M) procedures.**
    To properly code E/M services, the medical assistant must understand important differences, or variations, from the basic steps. Assigning the correct E/M code includes identifying the section, subsection, category, and subcategory of the procedure or service; reviewing the reporting instructions and guidelines for the code chosen; reviewing the level of E/M service; determining the extent of the history obtained and examination performed; and determining the complexity of medical decision making.

12. **Identify common CPT coding guidelines for Anesthesia procedures.**
    Anesthesia coding differs from any other form of coding in the way anesthesia services are billed. A standard formula has been established for payment of anesthesia services: Basic unit values (B) + Time units (T) + Modifying units (M) + Physical Status (PS): B + T + M + PS. The total number of units is then multiplied by the conversion factor.

13. **Identify common CPT coding guidelines for surgical procedures.**
    Specific guidelines and notes related to surgery coding must be considered when assigning a CPT code. Always review the current year's guidelines in the Surgery section for the most up-to-date information.

14. **Discuss coding factors for the integumentary system and muscular system, and for maternity care and delivery.**
    Excision of benign lesions includes a simple closure and anesthesia. Different instructions are provided for each type of wound repair. Fractures are handled according to the type. The services normally provided

Continued

SUMMARY OF LEARNING OBJECTIVES—*continued*

in uncomplicated maternity cases include antepartum care, delivery, and postpartum care.

15. Identify common CPT coding guidelines for Radiology, Pathology and Laboratory, and Medicine sections.

Assigning accurate CPT codes for the Radiology section is similar to the process for the Surgery section. The Radiology section contains all diagnostic imaging codes, including x-ray studies, ultrasound, magnetic resonance imaging (MRI), and nuclear medicine procedures, in addition to radiation oncology and several other types of diagnostic imaging procedures, services, and therapies.

Assigning accurate CPT codes for the Pathology and Laboratory section also is similar to the process for the Surgery section. The subcategories for the Pathology section include organ panels and disease panels, drug testing, therapeutic drug assays, evocative or suppression testing, consultations, urinalysis, chemistry, molecular diagnostics, infectious agents, microbiology, anatomic pathology, cytopathology, cytogenetic studies, and surgical pathology. In the Laboratory section, organ or disease panels are groupings of numerous tests performed to diagnose the health or disease status of specific organ systems.

The Medicine section contains codes for a variety of therapeutic procedures and diagnostic testing. This section also contains codes for Dialysis, Ophthalmology, Acupuncture, Chiropractic Manipulation, and Conscious Sedation. The steps for determining codes in the Medicine section are similar to those for determining codes in the Surgery section.

16. Do the following related to the HCPCS code set and manual:

- *Identify procedures and services that require HCPCS codes.*
  HCPCS is a collection of codes and descriptions that represent procedures, supplies, products, and services not covered by or included in the CPT coding system. HCPCS codes, like CPT codes, are updated annually by the Centers for Medicare and Medicaid Services (CMS). These codes are designed to promote standardized reporting and collection of statistical data on medical supplies, products, services, and procedures.

- *Describe how to use the most current HCPCS level II coding system.*
  Like the CPT manual, the HCPCS manual is divided into two parts: the Alphabetic Index and the Tabular List. As with the CPT, procedures and services are looked up in the Alphabetic Index, and the Tabular List then is used to confirm that the code is the most accurate and appropriate one. The HCPCS manual has no subsections, categories, or subcategories; it has only sections. An appendix contains all the HCPCS modifiers and their descriptions. The coding steps for HCPCS are almost identical to those for CPT Category I codes.

17. Perform procedural coding for an office visit and an immunization.

To code an office visit, the coder first must determine the level of all key components, which include the history, examination, and medical decision making. (See Procedure 15-2, part A.)

An immunization procedure is coded using the HCPCS code set. Coding for HCPCS is almost identical to coding for CPT because both manuals have an Alphabetical Index and a Tabular List. After searching the Alphabetic Index, the coder turns to the appropriate codes in the Tabular List to perform the final coding steps. The coder reads the section thoroughly to determine the most accurate code to assign to the procedure or service, and then codes the procedure or service. (See Procedure 15-2, part B.)

18. Summarize common HCPCS coding guidelines.

Ambulance Transport codes require specific modifiers to ensure code specificity. The HCPCS manual provides some figures that offer guidance as to what the medical and surgical supplies look like so they can be billed properly. Medical assistants can only bill for surgical supplies that were purchased by the medical office. The medical office can purchase the medical equipment wholesale but still bill patients and/or their insurance companies for the retail value of the equipment. When the insurance company is billed, it is vital that the medical assistant fill in the "Number of Units" box on the health insurance claim form for equipment provided to the patient.

CONNECTIONS

📖 Study Guide Connection: Go to the Chapter 15 Study Guide. Read and complete the activities.

evolve Evolve Connection: Go to the Chapter 15 link at *evolve.elsevier.com/kinn* to complete the Chapter Review Quiz. Check out the other resources listed for this chapter to make the most of what you have learned from the Basics of Procedural Coding.

BASICS OF HEALTH INSURANCE

SCENARIO

Jodie Bimmell, a registered medical assistant (RMA), has worked for Dr. Ted Crawford, an endocrinologist, for 3 years. Jodie started with Dr. Crawford as a receptionist; Dr. Crawford recognized that Judy was very detail-oriented, so he promoted her to take charge of the health insurance policies and procedures manual for the practice 2 years ago. Jodie trains all new medical assistants on how to verify patient health insurance coverage and eligibility. Because Jodie has learned quite a bit about health insurance, she can answer most of the patients' questions about their coverage, benefits, and/or exclusions of their policies. She knows where to direct patients who have more complicated ques-

tions and how to follow up—one of the most important duties of a professional medical assistant. She has a great attitude about assisting patients with insurance questions and does not hesitate to call the third-party payer on the patient's behalf. She provides patients with exceptional customer service. When patients call her for assistance, she responds within 24 hours (often within 1 hour) with answers to their questions or a resource to help them. Jodie is willing to help any staff member with other duties when necessary and prides herself on being a patient advocate. She is an enthusiastic team player who puts patients first.

While studying this chapter, think about the following questions:

- How important is the verification of services and benefits for reimbursement?
- How are privately sponsored health insurance plans and government-sponsored health insurance plans different?
- What is the Affordable Care Act and how does this legislation affect healthcare facilities?

- Why is it important to verify eligibility and preauthorize services before the patient appointment is scheduled?
- Is preauthorization necessary for patients who have a managed care health plan? Why or why not?
- Why is it important to educate patients on their health insurance benefits?

LEARNING OBJECTIVES

1. Define, spell, and pronounce the terms listed in the vocabulary.
2. Discuss the purpose of health insurance and explain the health insurance contract between the patient and the health plan.
3. Identify types of third-party plans.
4. Discuss the Affordable Care Act's effect on patient healthcare access.
5. Summarize the different health insurance benefits available and interpret information on a health insurance identification (ID) card.
6. Explain the importance of verifying eligibility and be able to verify eligibility of services, including documentation.
7. Explain the health insurance contract between the healthcare provider and the health insurance company.

8. Explain how insurance reimbursements are determined and discuss the effect health insurance has on provider reimbursements.
9. Summarize privately sponsored health insurance plans.
10. Differentiate among the different types of managed care models.
11. Outline managed care requirements for patient referral and obtain a referral with documentation.
12. Describe the process for preauthorization and how to obtain preauthorization including documentation.
13. List and discuss various government-sponsored plans.
14. Review employer-established self-funded plans.

VOCABULARY

beneficiary A recipient of health insurance benefits.
capitation A contract between the health insurance plan and the provider for which the health insurance plan will pay an agreed-upon monthly fee per patient and the provider agrees to provide medical services on a regular basis.
explanation of benefits (EOB) A document sent by the insurance company to the provider and the patient explaining

the allowed charge amount, the amount reimbursed for services, and the patient's financial responsibilities.
fee-for-service A reimbursement model in which the health plan pays the provider's fee for every health insurance claim.
gatekeeper The primary care provider, who can approve or deny when the patient seeks additional care via a referral to a specialist or further medical tests.

government-sponsored health insurance Health insurance programs that are sponsored by the government and offer coverage for the elderly, disabled, military, and indigent.

online provider insurance Web portal An online service provided by various insurance companies for providers to look up patient insurance benefits, eligibility, claims status, and explanation of benefits.

privately sponsored health insurance Health insurance companies that operate for profit and use managed care plans to reduce the costs of healthcare.

qualified Medicare beneficiaries (QMB) Low-income Medicare patients who qualify for Medicaid for their secondary insurance.

third-party administrator (TPA) The intermediary and administrator who coordinates patients and providers, as well as processes claims, for self-funded plans.

subscriber The person who is the signer on the health insurance policy.

utilization management A process of managing healthcare costs by influencing patient care decision making through case-by-case assessments of the appropriateness of care.

waiting period The amount of time a patient waits for disability insurance to pay after the date of injury.

PURPOSE OF HEALTH INSURANCE

Health insurance is a third-party payer system that reimburses a provider when services are rendered for an insured patient. A monthly *premium,* or payment, is paid for a list of health insurance benefits detailed in the contract; the premium can be paid by the employer if the **subscriber** is employed with benefits, or it is paid by the patient for individual coverage. The patient provides evidence of the health insurance contract to the healthcare provider in the form of an insurance identification (ID) card. The provider then submits a claim to the health insurance company for services rendered. The third party then *reimburses,* or pays, the claim to the healthcare provider for services already rendered.

To understand the specifics of the insurance plan, it is vital to review the terms of the health insurance contract with the patient and the healthcare provider.

CONTRACT WITH PATIENTS

To obtain health insurance coverage, applicants need to apply either through their employer or privately. There are two types of health insurance plans in the United States: **privately sponsored health insurance plans** and **government-sponsored health insurance plans**. Health insurance plans typically cover health services and procedures that are deemed *medically necessary,* or health services that are necessary to improve the patient's current health condition. Most insurance policies do not cover *elective procedures,* or medical procedures that are not deemed medical necessary, or needed to improve the patient's current health, such as a facelift. Most of today's health insurance policies cover *preventive care,* which includes services provided to help prevent certain illnesses or that lead to an early diagnosis. Some preventative care services include yearly routine vaccinations, blood tests, urine analysis, and hearing and vision testing; preventative coverage depends on the insurance policy.

HEALTH INSURANCE PLANS
Government-Sponsored Health Insurance Plans

Government-sponsored health insurance plans are federal- or state-sponsored plans that require patients to pay minimal to no monthly premiums. In order to qualify, patients must meet the program requirements such as age, disability, income level, or occupation. However, these health insurance plans offer benefits and healthcare access is limited to healthcare providers that are contracted with them.

Employer-Sponsored Group Policies

In the recent past, businesses have offered their eligible full-time employees health insurance as a *group policy,* a privately sponsored health insurance plan purchased by an employer for a group of employees. The employer exercises the right to establish how much their employees pay for health insurance coverage for themselves, their spouse (i.e., domestic partner), and children. Employers usually sponsor a percentage of the monthly premium, thus making health insurance coverage more affordable for their employees. Employers also determine the health insurance benefits under the group policy. Health insurance monthly premiums and benefits can vary from employer to employer. For example, the health insurance plan for Employer A covers chiropractic care but the health insurance plan for Employer B does not. Group policies usually provide greater benefits at lower premiums because of the large pool of employees. Often the employee shares the cost of the monthly premium through payroll deductions.

Individual Health Insurance Plans

Not so long ago it was very difficult for individuals who did not work full time to obtain affordable health insurance coverage if they did not qualify for a government-sponsored health insurance plan. Although there were individual insurance health plans, health insurance not sponsored by an employer, these were very difficult to qualify for. If an applicant had a preexisting condition, which is a health condition that existed before the application that needed ongoing medical care, the health insurance plan exercised the right to deny coverage or charged exorbitant monthly premiums.

The Affordable Care Act

In the early 2000s it became clear that a large number of Americans lacked basic health insurance. *Preexisting conditions* made it difficult for Americans who did not work full time or were self-employed to obtain health insurance. In addition, the health insurance market was discriminating against young adults of 18+ years that may not have been qualified to receive health benefits because they could not find full-time employment.

In 2010 the Patient Protection and Affordable Care Act, which is also known as the *Affordable Care Act* and also Obamacare, was enacted. It increased the quality, availability, and affordability of private and public health insurance for more than 44 million uninsured Americans. The legislation includes new qualifying regulations, taxes, mandates, and subsidies. The federal mandate not only opens opportunities for more Americans to obtain affordable health insurance, but also works to reduce overall healthcare spending in the long run. Other patient protections and provisions under the Affordable Care Act include:

- Insurance companies are prohibited from dropping patient health coverage if the individual gets sick or makes an unintentional mistake on the health insurance application
- Eliminates preexisting conditions and gender discrimination so patients cannot be charged more based on their health status or gender
- Young adults can remain on their parent's or guardian's insurance policy until age 26
- Creates *Health Insurance Marketplaces* where low-to-middle-income Americans can compare plans and lower their costs on healthcare coverage
- States will expand Medicaid coverage to 15.9 million Americans to include those who qualify for cost assistance through the marketplace
- Requires all Americans to obtain and maintain minimum essential insurance coverage through the year or there will be a monthly tax penalty imposed. For those who cannot afford health insurance based on their household income, tax deductions and payment subsidies are available
- Individuals seeking health insurance can only apply during the open enrollment period, which is established by each state

With more Americans having health insurance, the number of office visits to providers across the country is expected to increase. Refer to Box 16-1 for the Affordable Care Act essential health benefits. Thus efficient health insurance management policies should be instituted to meet the new demand for services.

Box 16-1   Essential Health Benefits Outlined by the Affordable Care Act

Ambulatory patient services
Emergency services
Hospitalization
Maternity and newborn care
Mental health and substance abuse disorder services, including behavior health services
Prescription drugs
Rehabilitative and habilitative services and devices
Laboratory services
Preventive services and wellness services; chronic disease management
Pediatric services, including oral and vision care

Affordable Care Act Navigators Program

Affordable Care Act Navigators are certified enrollment counselors who assist consumers through a variety of outreach, education, enrollment, postenrollment, and renewal support services including, but not limited to, the following:

- Inform eligible consumers of the availability and benefits of obtaining healthcare coverage
- Promote the value of purchasing healthcare coverage
- Motivate consumers to act
- Help consumers to shop and compare plans
- Facilitate enrollment into respective health insurance marketplaces
- Assist consumers with the eligible renewal process
- Provide postenrollment outreach and support to eligible consumers

The Navigators Program is federally mandated for all state health exchanges. The navigators help consumers, small businesses, and employees as they look for health coverage options through the marketplace, including completing eligibility and enrollment forms. These individuals and organizations are required to be unbiased. Their services are free to consumers.

BENEFITS

Every health insurance contract is tailored to the needs of each individual or group policy, and the combinations of benefits are limitless. Benefits cover the *amount loss,* or the amount that should be paid to the healthcare provider for services rendered. Employers can pick and choose the benefits they want for their employees; this is also called "cafeteria style." A policy may contain one or any combination of the benefits found in Table 16-1. Medical assistants should be familiar with how to look up patient benefit information to inform patients of their financial responsibilities before scheduling an appointment.

Hospitalization

Hospital coverage pays the cost of all or part of the patient's hospital room and board including specific hospital services, such as the hospital surgical room fee or a hospital stay of less than 30 days. Hospital insurance policies frequently set a maximum amount payable per day and a maximum number of days of hospital care; these policies and procedures are established by the health insurance plan.

Surgical

Surgical coverage pays all or part of a surgeon's fee; some plans also pay for an assistant surgeon. Surgery may be performed in a hospital, provider's office, or outpatient surgery center. The insurance company frequently provides the guarantor with a surgical fee schedule that establishes the amount they will pay for commonly performed procedures.

Basic Medical

Basic medical coverage pays all or part of a healthcare provider's fee for nonsurgical services, including hospital, home, and office visits and consultations. Payments are made for many different types of

TABLE 16-1   Types of Health Insurance and Plan Benefits

BENEFIT	COVERED	PAYS	BENEFIT	COVERED	PAYS
Hospitalization	Cost of all or part of the hospital room and board; and specific hospital services (i.e., costs involved in having surgery in a hospital)	Maximum amount per day and maximum number of days	Dental care	Preventive care; treatment and repair of teeth and gums	Typically pays 100% for preventive care, 50% for repair and treatment
Surgical	Any surgical procedure, including but not limited to incision or excision; removal of foreign bodies; aspiration; suturing; reduction of fractures	Surgeon's fee Assistant surgeon's fee	Vision care	Eye examination and glasses or contacts	Set benefit amount, depending on vision care policy for examination and glasses
Basic medical	Outpatient and provider office procedures and services	Provider's fees; diagnostic, radiologic, laboratory, and pathology fees	Medicare supplement	Deductible and co-insurance amounts unpaid by Medicare	Deductible and co-insurance amounts unpaid by Medicare
Major medical	Catastrophic or prolonged illness or injury	Takes over when basic medical, hospitalization, and surgical benefits end	Life insurance	Loss of life	Usually a lump sum payment of the life insurance benefit
Disability	Accident or illness resulting in an inability for patient to work; can be paid whether work-related or not	Cash benefits paid in lieu of salary while patient is unable to earn an income	Long-term care	Long-term skilled nursing or rehabilitation care	Set amount determined by policy benefits

healthcare professional's visits including nurses, physical therapists, and occupational therapists. The insurance plan may include a provision for diagnostic laboratory, radiology, and pathology expenses. Basic medical covers a percent of the fee schedule's allowed cost; it is common for the insurance plan to cover 80%, with the additional 20% being the patient's financial responsibility.

Disability (Loss of Income) Protection

Disability insurance is a form of insurance that insures the beneficiary's earned income against the risk that a disability will make working uncomfortable (e.g., psychological disorders), painful (e.g., back pain), or impossible (e.g., coma). It encompasses paid sick leave, short-term disability benefits, and long-term disability benefits.

Weekly or monthly cash benefits are provided to employed policyholders who become unable to work as a result of an accident or illness. Many disability policies have a **waiting period** until benefits can be paid. Payments are made directly to the **beneficiary** and are intended to replace lost income resulting from an illness or other disability. It is not intended for payment of specific medical bills, and it should not be confused with a regular health insurance plan.

Dental Care

Dental benefits offer a variety of options in the form of either fee-for-service or managed care plans that reimburse or discount a portion of a patient's dental expenses.

Most dental plans have preventive dental care (e.g., cleaning and x-ray films) covered 100% twice a year, with most other services covered at a discount.

Vision Care

Vision care insurance usually provides coverage of a yearly eye examination and a discount on frames, lenses, and contact lenses. Some vision plans also pay for corrective procedures, such as laser eye surgery.

Medicare Supplement

Basic medical coverage for Medicare Part B is 80% after the deductible; this means that all Medicare patients are financially responsible for 20%. So some Medicare beneficiaries choose to purchase a privately sponsored supplemental health insurance policy to help cover the 20% medical cost incurred; these supplemental health insurance plans are known as *Medigap* policies. Medigap policies cover the difference between Medicare reimbursement and patient financial responsibilities. Federal regulations now require Medicare supplement policy benefits to be uniform to avoid confusion for the purchaser.

Liability Insurance

Liability insurance covers losses to a third party caused by the insured. There are many types of liability insurance, including automobile, business, and homeowners' policies. Liability policies often include benefits for medical expenses resulting from traumatic injuries, lost wages, and sometimes pain and suffering payable to victims injured by the insured person's home or car, without regard to the insured person's actual legal liability for the accident.

Life Insurance

Life insurance provides payment of a specified amount upon the insured's death, either to his or her estate or to a designated beneficiary. A subtype of life insurance, an endowment policy, allows the policyholder to build up funds to be dispersed on a specified schedule during his or her lifetime. Annuity life insurance policies provide monthly cash benefits if the policyholder becomes permanently and totally disabled. Sometimes the proceeds from life insurance are used to meet the expenses of the insured person's last illness.

Long-Term Care Insurance

Long-term care insurance is a relatively new type of insurance that covers a broad range of maintenance and health services for chronically ill, disabled, or developmentally delayed individuals. Medical services may be provided on an inpatient basis (e.g., at a rehabilitation facility, nursing home, or mental hospital), on an outpatient basis, or at home.

CRITICAL THINKING APPLICATION   **16-1**

Michael Sherman, an elderly patient, called to make an appointment, but was unsure what his benefits were. How can Jodie find out what benefits he qualifies for? Is it appropriate for Jodie to educate Michael on his health insurance benefits? Why or why not?

Premiums

Patients covered by an *employer-sponsored group health insurance plan,* or health insurance offered by their employer, typically share the cost for the monthly premium. Individual health insurance plans offered through federal- and state-sponsored health insurance marketplaces make monthly premium payments. Indigent, elderly, federally employed, or military patients who seek healthcare from the government have little or no monthly premiums.

Health Insurance Identification Card

As proof of health insurance coverage, patients are issued a health insurance ID card with the health insurance company, health plan name, health plan type, patient's name, subscriber ID, and health plan contact phone numbers. Review Figure 16-1 for a sampling of different insurance ID cards for common third-party payers. Refer to Procedure 16-1 on how to interpret information on the health insurance ID card.

PROCEDURE 16-1   Interpret Information on an Insurance Card

Goal: *To identify essential information on the health insurance identification (ID) card to confirm co-payment obligations and send accurate health insurance claims for reimbursement.*

EQUIPMENT and SUPPLIES

- Scanned copy of patient's health insurance ID, both sides
- Scanned copy of patient's state-issued ID card

PROCEDURAL STEPS

1. Review the scanned copy of the patient's health insurance ID card and state-issued ID card in the electronic health record (EHR). If the patient is a minor, then scan a copy of the insured's state-issued ID card.
   PURPOSE: To confirm the patient's identity is the name on the health insurance ID card.
2. Identify the subscriber on the health insurance ID card with the patient's name. If the patient is different than the insured name on the card, then obtain the relationship with the insured and the insured's date of birth and gender.
   PURPOSE: To submit an accurate health insurance claim, the insured's date of birth and gender is required.
3. Identify the insurance plan and health maintenance organization (HMO) network, if present.

   PURPOSE: To confirm that the provider is a participating provider for the insurance plan or the HMO network. If the provider is out of network, the patient should be informed that they would either have to pay more out of pocket or the medical services rendered will not be covered by the insurance plan.
4. Identify the insured's policy number and group number.
   PURPOSE: To accurately submit the health insurance claim under the correct insurance policy number and group number.
5. Identify the patient's co-payment, which is due before the appointment. Collect the correct amount. For example, if the provider is a general practitioner, then collect the co-payment for the primary care provider (PCP).
   PURPOSE: To ensure the proper co-payment is paid by the patient.
6. On the back of the health insurance ID card, ensure that a customer service phone number and medical claims address is present.
   PURPOSE: To ensure that the provider can contact customer service and has the correct mailing address.

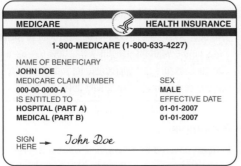

Medicare: The Medicare card uses the patient's social security number as the ID number. The card also details the plan coverages, in this case Part A and Part B.

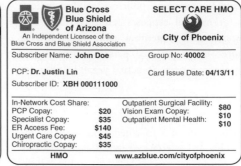

HMO ID Card: Notice the Health Insurance Plan and the HMO Plan are both listed. Common copayments are listed are also listed. HMO members are required to choose PCP which is designated on their health ID card.

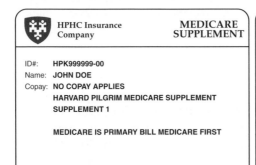

Medicare Secondary Insurance: The ID card states that it is a supplement to Medicare, thus Medicare should be billed as the primary. The ID number does not match the Medicare card.

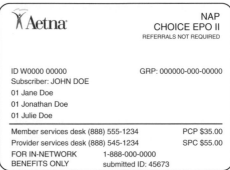

EPO Plan ID Card: Members are not required to choose a PCP, but can only use their benefits for in-network providers and facilities. Notice the ID number stays the same for the insured and all family members listed.

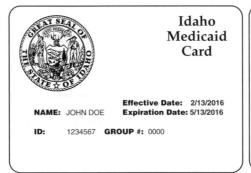

Medicaid: Medicaid cards have the state seal printed on them indicating that services can only be performed by the sponsoring state. These cards contain a effective and expiring date. If a patient presents a card with an expired date, contact Medicaid to confirm their benefits have been extended.

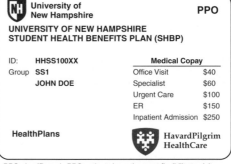

PPO plan ID card: PPO patients have the most flexibility to visit whichever provider, primary care of specialist they choose. Notice the medical copays are slightly higher than HMO copayments.

FIGURE 16-1 A variety of different health insurance identification cards.

VERIFYING ELIGIBILITY OF SERVICES

Verification of eligibility is the process of confirming health insurance coverage for the patient for the medical service on the date of service. It is vital for the healthcare facility to ensure that the patient who is seeking healthcare is in the provider's network of contracted health insurance plans. Before scheduling the appointment, health insurance information should be collected over the phone (unless it is an emergency situation). The medical assistant should verify the *effective date,* or date the insurance coverage began, and confirm that the patient is covered on the date the medical services will be rendered. The medical assistant should make it a practice to review the **online insurance Web portal**, which can verify insurance eligibility, benefits, and exclusions prior to the patient's appointment. If the online insurance provider portal is not available, the medical assistant should contact the provider services desk; the phone number should be listed on the back side of the patient's health insurance ID card. Refer to Procedure 16-2 on how to verify eligibility of services, including documentation.

Online Insurance Provider Portals

In the recent past, the medical assistant would have to call the health insurance company to verify eligibility for each and every patient. Each call to the health insurance company automated system would take at least 5 minutes and the medical assistant would not have access to all of the patient's benefit information unless he or she spoke to a member services agent, which would take even more time. Today, most privately sponsored health insurance plans have offered online insurance provider portals, which allows for quick and easy verification of eligibility (Figure 16-2). The healthcare facility will have to apply for access to the online insurance provider portal. Once approved, patient benefits can be looked up in their entirety in seconds instead of minutes. Patient benefit plan information can be uploaded to the electronic health record (EHR) very quickly; this process reduces the use of paper in the healthcare facility.

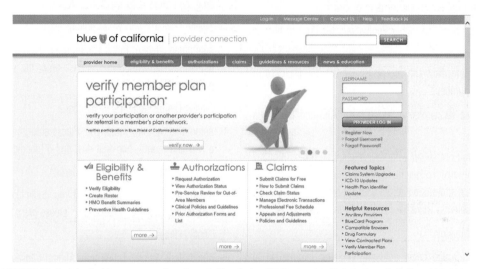

FIGURE 16-2 Online health insurance provider web portal. (From Fordney MT: *Insurance handbook for the medical office*, ed 14, St. Louis, 2017, Elsevier.)

PROCEDURE 16-2   Verify Eligibility of Services, Including Documentation

Goal: *To confirm that the patient's insurance is in effect; to determine the benefits covered, exclusions, and noncovered procedures and services; and to determine whether preauthorizations are included or required.*

EQUIPMENT and SUPPLIES

- Patient health record
- Patient's health insurance identification (ID) card

PROCEDURAL STEPS

1. When a patient calls for an appointment, identify the patient's insurance plan. Ask for information on the patient's ID card including the subscriber number, the group number, and the phone number for provider services. Choose a partner and read the following scripted scenario between Shelly the medical assistant and Amy the patient.

   Shelly: Hello, you've reached Dr. Crawford's office, how can I help you?

   Amy: Yes, I would like to make an appointment to see Dr. Crawford.

   Shelly: Have you been seen by us before?

   Amy: No, this is the first time.

   Shelly: Well, welcome to our office! The first available appointment we have for new patients is next Monday at 9 AM; does that work for you?

   Amy: Sure.

   Shelly: Ok, please tell me your full name, last name first.

   Amy: Palmer, Amy.

   Shelly: Great, and now your date of birth.

   Amy: 11/12/1964.

   Shelly: Can I have your home address?

   Amy: 3434 Homestead Place, Wichita, Kansas, 39493.

   Shelly: And phone number?

   Amy: 585 896-5632.

   Shelly: Great! Now will you be using your health insurance?

   Amy: Yes, I have Blue Shield.

   Shelly: Amy, do you know if it is a PPO or an HMO plan?

   Amy: It is an HMO plan.

PROCEDURE 16-2   *—continued*

Shelly: Ok, if you have the card in front of you, can you please tell me the HMO plan name?

Amy: It is the Wichita Community IPA.

Shelly: Great, we are contracted with them. Are you the insured? Or are you a dependent?

Amy: This is my husband's insurance.

Shelly: Ok, can I get his full name and his date of birth?

Amy: Yes, his name is David Christopher Palmer and his date of birth is 8/1/1962.

Shelly: Thanks for that info. Now can you please tell me the insurance ID number and the group number?

Amy: Yes, the insurance ID number is XEA900000900 and the group number is X0009000.

Shelly: Thanks! Amy, you are all set with your appointment next Monday at 9 AM. Please come at least 15 minutes early to fill out any paperwork. I will verify your insurance information before your appointment and contact you if there are any problems. Thanks for calling, have a great day!

Amy: Thanks, see you Monday.

PURPOSE: To prepare for and begin gathering required information to perform both insurance verification and insurance claim completion procedures.

2. At the time of the appointment, obtain and photocopy both sides of the patient's health insurance ID card(s) and a state-issued ID card.
   PURPOSE: To ensure that the correct ID, group, and policy numbers are obtained, in addition to the name, address, and phone number of the insurance carrier or carriers. The state-issued ID card is used to confirm the patient's identity.

3. Call the health insurance company with the contact number listed on the back of the patient's health insurance ID card or you can log into the online provider insurance Web portal when you have access. Use the following script to initiate a verification of eligibility encounter with the health insurance plan's automated phone system.

Automated System: Thank you for calling Anthem Blue Cross of California. Please choose from one of the following options: Press 1 for verification of eligibility; press 2 to request a referral; press 3 to request an authorization of a medical service; press 5 to request an authorization of a formulary drug; and press 0 to speak to a representative.

Shelly: (Presses 1 to verify patient eligibility.)

Automated System: Thank you for using the Anthem Blue Cross of California automated verification line. Please enter the subscriber's ID number and press the # key.

Shelly: (Enters patient's ID number.)

Automated System: Thank you. Please enter the patient's date of birth with a two-digit month, two-digit day, and a four-digit year.

Shelly: (Enters patient's date of birth.)

Automated System: Thank you. If you would like to hear eligibility information for the patient "Miriam Cho" please press 1.

Shelly: (Presses 1.)

Automated System: Thank you. Miriam Cho has a PPO and is eligible for benefits for (today's date). Would you like to hear the co-payment and deductible amount? Press 1 for yes; hang up if you are finished.

Shelly: (Presses 1.)

Automated System: Thank you. The patient has a co-pay of $30 for the PCP, $50 for the specialist, and $60 for urgent care. The plan has a $4000 deductible, of which $2200 has been met as of (today's date). If you are done, please hang up. If you would like more benefit information, please press 0 for a customer service representative.

Shelly: (Records benefit information and hangs up the phone.)

ACCESSING HEALTHCARE

When the insured patient seeks medical care, a healthcare provider renders medical services at any *in-network* healthcare facility, which are locations that are contracted in the patient's health insurance plan, including medical offices, urgent care centers, and hospitals. In-network healthcare providers and facilities are contracted with the health insurance plan and have agreed to provide health services at a reduced fee. Many health insurance plans do not reimburse for healthcare services provided at *out-of-network* facilities; so prior to the appointment scheduled, the medical assistant should verify that the provider and the healthcare facility are in-network of the patient's insurance plan.

Participating Provider Contracts

With all government-sponsored health plans and most privately sponsored health plans, healthcare providers must become *participating providers* (PARs): These providers are contracted with the insurance plan and have agreed to accept the contracted fee schedule. Healthcare providers can apply to become PARs through a process called *credentialing*. Credentialing is the process of confirming the healthcare provider's qualifications, including the healthcare provider's license to practice medicine, affiliated organizations, and his or her education and professional background.

Once the healthcare provider is credentialed, the health insurance plan issues a contract to become an in-network PAR. The contract includes a fee schedule that the health insurance company will use to reimburse the provider for health services rendered; by signing the contract, the provider agrees to accept the health insurance plan's fee schedule, even if it is lower than their fee schedule.

Contracted Fee Schedules

In the United States payment for services is typically made after the health services are rendered. In other words, healthcare providers are paid weeks, sometimes months, after medical services have been provided to the patient. Once the service is provided to the patient, the healthcare provider must submit a health insurance claim, which includes the diagnosis and procedure codes and total charges. Although the healthcare provider establishes their own fee schedule, or list of charges associated with various medical services provided, health insurance plans maintain their own rates at which they reimburse.

A healthcare provider has three commodities to sell: time, expertise, and services. In every case, healthcare providers must place an estimate on the value of these services. Fees for medical procedures and services differ from office to office based on the type of practice and the needs of the facility. Providers establishing the practice normally set the fees for procedures and services. In the past, most providers worked on a **fee-for-service** basis; that is, patients were charged for the provider's service based on each individual service performed.

In recent years, health insurance plans, particularly government-sponsored and managed healthcare organizations, have greatly influenced what healthcare providers can be reimbursed by establishing the allowable charge. The *allowable charge* is the maximum that third-party payers will pay for a procedure or service. The patient cannot be charged for the amount above the allowable charge if the provider and/or the healthcare facility are contracted in-network.

How Reimbursements Are Determined

Insurance benefits may be determined and paid in one of several ways:

- Determination of the usual, customary, and reasonable (UCR) fees
- Indemnity schedules
- Service benefit plans
- Resource-based relative value scale (RBRVS)

Usual, Customary, and Reasonable Fees

Some insurance companies agree to pay on the basis of all or a percentage of a UCR fee. Charges for a specific service are compared with a database showing (1) charges to other patients for the same service by the same type of provider and (2) charges to patients by other providers performing the same or similar services in the same geographic area. The insurance company determines whether the provider's charge is UCR, and sets the allowed charges.

Indemnity Schedules

Indemnity plans are traditional health insurance plans that pay for all or a share of the cost of covered services, regardless of which provider, hospital, or other licensed healthcare provider is used. Because providers and other providers are paid for each office visit, test, procedure, or other service they deliver, indemnity plans are often called fee-for-service plans.

An indemnity health insurance plan, also known as *major medical,* is a more flexible yet more costly option. Many people refer to this as a traditional plan because it preceded the advent of managed care (e.g., health maintenance organizations [HMOs], preferred provider organizations [PPOs], and point of service [POS] plans).

Policyholders of indemnity plans and their dependents choose when and where to get healthcare services. When the policy is purchased, the subscriber is often given a schedule of indemnities (i.e., a fee schedule), which explains the benefit payment amounts. Indemnity benefits are usually paid to the person insured unless that person has authorized payment directly to the provider, which is a common practice.

Service Benefit Plans

In *service benefit plans,* the health insurance company agrees to pay for certain surgical or medical services without additional cost to the person insured. There is no set fee schedule. In a service benefit plan, surgery with complications would warrant a higher fee than an uncomplicated procedure. Premiums are sometimes higher for this type of coverage, but reimbursements are also larger. Benefit payments are sent directly to the provider and are considered full payment for services rendered. Consider this example: the service benefit plan states that it will pay $900 for a cholecystectomy. If Dr. Jones charges $1500 for this procedure, he must accept the $900 as payment in full and write off the difference.

Resource-Based Relative Value Scale

The *RBRVS* is one of the outcomes of the Medicare Physician Payment Reform that was enacted in the Omnibus Budget Reconciliation Act of 1989 (*OBRA '89*). Originally, Medicare Part B had paid providers using a fee-for-service system based on UCR charges. However, implementation of the RBRVS in 1992 changed this system to a fee scale consisting of three parts:

- Provider work
- Charge-based professional liability expenses
- Charge-based overhead

The provider work component includes the degree of effort invested by a provider in a particular service or procedure and the time it consumed. The professional liability and overhead components are computed by the Centers for Medicare and Medicaid Services (CMS).

The RBRVS fee schedule is designed to provide nationally uniform payments after adjustment to reflect the differences in practice costs across geographic areas. The fee schedule includes a conversion factor, which is a single national number applied to all services paid under the fee schedule. Conversion factors are changed by Congress, usually annually, at the request of the CMS.

Depending on the contract between the provider and the insurance carrier (especially Medicare, Medicaid, and other government programs), the provider either writes off the difference between the RBRVS schedule and his or her fee.

Contracts between the provider of service and the insurance payer vary greatly, depending on the insurance or third-party payer. It is important for the medical assistant to know the contract terms for each third-party payer and, upon receipt of payment, to examine the **explanation of benefits (EOB)** from the insurance carrier closely to ensure that all benefits have been reimbursed appropriately and correctly.

PRIVATELY SPONSORED HEALTH INSURANCE PLANS

Privately sponsored health insurance plans, also known as commercial insurance plans, are for-profit organizations. As such, health insurance companies make annual changes to the participating provider contract to negotiate lower reimbursements. Most privately sponsored plans use managed care to reduce the costs of delivering quality healthcare.

Blue Cross/Blue Shield

Blue Cross and Blue Shield (BC/BS) are America's oldest and largest system of privately sponsored insurers. BS began in 1900 from the lumber and mining camps of the Pacific Northwest. BC began in 1929 when an executive at Baylor University came up with a plan for teachers to budget for their future hospital bills. Both BC and BS set the precedent for monthly prepaid healthcare.

BC/BS offers incentive contracts to healthcare providers. PARs agree to write off the difference or balance between the amount charged by the provider and the approved fee established by the insurance plan. They also agree to bill the patient only for the deductible and co-pay/co-insurance amounts that are based on BC/BS allowed rates, and the full charge for any uncovered services.

Other Commercial Insurances

Most Americans seeking health insurance from the Health Insurance Marketplace are covered by health insurance sponsored by private insurance companies (e.g., Aetna, BC, BS, CIGNA, Kaiser Permanente, Metropolitan, and Prudential). Private insurance companies operate to make a profit, and therefore have established protocols to reduce healthcare costs. To control how patients receive medical care, private insurance companies have established *managed care organizations* (MCOs).

MANAGED CARE ORGANIZATIONS

MCOs are a type of healthcare organization which contracts with various healthcare providers and medical facilities at a reduced payment schedule for their insurance members. Patient care is coordinated through a diverse network of providers and hospitals. There are different types of managed care plans such as *health maintenance organizations* (HMOs) and *preferred provider organizations* (PPOs) that provide healthcare in return for scheduled payments and that coordinate healthcare through a defined network of primary care providers (PCPs), hospitals, and other providers.

The goal of MCOs is to reduce the cost of delivering quality care to patient members. MCOs negotiate reduced rates with contracted providers; in return, the managed care plan increases the provider's patient care load. Managed care plans also require *referrals* for their patients to be treated with a specialist provider, thus limiting patient access to more expensive care. The *preauthorization* process can further control patient care costs; medical care, testing, and medication therapy is only provided when it is justified to the health insurance plan. It is important that medical assistants be well versed in the various models of managed care to fully understand their effects on healthcare costs (Table 16-2).

TABLE 16-2 Advantages and Disadvantages of Managed Care

ADVANTAGES	DISADVANTAGES
Healthcare costs are usually controlled	Access to specialized care and referrals can be denied or limited
Contracted and agreed-upon fee schedule	Providers' choices in the treatment of patients can focus more on cost effectiveness instead of necessity of treatment
Authorized services are usually paid for	More paperwork may be required
Most preventive medical treatment is covered	Treatment may be delayed because of preauthorization requirements
Patients' out-of-pocket expenses tend to be less than with traditional insurance	Reimbursement historically is less than with traditional insurance

Models of Managed Care Plans

Health Maintenance Organization

The passage of the Health Maintenance Organization Act in 1973 provided for federal aid to health insurance prepayment plans that met certain criteria, this legislation brought about a rapid growth in HMOs. HMOs are state-licensed health plans that are regulated by HMO laws that require them to include preventive care, such as routine physical examinations and other services, as part of their benefits package. The goal of the HMO health insurance plan is to reduce the cost of healthcare. HMO plans typically have the lowest monthly premiums among other health insurance plans, with lower patient financial responsibility. Patients are required to select a *primary care physician* (PCP), a general practitioner who acts as the **gatekeeper** to more specialized care. The insurance plan will not pay for services that are not in their provider network; patients are 100% financially responsible for medical expenses incurred outside the HMO network of providers. For example, patients wanting to visit the dermatologist for eczema must visit their PCPs first; they would be fully financially responsible if they made an appointment with a dermatologist directly. The PCP can either offer the patient a medication therapy or refer them to the specialist.

PCPs receive financial incentives when they reduce the cost of patient care. In the earlier example, prescribing medicine to the patient is more cost effective than referring the patient to the specialist. HMOs always require referrals from the PCP to specialists, for precertification and preauthorization, for hospital admissions, outpatient procedures, and treatments. There are several different types of HMO models.

Independent Physician Association

An independent physician association (IPA) is an independent group of providers and other healthcare professionals who are under contract to provide services to members of different HMOs, in addition to other insurance plans, usually at a fixed fee per patient. The providers in the IPA, who usually have separately owned practices, formally organize a physician association and continue to practice in their own offices. A healthcare provider may be contracted with several IPAs. Payments to providers by an IPA can be structured either as **capitation** or fee-for-service fee schedule.

Staff Model

A staff model HMO hires salaried healthcare providers. Rather than contracting with providers to create a network, the HMO owns the network. Medical care is authorized by the patient's PCP. No capitation or fee-for-service payment structure is used with the staff model; however, the providers may receive bonuses biannually or annually based on the number of patients treated or the cost savings.

Group Model

A group model HMO contracts with a multispecialty medical group to deliver care to its members. The HMO reimburses the providers' group, which is responsible for reimbursing provider members and contracted healthcare facilities. This arrangement is similar to an IPA in that the multispecialty group may organize a physician association; however, the group members typically practice together in one facility. The payment structure to the providers can be either capitation or fee-for-service. Refer to Table 16-3 to compare the different types of HMOs.

CRITICAL THINKING APPLICATION   **16-2**

Stephanie Hudson is a patient who called to make an appointment with the endocrinologist because she was having trouble managing her diabetes. She told Jodie over the phone when she was making the appointment that she has Aetna HMO. Will Jodie be able to schedule Miss Hudson's appointment with the endocrinologist? Why or why not? What would she need to make an appointment?

TABLE 16-3 Health Maintenance Organization Models

MODEL	STRUCTURE	CONTRACT TYPE
IPA	General or family practice provider or provider group that practices independently and may contract with several IPAs	Capitation or fee-for-service
Staff	One or more providers hired by an HMO	Salaried
Group	Multispecialty group with or without a PCP (i.e., gatekeeper); may contract with several IPAs	Capitation or fee-for-service

Preferred Provider Organization

A PPO is a managed care network that contracts with a group of providers; the providers agree on a predetermined list of charges for all services, including those for both normal and complex procedures. The PPO model of managed healthcare preserves the fee-for-service concept that many providers prefer. Typically, the patient's financial responsibilities represent on average 20% to 25% of the allowed charge, but this depends on the patient's health insurance benefits. A provider who joins a PPO does not need to alter the manner of providing care and continues to treat and bill the patients on a fee-for-service basis. When a patient covered under a PPO plan comes for treatment, the provider treats the patient and bills the PPO. Patients do not need to visit their PCP to obtain a referral to a specialist for more specialized care and they have more control over healthcare choices.

PPOs furnish their subscribers with a list of participating providers and healthcare facilities from which they can access in-network healthcare at PPO reduced rates. Rates are quite often lower than those charged to non-PPO patients.

Although patients have the option to visit a specialist when they feel the need, they are still required to obtain preauthorization for referrals for more expensive medical therapy such as formulary medication and some medical testing.

CRITICAL THINKING APPLICATION   **16-3**

Henry Hudson called Jodie; he was upset because he received a patient statement balance. He told Jodie that he has full coverage insurance through his employer and did not know why he had a balance. What information can Jodie share with Henry to explain his financial responsibility?

Exclusive Provider Organization

An EPO combines features of an HMO (e.g., an enrolled group or population, PCPs, and an authorization system) and a PPO (e.g., flexible benefit design and fee-for-service payments). Patients with EPO coverage will not be covered for services outside the designated network of providers (unless there is an emergency), but may not need to obtain a referral for specialized care. EPO plan members are not required to choose a PCP as HMO members are.

Professional Courtesy

Professional courtesy occurs when the health provider decides to reduce or eliminate the patient's financial obligations for healthcare provided. Providers used professional courtesy to eliminate the patient's financial responsibility because they either had a personal relationship with or had made financial arrangements before the service. However, the onset of strict managed care policies and procedures have all but eliminated professional courtesy. Managed care plans want to ensure that patients meet their financial responsibility to prevent fraud and to ensure quality care is delivered. Managed care contractors may request financial records, including patient account balance statements, confirming that healthcare providers are making an effort to collect payments from their patients.

Referrals

Patients seeking specialized care must first visit their assigned PCP to obtain a referral to a specialist or for more specialized therapy or care. Patients with HMO plans can only obtain a referral to the specialist by visiting their assigned PCP. HMOs will measure how many patients are referred to specialists by individual PCPs. Approval or denial of a referral can take anywhere from a few minutes to a few days. The three types of referrals are as follows:

- A *regular referral* usually takes 3 to 10 working days for review and approval. This type of referral is used when the provider believes that the patient must see a specialist to continue treatment.
- An *urgent referral* usually takes about 24 hours for approval. This type of referral is used when an urgent but not life-threatening situation occurs.
- A *STAT referral* can be approved online when it is submitted to the utilization review department through the provider's

Web portal. A STAT referral is used in an emergency situation as indicated by the provider.

A *regular referral* is the most common type and can be inconvenient for the patient. With most managed care plans, preauthorization needs to be obtained for a referral (Procedure 16-3). Remember this cardinal rule: never tell the patient the referral has been approved unless you have a hard copy of the authorization. A referral is authorized after the approval has been received. When a referral is approved the PCP's office and the patient should receive a copy of the authorization. Always review the authorization thoroughly and confirm details such as approved diagnosis and procedure codes and the exact period of time the authorization lasts. The patient will receive a letter with an authorization number and details regarding the approved services. The patient must bring the authorization to the specialist's office on the date of their appointment.

PROCEDURE 16-3   Obtain a Referral with Documentation

Goal: *To obtain a referral from a health plan's provider services desk phone number listed on the back of the patient's health insurance ID card.*

EQUIPMENT and SUPPLIES

- Patient health record
- Preauthorization form (Figure 16-3)
- Patient's insurance identification (ID) card

PROCEDURAL STEPS

1. Assemble the necessary documentation such as the patient ID card, the verification of eligibility, and the online insurance provider Web portal log-in information.
   PURPOSE: To avoid wasting time searching for information needed to perform the task.
2. Examine the patient's health record and determine the service or procedure for which preauthorization is being requested, including, if applicable, the specialist's name and phone number and the reason for the request.
   PURPOSE: To correctly complete the required form for gaining authorization from the patient's insurance carrier for the specified treatment.
3. Fill out the preauthorization form providing all information requested, which may include the following:
   - The patient's demographic and insurance information

- If the patient is a dependent: Information about the guarantor, such as name, date of birth, and gender.
- The provider's identification information, including the National Provider Identifier (NPI) and group ID number(s)
- The diagnosis and planned procedure or treatment, or the name and contact information of the provider to whom the patient is being referred.

NOTE: This can also be completed through the online insurance provider Web portal.

4. Proofread the completed form.
   PURPOSE: To ensure the accuracy of the information.
5. Attach a copy of the preauthorization submission confirmation to the patient's health record. This information should include the following:
   - A letter that preauthorizes the specified treatment
   - An authorization number
   - Confirmation of the specific number of procedures, services, or treatment sessions allowed; authorization for referral of the patient to a specialist

---

Preauthorization for Surgical Procedures

Many insurance companies require preauthorization, usually within 24 hours, if a patient is to be hospitalized or undergo certain medical procedures. Insurance claims for payment will be denied if proper preauthorization is not obtained. Refer to Procedure 16-4 on how to perform a preauthorization for surgery.

All managed care plans, including HMOs, PPOs, and EPOs, require preauthorization for medical services such as surgery,

expensive medical tests, and medication therapy. Preauthorization may be requested by calling the health insurance plan provider desk services number listed on the patient's health insurance ID card and by submitting a completed request for a preauthorization form (Figure 16-3). A preauthorization provides the following information:

- An authorization code, which may be alphabetic, numeric, or alphanumeric

- The date on which the referral request was received by the utilization review department
- The date on which the referral was approved and its expiration date
- The exact time period the authorization is valid.
- Authorized diagnosis and procedural codes
- The name, address, and telephone number of the contracted specialist where the authorized services will be provided
- The comments section: This is the most critical area of a referral because this area designates the services that have been approved.
- The specified number of authorized visits to the specialist
- An authorization may be issued for (1) evaluation only, (2) evaluation and treatment plan, (3) evaluation and biopsy, (4) evaluation and one injection, and so on.

Notes about the authorization process:

- If the authorization expires and services have not been provided, an extension may be requested. **Utilization manage-**

ment will need to extend the expiration date and this will generate a new authorization with a new number. Be sure to update the authorization number for dates of services beyond the original authorization time window.

- If services are provided after the preauthorization's expiration date, the claim will be denied. If this happens, contact utilization management to request approval. Sometimes the patient, the specialist's office, or both must be involved in this process.
- Always ensure that any specialist to whom the provider refers a patient is contracted with the same managed care plan as the PCP.
- The medical assistant should explain to the patient specifically which services were approved.
- The PCP's office and/or the patient are notified if a referral is denied because of insufficient information or lack of medical necessity. When the PCP's office provides the utilization management committee with the necessary information, the referral can be reviewed again (Figure 16-3).

Preauthorization Request Form

TO BE COMPLETED BY PRIMARY CARE PHYSICIAN OR OUTSIDE PROVIDER

☐ Medicare ☑ Blue Cross/Blue Shield ☐ Tricare ☐ Health Net
☐ Medicaid ☐ Aetna ☐ Cigna ☐ Other
Group No.: 54098XX

Name: (First, Middle Initial, Last) Louann Campbell   Date: 7-14-20XX
☐ Male ☑ Female   Birthdate: 4-7-1952   Home Telephone Number: (555) 450-1666
Address: 2516 Encina Avenue, Woodland Hills, XY 12345-0439
Primary Care Physician: Gerald Practon, MD
Referring Physician: Gerald Practon, MD
Referred to: Raymond Skeleton, MD   Office Telephone number: (555) 486-9002
Address: 4567 Broad Avenue, Woodland Hills, XY 12345
Diagnosis Code: M54.5   Diagnosis: Low back pain
Diagnosis Code: M51.27   Diagnosis: Sciatica
Treatment Plan: Orthopedic consultation and evaluation of lumbar spine; R/O herniated disc L4-5
Authorization requested for: ☐ Consult only ☐ Treatment Only ☐ Consult/Treatment
☑ Consult/Procedure/Surgery ☐ Diagnostic Tests
Procedure Code: 99244   Description: New patient consultation
Procedure Code: ___   Description: ___
Place of service: ☑ Office ☐ Outpatient ☑ Inpatient ☐ Other   Number of visits: 1
Facility: ___   Length of stay: ___
List of potential future consultants (i.e., anesthetists, surgical assistants, or medical/surgical):
Physician's Signature: *Gerald Practon, MD*

TO BE COMPLETED BY PRIMARY CARE PHYSICIAN
PCP Recommendations: See above   PCP Initials: *GP*
Date eligibility checked: 7-14-20XX   Effective Date: 1-15-20XX

TO BE COMPLETED BY UTILIZATION MANAGEMENT
Authorized: ___   Auth. No. ___   Not Authorized: ___
Deferred: ___   Modified: ___
Effective Date: ___   Expiration Date: ___

FIGURE 16-3 Preauthorization Request Form.

Utilization Management/Utilization Review

Utilization management is a form of patient care review by healthcare professionals who do not provide the care but are sponsored by health insurance companies. It is a necessary component of managed care to control costs. A *utilization review committee* reviews individual cases to make certain that medical care services are medically necessary (the specificity of diagnosis coding is critical) to ensure that providers are using their resources efficiently. This committee also reviews all provider referrals and cases of emergency department visits and urgent care. For referrals, the committee reviews the referral and either approves or denies it, so it is important to submit accurate documentation. The medical assistant should contact the utilization review department directly; it should never be left to the patient to contact this department.

PROCEDURE 16-4 | **Obtain Preauthorization for a Surgical Procedure with Documentation**

Goal: *To obtain preauthorization from a patient's managed care organization (MCO) for requested services or procedures with documentation.*

EQUIPMENT and SUPPLIES

- Patient health record
- Preauthorization form (Figure 16-3)
- Patient's insurance identification (ID) card

PROCEDURAL STEPS

1. Assemble the necessary information such as the patient ID card, the verification of eligibility, and the health plan's provider services desk phone number listed on the back of the patient's health insurance ID card.
   PURPOSE: To avoid wasting time searching for information needed to perform the task.
2. Examine the patient's health record to determine the procedure for which preauthorization is being requested and assign the appropriate diagnosis and procedural codes for the surgical procedure.
3. Fill out the preauthorization form, providing all information requested, which may include the following:
   - The patient's demographic and insurance information

- If the patient is a dependent: Information about the guarantor, such as name, date of birth, and gender
- The provider's identification information, including the National Provider Identifier (NPI) and group ID number(s)
- The facility, including the NPI number and address

NOTE: This can also be completed through the online insurance provider Web portal.

4. Proofread the completed form.
   PURPOSE: To ensure the accuracy of the information.
5. Attach a copy of the preauthorization submission confirmation to the patient's health record. This information should include the following:
   - A letter that preauthorizes the surgery
   - An authorization number
   - Confirmation of the authorization to schedule the surgery
   PURPOSE: To document in the patient's health record the authorization for the procedure.
6. Call the patient to schedule the surgery.

GOVERNMENT-SPONSORED PLANS

Government-sponsored health insurance plans provide health insurance coverage with reduced or no monthly premiums for the indigent, the elderly, the military, and government employees. There are a variety of different insurance plans, but patients need to qualify either by age, income, government occupation, or health condition. A patient who is age 65 or older can qualify for *Medicare* insurance coverage. A low-income patient may be eligible for *Medicaid*. Dependents of military personnel are covered by *TRICARE*; and surviving spouses and dependent children of veterans who died in the line of duty are covered by the *Civilian Health and Medical Program of the Veterans Administration* (CHAMPVA). Some wage earners are protected against the loss of wages and the cost of medical care resulting from an occupational accident, disease, or disability through *workers' compensation insurance.*

Medicare

Established in 1966, Medicare is a federal health insurance program that provides healthcare coverage for individuals age 65 and older, the disabled, and patients with diagnosed end stage renal disease (ESRD). Today Medicare is the world's largest insurance program. In 2015 there were more than 55 million beneficiaries. The Medicare program was developed by the Healthcare Financing Administration (HCFA) as part of Title XVIII of the Social Security Act. HCFA now is known as the Centers for Medicare and Medicaid Services (CMS), a division of the Department of Health and Human Services (DHHS). Laws enacted by Congress regulate the Medicare program.

The Medicare plan is divided into four parts: Part A, Part B, Part C, and Part D (Table 16-4). Part A is hospital insurance for qualified Medicare participants and is financed with special contributions deducted from employed individuals' salaries, with matching contributions from their employers. These sums are collected, along with regular Social Security contributions, from wages and self-employment income earned during a person's working years, so there is no monthly premium paid. Part B is medical insurance for ambulatory care, including primary care and specialists for which patients are required to pay a monthly premium; Part B functions similar to a PPO in that patients can visit any specialist without a referral. Part C is an option for Medicare-qualified patients to turn their Part A and Part B benefits into a privately sponsored plan that can offer some additional benefits. Part D is a prescription drug program offered to Medicare-qualified individuals that requires an additional monthly premium. Optional Medigap policies pay the deductible and the 20% co-payment for those who choose to pay for the additional coverage.

TABLE 16-4	Comparing Medicare Plans		
	COVERED SERVICES	MONTHLY PREMIUM	DEDUCTIBLE
Part A	Inpatient hospital care, skilled nursing facilities, home healthcare, and hospice services	$0	$1288 deductible for each benefit period; Days 1-60: $0 co-insurance for each benefit period; Days 61-90: $315 co-insurance per day of each benefit period; Day 91 and beyond: $630 co-insurance per each "lifetime reserve day" after day 90 for each benefit period (up to 60 days over a lifetime)
Part B	Outpatient hospital care, durable medical equipment, provider's services, and other medical services	$104.90	$166, plus 20% co-insurance for all medical services
Part C	Expanded inpatient hospital and outpatient hospital care benefits	Varies by plan	Varies by plan
Part D	Prescription drugs	Varies by income	Varies by plan

CRITICAL THINKING APPLICATION   **16-4**

Beatrice Hampton is a Medicare patient who has Part A and Part B coverage. Will Medicare cover her office visit with the endocrinologist? What percent of the bill will she be financially responsible for?

Medicaid

In 1965 the federal government provided for the medically indigent through a program known as Medicaid. Title XIX of Public Law 89 to 97, under the Social Security Amendments of 1965, provided for agreements involving cost sharing between federal and state governments to provide medical care for people meeting specific eligibility criteria. All states and the District of Columbia have Medicaid programs, but these programs vary by state. A person eligible for Medicaid in one state may not be eligible in another state, and covered medical services may differ.

The federal government provides funding to the state for Medicaid programs and the states individually decide whether to provide funds for extension of benefits. The state determines the type and extent of medical benefits that will be covered within the minimum standards established by the federal government; the Affordable Care Act has amended these standards.

A medical office has the right to limit the number of Medicaid patients they accept to their practice for financial reasons. The Medicaid Fee Schedule is the lowest of all insurance companies and it may not be in the medical office's financial interest to accept Medicaid patients. The provider who does accept Medicaid patients automatically agrees to accept Medicaid payments as payment in full for covered services. The patient cannot be billed for the difference between the Medicaid payment and the amount the provider charged. Eligibility for benefits is determined by the respective states, but most Medicaid recipients also are some or all of the following:

- Individuals who are medically needy
- Recipients of Aid to Families with Dependent Children (AFDC)

- Individuals who receive Supplemental Security Income (SSI)
- Individuals who receive certain types of federal and state aid
- Individuals who are **qualified Medicare beneficiaries (QMBs)**—Medicaid pays for Medicare Part B premiums, deductibles, and co-insurance for qualified low-income elderly individuals
- Individuals in institutions or receiving long-term care in nursing facilities and intermediate-care facilities

Government-Sponsored Health Maintenance Organization Plans

In an effort to reduce costs and increase the delivery of care efficiently, many Medicare and Medicaid state programs have provided their members options to join a health maintenance organization (HMO) plan. Medicare or Medicaid may sponsor these patients, but they may have a privately sponsored insurance card. These insurance identification (ID) cards state that they are government sponsored, which means that they may not cover all medical services as privately sponsored insurances do. Medical assistants should be diligent about patient verification to ensure what medical services will be covered and share this information with the patient before services are provided.

Children's Health Insurance Program

Children's Health Insurance Program (CHIP) is a state-funded program for children whose family income is above the Medicaid qualifying income limits. CHIP premiums are typically 5% of the family monthly income. State CHIP programs cover routine checkups, immunizations, doctor visits, prescriptions, dental care, vision care, inpatient and outpatient hospital care, laboratory tests, x-rays, and emergency services. CHIP programs are similar to HMO plans in that care is only covered through the designated network of providers. There are smaller co-payments for medical services for CHIP patients.

TRICARE

After World War II and the Korean War, there were a large number of military veterans who did not have access to effective healthcare during peacetime. To address this problem, Congress passed the Dependents Medical Care Act of 1956 and the Military Medical Benefits Amendments of 1966, which allowed the Secretary of Defense to contract with civilian healthcare providers. This civilian healthcare program became known as the Civilian Health and Medical Program of the Uniformed Services (CHAMPUS) in 1966. The program administering these benefits became CHAMPUS, which today is known as TRICARE. TRICARE is now the comprehensive healthcare program for all seven uniformed services:

the Army, Navy, Marine Corps, Air Force, Coast Guard, Public Health Service, and the National Oceanic and Atmospheric Administration. TRICARE also covers family members of active duty personnel, military retirees and their eligible family members under the age of 65, and the survivors of all uniformed services.

The TRICARE program is managed by the military in partnership with civilian hospitals and clinics. It is designed to expand access to healthcare, ensure high-quality care, and promote medical readiness. All military hospitals and clinics are part of the TRICARE program and offer high-quality healthcare at low cost to plan users. TRICARE offers three types of plans: TRICARE Prime, TRICARE Extra, and TRICARE Standard. Review Table 16-5 for a comparison of the different TRICARE plans.

TABLE 16-5   Comparing TRICARE Plans

ACTIVE FAMILY DUTY MEMBERS			
	TRICARE PRIME	**TRICARE EXTRA**	**TRICARE STANDARD**
Annual deductible	None	$150/individual or $300/family for E-5 & above; $50/$100 for E-4 & below	$150/individual or $300/family for E-5 & above; $50/$100 E-4 & below
Annual enrollment fee	None	None	None
Civilian outpatient visit	No cost	15% of negotiated fee	20% of allowed charges for covered service
Civilian inpatient admission	No cost	Greater of $25 or $13.90 a day	Greater of $25 or $13.90 a day
Civilian inpatient mental health	No cost	$20/day	$20/day
Civilian inpatient skilled nursing facility care	$0 per diem charge per admission; no separate co-payment/cost-share for separately billed professional charges	$11/day ($25 minimum) charge per admission	$11/day ($25 minimum) charge per admission
RETIREES (UNDER 65), THEIR FAMILY MEMBERS, AND OTHERS			
	TRICARE PRIME	**TRICARE EXTRA**	**TRICARE STANDARD**
Annual deductible	None	$150/individual or $300/family	$150/individual or $300/family
Annual enrollment fee	$260/individual or $520/family	None	None
Civilian co-pays		20% of negotiated fee	25% of allowed charges for covered service
Outpatient emergency care mental health visit	$12 $30 $25 $17 (group visit)		
Civilian inpatient cost share	$11/day ($25 minimum) charge per admission	Lesser of $250/day or 25% of negotiated charges plus 20% of negotiated professional fees	Lesser of $512/day or 25% of billed charges plus 25% of allowed professional fees
Civilian inpatient skilled nursing facility care	$11/day ($25 minimum) charge per admission	$250 per diem co-payment or 20% cost-share of total charges for institutional care, whichever is less, plus 20% cost-share of separately billed professional charges	25% cost-share of allowed charges for institutional services plus 25% cost-share of allowable separately billed professional charges

Civilian Health and Medical Program of the Veterans Administration

CHAMPVA, a health benefits program similar to TRICARE, was established in 1973 for the spouses and dependent children of veterans suffering total, permanent, service-connected disabilities and for surviving spouses and dependent children of veterans who died as a result of service-related disabilities. The Department of Veterans Affairs (VA) shares with eligible beneficiaries the cost of certain healthcare services and supplies.

Workers' Compensation

Workers' compensation is an insurance plan for individuals who are injured on the job either by accident or an acquired illness. An example of an acquired illness would be mesothelioma from inhaling asbestos while on the job. The insurance plan covers all healthcare expenses related to the injury or illness and also includes monetary compensation for loss of income. Compensation benefits include medical care and rehabilitation benefits, weekly income replacement benefits for temporary disability, permanent disability settlements, and survivor benefits when applicable. The provider accepts the workers' compensation reimbursements as payment in full and does not bill the patient. Time limitations are set for the prompt reporting of workers' compensation cases. The employee is obligated to promptly notify the employer; the employer, in turn, must notify the insurance company and must refer the employee to a source of medical care.

State legislatures in all 50 states have passed workers' compensation laws to protect workers against the loss of wages and the cost of medical care resulting from an occupational accident or disease, as long as the employee was not proven negligent. State laws differ as to the classes of employees included and the benefits provided by workers' compensation insurance. Federal and state legislatures require employers to maintain workers' compensation coverage to meet minimum standards, covering a majority of employees, for work-related illnesses and injuries. The purpose of workers' compensation laws is to provide prompt medical care to an injured or ill worker so that the person may be restored to health and return to full earning capacity in as short a time as possible.

EMPLOYER-ESTABLISHED SELF-FUNDED PLANS

Many large companies or organizations have enough employees that they can fund their own insurance program. This is called a *self-funded plan*. Technically, a self-funded plan is not insurance by true definition. The employer pays employee healthcare costs from the funds collected from employee monthly premiums. Usually the costs of benefits and premiums for self-funded plans are similar to those for group plans. Self-funded plans tend to work best for companies that are large enough to offer good benefit coverage and reasonable premium rates and are able to pay large claims for expensive medical services. Often a **third-party administrator (TPA)** handles paperwork and claim payments for a self-insured group.

Self-funded healthcare is an arrangement in which an employer provides health or disability benefits to employees with its own funds.

This is different from fully insured plans, in which the employer contracts an insurance company to cover the employees and dependents. In self-funded healthcare, the employer assumes the direct risk for payment of the claims for benefits. The terms of eligibility and coverage are set forth in the insurance plan document, which includes provisions similar to those found in a typical group health insurance policy.

CLOSING COMMENTS

Health insurance and benefits coverage can be confusing to the patient, so medical assistants should educate themselves on the specific details of all plans accepted at the healthcare facility. The Affordable Care Act allows health insurance to be accessible to more Americans than any other time in history, so the demands on the current healthcare system will greatly increase over the next few years. Managed care has often been criticized in the media for its cost-saving practices; however, extra efforts made by medical assistants to overcome these challenges and educate their patients on how to use their health insurance plans will improve the quality of care delivered to their patients. Providers and healthcare facilities need to evaluate their ability to accept the fee schedule of insurance plans they are contracted with, especially since Medicaid's fee schedule is the lowest in the industry.

Patient Education

It is important for patients to understand how their insurance works. Many people, especially elderly individuals, believe that if they have health insurance, all charges for their healthcare will be covered. The responsibilities of a medical assistant include keeping the patient informed of his or her financial responsibilities and answering questions about their benefits and exclusions. Often healthcare facilities provide their patients with informational brochures that explain how health insurance and reimbursement work and provide definitions of some of the more common terms used in the insurance claims process. If patients are well advised and comfortable with insurance facts before treatment begins, the medical experience will go more smoothly, and collection of their financial responsibilities will be easier. The medical assistant must practice good communication skills, patience, and tact when discussing reimbursement and financial responsibilities issues with patients.

Legal and Ethical Issues

Verification of eligibility is a process that is important not only to ensure the insurance plan is valid at the time of service, but to ensure patient identity. Falsifying one's identity to use someone else's health insurance benefits is a common fraudulent practice. The only way to prevent this type of health insurance fraud is to diligently verify all patients when they schedule appointments with the healthcare facility. A state issued ID should be presented with the patient's health insurance ID to verify identity. If the medical assistant suspects fraud, he or she should report it to the health insurance plan immediately and the patient should be informed that they cannot be seen by the medical professional until issues relating to the health insurance are resolved.

Professional Behaviors

Patients can be confused or angered when insurance companies deny authorization of services or referrals. Although these decisions are made by insurance companies, many times the blame is put on the medical front office assistants. In situations like these, it is important for medical assistants to stay calm and listen to the patient's concerns. In most cases, the patient will come to realize that there is nothing the medical assistant can do, but the patient may need to express frustration. Once the patient has calmed down, the medical assistant can then recommend options such as paying cash, making payment arrangements, or bringing attention to the patient's insurance member services hotline. Compassionately assure patients that their health is most important and that you will do what you can so they can receive the appropriate medical treatment.

If the patient continues to escalate the situation and/or becomes belligerent, excuse yourself from the discussion and ask either an office manager or another medical assistant to step in. A medical assistant should never return anger and/or frustration to the patient. Remember, the patient may be mentally compromised and frustrated from extensive health care problems, so don't exacerbate the situation by releasing your own anger. If the patient's health is made the primary concern, the healthcare facility can work with the insurance company so the patient can receive appropriate medical care.

SUMMARY OF SCENARIO

Although she initially was nervous about explaining fees to patients and asking for payment, Jodie has become more comfortable in doing this aspect of her job because she understands the business aspect of the practice. The provider is operating the practice to make a profit and support his family, and the practice also is a source of support for the employees' families. Patients understand that providers must charge for their services, and have become accustomed to co-payments and co-insurance amounts. Many times, these fees are collected in advance, before the patient sees Dr. Crawford. This practice saves time on checkout, and most patients believe that the co-pay is a small cost compared with the entire fee that providers charge to manage their care in one office visit.

Jodie has noticed that the usual, customary, and reasonable fees that Dr. Crawford charges his patients directly affect the reimbursements that are paid by various insurance and managed care companies. Jodie has attended several health insurance billing seminars sponsored by Medicare and Blue Cross/Blue Shield and has noticed a drop in health insurance claim rejections. Dr. Crawford commented that he uses professional courtesy much less frequently than in the past because of the many rules and regulations placed on providers by managed care companies. He still offers the occasional patient a professional discount when it does not violate the managed care contract that he holds with the insurer or managed care company.

SUMMARY OF LEARNING OBJECTIVES

1. **Define, spell, and pronounce the terms listed in the vocabulary.**
   Spelling and pronouncing medical terms correctly bolster the medical assistant's credibility. Knowing the definitions of these terms promotes confidence in communication with patients and co-workers.
2. **Discuss the purpose of health insurance and explain the health insurance contract between the patient and the health plan.**
   Health insurance is a third-party payer system that reimburses a healthcare provider when services are rendered for an insured patient. A monthly premium is paid for a list of health insurance benefits detailed in the contract. The patient then provides evidence of the health insurance contract to the healthcare provider. The provider then submits a claim to the health insurance company for services rendered. The third party then reimburses the healthcare provider.

   Health insurance is a contract between a guarantor and a third-party payer. The guarantor agrees to pay a monthly premium to the health insurance company for health services coverage. When the guarantor or any of their dependents seeks health services, the health insurance will pay for all medically necessary services on the guarantor's behalf as detailed in the health insurance contract.
3. **Identify types of third-party plans.**
   There are two types of health insurance plans in the United States: privately sponsored health insurance plans and government-sponsored health insurance plans. Health insurance plans typically cover health services and procedures that are deemed medically necessary, or health services that are required to improve the patient's current health condi-

tion. Most insurance policies do not cover elective procedures, or medical procedures that will not improve the patient's current health, such as a facelift. Most of today's health insurance policies cover preventive care, which includes services provided to help prevent certain illnesses or that lead to an early diagnosis.
4. **Discuss the Affordable Care Act's effect on patient healthcare access.**
   In 2010, the Patient Protection and Affordable Care Act was enacted, which is also known as the *Affordable Care Act* or Obamacare. It increased the quality, availability, and affordability of private and public health insurance for more than 44 million uninsured Americans. The legislation includes new qualifying regulations, taxes, mandates, and subsidies. The federal mandate not only opens opportunities for more Americans to obtain affordable health insurance, but also works to reduce overall healthcare spending in the long run.
5. **Summarize the different health insurance benefits available and interpret information on a health insurance identification (ID) card.**
   Insurance packages are often tailored to the needs of each individual or group, and the ways to combine benefits are limitless. Health insurance policies normally contain a combination of the different benefits, such as surgical, medical, hospitalization, and major medical.

   As proof of health insurance coverage, patients are issued a health insurance ID card with the health plan name, patient's name, subscriber ID, and health plan contact information (Figure 16-1). Refer to Procedure 16-1 on how to interpret information on the health insurance ID card.

SUMMARY OF LEARNING OBJECTIVES—*continued*

6. **Explain the importance of verifying eligibility and be able to verify eligibility of services, including documentation.**

It is important to verify insurance benefits before providing services to patients. Verifying benefits is necessary to ensure that the patient is covered by insurance and to determine what benefits will be paid for routine and special procedures and services. Verification protects the provider and the patient against unexpected medical care costs.

Many problems for both the patient and the medical office can be prevented if the medical assistant develops and follows a procedure for verifying insurance benefits before services are rendered. This procedure includes gathering as much information as possible about the demographics of the patient and his or her insurance coverage. A pragmatic and tactful discussion with all new patients to explain the facility's established policy on insurance claims processing and the collection of fees not covered by the patient's policy will pay off. Refer to Procedure 16-2 on how to verify eligibility with documentation.

7. **Explain the health insurance contract between the healthcare provider and the health insurance company.**

In the United States payment for services is typically after the health services are rendered. In other words, healthcare providers are paid weeks, sometimes months, after medical services have been provided to the patient. Once the service is provided to the patient, the healthcare provider must submit a health insurance claim, which includes the diagnosis, the procedure, and total charges. Although the healthcare provider establishes their own fee schedule, or list of charges associated with various medical services provided, health insurance plans maintain their own rates at which they reimburse.

8. **Explain how insurance reimbursements are determined and discuss the effect health insurance has on provider reimbursements.**

Benefits are determined and paid in one of several ways: indemnity schedules; service benefit plans; usual, customary, and reasonable (UCR) fees; and the resource-based relative value scale (RBRVS). Medical assistants should become familiar with each of these methods and be able to differentiate the types of schedules, fees, and scales to determine which insurance payer uses them and how they affect reimbursement to the provider.

Healthcare providers have three commodities to sell: time, judgment (i.e., expertise), and services. In every case healthcare providers must place an estimate on the value of these services. However, in recent years health insurance plans, particularly government and managed healthcare organizations, have greatly influenced what healthcare providers can charge by establishing the allowable charge. The allowable amount is the maximum that third-party payers will pay for a particular procedure or service.

9. **Summarize privately sponsored health insurance plans.**

Privately sponsored health insurance plans, also known as commercial insurance plans, are for-profit organizations. As such, health insurance companies make annual changes to the participating provider contract to negotiate lower payments. Most privately sponsored plans use managed care to reduce the costs of delivering quality healthcare.

10. **Differentiate among the different types of managed care models.**

Managed care is a broad term used to describe a variety of healthcare plans developed to provide healthcare services at lower costs. It is important for the medical assistant to be familiar with various plan types such as the health maintenance organization (HMO), preferred provider organization (PPO), and exclusive provider organization (EPO) and to understand the policies of each one.

11. **Outline managed care requirements for patient referral and obtain a referral with documentation.**

Obtaining preauthorization for making referrals must be done according to the guidelines of the individual insurance companies. If the medical assistant is uncertain about the procedure, he or she should always refer to the insurance plan's policies and procedures manual.

The medical assistant should refer to the insurance plan's policies and procedures to accurately obtain preauthorization for a referral. Refer to Procedure 16-3 on how to obtain a referral with documentation.

12. **Describe the process for preauthorization and how to obtain preauthorization with documentation.**

Managed care plans, including HMOs, PPOs, and EPOs, require preauthorization for medical services such as surgery, expensive medical tests, and medication therapy. Preauthorization may be requested by calling the health insurance plan, which should be documented in the patient's electronic health record (EHR).

Many insurance companies require preauthorization, usually within 24 hours, if a patient is to be hospitalized or undergo certain medical procedures. Insurance claims for payment will be denied if proper preauthorization is not obtained. Refer to Procedure 16-4 on how to perform a preauthorization for surgery.

13. **List and discuss various government-sponsored plans.**

Government-sponsored health insurance programs include Medicare, Medicaid, TRICARE, CHAMPVA, CHIPS, and worker's compensation. The elderly, disabled, military, indigent, and those injured at work may qualify for one of these programs. Because these programs are sponsored by the government, participating providers (PARs) must accept a lower fee schedule for reimbursements.

14. **Review employer-established self-funded plans.**

Self-funded healthcare or self-insurance is an arrangement in which an employer provides health or disability benefits to employees with its own funds. This is different from fully insured plans, in which the employer contracts with an insurance company to cover the employees and dependents. In self-funded healthcare, the employer assumes the direct risk for payment of the claims for benefits.

CONNECTIONS

📖 Study Guide Connection: Go to Chapter 16 Study Guide. Read the Case Study and Workplace Applications and complete the assignments. Do online research for answers to the questions in the Internet Activities associated with the basics of health insurance.

*e*volve Evolve Connection: Go to the Chapter 16 link at *evolve.elsevier.com/ kinn* to complete the Chapter Review Quiz. Check out the other resources listed for this chapter to make the most of what you have learned from Basics of Health Insurance.

17

MEDICAL BILLING AND REIMBURSEMENT

The instructor in Ann Snyder's administrative medical assistant class, Grant Wilson, knows that working with health insurance can be quite rewarding. Mr. Wilson works with Ann and her classmates, answering their questions and helping them to see that medical insurance is not as complicated as it may seem.

A medical assistant who is detailed oriented enjoys billing and coding activities. The individual who performs these duties in the provider's office is a critical staff member because tasks related to billing have a significant effect on the provider's income. That income is used to pay the clinic's expenses,

including payroll, so the facility staff indirectly counts on accurate and timely billing. Medical assistants who continually develop their coding skills are assets to the practice and can look forward to a long and rewarding career.

Mr. Wilson is sure to show the students several different Explanation of Benefits (EOBs) from a variety of insurance companies so that the students can learn how the reimbursement process works for a variety of health insurance plans. Ann will learn about the importance of verifying patient billing information and the steps for obtaining precertification for medical procedures; she also will learn how to discuss the patient's billing record professionally.

While studying this chapter, think about the following questions:

- Why is it important for Ann to obtain accurate patient billing information?
- Why is it important to verify insurance eligibility and process precertification before the patient receives medical services?
- How can Ann complete a CMS-1500 Health Insurance Claim Form?

- Will Ann be able to read an EOB to determine the patient's financial responsibility?
- How can Ann successfully inform patients of the financial responsibilities they face as a result of third-party requirements?

LEARNING OBJECTIVES

1. Define, spell, and pronounce the terms listed in the vocabulary.
2. Identify steps for filing a third-party claim
3. Identify the types of information contained in the patient's billing record.
4. Apply managed care policies and procedures, describe processes for precertification, and obtain precertification, including documentation.
5. Explain how to submit health insurance claims, including electronic claims, to various third-party payers.
6. Review the guidelines for completing the CMS-1500 Health Insurance Claim Form, and complete an insurance claim form.
7. Differentiate between fraud and abuse.
8. Discuss the effects of upcoding and downcoding.

9. Discuss methods of preventing the rejection of claims, and display tactful behavior when speaking with medical providers about third-party requirements.
10. Describe ways of checking a claim's status.
11. Review and read an Explanation of Benefits.
12. Discuss reasons for denied claims.
13. Define "medical necessity" as it applies to diagnostic and procedural coding; also, apply medical necessity guidelines.
14. Explain a patient's financial obligations for services rendered, and inform a patient of these obligations.
15. Show sensitivity when speaking with patients about third-party requirements.

VOCABULARY

audit A process done before claims submission to examine claims for accuracy and completeness.

capitation agreement A contract between a provider and an insurance company in which the health plan pays a monthly fee per patient, while the provider accepts the patient's copay as payment in full for office visits.

claims clearinghouse An intermediary that accepts the electronic claim from the provider, reformats the claim to the

specifications outlined by the insurance plan, and submits the claim.

CMS-1500 Health Insurance Claim Form (CMS-1500) Form used by most health insurance payers for claims submitted by providers and suppliers.

coinsurance A policy provision in which the policyholder and the insurance company share the cost of covered medical services in a specified ratio.

copayment A patient financial responsibility, which is due at the time of the office visit.

deductible A patient financial responsibility that the subscriber for the policy is contracted per year to pay toward his or her health care before the insurance policy reimburses the provider.

downcoding When a lower specificity level, or more generalized code, is assigned.

explanation of benefits (EOB) A form that is sent by the insurance company to the provider who submitted the insurance claim, which accompanies a check or a document indicating that funds were electronically transferred.

intentional Determining whether fraudulent medical billing practices were done with purpose or by accident.

medical necessity A health insurance carrier's decision that the CPT and HCPCS codes (services or supplies) used to treat the patient's diagnosis (indicated by the ICD code) meet the accepted standard of medical practice.

National Provider Identifier An identifier assigned by the Centers for Medicare and Medicaid Services (CMS) that classifies the healthcare provider by license and medical specialties.

participating provider A healthcare provider who has signed a contract with a health insurance plan to accept lower reimbursements for services in return for patient referrals.

precertification The process of obtaining the dollar amount approved for a medical procedure or service before the procedure or service is scheduled.

release of information A form completed by the patient that authorizes the medical office to release medical records to the insurance company for health insurance reimbursement.

remark codes The area on the EOB where the payer indicates the conditions under which the claim was paid or denied.

upcoding When the provider may be inclined to code to a higher specificity level than the service provided actually involved.

Medical billing and reimbursement represent the financial lifeline of the healthcare facility. Collecting accurate patient health insurance information is essential to submit accurate health insurance claims. Each health insurance company has its own claims submission policies and procedures for timely reimbursement. A successful medical assistant in insurance billing learns the various insurance company requirements and submits accurate claims. Many health insurance companies have setup online provider webportals, and this has made the process of checking the status of a claim quick and easy. The medical assistant also needs to interpret the **explanation of benefits (EOB)** to determine the patient's **coinsurance** and/or **deductible**. Clear communication with the patient about his or her financial responsibilities takes patience and sensitivity.

STEPS IN MEDICAL BILLING

Medical billing tasks begin when the patient seeks medical services from the provider, usually when an appointment is made. If you plan to work in this area in the healthcare facility, you typically would follow these steps in performing insurance billing tasks.

- Collect patient information when the patient calls to schedule an appointment. This includes information about the insured, his or her employer, demographic information, and health insurance data. When the patient arrives for the appointment, you should inform the patient of his or her **copayment** responsibility and collect it before medical services are provided.
- At the time of the appointment, make a copy or scan of both sides of the patient's insurance card and also of a government-issued picture ID.
- Verify the patient's eligibility, confirming that the patient's contract with the insurance company is valid for the date of service. Patient eligibility can be confirmed by calling the provider services desk phone number on the back of the health insurance ID card, or by using the provider Web portal sponsored by the patient's health insurance company. Review patient benefits and exclusions for certain medical procedures and services.

- If **precertification** is needed, contact the health insurance company's representative to request it.
- After services have been rendered to the patient, code the diagnosis and procedures and review the encounter form/superbill for completeness. The charges for the procedure or procedures should be provided automatically by the medical billing software.
- Complete the **CMS-1500 Health Insurance Claim Form (CMS-1500)** (see Figure 17-8) or an electronic claim form. Submit the form to the insurance company or **data clearinghouse**.
- Review the electronic claims submission report to ensure that the claim was submitted accurately. Correct any discrepancies through the claims clearinghouse and resubmit denied claims.
- Meet the timely filing requirements of each of the different health insurance carriers. Health insurance companies do not pay claims submitted after the established filing period, and this balance cannot be billed to the patient.
- Post payments in the patient's account using the EOB to identify the line items that were paid, reduced, or denied. Patient account statements for their financial responsibility should be mailed out. Health insurance claims for patient accounts with secondary insurance should be submitted.
- Each payment for a procedure line item must be posted correctly in the patient's account. Patient accounts should reflect that the amount above the contracted allowed amount needs to be adjusted per line item.

CRITICAL THINKING APPLICATION   **17-1**

The medical billing manager informs Ann that she has noticed an increase in the number of insurance claim rejections that state the patient cannot be identified. Which step of the medical billing process might be addressed to resolve this problem?

TYPES OF INFORMATION FOUND IN THE PATIENT'S BILLING RECORD

The claim submission process begins after the patient receives services from the provider. When the first appointment is made for a patient, it is routine to ask the patient for all pertinent insurance billing information. Much of this information is collected on the patient registration/intake form, which is completed when the patient comes to the medical office for the initial visit (Figure 17-1). This information should always be collected from every new patient seen by the provider. Returning or established patients should be asked before every visit whether any changes have been made to their health insurance plan and whether their insurance information is complete and up-to-date.

Obtaining accurate patient information for submitting a health insurance claim is important, but a medical release of information form, signed by the patient, also should be kept in the person's health record. The release form allows the authorized release of medical information to the health care insurer. Even though the patient expects the insurance form to be filled out and submitted for

---

Patient Registration Form

PATIENT INFORMATION (Please print clearly)   Social Security# 123-45-6789

Please check one: ☐ Married   ☑ Single   ☐ Divorced   ☐ Separated   ☐ Widowed

Patient's Full Name _____ Rose Dawson _____ Age 81 DOB 02/17/XX Sex F

Address 123 Titanic Place

City New York   State NY   Zipcode 10001

Home Phone (212) 545-1212   Driver's License # N/A

Occupation Retired

Patient's Employer None   Phone Number

Address

City _____ State _____ Zipcode

Spouse None   Social Security #

Address

City _____ State _____ Zipcode

Occupation   Driver's License Number

Family Physician Robert Wilson, MD   Referred by

In case of emergency, contact Marie Dawson   Relationship daughter

Address 123 Titanic Place

City New York   State NY   Zipcode 10001

INSURANCE INFORMATION

Primary Coverage, Name of Carrier: Medicare

   Identification # 123-45-6789A

   Group #

   Subscriber   Rose Dawson

   Effective Date 2/17/20XX

Secondary Coverage Name of Carrier: AARP Secondary Policy

   Identification # 123-45-6789A

   Group #

   Subscriber   Rose Dawson

   Effective Date 2/17/20XX

PAYMENT AUTHORIZATION

Although covered by insurance, I am aware that I am personally responsible for all charges. An electronic copy of this authorization will be as valid as the original.

Rose Dawson

Signature of Patient   12/15/20XX

     Date

FIGURE 17-1 Completed patient registration/intake form.

payment, this cannot be done without a signature in the patient's health record granting permission.

MANAGED CARE POLICIES AND PROCEDURES

Medical billers should familiarize themselves with procedures commonly used by managed care organization (MCO) health plans, such as precertification. Medical assistants must keep in mind that services provided to patients who are sponsored by an MCO plan may not be reimbursed if the policies and procedures specific to the insurance plan are not followed. For example, pain management services typically require a preauthorization. If a pain management facility were to provide these services to the patient without preauthorization, the MCO would deny all insurance claims. To submit accurate health insurance claims, medical assistants should establish office procedures for applying MCO policies and procedures (Procedure 17-1). To find out more about training offered by MCOs for medical billing purposes, review the following box.

Health Plan–Sponsored Training in Medical Billing

Some major health plans offer annual training in newly implemented medical billing policies and procedures. These sessions usually are held in a metropolitan area, and training can range from 1 day to a week of informative seminars. Although these training sessions can be expensive, the knowledge gained from them ensures that the most accurate health insurance claims are submitted for reimbursement. The experts conducting the seminars also can answer questions about specific medical billing situations, which can prove valuable for future claims submissions. Medical billers should visit the insurance company's website to see whether any training sessions are scheduled that they can attend. It is wise for an office representative to attend a workshop at least once a year for most of the insurance companies to which the practice submits claims.

PROCEDURE 17-1	Show Sensitivity When Communicating With Patients Regarding Third-Party Requirements

Goal: *To demonstrate sensitivity through verbal and nonverbal communication when discussing third-party requirements with patients.*

Scenario: *Ken Thomas saw Jean Burke N.P. for his asthma today. He was prescribed a fluticasone inhaler 220 mcg and a refill on his Albuterol inhaler. When Ken stops at the check-out desk, to make a follow-up appointment, he looks concerned. You inquire how you can help him and he states that he is wondering if his new insurance will pick up the fluticasone inhaler. He further explains that he has used it in the past with great results, but he recently switched insurance plans and he is finding it doesn't have the same coverage as his old plan.*

Role play #1: You call the insurance company and discuss the coverage with the insurance carrier's representative. The representative tells you that the fluticasone inhaler is not covered. The representative gave you names of two other inhalers that would be covered.

Role play #2: You must explain to Ken, who is upset with his insurance coverage, that he would have to cover the $250 inhaler.

EQUIPMENT and SUPPLIES

- Copy of patient's health insurance ID card
- Prescription for new medication

PROCEDURAL STEPS

1. Gather a copy of the patient's health insurance ID card and the prescription for the new medication.
   PURPOSE: Having the required documents will help you to be more efficient as you perform the task.
2. Review the insurance card for coverage information and the phone number for providers.
   PURPOSE: You will need the phone number from the ID card to call the insurance carrier. You will also need to provide the insurance representative the patient's information.
3. Call (use role play #1) the insurance company and clearly state the patient's information, the patient's question, and the new medication.

PURPOSE: The insurance representative will need the patient's information and the question to assist you. Speaking clearly as you provide the information will help the listener understand what you are asking.

4. Demonstrate professionalism through verbal communication skills, by stating a respectful, clear, organized message while pronouncing medical terminology and medications correctly.
5. Explain to the patient (use role play #2) the message from the insurance representative using language that can be understood by the patient.
   PURPOSE: For the patient to understand your message, you need to use language that he can understand.
6. Demonstrate sensitivity to the patient by paying attention to and responding appropriately to the patient's nonverbal body language and verbal message.
   PURPOSE: Demonstrating sensitivity can come from verbal messages and body language. Paying attention to the patient and responding appropriately to the patient's message and nonverbal communication is important.

PROCEDURE 17-1 —*continued*

---

7. Demonstrate sensitivity to the patient by showing empathy and clarifying that you understand what the patient is stating. Give the patient your full attention during the conversation and reserve judgment.

8. Demonstrate sensitivity to the patient by using a pleasant, courteous tone of voice. Use body language to communicate respect (e.g., eye contact if culturally appropriate, keep arms uncrossed and relaxed).
   PURPOSE: As the person's frustration and anger increase, it is important to use a pleasant, courteous, and normal tone of voice. Keeping your body

appearance relaxed (e.g., arms uncrossed, hands relaxed) will help to show the patient you are calm.

9. Provide the patient with options if appropriate.
   PURPOSE: Providing the patient with choices also shows the patient that you care.

Precertification

In an effort to control costs, many MCOs require precertification for specialized medical services. Precertification is the process of obtaining the dollar amount approved for a medical procedure or service before the procedure or service is scheduled. To obtain precertification, the medical assistant typically calls the provider services desk phone number on the back of the patient's health insurance ID card. Precertification does not guarantee payment of services after submission of the health insurance claim; however, the process ensures that both the healthcare provider and the patient are informed of the amount that will be reimbursed and the amount the patient will have to pay.

The policies and procedures for each individual health plan determine whether precertification is required before a procedure is scheduled. Almost every health maintenance organization (HMO) insurance plan requires precertification, but medical assistants must confirm the requirement by contacting provider services. Successful medical billers are diligent in obtaining precertification.

The precertification process (Procedure 17-2) is very similar to the preauthorization process in that the health insurance plan is contacted after the primary care provider (PCP) recommends the specialized medical procedure or service. In fact, many health insurance companies use the terms precertification and preauthorization interchangeably. However, precertification specifically determines the dollar amount approved for the medical procedure, whereas preauthorization gives the provider approval to render the medical service.

Using a Health Insurance Company's Online Web Portal to Apply for Precertification

Typically in modern healthcare facilities, the medical assistant can request precertification online through the health insurance company's online Web portal. Consider this case, which is laid out in stepwise fashion to make it easier for you to follow the events:

1. Dr. Thomas Shea is the primary care provider (PCP) for Mary Tolbert, who has heartburn that has not improved with medication.

2. Because Ms. Tolbert's condition is not improving, Dr. Shea requests preauthorization for her to see Dr. Eduard Hamilton, a gastrointestinal (GI) specialist. Ms. Tolbert is insured by a health management organization (HMO).

3. The HMO plan authorizes Ms. Tolbert to see Dr. Hamilton; this authorization is sent to Ms. Tolbert, Dr. Shea, and Dr. Hamilton. When Ms. Tolbert receives the authorization, she schedules an appointment with Dr. Hamilton.

4. After evaluating Ms. Tolbert, Dr. Hamilton orders a colonoscopy. However, Ms. Tolbert is concerned about her financial responsibility. Therefore, Dr. Hamilton's office requests precertification for the colonoscopy on Ms. Tolbert's behalf.

5. The HMO plan notifies Dr. Hamilton that the plan would reimburse a total of $1,500, and Ms. Tolbert would be financially responsible for $400. The precertification is sent both to Dr. Hamilton and Ms. Tolbert, who agree to its financial terms and schedule the procedure.

PROCEDURE 17-2   **Perform Precertification with Documentation**

Goal: *To obtain precertification from a patient's insurance carrier for requested services or procedures.*

EQUIPMENT and SUPPLIES

- Paper method: Patient's health record, Prior Authorization (Precertification) Request form, copy of patient's health insurance ID card, a pen
- Electronic method: SimChart for the Medical Office (SCMO)

PROCEDURAL STEPS

1. For the paper method, gather the health record, precertification/prior authorization request form, copy of the health insurance ID card, and a pen. For the electronic method, access the Simulation Playground in SCMO.

PROCEDURE 17-2 —continued

2. Using the health record, determine the service or procedure that requires precertification/preauthorization.

3. For the paper method, complete the Precertification/Prior Authorization Request form using a pen. For the electronic method, click on the Form Repository icon in SCMO. Select Prior Authorization Request from the left INFO PANEL. Use the Patient Search button at the bottom to find the patient. Complete the remaining fields of the form.
PURPOSE: This provides information on the ordered procedure or service to the insurance carrier, who will then notify the provider's representative if it will be covered under the plan.

4. Proofread the completed form and make any revisions needed.
PURPOSE: To ensure the accuracy of the information.

5. Paper method: File the document in the health record after it is faxed to the insurance carrier. Electronic method: Print and fax or electronically send the form to the insurance carrier and save the form to the patient's record.
PURPOSE: Copies of all forms completed for the patient need to be maintained in the health record.

SUBMITTING CLAIMS TO DIFFERENT THIRD-PARTY PAYERS

All health insurance companies accept the CMS-1500 as the standard for submitting professional and technical claims for a variety of healthcare facilities. However, each health insurance plan has its own policies and procedures for the submission of claims.

Visit Medicare and Medicaid administrator websites for specific guidelines on submitting accurate claims in the provider's state. The MCO-sponsored insurance plans associated with **capitation agreements** have specific guidelines on the types of medical services that are billable. Privately sponsored health insurance plans have their own policies and procedures for submitting claims, and the medical assistant should research those of the health plans commonly seen in the practice.

The medical assistant can successfully manage the requirements of the different insurance plans by keeping a medical billing manual. The manual should contain the billing policies and procedures for most common third-party payers for the healthcare facility. The individual in charge of the manual should make sure that every medical biller has a copy and that the policies and procedures are up-to-date. For example, the date for Medicare's annual billing procedures and policies is October 1. Whenver an update is released, the medical billing manual also should be updated.

GENERATING ELECTRONIC CLAIMS

Since 2006 Medicare has required that all health insurance claims be sent electronically, and most health insurance plans have followed the same practice. If more than 90% of health insurance claims are submitted electronically, why is it important to learn the different fields of the CMS-1500 paper form? Electronic claims are submitted as a collection of data, and the data fields are identical to those on the CMS-1500. Therefore, a medical assistant who is familiar with a paper CMS-1500 will have no problem collecting data for an electronic health insurance claim.

Electronic claims are insurance claims that are transmitted over the Internet from the provider to the health insurance company through *electronic data interchange*. Electronic data interchange is the electronic transfer of data between two or more entities. When submitting electronic health insurance claims, a healthcare facility transmits the data for the claim, and the health insurance company accepts it. A *transmitter ID,* which is found on the patient's health insurance ID card, is needed to identify the specific health plan to which the claim should be submitted. Most medical billing software is designed to generate electronic claims.

Just as for paper claims, when electronic claims are submitted, accurate data are essential. When the medical assistant reviews the claim for accuracy, the claim is prepared for submission.

Electronic Claims Submission

Electronic claims are submitted in the HIPAA 5010 format and can be transmitted directly to the insurance carrier or to a claims clearinghouse.

Direct Billing

Direct billing is the process by which an insurance carrier allows a provider to submit insurance claims directly to the carrier electronically. Most major insurance carriers, including Medicare and Medicaid, provide software packages to providers that are used to enter patient and insured information, charges, and provider details. Many carrier-direct systems are supplied free of charge to the provider, but the direct system can transmit only to specific carriers. A transmitter ID is not needed when electronic claims are submitted through direct billing.

Clearinghouse Submissions

A claims clearinghouse is a healthcare entity that acts as an intermediary between the healthcare facility and the health insurance company. The clearinghouse accepts electronically submitted claims from healthcare agencies, **audits** the claims for completeness, and reformats them to meet the insurance companies' specifications. The claims are sorted by insurance plans and then sent in batches electronically to the appropriate insurance carriers. The insurance companies then send a report through the data clearinghouse to confirm the receipt of claims, claim status on previously submitted claims, and claim payment notification. A clearinghouse charges the healthcare facility a small fee for the service of sending and receiving claims transmissions, checking and preparing the claims for processing, consolidating claims so that one transmission can be sent to each carrier, and submitting claims in correct data format to the appropriate insurance payer. A typical fee is 25¢ per submitted claim. Other services that clearinghouses typically provide include:

- Reporting the number of claims submitted, and the number of errors and their specifics
- Forwarding claims to insurance carriers that accept electronic claims (e.g., Medicare, Medicaid, Blue Cross/Blue Shield, and others) or to another clearinghouse that may hold the contracts with specific payers
- Keeping provider offices updated as new carriers are added to the database
- Generating informative statistical reports

Medical Documentation with Electronic Claims

The electronic submission process sends only health insurance claim information; no other medical documentation can be sent at this time. If a health insurance company requires additional documentation, it notifies the medical office to provide specific documentation. Reimbursement is suspended until the documentation has been received and reviewed by the health insurance plan. Medical assistants should look through mail for documentation requests from insurance companies to facilitate faster reimbursements.

COMPLETING THE CMS-1500 HEALTH INSURANCE CLAIM FORM

The CMS-1500 Health Insurance Claim Form is used by most health insurance payers for claims submitted by providers and suppliers. The form has 33 blocks. These blocks are divided into three sections:

- *Section 1: Carrier.* The first section indicates the type of insurance plan to which the claim is being submitted; this section includes only Block 1.
- *Section 2: Patient and Insured Information.* The second section contains information about the patient and the insured; it includes Blocks 1a through 13.
- *Section 3: Physician or Supplier Information.* The third section contains information about the provider or supplier; it includes Blocks 14 through 33.

Table 17-1 presents a summary of the information needed to complete the CMS-1500 accurately.

Section 1: Carrier—Block 1 (Figure 17-2)

This block shows the type of insurance the patient has. Indicate the type of health insurance coverage applicable to this claim by putting an X in the appropriate box, marking only one box. This information directs the claim to the correct payer.

Section 2: Patient and Insured Information—Blocks 1a to 13 (Figure 17-3)

The CMS-1500 distinguishes between the patient and the insured. The insured is the individual who is directly contracted with the insurance company. For example, if an insurance claim for Sabrina Rudman is submitted and Blue Cross covers her through her employer, she is both the patient and the insured. However, if the insurance claim is for Chris Rudman, her son, Sabrina Rudman is the insured, and Chris Rudman, her dependent, is the patient. Every CMS-1500 requires the name, gender, and birth date of both the insured and the patient, even if they are different individuals. The blocks in Figure 17-3 highlighted in yellow are for the patient's information, and the blocks highlighted in blue are for the insured's information.

Blocks 1a, 4, 7, and 11(a-d)

Information required for the insured individual includes the person's health plan ID number, name, address, policy group number, birth date, gender, employer's name (if applicable), the name of the insurance plan, and whether the insured has another health benefit plan.

Blocks 2, 3, 5, 6, and 10 a-c

Required information for the patient includes the person's name, birth date, gender, address, relationship to the insured, patient status, and whether the patient's condition is related to his or her job, an automobile accident, or some other accident.

CRITICAL THINKING APPLICATION   17-2

Ann is preparing an insurance claim to bill to Blue Cross. She notes that the patient is the dependent of the insured, so she reviews the patient registration intake form and finds that the date of birth for the insured is not present. Can Ann accurately complete the CMS-1500?

Block 9

Block 9 is for recording information about any secondary insurance plan that may be applicable. The data required include the other insured person's name, policy or group number, birth date, gender, and employer (if applicable), and the name of the other insurance plan.

HEALTH INSURANCE CLAIM FORM

APPROVED BY NATIONAL UNIFORM CLAIM COMMITTEE (NUCC) 02/12

CARRIER →

PICA							PICA

1. MEDICARE	MEDICAID	TRICARE	CHAMPVA	GROUP	FECA	OTHER
☐ (Medicare #)	☐ (Medicaid #)	☐ CHAMPUS (Sponsor's SSN)	☐ (Member ID#)	☐ HEALTH PLAN (SSN or ID)	☐ BLK LUNG (SSN)	☐ (ID)

FIGURE 17-2 Section 1: Carrier (Block 1).

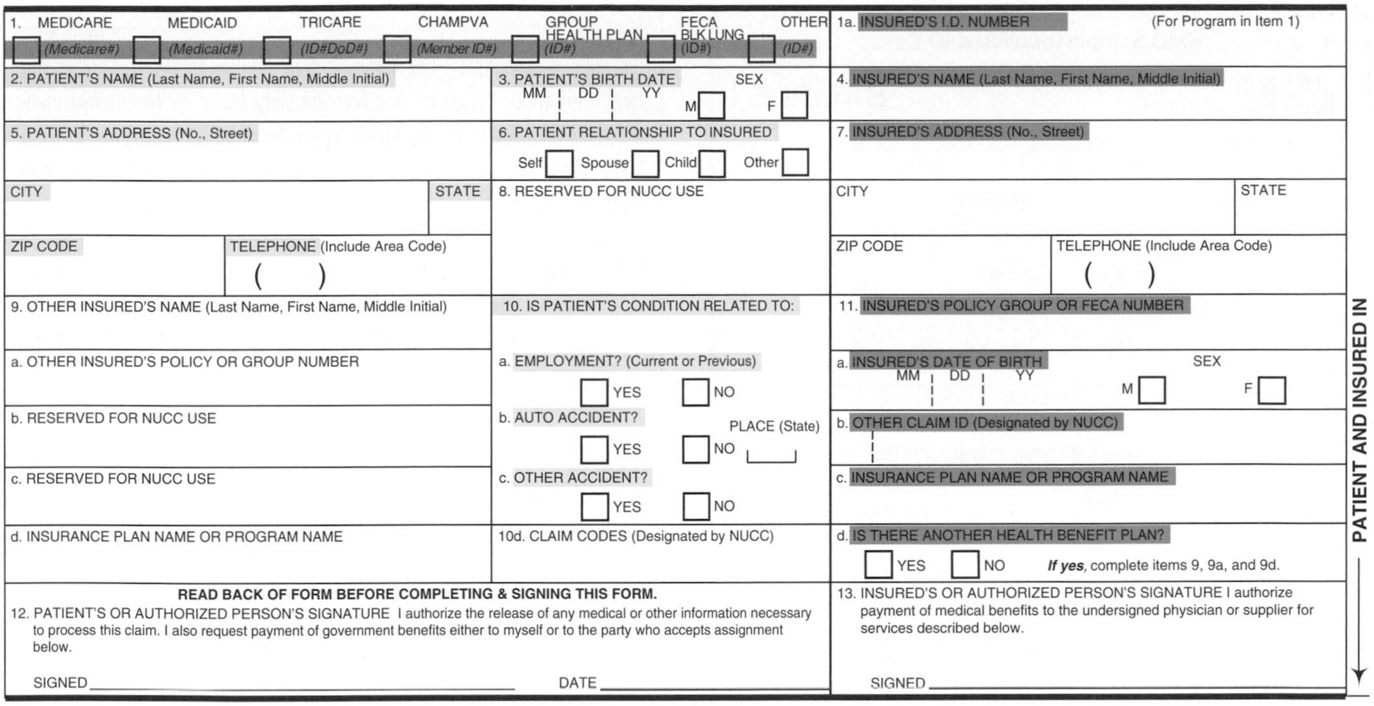
1. MEDICARE (Medicare#) MEDICAID (Medicaid#) TRICARE (ID#DoD#) CHAMPVA (Member ID#) GROUP HEALTH PLAN (ID#) FECA BLK LUNG (ID#) OTHER (ID#)
1a. INSURED'S I.D. NUMBER (For Program in Item 1)
2. PATIENT'S NAME (Last Name, First Name, Middle Initial)
3. PATIENT'S BIRTH DATE MM DD YY SEX M F
4. INSURED'S NAME (Last Name, First Name, Middle Initial)
5. PATIENT'S ADDRESS (No., Street)
6. PATIENT RELATIONSHIP TO INSURED Self Spouse Child Other
7. INSURED'S ADDRESS (No., Street)
CITY STATE
8. RESERVED FOR NUCC USE
CITY STATE
ZIP CODE TELEPHONE (Include Area Code) ( )
ZIP CODE TELEPHONE (Include Area Code) ( )
9. OTHER INSURED'S NAME (Last Name, First Name, Middle Initial)
10. IS PATIENT'S CONDITION RELATED TO:
11. INSURED'S POLICY GROUP OR FECA NUMBER
a. OTHER INSURED'S POLICY OR GROUP NUMBER
a. EMPLOYMENT? (Current or Previous) YES NO
a. INSURED'S DATE OF BIRTH MM DD YY SEX M F
b. RESERVED FOR NUCC USE
b. AUTO ACCIDENT? PLACE (State) YES NO
b. OTHER CLAIM ID (Designated by NUCC)
c. RESERVED FOR NUCC USE
c. OTHER ACCIDENT? YES NO
c. INSURANCE PLAN NAME OR PROGRAM NAME
d. INSURANCE PLAN NAME OR PROGRAM NAME
10d. CLAIM CODES (Designated by NUCC)
d. IS THERE ANOTHER HEALTH BENEFIT PLAN? YES NO *If yes*, complete items 9, 9a, and 9d.
READ BACK OF FORM BEFORE COMPLETING & SIGNING THIS FORM.
12. PATIENT'S OR AUTHORIZED PERSON'S SIGNATURE I authorize the release of any medical or other information necessary to process this claim. I also request payment of government benefits either to myself or to the party who accepts assignment below.
SIGNED DATE
13. INSURED'S OR AUTHORIZED PERSON'S SIGNATURE I authorize payment of medical benefits to the undersigned physician or supplier for services described below.
SIGNED
PATIENT AND INSURED IN

FIGURE 17-3 Section 2: Patient and Insured Information (Blocks 1a to 13).

Primary and Secondary Insurance Determination

In most cases, Medicare is usually the primary insurance, and there is a secondary policy to cover the 20% financial responsibility. In some cases, however, Medicare can be the patient's secondary insurance. This typically happens when a Medicare patient is still covered under an employer-sponsored group policy because the patient works full time. In other cases, a patient may have two insurance coverages, such as when both the patient and his or her spouse have employer-sponsored group insurance.

In the case of a child whose mother and father both carry the child as a dependent on their employer-sponsored health insurance plans, primary and secondary insurance status is determined by the birthday rule: whichever parent's birth date falls first in a calendar year is considered to have the primary insurance. The year of the parent's birth is not used. Therefore, if the mother's birth date is February 20 and the father's birth date is May 1, the mother's insurance is the primary insurance and the father's insurance is the secondary insurance.

Blocks 12 and 13

Block 12 requires the signature of the *patient* or an authorized person, and Block 13 requires the signature of the *insured* or an authorized person. In Block 12, the signature authorizes the release of any medical or other information necessary to process or adjudicate the claim. In block 13, the signature affirms that the insured has a signature on file authorizing payment of medical benefits directly to the provider (whose name appears in Block 31). The phrase "Signature on File" may be entered in these fields.

Billing for HMO Health Plans

Health insurance ID cards for members of health maintenance organizations (HMOs) show two names: the name of a sponsoring health insurance company, and a separate name for the HMO health insurance plan (Figure 17-4). This can make it confusing for a medical assistant to identify where the claim should be submitted. The first step is to call the HMO plan and ask where the medical claim should be sent. Some HMOs require that insurance claims for medical office procedures be sent to the address for the HMO insurance plan, whereas claims for hospital procedures are sent to the sponsoring health insurance. Because medical billing policies and procedures change with every HMO plan, it is wise to keep this process up-to-date in the office billing manual.

Assignment of Benefits

In the health insurance contract between the third-party payer and the patient, the patient receives the benefit when a claim is submitted. For the medical practice to receive the benefit reimbursement directly from the insurance company, the patient must sign an *assignment of benefits* (Figure 17-5). The assignment of benefits transfers the patient's legal right to collect benefits for medical expenses to the provider of those services, authorizing the payment to be sent directly to the provider. In other words, the assignment of benefits authorizes the provider to not only submit the insurance claim on behalf of the patient, but also to be reimbursed directly by the third-party payer. When the patient has signed the assignment of benefits, the medical assistant completes Blocks 12 and 13 on the CMS-1500 with the statement "Signature on File" and the claim filing date.

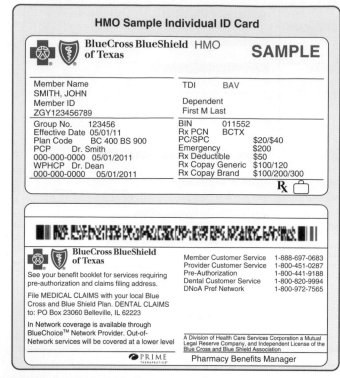

FIGURE 17-4 Patient HMO Health Insurance ID Card. (From Fordney MT: *Insurance handbook for the medical office*, ed 14, St Louis, 2017, Saunders.)

Section 3a: Physician or Supplier Information—Blocks 14 to 23 (Figure 17-6)

Block 14

Date of Current Illness, Injury, or Pregnancy (LMP). Block 14 requires the date of the current illness, injury, or pregnancy. The date should be the date on which the current illness or condition began; the date an injury occurred; or, in the case of pregnancy, the date of the last menstrual period (LMP).

Block 15

Other Date. If the patient had the same or a similar illness or condition before the current one, enter the date of onset of the earlier condition.

Block 16

Dates Patient Unable to Work in Current Occupation. These dates are used to help determine an employee's long- or short-term disability payments.

Block 17 and 17b

Name of Referring Provider or Other Source. If the patient was referred by another provider, that provider's name goes in Block 17 and his or her **National Provider Identification (NPI)** number is entered in Block 17b.

National Provider Identification

Most government-sponsored insurance claims require that the National Provider Identifiers (NPIs) for the referring and rendering providers be printed in Blocks 17b and 24J, respectively. Every healthcare entity is required to have an NPI. The NPI is an identifier assigned by the Centers for Medicare and Medicaid Services (CMS) that classifies the healthcare provider by license and medical specialties. The Administrative Simplification provisions of the Health Insurance Portability and Accountability Act of 1996 (HIPAA) mandated the adoption of standard unique identifiers for healthcare providers and health plans. The purpose of these provisions is to improve the efficiency and effectiveness of the electronic transmission of health information.

Some privately sponsored insurance companies may require claims to be submitted with the NPI. However, each privately sponsored insurance plan in each state has its own policies and procedures, so medical assistants will find that some third-party payers require NPIs, whereas others do not.

Block 18

Hospitalization Dates Related to Current Services. Block 18 is not used for claims from an ambulatory care practice.

Block 19

Additional Claim Information (Designated by NUCC). Some insurance plans ask for specific identifiers in Block 19. The medical assistant should check the instructions from the applicable third-party payer.

Block 20

Outside Lab?/$Charges. Applies to diagnostic laboratory services provided by an independent or a separate provider (who is listed in Block 32). Put an X in the YES box to indicate that the diagnostic test was performed by an entity other than the provider billing for the service (i.e., the provider listed in Block 33), and that the provider in Block 33 paid the laboratory directly. Include the amount the provider was charged by the diagnostic laboratory.

Block 21

Diagnosis or Nature of Illness or Injury. The ICD-10-CM diagnosis code or codes are entered. Enter one code for each of the 12 fields; the primary diagnosis should be recorded in the first field.

Block 22

Resubmission Code/Optional Reference Number. Both the resubmission code and the original reference number assigned by the insurance payer must be entered in this block.

Block 23

Prior Authorization Number. The preauthorization number obtained from the insurance company is entered.

Section 3b: Physician or Supplier Information—Blocks 24 to 33 (Figure 17-7)

Procedure codes, such as the Current Procedural Terminology (CPT) codes and/or the Healthcare Common Procedure Coding System (HCPCS) codes, are listed in Block 24. Each procedure code is considered a line item; the line numbers are found to the left of Block 24. The insurance claim form is read horizontally; therefore, all data in one line belongs to the coordinated CPT/HCPCS code. For claims that require more than six line items, a second CMS-1500 should be generated. Check with the insurance company to confirm how to indicate that the claim has multiple pages; some insurance

Assignment of Benefits

IMPORTANT: Please Fill-Out This Form Completely and Legibly (Do not leave anything blank)

Patient Name: *Rose Dawson*   DOB *02/17/XX*

Insurance Policy # *123-45-6789A*   Group # _____

Insured Name (if other than patient): _____   Insured DOB _____

Insured's Social Security# *123-45-6789*   Insured's Employer *None*

Your relationship to the Insured: (Self) Parent   Spouse   Other: _____

I hereby instruct and direct my health insurance policy to pay by check made out and mailed to:

Feel Better Family Practice, 101 Jack Place, New York, NY 10001

If my current health insurance policy prohibits direct payment to the clinic, please sign over the insurance check directly to the Feel Better Family Practice or Robert Wilson, MD and **mail it to the above address** as payment toward the total charges for the professional services rendered.

This is a direct Assignment of my rights and benefits under this insurance policy.

(Check each box and sign at the bottom)

☑ A copy of this Assignment that has been signed shall be considered as effective and valid as the original.

☑ I authorize the release of any health information related to the claim for my insurance company, payment adjuster, or attorney involved for the purpose of processing claims and reimbursements for services rendered.

☑ I authorize the use of my signature on all insurance submissions.

☑ I understand that I am financially responsible for all charges whether or not paid by insurance.

Dated this ___*15*___ day of ___*December*___, 20 *XX* .

Rose Dawson
_____   _____
Signature of Insured   Witness

_____
Signature of Patient, If other than Policyholder

FIGURE 17-5 Completed Assignment of Benefits form.

14. DATE OF CURRENT ILLNESS, INJURY, or PREGNANCY(LMP) MM | DD | YY QUAL.	15. OTHER DATE QUAL.| | | MM | DD | YY	16. DATES PATIENT UNABLE TO WORK IN CURRENT OCCUPATION MM | DD | YY MM | DD | YY FROM | | TO | |
17. NAME OF REFERRING PROVIDER OR OTHER SOURCE	17a. | 17b. | NPI |	18. HOSPITALIZATION DATES RELATED TO CURRENT SERVICES MM | DD | YY MM | DD | YY FROM | | TO | |
19. ADDITIONAL CLAIM INFORMATION (Designated by NUCC)		20. OUTSIDE LAB? $ CHARGES ☐ YES ☐ NO
21. DIAGNOSIS OR NATURE OF ILLNESS OR INJURY Relate A-L to service line below (24E) ICD Ind. | |		22. RESUBMISSION CODE ORIGINAL REF. NO.
A. |_____ B. |_____ C. |_____ D. |_____		
E. |_____ F. |_____ G. |_____ H. |_____		23. PRIOR AUTHORIZATION NUMBER
I. |_____ J. |_____ K. |_____ L. |_____		

FIGURE 17-6 Section 3a: Physician or Supplier Information (Blocks 14 to 23).

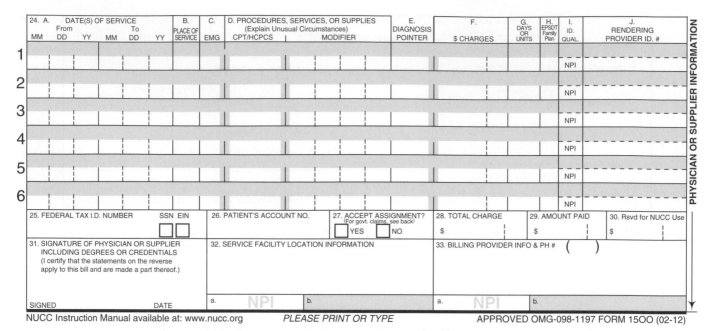

FIGURE 17-7 Section 3: Physician or Supplier Information (Blocks 24 to 33).

companies require the statement "Continued" or "Page 1 of 2" in Box 28, Total Charges.

Block 24

Procedures and Charges. Look at Block 24, line 1, in Figure 17-7. Note that the date of service (Block 24A) is the same for both From and To. This indicates that the patient was discharged after the procedure, so there was no inpatient stay. If the patient had had a hospital stay, the dates would be different.

The place of service (POS) code is entered in Block 24B. For services provided in an ambulatory care setting, the POS code is 24. As shown in Table 17-2, this two-digit code indicates that the procedure took place in an Ambulatory surgical center.

If Block 24C (EMG [emergency]) does not contain a Y, the procedure most likely was scheduled.

Block 24D (CPT/HCPCS and Modifier) provides room for a single five-digit code and up to four separate two-digit modifiers. Turning again to Figure 17-7, note that the CPT code is 19100. According to the CPT code set, the description for code 19100 is "biopsy of breast; percutaneous, needle core, not using imaging guidance." Modifier -50 indicates a bilateral procedure, so we can assume that both breasts were biopsied. The medical assistant should always check with the insurance company to determine whether the plan's medical billing policies and procedures require additional modifiers. No space is provided for a written description of the code; only the code is required. As Block 24D indicates, any unusual circumstances that affected the ability to choose an accurate CPT or HCPCS code should be explained beyond the CMS-1500.

The diagnosis pointer (Block 24E) indicates which diagnosis is used for each line item. Figure 17-7 shows only one diagnosis (N63 Unspecified lump in breast), so the diagnosis pointer is A. If more than one diagnosis is required, the pointer block separates the numbers with a comma.

In Block 24F ($ Charges), the dollar amount of the provider's fee for the service is entered. This fee is calculated in the office based on

work, expertise, and time. If a series of services was performed on any one line, multiply the number of days or units (Block 24G) by the charge for one procedure or service and enter the total amount for all days or units. This field is most commonly used for multiple visits, units of supplies, or anesthesia units.

Block 24H (EPSDT/Family Plan) identifies specific services covered under state health insurance plans. Refer to the appropriate insurance payer's guidelines (typically Medicaid or the Medicaid intermediary) for instructions on completing this block. Leave this block blank for Medicare; TRICARE and CHAMPVA (military insurance plans); group health plans; Federal Employees Compensation Act (FECA)/Black Lung; and most other types of insurance. (EPSDT stands for Early and Periodic Screening, Diagnosis, and Treatment, the child health program under Medicaid).

In Block 24I (Rendering Provider ID Qualifier) and Block 24J (Rendering Provider ID Number), enter the NPI of the provider who rendered the service, as identification.

Block 25 to 33

Facility Information. The Federal Tax ID Number (Block 25) of the provider filing the claim can be listed as a Social Security number (SSN) or an Employer Identification Number (EIN); mark the appropriate box with an **X**.

In Block 26 (Patient's Account No.), enter the account number or medical record number assigned to the patient by the provider of the service.

In Block 27 (Accept Assignment?), put an **X** in the YES box if the provider will accept assignment; this means that he or she is a **participating provider** and agrees to abide by the terms of the agreement with the insurance company to accept what the plan pays on the contracted fee schedule.

Block 28 (Total Charge) shows the amount billed on the claim form for all services rendered. To arrive at this amount, add up the charges reported in Block 24F for all the lines of service on the claim form.

Block 29 (Amount Paid) is the amount received from the patient or other payers.

Block 30 (Reserved for NUCC Use). Some secondary insurance claims use this box for the claim amount due after the primary insurance has paid.

Block 31 (Signature of Physician or Supplier) is the provider's signature, verifying that he or she provided the services listed, and they have been checked for accuracy.

In Block 32 (Service Facility Location Information), enter the name, address, city, state, and ZIP code for the site where the services listed in the claim were rendered. Enter the facility's NPI in Block 32a.

In Block 33 (Billing Provider Info & PH #), enter the address and phone number of the provider asking to be paid on this claim. In Block 33a, enter the same NPI number listed in Block 24J.

Procedure 17-3 shows how to complete a health insurance claim form using the information from an insurance card and an encounter form.

CRITICAL THINKING APPLICATION 17-3

Ann is reviewing an encounter form that has one CPT code and two HCPCS codes with one diagnosis code for the same office visit. How many lines in Box 24 of the CMS-1500 will she need to use? Will all three CPT/HCPCS codes point to the same diagnosis? Why or why not?

TABLE 17-1   Information Required for Completion of the CMS-1500 Health Insurance Claim Form

BLOCK	INFORMATION NEEDED	BLOCK	INFORMATION NEEDED
	Completed patient registration/intake form	10a-c	If patient's condition or illness is related to employment, auto accident, or some other type of accident, make sure information is obtained as outlined in Block 1
	Photocopy of insurance card or cards (front and back)		
	Encounter form	10d	Claim codes as designated by NUCC
	Preauthorization or precertification number (when applicable)	11	Insured's policy, group, or FECA number (primary insurance)
SECTION 1: CARRIER		11a	Primary insured's date of birth and gender
1	Type of insurance	11b	Other claim ID designated by NUCC
SECTION 2: PATIENT AND INSURED INFORMATION		11c	Primary insured's insurance plan or program name
1a	Insured's identification (ID) number (primary insurance)	11d	Determine whether the patient also is covered by a secondary health insurance plan
2	Patient's full name	12	Confirm that the patient's release of information form has been signed dated and is in the patient's record
3	Patient's date of birth and gender		
4	Insured's name (primary insurance)	13	Confirm that the insured's authorization of benefits form has been signed dated and is in the patient's record
5	Patient's address and telephone number • Permanent address (including apartment number if appropriate) • City, state, ZIP code • Telephone number		
		SECTION 3: PHYSICIAN OR SUPPLIER INFORMATION	
		14	Date current illness, injury, or pregnancy began
6	Patient's relationship to insured	15	Determine whether patient has had the same or similar symptoms
7	Insured's address and telephone number • Permanent address (including apartment number if appropriate) • City, state, ZIP code • Telephone number	16	From-To dates if patient was unable to work at current occupation
		17	Name of ordering or referring provider
		17a	Not required
		17b	Ordering or referring provider's NPI
9	Other insured's name (secondary insurance)*	18	From-To dates if patient encounter included an inpatient hospital stay
9a	Policy or group number (secondary insurance)*		
9b	Secondary insured's date of birth and gender*	19	Determine whether insurance carrier in carrier block and Block 1 requires any information to be entered in this field
9c	Secondary insured's employer or school name*		
9d	Secondary insured's insurance plan or program name*	20	Determine whether an outside laboratory was used; if so, enter charges billed to provider for outside lab services

Continued

TABLE 17-1   Information Required for Completion of the CMS-1500 Health Insurance Claim Form—*continued*

BLOCK	INFORMATION NEEDED	BLOCK	INFORMATION NEEDED
21	ICD-10-CM code or codes for patient's condition, illness, or injury (maximum of four per claim)	24I	Qualifier ID code (if no NPI available)
22	Is Medicaid claim being resubmitted? If yes, provide reference number from original Medicaid claim submitted	24J	Rendering (treating) provider's NPI—unshaded field PIN (if no NPI is available)—shaded field
		25	Rendering provider's federal tax ID number (EIN or SSN)
23	If prior authorization and/or referral is required, provide authorization (approval) number from insurance payer (preauthorization or precertification number)	26	Patient's account number with rendering provider
		27	Determine whether contract or agreement between provider and insurance carrier allows provider to accept assignment
24A	From-To dates of service for current encounter	28	Total charges from Block 24F, lines 1-6
24B	Place of service (POS) code	29	Amount paid by patient, insured, or other insurance
24C	If an emergency, put a Y in this box	30	Balance due (if any amount paid is shown in Block 29)
24D	CPT and/or HCPCS code CPT and/or HCPCS modifier(s) (maximum of four per charge line)	31	Signature of provider performing service or procedure
		32	Address of facility where services were rendered
24E	Block 21 field or reference number (1, 2, 3 and/or 4)	32a	NPI number of service facility listed in Block 32
24F	Total charge for CPT- or HCPCS-coded services listed in Block 24D • If more than 1 day or unit is indicated in Block 24G, multiply the charge for the service(s) coded in Block 24D by the number of days/units in Block 24G; enter the result in Block 24F	32b	Qualifier ID number and PIN of facility listed in Block 32 (if no NPI available)
		33	Name, address, and phone number of performing (rendering) provider
		33a	NPI of provider listed in Block 33
24G	Total number of days or units	33b	Qualifier ID number and PIN of provider listed in Block 33 (if no NPI available)
24H	EPSDT or Family Plan code (Medicaid or AFDC)		

*Only required if a secondary insurance exists and is to be submitted to the insurance carrier.

AFDC, Aid to Families with Dependent Children; *CPT,* Current Procedural Terminology coding system; *EIN,* Employer Identification Number; *EPSDT,* Early and Periodic Screening, Diagnosis, and Treatment; *FECA,* Federal Employees Compensation Act; *HCPCS,* Health Care Common Procedural Coding System coding method ; *ICD-10-CM,* International Classification of Diseases, Tenth Revision, Clinical Modification coding method; *NPI,* National Provider Identifier; *PIN,* personal identification number; *POS,* place of service.

TABLE 17-2   Place of Service Codes

CODE	DESCRIPTION	CODE	DESCRIPTION
11	Doctor's office	33	Custodial care facility (domiciliary or rest home services)
12	Patient's home	34	Hospice (domiciliary or rest home services)
21	Inpatient hospital	35	Adult living care facilities (residential care facility)
22	Outpatient hospital	41	Ambulance—land
23	Emergency department—hospital	42	Ambulance—air or water
24	Ambulatory surgical center	50	Federally qualified health center
25	Birthing center	51	Inpatient psychiatry facility
26	Military treatment facility/uniformed service treatment facility	52	Psychiatric facility—partial hospitalization
31	Skilled nursing facility (swing bed visits)	53	Community mental health care (outpatient, 24-hour/day services, admission screening, consultation, and educational services)
32	Nursing facility (intermediate/long-term care facilities)		

TABLE 17-2   Place of Service Codes—*continued*

CODE	DESCRIPTION	CODE	DESCRIPTION
54	Intermediate care facility/mentally retarded	65	End-stage renal disease treatment facility
55	Residential substance abuse treatment facility	71	State or local public health clinic
56	Psychiatric residential treatment center	72	Rural health clinic
60	Mass immunization center	81	Independent laboratory
61	Comprehensive inpatient rehabilitation facility	99	Other unlisted facility
62	Comprehensive outpatient rehabilitation facility		

PROCEDURE 17-3   Complete an Insurance Claim Form

Goal: *To accurately complete a CMS-1500 Health Insurance Claim Form (see Figure 17-8).*

EQUIPMENT and SUPPLIES

- Patient's health record
- Copy of patient's insurance ID card or cards
- Patient registration/intake form
- Encounter form
- Insurance claims processing guidelines
- Blank CMS-1500 Health Insurance Claim Form

PROCEDURAL STEPS

Background: Almost all medical billing is done electronically through a practice management billing software. The paper CMS-1500 Health Insurance Claim Form is provided only to help students practice and develop their medical billing skills.

Complete each block (as appropriate) of the CMS-1500 (see Table 17-2 for block descriptions).

1. Gather the documents required to complete the claim form.
2. Complete the claim form using a pen. Use capital letters. Do not use punctuation (commas or dollar signs) unless indicated in the insurance manual or guidelines. Use a hyphen to hyphenate last names.
3. Using the patient's health insurance ID card, determine the type of insurance, and the insurance ID number. Enter this information into block 1 and 1a.
   PURPOSE: After selecting the appropriate type of health insurance, the medical assistant can refer to the claims processing guidelines for that plan.
4. Using the ID card, the encounter form, and the registration/intake form, determine the patient's information and insured individual's information. Accurately complete blocks 2, 3, 5, 6, 9, and 10 a-c by entering in the patient's information. Complete 4, 7, and 11, a-d with the insured's information.
   PURPOSE: By distinguishing between the patient and the insured, the medical biller can determine whether the insurer requires additional information for submission of an accurate claim.
5. Complete blocks 12 and 13, by entering "signature on file" and the date.

NOTE: The assignment of benefit form should have been signed by the patient and/or the insured at registration. Enter the dates in either the six (6)–digit format (MM/DD/YY) or the eight (8)–digit format (MM/DD/YYYY).
PURPOSE: To submit an insurance claim, the medical practice must be authorized to release the service information on behalf of the patient or the insured.

6. Accurately enter the physician or supplier information by completing blocks 14-23. Use the eight (8)–digit format (MM/DD/YYYY) when needed.
7. Using the encounter form, complete blocks 24 and the appropriate blocks from 24A through 24H.
   NOTE:
   - Block 24A: Enter the dates of service, both From and To. For ambulatory services, enter the same date in the FROM and TO fields. Enter a date for each procedure, service, or supply in eight (8)–digit format (MM/DD/YYYY).
   - Block 24F: Enter the charge for the listed service or procedure. *Do not use commas when reporting dollar amounts.* The cents column is the small column to the right.
   - Block 24G: Enter the number of days or units. This block is usually used for multiple visits, units of supplies, anesthesia units or minutes, or oxygen volume. If only one service is performed, enter 1.
8. Complete blocks 24I through 27 by entering information on the provider's or healthcare facility where the service was provided and the patient's account number. Check the correct box to indicate acceptance of assignment of benefits.
9. Complete blocks 28 – 29 by entering the total charges, total amount paid, and the total amount due. Complete blocks 31-33a by entering in the provider's and facility's information.
10. Review the claim for accuracy and completeness before submitting. Correct any errors or missing information.
    NOTE: Before sending the claim, make a copy of the form and file the copy in the patient's insurance claim file.
    PURPOSE: It is important to double-check the form for accuracy and missing required information.

ACCURATE CODING TO PREVENT FRAUD AND ABUSE

Accurate coding in any healthcare environment is essential to prevent fraud and abuse in reimbursement (Box 17-1). According to the Health Insurance Portability and Accountability Act (HIPAA):

> Fraud is defined as knowingly and willfully executing or attempting to execute a scheme to defraud any healthcare benefit program or to obtain by means of false or fraudulent pretenses, representations, or promises any of the money or property owned by any healthcare benefit program.

Abuse in medical billing can be likened to actions that are contrary to ethical standards in the medical office. Unlike fraud, abuse is an inadvertent action that directly or indirectly results in an overpayment to the healthcare provider. Abuse is similar to fraud, except that it is unclear if the unethical practice was committed deliberately. The term **intentional** is important when determining whether fraudulent medical billing practices were done with purpose or accident.

Violations of the laws governing reimbursement may result in nonpayment of claims, civil monetary penalties (CMPs), exclusion from the payer program, criminal and civil liability, and in extreme cases, jail time. These laws may be changed or updated, so the person who is responsible for coding must pay close attention to detail and act as a sort of "medical detective" to build a case against a provider or clinic. The ICD-10-CM manual is updated annually. The *Federal Register* announces most changes, and new coding manuals often have a few pages dedicated to the updates for that particular year. Accurate use of the ICD-10-CM manual is essential for correct translation of the diagnostic statements in the health record into alphanumeric codes.

UPCODING AND DOWNCODING

Because diagnostic coding is directly related to insurance reimbursements, providers may be inclined to code to a higher specificity level than the service provided actually involved. This practice is called **upcoding,** and when it is performed regularly, it is a type of fraud and abuse. An example of upcoding would be to include a diagnosis of hyperlipidemia for an otherwise healthy person to justify a higher evaluation and management (E/M) procedure code. The medical assistant should respectfully inform the provider that this is a fraudulent practice and that fines and other penalties can be associated with this course of action.

In **downcoding,** a lower specificity level, or more generalized code, is assigned. Downcoding can be done by a variety of different stakeholders, including the coder, the insurance company, and/or a coding auditor. A coder may downcode a diagnosis to a not otherwise specified (NOS) code to avoid taking the time to look up a more accurate code. An insurance carrier may downcode a diagnosis and/or a procedure code after reviewing requested medical documentation, thus lowering the amount reimbursed to the provider. A coding auditor may downcode diagnosis and/or procedure codes when auditing patients' health records. All downcoding results in lower reimbursements to the provider.

Box 17-1   Guidelines for Reviewing Claims before Submission

The following guidelines can help ensure that clean insurance claims are submitted.

- Proofread the form carefully for accuracy and completeness.
- Make certain any necessary attachments are included with the completed form.
- Follow office policies and guidelines for claim review and signatures.
- Forward the original claim to the proper insurance carrier either by mail or electronically.
- When creating a paper claim for a workers' compensation claim, scan a copy of the completed and signed claim form into the patient's health record.
- Make sure the patient's and/or insured's name, address, and ID, group, and/or policy number are identical to the information printed on the insurance card.
- Make sure the patient's birth date and gender are the same as in the medical record.
- Section 2, Patient and Insured Information **(Blocks 1-13):** Complete these blocks accurately, according to the insurance carrier's guidelines.
  - **Block 11:** Enter the word NONE if Medicare is the primary payer.
  - **Block 12:** Make sure the patient has authorized the **release of information**, and that Block 12 has a handwritten signature, the words "Signature on File," or the acronym SOF.

- **Blocks 17** and **17b:** If applicable, enter the referring, provider's name and National Provider Identifier (NPI) number.
- **Block 27** (Accept Assignment?): Put an X in the YES box if the provider is a participating provider (PAR) or has an agreement with the insurance carrier or payer to accept assignment.
- Make sure the diagnosis is not missing or incomplete.
- Check that the diagnosis has been coded accurately, according to the ICD-10-CM coding manual, and corresponds to the treatment.
- **Blocks 14–24J** (required fields for diagnosis and procedure): Make sure these blocks are completed accurately, according to the guidelines of the third-party payer or insurance company.
- List the fees for each charge individually; or, if more than 1 day or unit is entered in **Block 24G,** they must be computed correctly
- **Block 25:** Double-check the provider's federal Social Security number (SSN) or Employer Identification Number (EIN) to ensure accuracy.
- **Block 31:** Check for the provider's signature, which must be on the form.
- **Block 24J** and **Blocks 33a, 33b:** Make sure the provider's NPI, corresponding to the insurance carrier being billed, has been entered in Block 24J and again in Block 33a. When applicable, enter the provider's personal identification number (PIN) in Block 33b, with the qualifying number, when applicable.

PREVENTING REJECTION OF A CLAIM

It is important for the medical assistant to understand and comply with the specific guidelines for completing a CMS-1500 established by each third-party payer and insurance company; this prevents delays in reimbursement and denial of payment. The guidelines for Medicare, Medicaid, TRICARE, and workers' compensation can be found online at the websites for these healthcare insurers. Most practice management billing systems have built-in "claim scrubbers" (i.e., software that automatically corrects some common billing errors), which help in the process. If claims are sent electronically through a clearinghouse, claims auditing is done before the clearinghouse transmits the claim to the third-party payer. Claims without significant errors of any type are called *clean claims*. Claims with incorrect, missing, or insufficient data are called *dirty claims*.

Communicating with Providers About Third-Party Requirements

It can be challenging for a provider to keep up with the annual changes set forth by Medicare, private health insurance companies, and the ICD-10-CM updates. This is why healthcare practitioners do well to trust their medical office staff to keep well informed on the various changes in the health insurance industry.

Some providers may be so focused on patient care that they feel uncomfortable with change. This may be the case with the encounter form/superbill used in patient care. A provider may feel comfortable using the same form, but over time, some codes may have changed or become obsolete, or new medical services offered may not be listed on the form.

A medical coder should tactfully discuss with the provider the benefits of using an updated encounter form. If the provider is still reluctant to change the form, even though it is outdated, the medical coder may suggest that the form will not be changed, just the codes on it. Adjust the encounter form to include an open text box for the provider to add medical procedures that he performs occasionally.

When communicating with the provider about coding issues, you must always show a respectful attitude, even though you may be the expert on coding and medical billing. The many changes occurring in medical coding and billing can be overwhelming and confusing for some providers; the approach of coding professionals should be to guide them patiently through these changes.

CHECKING THE STATUS OF A CLAIM

The medical biller should keep track of every submitted claim to ensure timely reimbursement. Clearinghouses send a confirmation report right after submission of a claim. The medical biller should always reconcile the claims submitted through the medical billing software with the claims listed on the confirmation report. Medical assistants should maintain this practice to ensure that every claim is submitted correctly.

The claim submission confirmation report also indicates claims that were rejected because they were incomplete. These claims should be corrected and resubmitted electronically immediately. Often these claims are rejected for typographical errors, so the medical biller should compare the patient's account in the practice management software to the information on the patient's registration/intake form, to ensure accuracy.

It takes 10 to 14 business days for insurance companies to process insurance claims electronically, but allow up to 30 days. If no further response is received from the insurance company about the claim after a month, the medical biller can visit the company's provider Web portal or call the provider services number on the back of the patient's health insurance ID card to check the status of a claim. To confirm claim status, you must provide the insured subscriber's member number and birth date; the patient's name and birth date; and the date of service. The state insurance commission has standards that third-party payers must abide by, including claim processing times and payment guidelines. Medical assistants should keep the commission's contact information in the office medical billing manual as a reference in case a claim should be reported.

EXPLANATION OF BENEFITS

An **Explanation of Benefits (EOB)** is sent by the insurance company to the provider who submitted the insurance claim, which accompanies a check or a document indicating that funds were electronically transferred. Medicare sends a remittance advice (RA) with confirmation of electronic funds transfer; although it has a different name, the document is the same as the EOB. The medical practice cannot deposit the check and disregard the EOB, which provides detailed accounting for the submitted insurance claim. The EOB breaks down each line item charge from Block 24 on the CMS-1500 into the charged amount, the amount allowable, and the paid amount as shown in Figure 17-8.

Reading the Explanation of Benefits

The EOB contains essential information about the submitted health insurance claim. To apply payments to a patient's account properly, it is vital that the medical assistant understand all the elements of an EOB. Figure 17-8 shows a completed CMS-1500. When interpreting the EOB, review the following steps.

1. Verify that the EOB applies to the correct patient by comparing the account number and date of service on the EOB with the submitted CMS-1500.

HEALTH INSURANCE CLAIM FORM

APPROVED BY NATIONAL UNIFORM CLAIM COMMITTEE (NUCC) 02/12

☐☐☐ PICA | PICA ☐☐☐

| 1. MEDICARE | MEDICAID | TRICARE | CHAMPVA | GROUP HEALTH PLAN | FECA BLK LUNG | OTHER | 1a. INSURED'S I.D. NUMBER | (For Program in Item 1) |
| ☑ (Medicare#) | ☐ (Medicaid#) | ☐ (ID#/DoD#) | ☐ (Member ID#) | ☐ (ID#) | ☐ (ID#) | ☐ (ID#) | 123-45-6789A | |

| 2. PATIENT'S NAME (Last Name, First Name, Middle Initial) | 3. PATIENT'S BIRTH DATE | SEX | 4. INSURED'S NAME (Last Name, First Name, Middle Initial) |
| ROSE DAWSON | MM 02 DD 17 YY XX | M ☐ F ☑ | ROSE DAWSON |

| 5. PATIENT'S ADDRESS (No., Street) | 6. PATIENT RELATIONSHIP TO INSURED | 7. INSURED'S ADDRESS (No., Street) |
| 123 TITANIC PLACE | Self ☑ Spouse ☐ Child ☐ Other ☐ | 123 TITANIC PLACE |

| CITY | STATE | 8. RESERVED FOR NUCC USE | CITY | STATE |
| NEW YORK | NY | | NEW YORK | NY |

| ZIP CODE | TELEPHONE (Include Area Code) | | ZIP CODE | TELEPHONE (Include Area Code) |
| 10001 | ( ) | | 10001 | ( ) |

| 9. OTHER INSURED'S NAME (Last Name, First Name, Middle Initial) | 10. IS PATIENT'S CONDITION RELATED TO: | 11. INSURED'S POLICY GROUP OR FECA NUMBER |
| ROSE DAWSON | | 123-45-6789A |

| a. OTHER INSURED'S POLICY OR GROUP NUMBER | a. EMPLOYMENT? (Current or Previous) | a. INSURED'S DATE OF BIRTH | SEX |
| 123-45-6789 | ☐ YES ☑ NO | MM 02 DD 17 YY XX | M ☐ F ☑ |

| b. RESERVED FOR NUCC USE | b. AUTO ACCIDENT? PLACE (State) | b. OTHER CLAIM ID (Designated by NUCC) |
| | ☐ YES ☑ NO | |

| c. RESERVED FOR NUCC USE | c. OTHER ACCIDENT? | c. INSURANCE PLAN NAME OR PROGRAM NAME |
| | ☐ YES ☑ NO | MEDICARE |

| d. INSURANCE PLAN NAME OR PROGRAM NAME | 10d. CLAIM CODES (Designated by NUCC) | d. IS THERE ANOTHER HEALTH BENEFIT PLAN? |
| AARP SECONDARY POLICY | | ☑ YES ☐ NO *If yes*, complete items 9, 9a, and 9d. |

READ BACK OF FORM BEFORE COMPLETING & SIGNING THIS FORM.

12. PATIENT'S OR AUTHORIZED PERSON'S SIGNATURE I authorize the release of any medical or other information necessary to process this claim. I also request payment of government benefits either to myself or to the party who accepts assignment below.

SIGNED SIGNATURE ON FILE   DATE 01/14/20XX

13. INSURED'S OR AUTHORIZED PERSON'S SIGNATURE I authorize payment of medical benefits to the undersigned physician or supplier for services described below.

SIGNED SIGNATURE ON FILE

14. DATE OF CURRENT ILLNESS, INJURY, or PREGNANCY (LMP) MM DD YY QUAL.	15. OTHER DATE QUAL. MM DD YY	16. DATES PATIENT UNABLE TO WORK IN CURRENT OCCUPATION MM DD YY MM DD YY FROM TO
17. NAME OF REFERRING PROVIDER OR OTHER SOURCE ROBERT WILSON, MD	17a. 17b. NPI 11122233344	18. HOSPITALIZATION DATES RELATED TO CURRENT SERVICES MM DD YY MM DD YY FROM TO
19. ADDITIONAL CLAIM INFORMATION (Designated by NUCC)		20. OUTSIDE LAB? $ CHARGES ☐ YES ☐ NO

21. DIAGNOSIS OR NATURE OF ILLNESS OR INJURY Relate A-L to service line below (24E)   ICD Ind.

A. E11.22   B. ____   C. ____   D. ____
E. ____   F. ____   G. ____   H. ____
I. ____   J. ____   K. ____   L. ____

| 22. RESUBMISSION CODE | ORIGINAL REF. NO. |
| 23. PRIOR AUTHORIZATION NUMBER | |

| 24. A. DATE(S) OF SERVICE | | | B. PLACE OF SERVICE | C. EMG | D. PROCEDURES, SERVICES, OR SUPPLIES (Explain Unusual Circumstances) | | E. DIAGNOSIS POINTER | F. $ CHARGES | G. DAYS OR UNITS | H. EPSDT Family Plan | I. ID. QUAL. | J. RENDERING PROVIDER ID. # |
From MM DD YY	To MM DD YY				CPT/HCPCS	MODIFIER						
01 14 XX	01 14 XX		11		99213		1	$125 00	1		NPI	11122233344
											NPI	
											NPI	
											NPI	
											NPI	
											NPI	

| 25. FEDERAL TAX I.D. NUMBER | SSN EIN | 26. PATIENT'S ACCOUNT NO. | 27. ACCEPT ASSIGNMENT? (For govt. claims, see back) | 28. TOTAL CHARGE | 29. AMOUNT PAID | 30. Rsvd for NUCC Use |
| 098-76-5432 | ☐ ☑ | RW125638 | ☑ YES ☐ NO | $ 125 00 | $ 0 | |

31. SIGNATURE OF PHYSICIAN OR SUPPLIER INCLUDING DEGREES OR CREDENTIALS (I certify that the statements on the reverse apply to this bill and are made a part thereof.)	32. SERVICE FACILITY LOCATION INFORMATION	33. BILLING PROVIDER INFO & PH # ( )
Robert Wilson, MD 01/14/XX SIGNED DATE	Feel Better Family Practice 101 Jack Place New York, NY, 10001 (212) 555-1212	Robert Wilson, MD 101 Jack Place New York, NY, 10001 (212) 555-1212
	a. 22233344455 b.	a. 11122233344 b.

NUCC Instruction Manual available at: www.nucc.org   **PLEASE PRINT OR TYPE**   APPROVED OMB-0938-1197 FORM 1500 (02-12)

CARRIER

PATIENT AND INSURED INFORMATION

PHYSICIAN OR SUPPLIER INFORMATION

FIGURE 17-8 Completed CMS-1500 Health Insurance Claim Form.

2. Confirm that the EOB shows the same figures as the submitted CMS-1500 for the amount charged per line (Block 24F) and the number of lines (Block 24J); in other words, the line items and charges should match. Sometimes the EOB summarizes the entire claim in one charged amount. In this case, confirm that the total charged is the same as in Block 28.

3. Post the payment and adjusted amount per line item. In the practice management billing software, these are posted on the same line. The patient's responsibility, as determined by the primary insurance EOB, is calculated using the following equation:

Charged amount − Payment amount − Adjusted amount
= Patient's responsibility

4. Once the patient's responsibility has been determined, check the patient's health record to see whether a secondary insurance is listed. If one is, submit a health insurance claim with the balance due determined by the primary insurance EOB. If no secondary insurance is listed, the patient is billed for the balance due.

5. Review the **remarks codes** on the EOB for any additional messages or information about the claim. The remarks codes area is where the payer indicates the conditions under which the claim was paid. For example, code 01 states that the claim amount allowed was established by the contract between the health insurance plan and the provider. Other remarks codes give the reasons a claim was denied or rejected. Some remarks codes indicate that the claim is pending, awaiting specific information.

6. All remarks codes on pending or denied claims should be followed up immediately upon receipt of the EOB, to prevent further delay in payment for other claims.

Rejected Claims

The EOB provides detailed information on rejected claims. Just as payments on the EOB, rejected claims are presented as line items, just as in Block 24 of the CMS-1500. All rejected claims have a code, with a legend toward the bottom the page. Some of the reasons claims are rejected are:

- The interval specified for filing the claim had expired (check the insurance plan's billing policies manual for details).
- Incorrect ICD-10-CM, CPT, and/or HCPCS codes or combinations of codes were entered.

- The insurer claims that the ICD-10-CM code and the CPT/HCPCS codes do not match; that is, the claim lacks **medical necessity**.
- More than one CPT/HCPCS code was filed on the same date of service, and they are mutually exclusive when billed together.
- The claim was submitted to the wrong insurance plan.

Rejected claims should be corrected and resubmitted for payment electronically unless otherwise specified. Use Block 22 on the CMS-1500 according to insurance plan billing guidelines to indicate a resubmitted claim. These claims should be resubmitted as soon as possible to prevent further delay in reimbursement.

DENIED CLAIMS

The two main reasons for denial of payment are technical errors and insurance policy coverage issues. Technical errors include incorrect, incomplete information, typographic and/or mathematical errors. Common reasons for denial include:

- The patient was not covered by the insurance plan on the date of service.
- A listed procedure was not an insurance benefit.
- Preauthorization for the service was not obtained.
- Medical necessity

Medical Necessity

To obtain the correct reimbursement for a provider, the medical biller must submit the correct codes. The diagnosis code is the reason the medical procedure rendered was necessary. For example, if a claim submitted to the insurance company indicated, through coding error, that a bunionectomy was performed for a tonsillitis diagnosis, the insurer will deny the claim based on medical necessity. Therefore, maintaining accurate health records and efficient claims processing are possible only if *each and every* procedure and service provided during an office visit or encounter is justified.

If an insurance claim is denied for medical necessity, and the medical assistant believes that a payment should be made, an appeal letter should be sent to the insurance plan (Procedure 17-4). The appeal letter should not only identify the denied claim, but also include a statement from the provider detailing the medical reasoning for performing the procedure. Additional medical reports (e.g., laboratory reports, operative reports, and history and physical examination findings [H&P]) should be sent if they support the provider's treatment decision.

PROCEDURE 17-4 **Utilize Medical Necessity Guidelines: Respond to a "Medical Necessity Denied" Claim**

Goal: *To resolve the insurance company's denial of medical necessity by completing an accurate claim.*

Scenario: *You are working at Walden-Martin Family Medical Clinic, 1234 Anystreet, Anytown, AL 12345 (phone: 123-123-1234).*

You receive a letter indicating that Medicare has denied the following claim for not being medically necessary:

Patient: Norma B. Washington
Date of Service: 06/13/20XX
Provider: Julie Walden MD

DOB: 08/07/1944
ICD: G43.101 (Migraine)

Policy/ID Number: 847744144A
CPT: J3420 (B-12 injection)

PROCEDURE 17-4   *—continued*

You did some research and the information above was the only information sent to Medicare for that encounter. The following information was the correct information for the encounter:

Patient: Norma B. Washington   DOB: 08/01/1944   Date of Service: 06/15/20XX
ICD: G43.101 (Migraine)   CPT: J1885 (Toradol 15 mg—$15.50) and 90772 (Injection, Ther/
                                    Proph/Diag—$25.00)
ICD: D51.0 (Vitamin B12 deficiency anemia)   CPT: J3420 (B-12 injection—$24.00) and 90772 (Injection, Ther/
                                    Proph/Diag—$25.00)
To be billed to: Medicare, 1234 Insurance Road, Anytown, AL 12345-1234

EQUIPMENT and SUPPLIES

- Paper method: Patient's health record, copy of patient's insurance ID card or cards, patient registration/intake form, encounter form, blank CMS-1500 Health Insurance Claim Form, and a pen
- Electronic method: SimChart for the Medical Office
- Insurance denial letter or scenario (see above)

PROCEDURAL STEPS

1. Review the insurance denial letter (scenario) carefully. Compare the patient's information from the denial letter to the health record, claim, and encounter form. Look for errors in the patient's name and date of birth.
   PURPOSE: Errors in patient information can be a reason for denial.
2. Compare the insurance denial letter (scenario) to the health record, claim, and encounter form. Look for errors in the date of service, the diagnosis,

and the procedure codes. The procedure must be medically necessary for the diagnosis indicated.
   PURPOSE: Errors related to the encounter must be matching for the claim to be accepted. The procedure codes must indicate an acceptable standard of treatment for the diagnosis listed. In some cases, the encounter form may contain a diagnosis that did not make it into the original claim form. Review the patient's health record to determine whether the procedure was medically necessary.
3. Complete a claim (either CMS-1500 or an electronic claim using SimChart) by entering in the information about the carrier, patient, and insured.
4. Enter the information regarding the physician, procedures, and diagnosis. Make sure to include all of the information from the encounter.
5. Proofread the claim form for accuracy before submitting the claim.

The Patient's Financial Responsibility

Most MCO health insurance contracts require patients to pay a **copayment,** which is collected at the time of service (Table 17-3). Copayments usually range from $10 to $75 for office visits; they vary, depending on whether the patient is seen by a PCP or a specialist, in urgent care, or in the emergency department. Office visits and prescription copayments do not count toward the yearly contracted deductible. The medical assistant must make sure that the proper copayments are received and credited to patients' accounts.

A **deductible** is an amount that the policyholder for the policy is contracted per year to pay toward his or her healthcare before the insurance company begins to reimburse the healthcare provider. The deductible amount is stated in the insurance contract between the patient and the health insurance company.

Coinsurance is a policy provision in which the policyholder and the insurance company share the cost of covered medical services in a specified ratio. For example, the plan may set an 80/20 ratio; this means that after the yearly deductible has been met, the insurance carrier pays 80% of the cost of services, and the insured pays 20%. The patient's deductible, or coinsurance financial responsibility, is documented on the EOB.

To help patients understand their health insurance benefits, the medical assistant must be confident in defining the terms copayment, coinsurance, and deductible, taking on the role of patient navigator.

The medical office can contact the insurance company on the patient's behalf to determine the amount of the deductible and/or coinsurance the patient has already paid in the calendar year. The process of precertification enables the healthcare provider to inform patients of how much the procedure will cost them.

TABLE 17-3 Comparing Patient Financial Responsibilities		
PATIENT FINANCIAL RESPONSIBILITY	**WHEN PATIENT PAYS**	**AMOUNT PATIENT PAYS**
Copayment	At the time of medical service	Fixed amount, $10 to $75 per visit
Deductible	After the provider has been paid	Variable amount, up to 30%
Coinsurance	After the provider has been paid	Variable amount, up to 30%, but not to exceed deductible

Allowed Amount

For providers to become participating providers in an insurance network, they must agree to accept the insurance plan fee schedule as payment in full for services rendered. This means that all fees above the plan's allowed amount should be adjusted. The allowed amount may be all or part of a charge for a service or procedure. For example, a provider typically may charge $80 for a Level I office visit; however, the insurance plan's allowable amount may be only $60. If the provider is a participating provider, he or she is obligated to adjust the difference between these two amounts—$20. However, if the provider is not a participating provider, he or she can bill the patient for the $20 balance. Because contracts between third-party payers and providers vary greatly, it is important for the medical assistant to examine the EOB closely and to be knowledgeable about the contract provisions between the provider and all insurance carriers he or she uses to recognize the appropriate contracted amount.

CRITICAL THINKING APPLICATION   **17-6**

Ann is reviewing a Remittance Advice (RA) for a Medicare patient with no secondary insurance. The charge for the office visit was $100; the insurance company allowed 80%, of which the insurance company paid 50%. What did the insurance company reimburse and what is the patient's responsibility? What amount should be adjusted?

Calculating the Coinsurance and Deductible

Consider this example: Mrs. Anita Jones' health insurance plan has a $500 annual deductible, after which the insurance company pays 95% of all charges. Mrs. Jones, therefore, has a 5% coinsurance expense in addition to the deductible. She also has a $1,000 out-of-pocket expense maximum; this means that once Mrs. Jones has paid $1,000 total (which includes the deductible), the insurance company pays 100% of any balance remaining. Mrs. Jones has incurred a $10,000 charge for cardiac surgery performed by her provider. Now look at Figures 17-9 and 17-10.

- In Figure 17-9, Column A shows that Mrs. Jones' paid the $500 deductible, and 5% of $10,000 (i.e., an additional $500). The insurance company then paid the remaining balance of $9,000.
- In Figure 17-10, Column B shows that Mrs. Jones' cardiac surgery cost $20,000. Mrs. Jones' total out-of-pocket expense remains $1,000; therefore, in this case the insurance company is responsible for payment of the balance of $19,000. Because her maximum out-of-pocket expense, according to the plan, is $1,000, even though the charges were doubled, she still pays only the $1,000 total out-of-pocket expense.

Using the example in Figure 17-9, if the allowable amount for Mrs. Jones' $10,000 cardiac surgery is $8,500, the $1,500 difference between the provider's charge and the allowed amount (i.e. the additional $500 above Mrs. Jone's out-of-pocket expense) would be either written off or passed on to the patient as an out-of-pocket expense. In Column A, a line has been added to show the $8,500 allowable amount and that $1,500 has been billed to the patient. In Column B, the provider adjusts the charged amount above the contracted amount.

Discussing Patients' Financial Responsibility

Patients must understand that the guarantor is the person ultimately responsible for the entire bill. Remember, the insurance policy is a contract between the policyholder and an insurance plan. The provider is not a party to this contract.

Providers and their staff members, therefore, are not responsible for pursuing insurance payment for the patient's benefit. However, it is in the practice's best interest to actively assist patients if problems arise in securing payment. This is true for two reasons. First, the staff is almost always more knowledgeable than the patient about the health insurance business. Many patients do not even read their insurance policies and have no idea what is and is not covered. Some patients expect insurance to pay all costs simply because they are paying a premium. The medical assistant may need to educate these patients about their policies and offer advice on how patients can effectively work with their insurance company to get answers to questions and make sure they are receiving all the benefits to which they are entitled.

The second reason for helping patients understand their health insurance plan is that this helps ensure that the provider is compensated for his or her services. If the medical assistant acts as a patient navigator with the insurance company, his or her efforts usually result in regular reimbursements (Figure 17-11).

Medical assistants gain knowledge about the insurance industry when they actively assist patients with their concerns. The more experience a medical assistant has in working with insurance and third-party payers, the more helpful he or she can be to patients. As mentioned previously, medical assistants should keep a manual of medical billing policies and procedures for most of the insurances plans they handle; this can serve as an excellent source of guidance and suggestions for working with a particular payer.

Always be sure to obtain the guarantor's signature on an agreement to pay for services. Most patient information sheets have a

	Column A	Column B
Total charge	$10,000	$20,000
Deductible (paid by Mrs. Jones)	(500)	(500)
5% (Mrs. Jones' portion)	(500)	(500)
Total amount paid by Mrs. Jones	$1000	$1000
Total amount paid by insurance	$9000	$19,000

FIGURE 17-9 Calculation of deductible and coinsurance.

	Column A	Column B
Total charge	$10,000	$20,000
Deductible (paid by Mrs. Jones)	(500)	(500)
5% (Mrs. Jones' portion)	(500)	(500)
Allowable amount $8500	(1500)	
Allowable amount $8500 with write off		(1500)
Total amount paid by Mrs. Jones	$2500	$1000
Total amount paid by insurance	$7500	$17,500

FIGURE 17-10 Calculation of allowable amount.

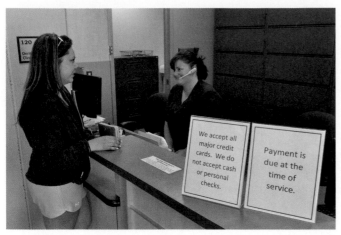

FIGURE 17-11 Medical assistant informing a patient of her financial responsibility.

section referring to the guarantor. A statement may be included, which the guarantor signs, that serves as an agreement to pay the costs of medical care. States have varying statutes that deal with guarantors, so be sure the office's policies comply with those laws. It is especially important to secure a written agreement to pay for services when the care will be long term for costly treatment or surgical procedures. Procedure 17-5 explains how to inform patients of their financial obligations for services rendered.

CRITICAL THINKING APPLICATION   **17-7**

The providers in the practice where Ann works are not in network of a preferred provider organization (PPO) that is often used in their geographic area. Many patients are confused when they have to pay a larger out-of-pocket fee for their medical services. How can Ann explain the reason for these higher fees to patients?

PROCEDURE 17-5 | **Inform a Patient of Financial Obligations for Services Rendered**

Goal: Inform patient of his/her financial obligation and to demonstrate professionalism when discussing the patient's billing record.

Scenario: During this role play, Christi Brown is meeting with you regarding the bill she received in the mail. When she called to make the appointment, she voiced her confusion about the bill, stating she thought her insurance covered everything. You check her record and see that she met her deductible and now needs to pay 20% of the billed amount. She owes $170.

EQUIPMENT and SUPPLIES

- Patient's account record
- Copy of patient's insurance card.

PROCEDURAL STEPS

1. Determine the patient's financial responsibility under the insurance plan by reviewing the copy of the patient's insurance card.
   PURPOSE: Having an understanding of the patient's financial responsibility from the insurance plan will help you to explain the terms to the patient.
2. Determine the amount the patient owes by reviewing the patient's account record.
   PURPOSE: It is important that when working with a patient that you are familiar with the facts of the situation.

3. Discuss the situation with the patient. (Role play the above scenario.)
4. Demonstrate professionalism when discussing the situation with the patient. Verbal and nonverbal communication should demonstrate patience, understanding, and sensitivity. The medical assistant should refrain from inappropriate and unprofessional behavior, including eye rolling, harsh words, disrespectful comments, and similar behaviors.
5. Demonstrate professionalism by respectfully providing the patient with payment options based on the clinic's policies and what the patient can pay on a monthly basis.
   PURPOSE: The medical assist should not force or harass the patient in paying. The medical assistant will be more successful if the communication with the patient is respectful.

Showing Sensitivity When Discussing Patients' Finances

Most patients use health insurance, but they do not always recognize that they will have financial obligations after the insurance plan pays its share. This is common among Medicare patients, who often feel that they should have all their medical expenses paid because they have government insurance. It usually falls to the medical assistant to inform patients of their coinsurance responsibilities.

Patients seeking medical care are not usually feeling like themselves because they may be (or have been) suffering through

pain and discomfort. As a result, their behavior may not be typical when the medical assistant suggests discussing their financial responsibilities.

Medical assistants should show patience and sensitivity when discussing a patient's financial obligations (Figure 17-12). Patients should never be harassed to make a payment or forced into payment arrangements. Medical assistants should always be courteous when discussing payments with patients. In addition, the medical practice should offer a variety of payment methods to meet patients' needs, including credit cards, and online payment options.

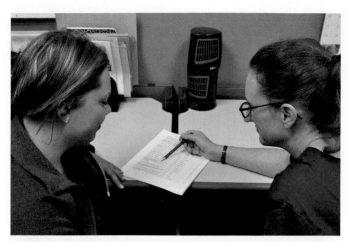

FIGURE 17-12 *Medical assistants must show respect and sensitivity when discussing financial issues with patients.*

CRITICAL THINKING APPLICATION   **17-8**

An elderly patient comes to the office and complains that Medicare did not pay her bill in full. "Medicare is supposed to pay 80% of all of my bills, and I have already paid my portion," she insists. What information does Ann need to get to the bottom on this problem? How can she explain situations like this to other patients?

CLOSING COMMENTS

Accurate insurance billing practices are essential for the financial success of every healthcare facility. Medical assistants are strong assets to the healthcare facility when they can submit claims electronically, manage denied and rejected claims, and discuss financial responsibilities with patients professionally. Medical assistants should always maintain a positive attitude toward patients and keep in mind that those who are ill or facing challenges are not always at their best and may not respond in a positive way when discussing their financial responsibilities.

Patient Education

Most patients are unaware of their benefits and coverages through their insurance policies. The medical assistant should encourage patients to read the entire policy to become familiar with its limitations and exclusions. Inform patients that when they call the insurance company with questions, they should always write down the date, the time, and the name of the person with whom they spoke. Using email is helpful because a record of the correspondence can easily be saved or printed. Making sure that patients have a general understanding of their health insurance coverage is well worth the effort.

Often patients do not dispute the decision or question the insurance company when a claim is rejected or not paid in the expected amount. Encourage them to call the company and question rejections if they do not understand why the claim was denied.

Legal and Ethical Issues

From time to time patients may ask for a reduced fee after the insurance has already paid. If the provider is a participating provider with the health insurance plan, he or she is obligated to follow the terms of contract. This includes collecting the patient's financial responsiblitiy detailed in the EOB. The insurance plan can penalize the healthcare facility if a concerted effort is not made to collect the patient's coinsurance and deductible amounts, thus not following the terms of the participating provider health insurance contract.

Professional Behaviors

Medical billers must have strong organizational skills. Not only are they responsible for submitting claims electronically in a timely manner, they also must manage claim denials and rejections. Denied and rejected claims need to be adjusted and rebilled for prompt payment. An organized medical biller ensures that all medical billing activities are worked on daily.

SUMMARY OF SCENARIO

Ann realizes that the best way to keep track of all the carriers is to keep an up-to-date manual that contains the addresses, phone numbers, and medical billing policies and procedures for each insurance plan the healthcare facility accepts. This manual can help prevent the rejection and denial of many claims because they will be submitted accurately the first time.

The medical assistant's understanding of how to calculate deductibles, coinsurance, and allowed amounts for procedures and services benefits both the provider and patient. The provider's productivity, income, and losses can be easily tracked, and the patient can be educated as to the exact amounts he or she is responsible for paying.

Ann also has learned the importance of being courteous to patients when discussing their financial obligations. She has learned how to use the Assignment of Financial Responsibility form to communicate what the patient owes in a clear, straightforward manner.

SUMMARY OF LEARNING OBJECTIVES

1. Define, spell, and pronounce the terms listed in the vocabulary.
   Spelling and pronouncing medical terms correctly reinforce the medical assistant's credibility. Knowing the definitions of these terms promotes confidence in communication with patients and co-workers.

2. Identify steps for filing a third-party claim.
   The medical assistant's medical billing tasks begin when the patient seeks medical services from the provider, usually when an appointment is made. Insurance billing and coding tasks typically completed by the

Continued

medical assistant include collecting accurate information and submitting a complete insurance claim.

3. **Identify the types of information contained in the patient's billing record.**

When the first appointment is made for a patient, it is routine to ask the patient for all pertinent insurance billing information. Much of this information is on the patient registration/intake form, which is completed when the patient comes to the medical office for the initial visit.

4. **Apply managed care policies and procedures, describe processes for precertification, and obtain precertification, including documentation.**

Medical assistants should be aware that services provided to patients who are sponsored by an MCO plan may not be reimbursed if the policies and procedures of the specific insurance plan are not followed. To submit accurate health insurance claims, medical assistants should establish office procedures for applying MCO policies and procedures. (See Procedure 17-1.)

In an effort to control costs, many MCOs require precertification of specialized medical services. The policies and procedures of each insurance plan determine whether precertification is required before a medical procedure is scheduled. Preauthorization helps the medical assistant ensure that the provider will be paid for procedures and services provided to the patient. The process for obtaining preauthorization (precertification) is outlined in Procedure 17-2.

5. **Explain how to submit health insurance claims, including electronic claims, to various third-party payers.**

Medical billers should familiarize themselves with the claim submission policies and procedures of the health insurance plans commonly seen in their office. A medical assistant can successfully manage the requirements of the different insurance plans commonly seen in the practice by keeping an up-to-date manual containing the billing policies and procedures of these third-party payers. Electronic claims are insurance claims that are transmitted over the Internet from the provider to the health insurance company. Most claims-processing software is designed to generate electronic claims.

6. **Review the guidelines for completing the CMS-1500 Health Insurance Claim Form, and complete an insurance claim form.**

The medical assistant should follow an established list of guidelines for completing the CMS-1500 Health Insurance Claim Form, including obtaining a signed assignment of benefits. The CMS-1500 has 33 blocks; except for specific blocks that require information about the patient and the insured, the requirements for completing the form vary from payer to payer. Accuracy in completing the CMS-1500 is vital. The process for completing claim forms accurately is outlined in Procedure 17-3.

7. **Differentiate between fraud and abuse.**

Abuse in coding can be likened to actions that are contrary to ethical standards in the medical office. Unlike fraud, abuse is an inadvertent action that directly or indirectly results in an overpayment to the healthcare provider. Abuse is similar to fraud, except that it is unclear whether the unethical practice was committed deliberately. The term "intentional" is important in defining fraud and abuse and in deciphering whether the coding practices were ethical or not.

8. **Discuss the effects of upcoding and downcoding.**

Medical coders have an ethical responsibility to prevent fraud and abuse resulting from upcoding. Coders also must be careful not to downcode, or assign codes that are not specific enough. Downcoding can be done by the coder, the insurance company, or even a coding auditor; it always results in lower reimbursements. When providers take the responsibility to assign either diagnostic or procedural codes, they should be guided on the importance of accurate codes and their relation to maximizing reimbursement.

9. **Discuss methods of preventing the rejection of claims, and use tactful behavior when speaking with medical providers about third-party requirements.**

It can be challenging for a provider to keep up with the annual changes published by Medicare, private health insurance companies, and the ICD-10-CM code set updates. Staff meetings to review third-party requirements should be conducted regularly by the medical billing supervisor. Medical assistants should be respectful to the healthcare provider when discussing third-party requirements that demand more effort on the provider's part. An understanding and patient attitude goes a long way. Rejection and delay of claims cost the medical facility time and money. Proven methods of preventing rejection and delay should be established and followed; these may include reviewing electronic claims submission reports and following up on aging reports.

10. **Describe ways of checking a claim's status.**

It is important to track health insurance claims once they have been submitted electronically. A regular practice of confirming submission of a claim with the health insurance plan or the clearinghouse is essential for prompt payment. If more than 2 weeks passes after a claim submission without a response from the insurance company, it is wise to follow up either through the online insurance provider Web portal or by phone.

11. **Review and read an Explanation of Benefits (EOB).**

The EOB is sent by the insurance company to the provider who submitted the insurance claim, along with a check or a document indicating that funds were transferred electronically. The EOB breaks down each line item charge into the amount allowable, how much the insurance plan paid, and how much the patient is contracted to pay to the provider.

12. **Discuss reasons for denied claims.**

The two main reasons for denial of payment are technical errors and insurance policy coverage issues. Technical errors include incorrect or incomplete information and typographic and/or mathematical errors.

13. **Define "medical necessity" as it applies to diagnostic and procedural coding; also, apply medical necessity guidelines.**

To ensure correct reimbursement, accurate diagnosis codes must be submitted, and they must be linked to the medical procedure code reported. The diagnosis code is the reason the medical procedure performed was necessary. If an insurance company denies a claim on the

SUMMARY OF LEARNING OBJECTIVES—*continued*

grounds that the medical treatment provided was not medically necessary, an appeal letter should be sent (Procedure 17-4). The appeal letter should not only identify the denied claim in question, but also include a statement from the provider detailing the medical reasoning for providing the billed treatment. Additional medical reports should be sent (e.g., lab reports, operative reports, H&P) if these documents support the provider's decision to treat the patient.

14. **Explain a patient's financial obligations for services rendered, and inform a patient of these obligations.**

    Patients must understand that the guarantor is the person ultimately responsible for the entire bill. The insurance policy is a contract between an insurance company or MCO and the policyholder, or a group of people (e.g., through an employer). The provider is not a party to this contract. Therefore, providers and their staff members are not responsible for pursuing insurance payment for the benefit of the patient. However, it is in the best interest of the staff to actively assist the patient if problems occur securing payment.

Always be sure to secure guarantors in writing (see Figure 17-11). Most patient information sheets have a section referring to the guarantor. A statement may be included for the guarantor sign, indicating an agreement to pay the costs of medical care. States have varying statutes that deal with guarantors, so be sure the office's policies reflect compliance with those laws. It is especially important to secure a written agreement to pay for services when the care will be long term or when a costly treatment or surgical procedure must be done. Procedure 17-5 explains how to inform patients of their financial obligations for services rendered.

15. **Show sensitivity when speaking with patients about third-party requirements.**

    Medical assistants should show patience and sensitivity when discussing a patient's financial obligations. Patients should never be harassed to make a payment or forced into payment arrangements. Medical assistants should always be courteous when discussing payments with patients.

CONNECTIONS

Study Guide Connection: Go to the Chapter 17 Study Guide. Read and complete the activities.

evolve Evolve Connection: Go to the Chapter 17 link at *evolve.elsevier.com/kinn* to complete the Chapter Review Quiz. To sharpen your test-taking skills, click on the Medical Assisting Exam Review and answer the practice questions. In addition, check out the other resources listed for this chapter to make the most of what you have learned from Medical Billing and Reimbursement.

18 PATIENT ACCOUNTS, COLLECTIONS, AND PRACTICE MANAGEMENT

SCENARIO

Brenda Newman works in patient accounts for Dr. Susan Wilkins, a neurologist. Among her responsibilities are posting all transactions to patient accounts, monitoring accounts receivable, negotiating patient accounts and making payment arrangements, making collection calls for outstanding patient accounts, and some simple bookkeeping for Dr. Wilkins. Dr. Wilkins also works with Grant Schmidt, a certified public accountant (CPA), who assists her with supervising her office bookkeeping, creating financial statements, and overall money management of her practice. Mr. Schmidt is always willing to offer advice to the clinic's staff if any bookkeeping questions arise.

The team effort involving Dr. Wilkins, Brenda, and Mr. Schmidt results in a balanced budget for the clinic, and as a result, staff members are able to enjoy more benefits and perks.

While studying this chapter, think about the following questions:

- Why is a continuous flow of income preferable to a once-a-month influx for a provider's office?
- Why is it important to post charges, payments, and adjustments in a timely manner?
- What should Brenda do when a patient wants to make payments on an outstanding patient account balance?
- What should Brenda do when patient accounts are outstanding for more than 90 days after the date of service?

LEARNING OBJECTIVES

1. Define, spell, and pronounce terms listed in the vocabulary.
2. Define bookkeeping and all the different transactions recorded in patient accounts.
3. Do the following related to patient account records:
   - List the necessary data elements in patient account records.
   - Discuss a pegboard (manual bookkeeping) system.
   - Explain when transactions are recorded in the patient account.
   - Perform accounts receivable procedures for patient accounts, including charges, payments, and adjustments.
4. Describe special bookkeeping procedures for patient account records, including credit balances, third-party payments, and refunds; explain how to interact professionally with third-party representatives.
5. Discuss payment at the time of service, and give an example of displaying sensitivity when requesting payment for services rendered.
6. Describe the impact of the Truth in Lending Act on collections policies for patient accounts.
7. Discuss ways to obtain credit information, and explain patient billing and payment options.
8. Review policies and procedures for collecting outstanding balances on patient accounts.
9. Do the following related to collection procedures:
   - Describe successful collection techniques for patient accounts.
   - Discuss strategies for collecting outstanding balances through personal finance interviews.
   - Describe types of adjustments made to patient accounts, including nonsufficient checks (NSF) and collection agency transactions.
10. Define bookkeeping terms, including *accounts receivable* and *accounts payable*.
11. Discuss patient education, in addition to legal and ethical issues, related to patient accounts, collections, and practice management.

VOCABULARY

accounts payable The management of debt incurred and not yet paid.

accounts receivable Money that is expected but has not yet been received. The amount charged on the encounter form becomes the account receivable for the healthcare facility.

adjustments Credits posted to the patient account record when the provider's fee exceeds the amount allowed stated on the EOB.

anti-kickback statute A criminal law that prohibits the exchange of anything of value to reward the referral of a patient sponsored by a government insurance plan.

bookkeeping The recording of financial transactions in the patient account. records.

cash on hand The amount of money the healthcare facility has in the bank that can be withdrawn as cash.

collections The process of using all legal resources available to collect payment for past due patient account balances.

credit A bookkeeping entry that increases accounts receivable; money owed to the provider.

descendant A family member who takes responsibility for the patient's estate after his or her death.

executor An individual assigned to make financial decisions about the estate of a deceased patient.

guarantor The individual who subscribes to an insurance plan and accepts financial responsibility for the patient.

intangible Something of value that cannot be touched physically.

invoice A list of products or services provided to the healthcare facility for payment.

medically indigent Patients that are in need of medical care, yet cannot pay.

nonsufficient funds check (NSF) When a patient pays a check without having sufficient funds in the bank to cover the payment so it is returned to the provider unpaid.

pegboard system A manual bookkeeping system that uses a day sheet to record all financial transactions for the date of service and maintains patient account balances by using physical cards.

plaintiff The party filing a complaint.

provider's fee schedule Fees established by the provider for services rendered.

refunds Payments returned to insurance companies for overpayments made on patient accounts.

small claims court A last resort option to collect payment from an outstanding patient account; in small claims court, the healthcare facility can sue the patient for the balance.

trustee The coordinator of financial resources assigned by the court during a bankruptcy case.

unsecured debt Debt that is not guaranteed by something of value; credit card debt is the most common type of unsecured debt.

Every patient encounter is a financial transaction for a healthcare facility. Transactions generated by the patient encounter include a variety of charges, payments, and adjustments that need to be accounted for on a daily basis. Financial management is essential if the owner of a healthcare practice is to pay his or her business operating expenses. If the expenses of operating the healthcare facility exceed the fees collected for services rendered, the business will be forced to close.

A *patient account,* a running balance of all financial transactions under the patient's account record, is created when the healthcare provider renders services. Charges are applied to the patient account when an *encounter form* (Figure 18-1) is completed during the office visit; this form lists all the procedures and charges for services rendered.

BOOKKEEPING IN THE HEALTHCARE FACILITY

Bookkeeping is the recording of financial transactions in the patient account records. Most healthcare facilities use practice management software for daily bookkeeping transactions. The charges documented on the encounter form are used to complete the health insurance claim form, which shows the diagnosis, procedures, and associated charges. *Payments* to the healthcare facility come as reimbursement from the insurance company or a patient payment. **Adjustments** are made to a patient's account when it is necessary to add or subtract an amount, which is not a payment, from the balance; for example, the difference between the provider's charged amount and the contracted insurance payment amount.

PATIENT ACCOUNT RECORDS

All charges and payments for professional services are posted to the patient's account record daily. In this way, the record becomes a

reliable source of information for answering all inquiries from patients about their financial responsibilities. The patient account record should include all information pertinent to collecting the account, such as:

- Name and address of the **guarantor**
- Insurance identification information
- Home and business telephone numbers
- Name of employer
- Any special instructions for billing
- Emergency or alternative contact information

The patient account statement (Figure 18-2) provides a running balance, the result of all of the different financial transactions performed in the account, including charges, payments, adjustments and **credits**.

Entering and Posting Transactions in Patient Accounts

When a practice management software system is used, charges are entered into the record automatically from the encounter form after the office visit.

When a pegboard system is used (see the Manual Bookkeeping box), transactions are initiated before the patient goes to the exam room. The patient account ledger card is inserted under the first or next available receipt, and the first available writing line of the card is aligned with the carbonized strip on the receipt. Enter the receipt number and the date; enter the account balance in the space labeled *previous balance;* and then enter the patient's name. A copy of the receipt is detached and clipped to the patient's chart to be routed to the provider.

Posting Charges

Whether practice management software or a pegboard system is used, the charges posted to the patient's account should be taken

STATE LIC.# C1503X
SOC. SEC. # 000-11-0000
PIN # _____

College Clinic
4567 Broad Avenue
Woodland Hills, XY 12345-4700

Phone: 555-486-9002

☐ Private ☒ Bluecross ☐ Ind. ☐ Medicare ☐ Medi-cal ☐ Hmo ☐ Ppo

Patient's last name	First		Account #:	Birthdate	Sex ☐ Male	Today's date
Smith	Lydia		13845	09/13/92	☒ Female	09/17/20XX
Insurance company	Subscriber			Plan #	Sub. #	Group
Blue Shield of CA	Lydia Smith			0473	186-72-10XX	849-37000

ASSIGNMENT: I hereby assign my insurance benefits to be paid directly to the undersigned physician, I am financially responsible for non-covered services.
SIGNED: Patient,
or parent, if minor *Lydia Smith*   Today's date 09/17/20XX

RELEASE: I hereby authorize the physician to release to my insurance carriers any information require to process this claim.
SIGNED: Patient,
or parent, if minor *Lydia Smith*   Today's date 09/17/20XX

✓	DESCRIPTION	CODE	FEE	✓	DESCRIPTION	CODE	FEE	✓	DESCRIPTION	CODE	FEE
	OFFICE VISITS	NEW EST.			Venipuncture	36415			OFFICE PROCEDURES		
	Blood pressure check	99211			TB skin test	86580			Anoscopy	46600	
	Level II	99202 99212			Hematocrit	85013			Ear lavage	69210	
	Level III	99203 99213			Glucose finger stick	82948			Spirometry	94010	
X	Level IV	99204 99214	$175		IMMUNIZATIONS				Nebulizer Rx	94664	
	Level V	99205 99215			Allergy inj. X1	95115			EKG	93000	
	PREVENTIVE EXAMS	NEW EST.			Allergy inj. X2	95117			SURGERY		
	Age 65 and older	99387 99397			Trigger pt. inj.	20552			Mole removal (1st)	17110	
	Age 40 - 64	99386 99396			Therapeutic inj.	96372			(2nd to 14th)	17003	
	Age 18 - 39	99385 99395			VACCINATION PRODUCTS				Flat warts (1st - 14th)	07110	
	Age 12 - 17	99384 99394			DPT	90701			15 or more	17111	
	Age 5 - 11	99383 99393			DT	90702			Biopsy, 1 lesion	11100	
	Age 1 - 4	99382 99392			Tetanus	90703			Addt'l. lesions	11101	
	Infant	99381 99391			MMR	90707			Endometrial Bx	58100	
	Newborn ofc	99432			OPV	90712			Skin tags to 15	11200	
	OB/NEWBORN CARE				Polio inj.	90713			Each addt'l. 10	11201	
	OB package	59400			Flu	90662			I & D abscess	10060	
	Post-partum visit N/C				Hemophilus B	90645			SUPPLIES/MISCELLANEOUS		
	LAB PROCEDURES				Hepatitis B vac.	90746			Surgical tray	99070	
	Urine dip	81000			Pneumovax	90670			Handling charge	99000	
	UA qualitative	81005			VACCINE ADMINISTRATION				Special report	99080	
X	Pregnancy urine	81025	20.00		Age: Through 18 yrs. (1st inj.)	90460			DOCTOR'S NOTES:		
	Wet mount	87210			Age: Through 18 yrs. (ea. addt'l. inj.)	90461					
	kOH prip	87220			Adult (1st inj.)	90471					
	Occult blood	82270			Adult (ea. addt'l. inj.)	90472					

DIAGNOSES ICD-10-CM		
_ Abdominal pain/unspec..R10.9	_ Colitis/unspec...........K51.90	_ FUO...................R50.9	_ Osteoarthritis (site)......M19._
_ Absess.................L02._	_ Confusion.............R41.0	_ Gastritis................K29.70	_ Otitis media...........H66.9_
_ Allergic reaction........T78.40_	_ CHF...................I50.9	_ Gastroenteritis (colitis)..K52.9	_ Parkinson's disease.....G20
_ Alzheimer's disease.....G30	_ Constipation...........K59.00	_ G.I. bleed.............K92.2	_ Pharyngitis, acute......J02.9
_ Anemia/unspec........D64.9	_ COPD.................J44.9	_ Gout/unspec..........M10.9	_ Pleurisy..............R09.1
_ Angina/unspec........I20.9	_ Cough.................R05	_ Headache.............R51	_ Pneumonia...........J18.9
_ Anorexia..............R63.0	_ Crohn's disease/unspec..K50.90	_ Health exam...........200._	_ Pneumonia, viral.......J12.9
_ Anxiety/unspec........F41.9	_ CVA..................I63.9	_ Hematuria/unspec......R31.9	_ Prostatitis/unspec......N41.9
_ Apnea, sleep..........G47.30	_ Decubitus ulcer........L89._	_ Herpes simplex........B00.9	_ PVD.................I73.9
_ Arrhythmia, cardiac.....I49.9	_ Dehydration...........E86.0	_ Herpes zoster.........B02.9	_ Radiculopathy........M54.1_
_ Arthritis, rheumatoid....M06.9	_ Dementia/unspec......F03	_ Hiatal hernia..........K44.9	_ Rectal bleeding........K62.5
_ Asthma/unspec........J45.909	_ Depression, major/unsp..F32.9	_ HTN (HBP)............I10	_ Renal failure..........N19
_ Atrial fibrillation........I48.0	_ Diab I, no complications..E10.0	_ Hyperlipidemia/unspec..E78.5	_ Sciatica..............M54.3_
_ B-12 deficiency.........E53.8	_ Diab II, no complications..E11.9	_ Hypothyroidism/unspec..E03.9	_ Shortness of breath.....R03.02
_ Back pain, low.........M54.5	_ w/kidney complic.....E11.2_	_ Impotentce...........N52._	_ Sinusitis, chr./unspec....J32.9
_ BPH.................N40	_ w/ophthalmic compl...E11.3_	_ Influenza, respiratory....J10.1	_ Syncope.............R55
_ Bradycardia/unspec.....R00.1	_ w/neurolog.compl.....E11.4_	_ Insomnia.............G47.0	_ Tachycardia/unspec.....R00.0
_ Broncitis, acute.........J20._	_ w/circulatory cmpl....E11.5_	_ IBS, diarrhea..........K58.	_ Tachy., supraventric....I47.1
_ Bronchitis, chronic......J42	_ Insulin use............Z79.4	_ Lupus, systemic erythim..M32.9	_ Tendinitis/unspec......M77.9
_ Bursitis/unspec.........M71.9	_ Diarrhea/unspec.......R19.7	_ MI, acute.............I21._	_ TIA.................G45.9
_ CA, breast............C50._	_ Diverticulitix..........K57.92	_ MI, old...............I25.2	_ Ulcer, duodenal/unspec..K26.9
_ CA, lung..............C34._	_ Diverticulosis.........K57.90	_ Migraine.............G43.9	_ Ulcer, gastric/unspec....K25.9
_ CA, prostate..........C61	_ Dizziness.............R42	_ Myalgia..............M79.1	_ Ulcer, peptic/unspec....K27.9
_ Cellulitis..............L03._	_ Dysuria...............R30.0	_ Neck pain............M54.2	_ URI/unspec...........J06.9
_ Chest pain/unspec......R07.9	_ Edema/unspec........R60.9	_ Neuropathy..........G62.9	_ UTI.................N39.0
_ Cirrhosis, liver/unspec...K74.60	_ Endocarditis..........I38	_ Nausea..............R11.1	_ Vertigo..............R42
_ Cold, common........J00	_ Esophageal reflux......K21.0	X Nausea/vomiting.......R11.0	_ Weight gain..........R63.5
	_ Fatigue (lethargy)......R53.83	_ Obesity/unspec.......E66.9	_ Weight loss..........R63.4

Diagnosis/additional description:
Pregnancy

Doctor's signature/date
Dr. B. Caesar   09-17-20XX

Return appointment information:	-with whom	Self other	Rec'd by:	Total today's fee	$195
Days Wks. Mos. 1 month			☐ Cash		
			☐ Check	Co-payment	$35
PLEASE RMEMBER THAT PAYMENT IS YOUR OBLIGATION, REGARDLESS OF INSURANCE OR OTHER THIRD PARTY INVOLVEMENT.			☐ Credit # _____	Amount rec'd. today	

FIGURE 18-1 Encounter form with charges. (Courtesy of Bibbero Systems, an InHealth Company, Petaluma, Calif.)

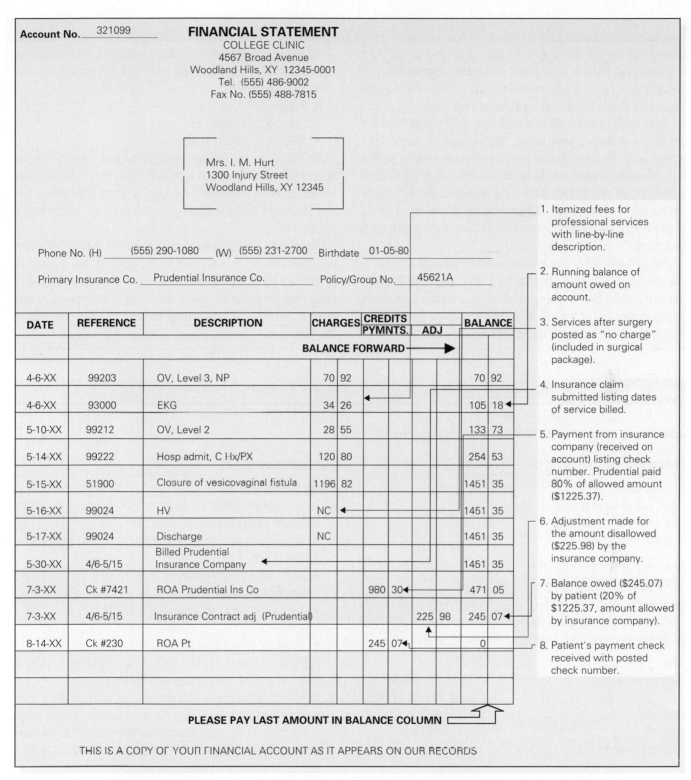

FIGURE 18-2 Patient account statement. (From Fordney WT: *Insurance handbook for the medical office*, ed 14, St. Louis, 2017, Elsevier.)

from the **provider's fee schedule**. Patient account management software systems automatically put in the correct fees or charges when a CPT/HCPCS* code is entered (Procedure 18-1).

When checking out a patient using a pegboard system, the medical assistant should insert the ledger card under the proper receipt and check the number previously entered to make sure the correct card is being used. Record the service by procedure code, post the charge from the fee schedule, enter any payment made, and write in the current balance. If there is no balance, place a zero or a straight line in the balance column.

CPT, Current Procedural Terminology; HCPCS, Healthcare Common Procedure Coding System.

Manual Bookkeeping

Although we live in a technology-savvy world, many providers still use a manual **pegboard system**. In many cases, providers who have been in practice for many years do not want to invest in a patient account software system because the manual system is so logical and practical to use.

Some certifying exams still include questions about manual systems. If the office experiences a power outage, the employees will have to use a manual system for the period in which patients are seen while the power is out. The medical assistant must be familiar with both manual and electronic patient account management systems. The pegboard is the most popular manual system for this purpose. It is simple to operate, and once a medical assistant learns the pegboard system, computer systems are much easier to understand.

The pegboard system gets its name from the lightweight aluminum or Masonite board that is used. This board has a row of pegs along the side or top that holds the forms in place. The patient account ledger cards are perforated for alignment on the pegs. All the forms used in any system must be compatible so that they can be aligned perfectly on the board.

The pegboard system generates all the necessary financial records for each transaction (by writing once with carbon paper) as follows:
- Encounter form
- Receipt
- Patient account ledger card
- Bookkeeping transaction entry

The system also may include a statement and bank deposit slip. It provides current accounts receivable totals and a daily record of bank deposits and **cash on hand**, in addition to the record of income and expenses. The need for separate posting to patient accounts is eliminated, and the chance for error is reduced.

The pegboard system allows the medical assistant to keep control over cash, collections, and receivables and ensures that every cent is accounted for and properly entered. It provides a record of every patient, every charge, and every payment, plus a daily recap of earnings—a running record of receivables and an audited summary of cash—and requires little time.

PROCEDURE 18-1 **Perform Accounts Receivable Procedures for Patient Accounts: Charges**

Goal: *To enter charges into the patient account record manually and electronically.*

EQUIPMENT and SUPPLIES

- Patient account ledger card
- SimChart for the Medical Office software
- Encounter form/Superbill
- Provider's fee schedule

Scenario 1: *Ken Thomas is a returning patient of Dr. Martin. He makes his $50 copayment at the time of the office visit.*

Scenario 2: *Martha Bravo is seeing Dr. Walden. He is being seen for hypertension (ICD-10-CM I10) for the first time for hypothyroidism (ICD-10-CM E03.9). She makes the $30 copayment at the time of the office visit.*

Name	Martha Bravo
Address	1234 Anywhere Station
	Anytown, Anystate 12345
Contact #1	(212) 555-1212
Contact #2	(212) 554-1313
Emergency Contact	John Bravo (212) 555-2627
DOB	1/23/56
SSN	111-22-3333
Health Insurance Information	Aetna
	Subscriber: Martha Bravo
	Subscriber DOB: 1/23/56
	ID #: XEK3332328748
	Group #: X1000
	Effective Date: 1/1/20-
Employer Information	Name: Malibu Gardening
	Contact: (212) 555-5151

PROCEDURAL STEPS

Posting Charges Manually

1. For new patients, create the patient account by entering the following information on a patient account ledger card:
   - Patient's full name, address, and at least two contact phone numbers
   - Date of birth
   - Health insurance information, including the subscriber number, group number, and effective date
   - Subscriber's name and date of birth (if the subscriber is not the patient)
   - Employer's name and contact information

   PURPOSE: To keep all insurance and collection information available with the patient account record balance for reference.

2. For returning patients, review the account record to see whether a balance is due. If there is a balance, bring this to the patient's attention when he or she comes for the appointment. Respectfully explain that the provider would appreciate a payment on the previous balance before he or she can care for the patient. Use the following dialogue:

   Brenda: Good morning, Ken. How are you feeling today?

   Ken: Not so good, I really need to see Dr. Martin again because my headaches have been getting worse.

   Brenda: I'm sorry to hear that. Let's get you in to see the doctor right away. I can collect the $50 copayment for today's visit, and here is a statement for your previous balance of $214. How would you like to take care of that today?

   Ken: Oh, I didn't know about the previous balance. Can I just pay the copayment today?

PROCEDURE 18-1   *—continued*

Brenda: Dr. Martin would like at least half of this previous balance paid before seeing you today, please. I know that medical bills can pile up pretty quick, but Dr. Martin would like to continue to provide you with quality care so you can feel back to yourself really soon.

Ken: Yes, I know you're right. I need to keep coming to see Dr. Martin. I can pay half of the $214 today, along with the copayment.

Brenda: Thanks, I know Dr. Martin really appreciates you as a patient. Would that be check or credit card?

Ken: Credit card, please.

Brenda: Okay, here is the credit card receipt and a copy of the updated statement. By the way, I'd like to document on your patient account when you will be able to pay the rest of this statement amount.

Ken: I'll pay the balance next month; is that okay?

Brenda: I'll let Dr. Martin know and put a note in your account. Thanks; you'll be called in shortly.

PURPOSE: To respectfully inform the patient of his or her financial obligations and the provider's intention of having the previous balance paid in full.

3. After seeing the patient, the provider completes the encounter form, which includes all procedures and the associated fee schedule. Using the completed encounter form (see Figure 18-1), enter the charges manually on the ledger card for the patient's account record. Total all the charges on the encounter form for the services rendered. Then subtract the copayment made from the total charges. The previous balance, if any, is added to this new total. Use the following worksheet to calculate the new balance. The new balance-due amount should be presented to the patient before he or she leaves the healthcare facility.

Total Charges	$_____
Amount paid (copayment)	$_____
+ Previous balance (if any)	$_____
= New Balance Due	$_____

PROCEDURAL STEPS

Posting Charges in SimChart for the Medical Office

1. After logging into SimChart, locate the established patient by clicking on Find Patient, enter the patient's name, verify DOB, and click on the radio button. This will bring you to the Clinical Care tab. If there is no encounter shown, create an encounter by clicking on Office Visit under Info Panel on the left, select a visit type, and click on Save. Once an encounter has been created, return to the Patient Dashboard and click on the Superbill link on the right (or click on the Coding and Billing tab).

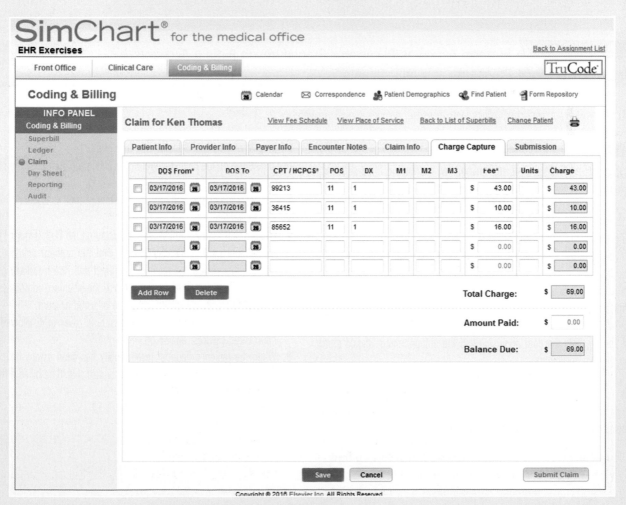

PROCEDURE 18-1 *—continued*

2. From the Superbill area, in the Encounters Not Coded section, click on the encounter (in blue). On page 1 enter the diagnosis in the Diagnosis field and document the services provided (additional services are found on pages 2-3 of the Superbill).
3. Complete the information needed on page 4 of the Superbill and submit.

4. Click on Ledger on the left and search for your patient. Once your patient has been located, click on the arrow across from the name in the ledger.
5. Enter the services provided and the payment received. Click on the Add Row button to continue to add services. The balance will be auto-calculated for you.

Posting Payments

All payments, including those received by mail or electronically, or when the patient pays the copay at the time of the appointment, are entered into the patient's account as a credit.

Payments should be posted by line item corresponding to the submitted health insurance claim (Procedure 18-2). All insurance payment amounts posted should match the total amount paid on the Explanation of Benefits (EOB) (Figure 18-3).

Posting Adjustments

Adjustments are credits posted to the patient account record when the provider's fee exceeds the amount allowed stated on the EOB. Adjustments should always be posted to the patient account record at the same time as the payment. Under the Health Information Technology for Economic and Clinical Health (HITECH) Act of 2009, healthcare providers may not discount the patient's financial responsibility after the health insurance has paid its portion;

PROCEDURE 18-2 Perform Accounts Receivable Procedures in Patient Accounts: Payments and Adjustments

Goal: *To process payments and adjustments to patient accounts records accurately.*

EQUIPMENT and SUPPLIES

- Patient account ledgers card, or SimChart for the Medical Office software
- Explanation of Benefits (EOB) (see Figure 18-3)

PROCEDURAL STEPS

Posting Payments and Adjustments Manually

1. Review the EOB for multiple patient accounts received by the healthcare facility.
2. Look up the ledger card for the patient account (or the patient ledger in SimChart) and compare the date of service on the EOB and with the date shown on the ledger card. Also, compare the amount charged for the dates of service; both the date of service and the amount charge should match on the two documents.
   PURPOSE: To confirm that the payment and adjustment posted are shown for the correct patient, date of service, and procedure.
3. Post the payment and adjustment line by line. To confirm the accuracy of the figures, the following formula can be used:

Total charged = Insurance payment amount + Amount adjusted
+ Patient responsibility or Secondary
insurance responsibility

Posting Payments and Adjustments in SimChart

Use a new line on the patient ledger in the patient account to post an insurance payment.

1. After one line on the EOB has been posted, post all subsequent lines on the EOB separately.
2. Confirm that the adjustment was necessary on the EOB (Figure 1). Review the amount paid. If there is concern that the amount adjusted was too much, either review the provider's contract with the insurance company's fee schedule to compare payments, or call the insurance company's provider services to inquire about the applicable adjusted amount.
   PURPOSE: Adjustments may be necessary in cases of disallowed charges, noncovered services, and so on.
3. When the patient's financial responsibility has been established, send the patient a statement. The secondary insurance should be billed if the patient is covered.

PROCEDURE 18-2   *—continued*

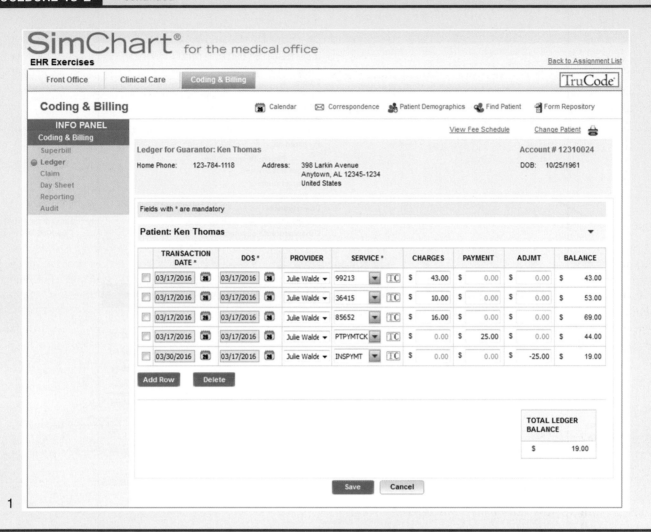

1

therefore, providers can adjust only the amount in the patient account approved by the health insurance company. The only other circumstance in which an adjustment can be made is when a patient or guarantor files for bankruptcy; the entire patient account balance then must be adjusted off the books.

The patient account record should have a column for the adjustment to be posted as a credit. <u>Remember, payments and adjustments are both credits</u>; however, payments are money that is received in the healthcare facility, and adjustments simply reduce the balance the patient owes on the account. When the payments and adjustments are subtracted from the charged amount, the balance is either the patient responsibility or the amount billed to the secondary insurance.

Before continuing to post to the next EOB line item, confirm that the payment amount, the adjusted amount, and the patient responsibility/secondary insurance balance match exactly the amounts calculated on the EOB (see Procedure 18-2).

Special Bookkeeping Entries for Patient Account Records

The following special bookkeeping entries are sometimes necessary to keep the patient account record in balance. They may be performed either with the practice management software or a pegboard system:

- Credit balances
- Third-party payments
- Refunds

Credit Balances

A *credit balance* occurs when a patient has paid in advance, or an overpayment or duplicate payment is made. For example, an overpayment occurs if the patient makes a partial payment and later the insurance allowance is more than the remaining balance. When this happens, the patient account will show a credit balance, or an amount that the provider owes. The medical assistant should

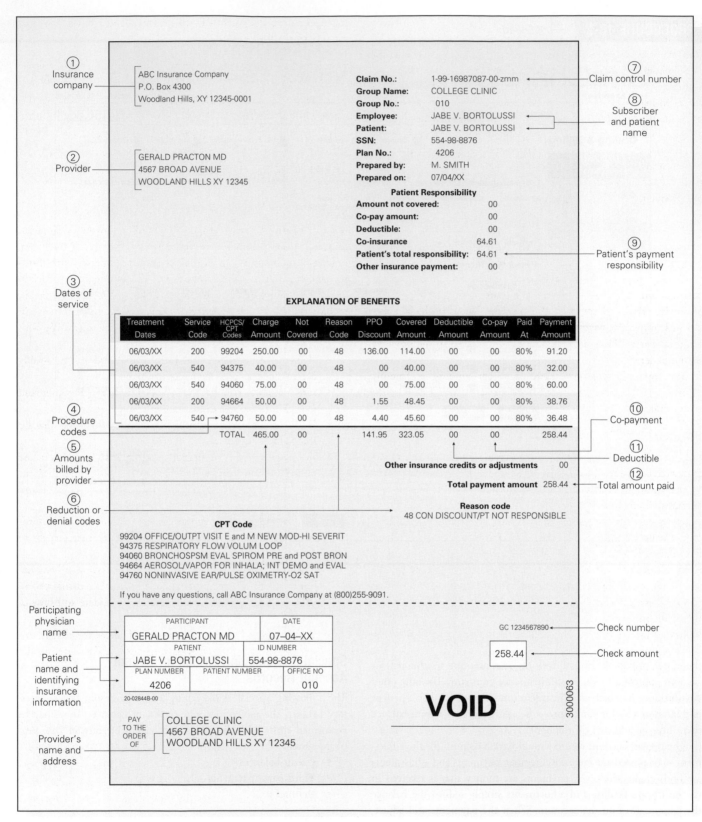

FIGURE 18-3 Explanation of Benefits (EOB). (From Fordney MT: *Insurance handbook for the medical office,* ed 14, St Louis, 2017, Elsevier.)

investigate to whom the credit balance is owed (i.e., the patient or the insurance company). The first place to investigate is the EOB from the insurance company; this document shows the exact amount of the patient's financial responsibility. The medical assistant should confirm that all the line items match the corresponding amounts on the EOB because many credit balances are created when an error is made in payment posting. If the patient's payment exceeded the amount indicated on the EOB, the provider must send a check for the balance to the patient. A credit balance creates a *debit* in the patient account, or an amount that is due by the provider to the patient or the insurance company, depending on which party made the overpayment.

Third-Party Payments

Third-party payments are reimbursement payments made by an insurance company that provides benefits for the patient. In other words, third-party payers pay the healthcare provider on behalf of the patient. Once the third party pays the insurance claim for the date of service, the total owed to the provider becomes the amount charged minus the payment amount and the amount adjusted by the third party. The remaining balance is still owed to the provider by the patient.

The total charged = insurance payment amount + amount adjusted + patient responsibility or secondary insurance responsibility.

Refunds

Just like credit balances, refunds create a credit in the patient account that needs to be accounted for. **Refunds** are returned payments made to the insurance companies for overpayments made on patient accounts. Sometimes overpayments occur if the health insurance company pays for the same patient, date of service, and procedures more than once by accident. The medical assistant should compare the original EOB to the second EOB to confirm that an overpayment has occurred. If both EOBs show the same payment for the same date of service, refund one payment. If the two EOBs show two different payments, call provider services for the health insurance plan to ensure proper payment to the patient account. The healthcare facility cannot keep the higher payment and return the lower payment. The medical assistant should contact provider services at the health insurance plan to confirm which payment they were supposed to receive and the reasoning behind the payment amount.

Once the amount of the refund has been confirmed, the medical office manager should send the insurance company a check, along with the necessary documentation confirming the refund amount, including a copy of both EOBs and a printout of the patient account ledger.

Most patient account management software can enter charges, payments, and adjustments. As discussed previously, charges increase what is owed to the provider, whereas payments and adjustments reduce what is owed to the provider. However, credit balances and refunds, if not handled properly, can reduce what is owed to the provider erroneously. A credit balance or refund is owed to the patient or to the insurance company; it does not belong to the healthcare facility. A note indicating that there is a refund on the patient account should be recorded, and the healthcare facility office

manager should document all credit balances and refunds in a separate electronic ledger file.

Interacting With Third-Party Representatives

Most health insurance plans sponsor an online provider Web portal for checking on verification of eligibility and claim status. However, in some circumstances medical assistants must interact with third-party representatives. This can be a time-consuming process involving waiting on hold on the telephone for long periods; nevertheless, medical assistants represent their healthcare facility, and they still must interact professionally. Here are some tips for interacting with third-party representatives:

- Before calling provider services, have all documents readily accessible to discuss the patient account
- Use headphones so that the music played while the phone call is on hold does not disturb the rest of the office
- If a long wait time is expected, work on other tasks that do not require phone use
- When the health insurance representative comes on the phone, refrain from telling him or her how long the wait was; representatives usually do not have much control over wait times
- Use the documents set aside for the phone call to confirm the patient's identity quickly so as to get to the purpose of the call
- Document the details of the phone conversation with the health insurance representative in the patient account record, including the representative's name and the date and time of the call
- If the conversation is a follow-up call, share the details collected from the previous call from notes documented in the patient account record

Payment at the Time of Service

Healthcare facilities accept the patient's health insurance card and copayment as good faith that the practice will be paid for the services rendered. For the most part, patients are expected to pay their copayment at the time of service unless previous arrangements have been made (Figure 18-4). Patients without health insurance should pay

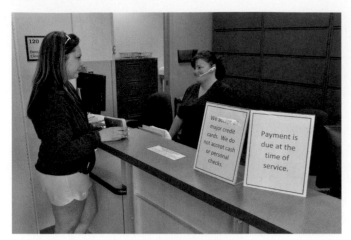

FIGURE 18-4 Most healthcare facilities display a sign informing patients that payments are due at the time of service.

after the charges for the day have been totaled. Patients should be informed when making an appointment that payment is expected at the time of service so that they are not surprised when asked for payment at the healthcare facility. The medical assistant may say, "Your charge for today is $25. Will that be cash, check, credit, or debit card?" If a patient asks to be billed, the medical assistant may say, "Our normal procedure is to pay at the time of service unless other arrangements are made in advance."

Displaying Sensitivity When Requesting Payment

The medical assistant must believe that the provider has a right to charge for the services rendered. Do not be embarrassed to ask for payment for the valuable services that have been provided. Remember that the practice is a business, and the provider must meet the obligations involved in keeping it fiscally healthy, including salary expenses. When tact and good judgment are used in billing and collecting, patients appreciate the service they receive and the help the medical assistant provides. Give each patient individual attention and personal consideration; also, be courteous and show a sincere desire to help the patient with financial problems.

CRITICAL THINKING APPLICATION   **18-3**

Adam Page comes to the front desk to pay his copay with a credit card. His card is declined. How can Brenda handle the situation? What options could be offered to Mr. Page to make a payment at the time of service?

Billing After a Payment Agreement Has Been Made

Most providers prefer payment before or at the time of service. However, if fees for surgery or long-term or expensive therapy are involved, payment arrangements become necessary, and a regular system of billing must be established. The medical assistant therefore must explain to the patient the professional fees, the services the charges cover, and the office credit policies. In most healthcare practices, the appropriate staff member sits down with the patient for a financial consultation before a payment arrangement contract is offered (Figure 18-5). The payment arrangement contract states the

monthly payment; how many months it must be paid; the payment due date; whether interest will be charged; and the penalties of nonpayment.

Using Credit for Medical Services

Some healthcare facilities distribute information about credit cards or loans available specifically for healthcare treatments. This is very popular for cosmetic surgeries, dental procedures, and laser eye surgeries. Offices that offer these types of procedures may want to investigate such alternative financing services. Although these options are valuable when used properly and repaid on time, they do create additional debt for the patient. As an alternative, the healthcare facility may allow the patient to split large healthcare expenses into two or three interest-free lump sum payments so that the patient does not incur credit card interest charges.

TRUTH IN LENDING ACT

When offering credit options for patients, the medical practice should be in compliance with Regulation Z of the Truth in Lending Act (TILA). TILA is enforced by the Federal Trade Commission (FTC) and is part of the Consumer Credit Protection Act. TILA requires that individuals be provided certain information when credit is extended, including the annual percentage rate (APR), the terms of the loan, and the total costs to the borrower. If an agreement exists between provider and patient that the practice will accept full payment in more than four installments, the practice must provide a Federal Truth in Lending Statement (Figure 18-6), even if no finance fees are charged. The statement is signed by the practice's representative and the patient.

Healthcare facilities occasionally allow their patients to pay in installments (although this practice is much less common than in the past). As long as no specific agreement has been made for payment to the provider in more than four installments and no finance charge is assessed, the account is not subject to TILA and does not require a signed Truth in Lending Statement.

OBTAINING CREDIT INFORMATION

Credit information is confidential. It should be guarded as carefully as confidential health information and should never be disclosed to unauthorized individuals. If a call is received about a patient's credit history, follow the healthcare facility's policy, based on regulations established by the Health Insurance Portability and Accountability Act (HIPAA) and legal guidelines in your state. When asking for credit information from patients in the office, do so in a private area where others cannot overhear the conversation. A patient should be able to complete a credit application in an area separate from the reception area, where the patient can sit in total privacy. Never access a credit report on patients unless it is necessary to process an application for credit privileges at the healthcare facility and the patient authorizes it.

MONTHLY PATIENT ACCOUNT STATEMENTS

Healthcare facilities should send monthly statements for all patient account records that have a balance due. These statements should be

PATIENT AGREEMENT

Patient's Name James Doland Soc. Sec. # 431-XX-1942

Address 67 Blyth Dr., Woodland Hills, XY 12345 Tel. No. 555-372-0101

WC Insurance Carrier Industrial Indemnity Company

Address 30 North Dr., Woodland Hills Telephone No. 555-731-7707

Date of illness 2-13-20XX Date of first visit 2-13-20XX

Emergency Yes X No

Is this condition related to employment Yes X No

If accident: Auto Other

Where did injury occur? Construction site

How did injury happen? fell 8 ft from scaffold suffering fractured right tibia

Employee/employer who verified this information Scott McPherson

Employer's name and address Willow Construction Company

Employer's telephone no. 555-526-0611

In the event the claim for workers' compensation is declared fraudulent for this illness or condition or it is determined by the Workers' Compensation Board that the illness or injury is not a compensable workers' compensation case, I James Doland , hereby agree to pay the physician's fee for services rendered.

I have been informed that I am responsible to pay any services rendered by Dr. Raymond Skeleton with regard to the discovery and treatment of any condition not related to the workers' compensation injury or illness. I agree to pay for all services not covered by workers' compensation and all charges for treatment and personal items unrelated to my workers' compensation illness or injury.

Signed James Doland Date 2-13-20XX

FIGURE 18-5 Patient payment agreement. (From Fordney MT: *Insurance handbook for the medical office*, ed 14, St Louis, 2017, Elsevier.)

computer generated at the beginning of each month for patient accounts that are 90 days past due or less. The patient account statement should make a visual impact, just as a letter does; therefore, the statement heads should be printed on clean, good-quality paper. Payment options such as check, e-check, online payments, and/or credit card should be presented clearly. The font on the statement should be large enough to be read easily and should provide itemized details on the following:
- Charges for the date of service
- Insurance payments and adjustments
- Patient payments, including copayments at the time of service

Envelopes should be imprinted with "Address Service Requested" in the appropriate place to maintain up-to-date mailing lists. A self-addressed return envelope included with the statement is convenient for the patient and encourages prompt payment. The statement should also indicate how old the balance is, such as "Balance now 30 days past due." For accounts that are more than 60 days past due, some offices apply neon-colored stickers to emphasize the need to pay the balance as soon as possible, thus avoiding further collection activity.

Medicare Advance Beneficiary Notices

Medicare does not cover some healthcare services so the *Advanced Beneficiary Notice* (ABN) is presented to patients in these circumstances. The ABN provides an option for patients to pay the provider's fee in full to receive services that Medicare does not cover. The patient decides whether he or she still wants to receive the services from the provider and completes the information on the form (Figure 18-7).

Professional Courtesy

In the past some providers did not charge professional colleagues or their close family members for medical care; this concept is called *professional courtesy*. However, this has led to fraud in the industry because some providers would recommend patients to auxiliary facilities from which the provider would receive compensation for the referral. The Stark law, which was passed to eliminate such fraud, imposes the following restrictions on professional courtesy:
- The professional courtesy must be extended to all members of the healthcare facility, not just a single provider
- The services provided must be routine for the healthcare facility extending the professional courtesy

LEONARD S. TAYLOR, M.D.
2100 West Park Avenue
Champaign, Illinois 61820

Telephone 351-5400

FEDERAL TRUTH IN LENDING STATEMENT
For professional services rendered

Patient _____ Joseph Brookhurst _____
Address _____ 353 West Terry Lane _____
_____ Birmingham, Alabama 35209 _____
Parent _____

1. Cash Price (fee for service)	$	1200.00
2. Cash Down Payment	$	200.00
3. Unpaid Balance of Cash Price	$	1000.00
4. Amount Financed	$	1000.00
5. FINANCE CHARGE	$	–0–
6. Finance Charge Expressed As Annual Percentage Rate		–0–
7. Total of Payments (4 plus 5)	$	1000.00
8. Deferred Payment Price (1 plus 5)	$	1200.00

"Total payment due" (7 above) is payable to Dr. Leonard S.
Taylor at above office address in five monthly installments
of $ 200.00 . The first installment is payable on May 1
19 xx , and each subsequent payment is due on the same
day of each consecutive month until paid in full.

4-15-2xxx   *Joseph Brookhurst*
Date   Signature of Patient; Parent if Patient is a Minor

FORM 9402 COLWELL SYSTEMS, INC., CHAMPAIGN, ILLINOIS

FIGURE 18-6 Truth in Lending Statement. (Courtesy Colwell Systems, Champaign, Ill.)

- The professional courtesy must be set forth in writing in advance by the healthcare facility's board of directors
- The professional courtesy cannot be extended to Medicare patients or other federal beneficiaries unless there is documentation of financial need
- The professional courtesy cannot violate any **anti-kickback statute** or state law

---

CRITICAL THINKING APPLICATION   **18-4**

Dr. Wilkins has just finished seeing Dr. James Franklin, who came to her as a patient. Dr. Franklin insists to Brenda that Dr. Wilkins always extends him professional courtesy. Brenda is not aware of an approved professional courtesy agreement with Dr. Franklin. However a professional courtesy agreement with Dr. Franklin is not on file. Whom should Brenda talk to?

Billing Minors

According to federal regulations, minors cannot be held financially responsible for their patient account balance unless they are emancipated. Bills for minors are usually addressed to a parent or legal guardian. If a bill is addressed to a minor, parents could take the attitude that they are not responsible because they never received a statement.

If the parents are separated or divorced, the parent who brings the child in for treatment is responsible for payment. Whatever financial agreement exists between the parents is strictly their personal business and should not concern the healthcare practice. The responsible parent should be so informed from the first appointment.

If a minor appears in the office and requests treatment, and you can ascertain that the person is legally emancipated, the minor can assume financial responsiblity. It may be wise to make a determination either with the office manager or with the provider as to whether the office wishes to treat an emancipated minor. Minors can be treated for certain conditions, such as sexually transmitted diseases (STDs), pregnancy, and birth control, without parental consent. In these cases, the medical assistant must determine where the patient account statement should be sent.

Medical Care for Those Who Cannot Pay

The medical profession traditionally has accepted the responsibility of providing medical care occasionally for individuals unable to pay for these services. Despite the increased scope of government-sponsored care for the **medically indigent,** providers still spend thousands of dollars each year providing services before securing some type of payment.

In many instances medical care of the indigent is available through social service agencies. Medical assistants should learn about local organizations and agencies that can aid patients in obtaining the necessary assistance. The provider can provide only medical services. Other agencies provide hospitalization, for example, or arrange for paying the costs of special therapy, rehabilitation, or medications. Unfortunately, another segment of the population consists of uninsured employees who are not eligible for public assistance, are not covered under a group policy, and cannot afford the high premiums for private medical insurance. Give special attention to helping these people arrange payment of their medical bills. If a provider accepts a case in advance for which a fee will not be paid, complete records must still be kept on the patient. The only deviation in procedure is that the financial record indicates no charge in the debit column.

Fees in Hardship Cases

Sometimes a healthcare practice is faced with the problem of deciding whether to reduce or cancel a fee in a hardship case. Before adjusting or canceling a fee, the provider or medical assistant should have a frank discussion with the patient about his or her financial situation. Find out whether the patient is entitled to or qualifies for medical assistance. For instance, if the patient's injuries are the result of a car accident, there may be medical insurance through the automobile policy. Circumstances may qualify the patient for local or state public assistance, such as crime victim assistance. Maintain information about such agencies that are available in the area and direct the patient to the appropriate one.

Discuss the fee in advance and make payment arrangements if the circumstances of hardship are known before services are rendered. The healthcare practice may suggest that a medically indigent patient seek care at a county hospital with public assistance. A provider should be free to choose his or her form of charity and should

A. Notifier: John Doe, MD, College Clinic, 4567 Broad Avenue, Woodland Hills, XY 12345 555-486-9002

B. Patient Name: Mary Judd   **C. Identification Number:** 0920XX7291

Advance Beneficiary Notice of Noncoverage (ABN)

NOTE: If Medicare doesn't pay for **D.** _B12 injections_ below, you may have to pay.
Medicare does not pay for everything, even some care that you or your health care provider have good reason to think you need. We expect Medicare may not pay for the **D.** _B12 injections_ below.

D.	E. Reason Medicare May Not Pay:	F. Estimated Cost
B12 injections	Medicare does not usually pay for this injection or this many injections	$35.00

WHAT YOU NEED TO DO NOW:
- Read this notice, so you can make an informed decision about your care.
- Ask us any questions that you may have after you finish reading.
- Choose an option below about whether to receive the **D.** _B12 injections_ listed above.
  Note: If you choose Option 1 or 2, we may help you to use any other insurance that you might have, but Medicare cannot require us to do this.

G. OPTIONS: Check only one box. We cannot choose a box for you.

☒ **OPTION 1.** I want the **D.** _B12 injections_ listed above. You may ask to be paid now, but I also want Medicare billed for an official decision on payment, which is sent to me on a Medicare Summary Notice (MSN). I understand that if Medicare doesn't pay, I am responsible for payment, but **I can appeal to Medicare** by following the directions on the MSN. If Medicare does pay, you will refund any payments I made to you, less co-pays or deductibles.

☐ **OPTION 2.** I want the **D.** _____ listed above, but do not bill Medicare. You may ask to be paid now as I am responsible for payment. **I cannot appeal if Medicare is not billed.**

☐ **OPTION 3.** I don't want the **D.** _____ listed above. I understand with this choice I am **not** responsible for payment, and **I cannot appeal to see if Medicare would pay.**

H. Additional Information:

This notice gives our opinion, not an official Medicare decision. If you have other questions on this notice or Medicare billing, call **1-800-MEDICARE** (1-800-633-4227/TTY: 1-877-486-2048).
Signing below means that you have received and understand this notice. You also receive a copy.

I. Signature: *Mary Judd*	J. Date: *March 20, 20XX*

According to the Paperwork Reduction Act of 1995, no persons are required to respond to a collection of information unless it displays a valid OMB control number. The valid OMB control number for this information collection is 0938-0566. The time required to complete this information collection is estimated to average 7 minutes per response, including the time to review instructions, search existing data resources, gather the data needed, and complete and review the information collection. If you have comments concerning the accuracy of the time estimate or suggestions for improving this form, please write to: CMS, 7500 Security Boulevard, Attn: PRA Reports Clearance Officer, Baltimore, Maryland 21244-1850.

Form CMS-R-131 (03/11)   Form Approved OMB No. 0938-0566

FIGURE 18-7 Advance Beneficiary Notice for Medicare patients. (From Fordney MT: *Insurance handbook for the medical office,* ed 14, St Louis, 2017, Elsevier.)

not feel obligated to substantially reduce or cancel a fee when the circumstances are known in advance.

The provider and the patient may agree on a fee, but special circumstances may subsequently arise that create a hardship. If the provider agrees to reduce the fee, the patient should be told that the reduction will be effective only after the adjusted amount is paid in full. For instance, if a fee of $500 is reduced to $350, the full amount of the $500 charge should appear on the ledger, and when $350 has been received, the remainder can be written off as an adjustment.

Pitfalls of Fee Adjustments

Problems can arise when a provider begins to reduce his or her fees. Patients may begin to expect fees to be reduced in all circumstances. Patients may even doubt the competency of a provider who habitually reduces fees. Make fee reductions the exception rather than the norm.

Take great care in reducing the fee for care of a patient who dies. The provider's sympathy is with the family in such instances, but generosity in reducing a fee could be misinterpreted and result in a suit for malpractice. The family may suspect that the fee was reduced because the provider knows he or she made an error.

If the provider agrees to settle for a reduced fee in a situation in which the patient is disputing the cost, ensure the negotiations are "without prejudice." By taking this precaution, the provider protects his or her right to collect the original sum should the patient refuse to pay the lowered fee. The discount offer, therefore, should be made in writing; should include the words "without prejudice"; and should state a definite time limit for making payment. Prepare two copies of the agreement and have the signatures witnessed by a staff member.

A fee should never be reduced because of poor results or as a means of obtaining payment to avoid the use of a collection agency. A fee reduction for these reasons degrades the provider and the practice of medicine.

COLLECTION PROCEDURES

When to Start Collection Procedures

Collection is the process of using all legal resources available to collect payment for past due patient account balances. Sometimes a patient may have difficulty meeting all of his or her financial obligations. The patient may have lost a job or insurance coverage. An emergency could arise that depletes finances. When patients must choose between paying their medical bills and having electricity, the provider often is forced to wait for payment. Although a few patients absolutely refuse to pay for their medical care, most are honest and willing to pay but may need help with a payment plan. Terms can be arranged for collecting payment in full when the office and the patient cooperate with each other. The medical assistant should attempt to work out a plan that the patient can abide by, and the patient should be expected to make promised payments.

Preparing Patient Accounts for Collection Activity

Sometimes it becomes necessary to aggressively attempt to collect the balances that patients owe the practice. Persuasive collection procedures include telephone calls, collection reminders and letters, and personal interviews.

Before you begin collection action, it is essential to determine which accounts have a balance due and how old the account balance is. Some accounts are grouped together, or "aged," according to the dates of the last payment activity, whereas others are grouped according to the original date of service. Patient account management software programs can create aging patient account reports that are grouped by month, beginning with the month the bill was first charged (Figure 18-8). Common account aging categories are:

- 0-30 days
- 30-60 days
- 60-90 days
- 90-120 days

Most bills with balances less than 30 days old are probably waiting for the health insurance to reimburse, so no collection action is needed. Patient account balances more than 90 or 120 days old require a final demand letter before the account is turned over to a collection agency. Always allow the provider to review and approve the list of patient accounts being sent to a collection agency. Once patient account balances are aged, follow the most appropriate collection activity, according to the practice's policy.

The medical assistant can use a variety of techniques to collect patient accounts, such as collection phone calls, collection letters, and skip tracing. Often more than one technique must be used to obtain payment. Always be courteous and kind when using all collection techniques.

Collection Phone Calls

A telephone call at the right time, in a negotiable demeanor, is more successful than notes, patient account statements, or collection letters. The personal contact call often prompts patients to mail in their payment or to make payments over the phone with a credit card. In the absence of time to make calls, the collection letter is the next best approach, but if collections are a serious problem, it may be worth an extra salary to hire a person to make the phone calls.

Always treat patients with the utmost respect on the telephone. Keep their financial record close by in case they have questions about their bill; also have their insurance company's phone number handy. Remember that some patients may not understand anything about insurance or third-party payers, so guide them to that understanding and be their advocate in getting as much reimbursement as possible so that the patient's share is smaller. Never simply insist that the insurance plan has paid and the patient's balance is due. This puts the patient in a negative mindset. Try using phrases such as the following:

- "Mrs. Diggs, it looks as if your insurance company paid late last month. I believe you have a co-insurance for your surgery which amounts to $450. Is that what you were expecting? Would you like to take care of the whole balance or split that into two payments? Let me review some of your payment options."
- "Mr. Hildebrand, we're showing that you have a balance due from your surgery. Your insurance has paid, and it looks as if you owe $700. We would be happy to help you by splitting that into two or three payments. When can I schedule that first payment for you?"
- "Mrs. Crumley, it seems that you have a balance due of $450 from your surgery, and I called to see whether I could help you budget that. You could pay $50 this week and split the remaining $400 into two payments over the next 2 months?"

Always abide by office policy when making payment arrangements in collection situations. Never be belligerent with a patient.

AETNA									
Patient Name	Acct #	Primary Insurance	Secondary Insurance	**Aging Analysis**					Total Balance
				0-30	31-60	61-90	91-120	over 120	
Bassett, Eleanor	75846	AETNA		$145.00	$0.00	$0.00	$0.00	$0.00	$145.00
Herron, John	83029	AETNA		$0.00	$42.41	$0.00	$0.00	$0.00	$42.41
Holt, Maxine	64739	AETNA	BLUE SHIELD	$145.00	$0.00	$0.00	$0.00	$0.00	$145.00
Kellog, Keenan	24537	AETNA		$0.00	$0.00	$145.00	$0.00	$0.00	$145.00
Lincoln, Frank	85940	AETNA		$0.00	$15.00	$0.00	$0.00	$0.00	$15.00
Markham, Melanie	14263	AETNA	MEDICARE	$0.00	$0.00	$0.00	$260.00	$0.00	$260.00
McDonald, Lydia	56374	AETNA		$260.00	$0.00	$0.00	$0.00	$0.00	$260.00
McLean, Mary	24395	AETNA		$0.00	$0.00	$0.00	$0.00	$260.00	$260.00
Aetna Aging Total :				**$550.00**	**$57.41**	**$145.00**	**$260.00**	**$260.00**	**$1,272.41**

FIGURE 18-8 Sample aging report. (From Fordney MT: *Insurance handbook for the medical office,* ed 14, St Louis, 2017, Elsevier.)

If he or she becomes irate, simply state that the person can call back when ready to discuss a solution for paying the account, say goodbye, and gently hang up the phone. Never listen to expletives or allow verbal abuse. Respectfully end the phone call by saying thank you and good bye; do not slam the phone.

Written notification is a must before making a final demand for payment indicating that legal or collection proceedings will be started. Each patient account should be handled individually on the basis of the experience with the patient involved.

General Rules for Telephone Collections

What to Do

- Call the patient when it can be done privately.
- Call only between 8 AM and 9 PM.
- Determine the identity of the person with whom you are speaking. If you ask, "Is this Mrs. Noble?" and she answers, "Yes," it could be the patient's mother-in-law or daughter-in-law, who is also "Mrs. Noble." Use the person's full name. Include suffixes, such as "Thomas Melborn, III." This may sound too formal, but it helps to ensure that the correct person is on the phone.
- Be dignified and respectful. One can be friendly and professional at the same time.
- Ask the patient whether it is a convenient time to talk. Unless you have the attention of the called party, there is little to be gained by continuing. If told that it is an inopportune time, ask for a specific time to call back or get a promise that the patient will call the office at a specified time.
- After a brief greeting, state the purpose of the call. Make no apology for calling, but state the reason in a friendly, business-like way. The provider expects payment, and the medical assistant is interested in helping the patient meet the financial obligation. Open the call with a phrase such as, "This is Alice, Dr. Crawford's medical assistant. I'm calling about your account." A well-placed pause at this point in the call sometimes gets an immediate response from the debtor with regard to the nonpayment.
- Assume a positive attitude. For example, convey the impression that the patient intended to pay, and it is only a matter of working out some suitable arrangements.
- Keep the conversation brief and to the point; do not make threats of any kind.
- Try to get a definite commitment—payment of a certain amount by a certain date.
- Follow up on promises made by the patient. This is best accomplished by using a tickler file or a note on the calendar. If the payment does not arrive by the promised date, remind the patient with another call. If the medical assistant fails to do this, the whole effort has been wasted.

What Not to Do

- Do not call between 9 PM and 8 AM. To do so may be considered harassment.
- Do not make repeated telephone calls on the same day.
- Do not call the debtor's place of work if the employer prohibits personal calls.
- If a call is placed to the debtor at work and the person cannot take the call, leave a message asking the debtor to "call Mrs. Black at 951-727-9238" without revealing the nature of the call; that is, do not state that the call is from "Dr. Crawford's office" or "Dr. Crawford's medical assistant."
- Refrain from showing any kind of hostility. An angry patient is a poorly paying patient. Insulted patients often do not pay at all.

Collection Letters

Some consultants believe that a printed collection letter or reminder enclosed with a statement is more effective than a personal letter. Their attitude is that a patient may be embarrassed by a personal letter and feel that he or she has been singled out for attention. An impersonal printed message will probably encourage the debtor to send a payment.

Letters that are friendly requests for an explanation of why payment has not been made are effective in most cases. These letters should indicate that the provider is sincerely interested in the patient's health and well-being and wants to help resolve the financial obligation. Invite the patient to the office to explain the reasons for nonpayment so that payment arrangements can be made. To lessen the patient's embarrassment, these letters can suggest that previous statements may have been overlooked.

When receiving these letters, most patients make some effort to explain their failure to make payment. If a patient really is having financial difficulties, he or she may be able to get public assistance. If it is a temporary financial problem, the provider and the patient may together be able to work out a satisfactory installment plan for payment.

The medical assistant often is given a free hand in designing collection patterns and composing collection letters. Many medical assistants compose a series of collection letters using example letters they have found effective. Such a series usually includes at least five letters in varying degrees of forcefulness.

Sometimes even a person with poor paying habits will pay if treated with respect and consideration. The medical assistant should never go beyond the authority granted by the provider in pursuing collections. If questions arise about special collection problems, always check with the provider before proceeding. This is particularly important with patients you do not know personally (e.g., patients the provider has seen in the hospital or at home and patients with no credit history). It is difficult to say whether the effects of pressing collections too hard (which can result in loss of patient good will) are more detrimental than the effects of not pursuing collections diligently enough (which can result in loss of revenue). The provider and the medical assistant should agree on general collection policies, as outlined earlier in this chapter, and the policies should be followed. In all cases in which an account is to be assigned to a collection agency, make sure the provider is aware of this and approves.

In most healthcare facilities, the medical assistant signs collection letters using his or her title, such as "Medical Assistant" below the typewritten signature. Do not list "Collections" below the name, because the patient may assume that the account has been placed with a collection agency. Some providers want to sign these communications personally, but generally the medical assistant who handles the patient accounts also signs the collection letters.

Personal Finance Interviews

Personal finance interviews with patients sometimes can be more effective than a whole series of collection letters. By speaking with a patient face to face, the medical assistant can come to an understanding of the problem more quickly, and an agreement about future payment plans can be reached (Figure 18-9).

Occasionally a patient may undergo a long course of treatment and yet make no attempt to pay anything on the account. Perhaps such a patient is only waiting for the provider or the medical assistant to suggest that a payment be made. When it is known in advance that the patient requires extensive treatment, the matter of payment should be discussed early in the course of treatment, the credit policy should be explained, and some agreement should be reached on a payment plan.

Because medical services are far more **intangible** than any commercial service, collection efforts must not be delayed too long. Any responsible, sincere patient will call the provider's office after receiving a second statement and explain the delay in payment or ask for a payment plan. This is best accomplished in a private, personal interview.

If the account ultimately must be referred to a collector, find a good agency with a high recovery rate. The value of medical accounts diminishes in direct proportion to the length of time that has elapsed since service was provided. All collection activity is costly. Know when to stop and call on the services of a professional agency.

Special Collection Situations

Tracing "Skips"

When a patient account statement is returned marked "Moved—no forwarding address," you may consider this account a "skip." This generally is accepted as an indication that the patient is attempting to avoid liability for debts, although some skips are innocent errors. The patient may have been careless in not leaving a forwarding address, or the mistake may have occurred in the healthcare facility. However, immediate action should be taken with regard to returned patient account statements. Do not wait until the next billing cycle to attempt to trace the debtor.

The Internet can be a valuable tool in tracing skips. You can use the online white pages to search for the patient's name.

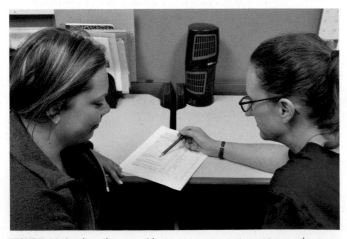

FIGURE 18-9 A face-to-face personal finance interview may motivate patients to take steps to settle their account balances.

Patients might even be found on social networking sites, such as Facebook, and that information may provide clues about the person's whereabouts. Investigate the search results carefully so that collection efforts are directed at the right person. If all attempts fail, turn the account over to a collection agency without delay. Do not keep a skip account too long because as time passes, the trail may become so cold that even collection experts will be unable to follow it.

Suggestions for Tracing Skips

- Examine the patient's original office registration card.
- Call the telephone number listed in the patient account record. Occasionally a patient may move without leaving a forwarding address but will transfer the old telephone number.
- If you are unable to contact the individual by telephone, make a few discreet calls to the references listed on the registration card to get leads.
- Check the Internet to secure the names and telephone numbers of neighbors or the landlord and contact these people to secure information about the debtor's whereabouts.
- Do not inform a third party that the patient owes money. Simply state that you are trying to locate or verify the location of the individual.
- Check the guarantor's place of employment for information. If the person is a specialist in his or her field of work, the local union or similar organizations may be contacted. Although they may not give you the person's current address, they will relay the message that you are seeking to contact him or her. Often people are stirred to pay if they think their employer may learn of their payment failure.
- Do not communicate with a third party more than once. This is specifically forbidden by law (Public Law 95-109, Sec. 804) unless the third party requests the collector to do so.

Claims Against Estates

The patient account record of a deceased patient may be handled a little differently from regular bills. Courtesy dictates that a bill not be sent during the initial period of bereavement, but do not delay longer than 30 days. The **executor** will expect to receive the statements from all healthcare providers. Use the following format to address the statement:

- Estate of (name of patient)
- c/o (spouse or next of kin, if known)
- Patient's last known address

Do not address the statement to a relative unless you have a signed agreement that that person will be financially responsible. If for some reason the statement cannot be addressed as just suggested (e.g., if the patient was in an assisted-living facility or a skilled nursing facility and no relative's name is available), seek information from the county where the estate is being settled.

A will generally is filed within 30 days of a death. The name of the executor usually can be obtained by sending a request to the Probate Department of the Superior Court, County Recorder's Office, in the county where the **decedent** lived. The time limits for filing an estate claim are determined by the state where the decedent resided.

After the name of the administrator or executor of the estate has been obtained, send a duplicate itemized statement of the account to that person by certified mail, return receipt requested. If no response is received in 10 days, contact the executor or the county clerk where the estate is being settled and obtain forms for filing a claim against the estate. This claim against the estate must be made within a certain time, which varies from 2 to 36 months, depending on the state where it is filed.

The executor of the estate either accepts or rejects the claim, and if it is accepted, sends an acknowledgment of the debt. Payment often is delayed because of the legal complications involved in settling an estate, but if the claim has been accepted, the provider eventually receives the payment. If the claim is rejected and there is full justification for claiming the bill, file a claim against the executor according to state laws. The time limit in such cases starts with the date on the letter of rejection sent in response to the original claim.

Because states have different time limits and statutes with regard to these issues, the medical assistant should contact the provider's attorney or the local court for the exact procedure to follow; or, the provider may prefer to turn such matters over to his or her legal counsel immediately.

Bankruptcy

Bankruptcy laws were passed to secure equal distribution of the assets of an individual among the individual's creditors. These are federal laws that apply in all the states. When notified that a patient has declared bankruptcy, do not send statements or make any attempt to collect on the account from the patient.

Chapter 8 bankruptcy usually is a "no asset" situation. Because the provider's charges are considered an **unsecured debt**, there is little purpose in pursuing collection. Chapter 15 is known as *wage-earner bankruptcy*, which means that the patient-debtor pays to a **trustee** a fixed amount agreed upon by the court. This money is passed on to the creditors. During this period, none of the creditors can attach the debtor's wages or otherwise attempt to collect the debt. However, the debts are paid in order, secured debts first; consequently, the provider may never receive payment from a debtor who has filed bankruptcy.

Using a Collection Agency

The medical assistant should try every means possible to collect on accounts before they become delinquent. As soon as the account is determined uncollectible through the office (i.e., the patient has failed to respond to the final letter or has failed to fulfill a second promise on payment), the provider should send the account to the collector. Skips should be assigned immediately.

Even though collection by an agency means sacrificing 40% to 60% of the amount owed, further delay only reduces the chances of recovery by the professional collector. If the agency finds that the case deserves special consideration, it will ask the provider's advice before proceeding further.

The collection agency chosen represents the healthcare practice. Therefore, the practice should ensure that its patients are treated with as much respect and dignity as possible through the collection process. There are many different collection agencies, so if one doesn't work out, prepare to switch to another that can better represent the healthcare practice.

CRITICAL THINKING APPLICATION   **18-5**

Brenda has had several complaints about the collection agency used by the office. Patients have called to report that the collectors are threatening and unprofessional. The collection agency's supervisor has been disrespectful to patients and has said that because they owe the money, the collection agency's job is to collect the account in whatever way necessary. How should the healthcare facility approach the collection agency about these complaints?

Working With the Collection Agency

A collection agency needs certain data to enable it to begin collection procedures on overdue accounts:

- Full name of the guarantor
- Name of the spouse
- Last known address
- Full amount of the debt
- Date of the last entry on account
- Occupation of the debtor
- Employer address and phone number

After an account has been released to a collection agency, the healthcare facility can make no further collection attempts. Once the agency has begun its work, a number of guidelines and procedures should be followed:

- Send no more patient account statements.
- The patient account record should be closed for activity because the account was forwarded to a collection agency.
- Refer the patient to the collection agency if he or she contacts the office about the account.
- Promptly report any payments made directly to your office to the collection agency and pay the collection agency's fee.
- Call the agency if any information is obtained that will be of value in tracing or collecting the account.

Making the Decision to Sue

The provider must decide whether he or she will benefit or suffer loss of good will by suing for a balance due rather than writing it off as a loss. Some providers believe it is unwise to resort to the court to collect medical bills unless extraordinary circumstances apply.

An account must be considered a 100% loss to the provider before legal proceedings are started. Remember never to threaten to begin legal proceedings unless the provider is prepared to carry out the threat and has decided to pursue legal action. If the provider decides in favor of a lawsuit, investigate thoroughly and obtain as much information as possible for the proceedings. Litigation to collect a balance due generally is in order when the following are true:

- The patient can afford to pay without hardship.
- The provider can produce office records that support the bill.
- The provider can justify the amount of the bill by comparing it with fee practices in the community.
- The patient's general condition after treatment is satisfactory.
- The persuasive powers of an ethical collection agency have been exhausted, and the agency advises suing.
- The patient can be given ample warning of the provider's intention to sue.

- The defendant (whether a patient or a parent or legal guardian) is legally liable for the services rendered to the patient.
- The statute of limitations has ruled out any possible malpractice action.
- The provider is neither indignant nor in a negative frame of mind.

Small Claims Court

Many healthcare practices find **small claims court** a satisfactory, inexpensive means of collecting delinquent accounts. The state law places a limit on the amount of debt for which relief may be sought in small claims court; this limit should be checked in local courts before recovery is sought in this manner.

Parties to small claims actions are not represented by an attorney at the hearing but may send another person to court on their behalf to produce records supporting the claim. Providers often send their medical assistant with records of unpaid accounts to show the judge.

If the court awards a judgment for the amount owed, the **plaintiff** in small claims court may also recover the costs of the suit. For a very small investment in time and money, the provider who uses this method saves the time of a civil court action and eliminates attorneys' fees.

After being awarded a judgment, the healthcare practice must still collect the money. The only person in a small claims action who has the right of appeal is the defendant. An appeal by the defendant may have the judgment set aside. The plaintiff cannot file an appeal in a small claims action; the decision of the court is final.

The necessary papers for filing action and full instructions on the course to follow may be obtained from the clerk of the local small claims court. It would be wise for a medical assistant who has never appeared in court to attend once as a spectator to preview the procedure; this should allow him or her to feel more at ease when appearing for the provider.

A collection agency to which an account may have been assigned may not file or handle a small claims action. It must either sue in the regular municipal or justice court or attempt to collect the debt in some other manner.

Special Bookkeeping Entries for Collections

Some patient accounts are difficult to collect on; the patient may send a bad check for payment or may lack the desire or ability to pay. These situations call for special bookkeeping entries to keep the patient account in balance. Such entries may be made either with the practice management software or a pegboard system:

- Nonsufficient funds checks (NSF)
- Collection agency transactions

Nonsufficient Funds Checks (NSF)

Nonsufficient funds (NSF) checks occur when a patient pays with a check without having sufficient funds in the bank to cover the payment. The bank will return the check to the healthcare practice marked NSF and will charge the practice's bank account a returned check fee. The payment posted to the patient account must be reversed. It is important to note that the original payment is not deleted; instead, a charge line item is added to the patient account record with the amount of the NSF check. The transaction description should read "NSF Date 02/23/20–". Many

medical offices add additional line items for NSF fee charges, but this is up to the discretion of the provider.

Posting Collection Agency Transactions

Collection agencies charge the healthcare practice different percentages of the amount owed to collect delinquent accounts; the agency with the cheapest fee is rarely the most effective. Agencies pay the *net back,* which is the amount of money paid to the practice after the agency has been paid its fee. The net back is the figure that should be considered when a collection agency is used, not simply the fee percentage. If a patient sends a payment after the account has been turned over to a collection agency, the payment must be recorded in the patient account record. Because the agency charges a fee for their collection efforts, the amount sent to the healthcare facility might be less than the actual payment amount. For instance, if the agency charges 25%, a $100 payment results in a $75 payment to the healthcare facility and the agency keeps $25. When posting the payment, the patient account must credit the full amount paid to the collection agency. This would be done by posting a $75 payment and $25 adjustment.

MANAGING FUNDS IN THE HEALTHCARE FACILITY

As mentioned previously, the purpose of financial management is to ensure that the healthcare facility earns enough money to cover its operating expenses. The financial records of the healthcare facility should show the following at all times:

- How much money was earned in a given period
- How much money was collected
- How much money is owed
- The distribution of all operational expenses

An accountant hired by the healthcare facility can prepare monthly and annual financial records from daily bookkeeping records. Periodic analyses of financial resources result in improved business practices, improved time management, elimination of unprofitable services, and more efficient expense budgeting. For the medical assistant, it is crucial to understand the difference between accounts receivable and accounts payable.

Accounts Receivable (A/R)

Accounts receivable is money that is expected but has not yet been received. The amount charged on the encounter form becomes the account receivable for the healthcare facility. When the payment on the patient account record is made, the received payment becomes cash on hand.

To disclose any discrepancies between the balance in all patient accounts and the current account receivable balance, a *trial balance* should be performed monthly, using the following computation:

Accounts receivable at first of month	$ _____
Plus total charges for month	$ _____
Subtotal	$ _____
Less total payments for month	$ _____
Subtotal	$ _____
Less total adjustments for month	$ _____
Accounts receivable at end of month	$ _____

The end of the month accounts receivable figure must agree with the figure arrived at by adding all the patient account balances. The accounts are then said to be *in balance*. If the two totals do not agree, this discrepancy should be brought to the attention of the accountant for resolution.

Accounts Payable (A/P)

Accounts payable is the management of debt incurred and not yet paid. All invoices, statements, and operational expenses are included in accounts payable. When expenses have been paid, they are no longer categorized as accounts payable.

Invoices and Statements

If delivered products are not paid for at the time of purchase, the vendor usually includes an **invoice** for payment with delivery of the merchandise. An invoice describes the products delivered and shows the amount due. Always check to verify that the items listed on the packing slip and invoice are included in the delivery.

Invoices should be placed in a designated accounts payable folder until paid. The healthcare facility may make more than one purchase from the same vendor during the month and send only a single payment at the end of the month for all deliveries.

Paying for Purchases

At the time of payment, compare the statement with the invoice to verify its accuracy. Then, fasten the statement and invoice together, write the date, the amount paid, and the check number on the statement, and place it in the Paid file.

CRITICAL THINKING APPLICATION   18-6

Brenda does not recall ordering a certain item from the office supply company. However, it was included in her last shipment and was shown on the packing list. How can she determine whether the item was ordered?

CLOSING COMMENTS

Patient accounts management and collections are critical responsibilities in the healthcare facility, and a responsible medical assistant is a great asset in this important area. Always maintain a positive attitude with patients when discussing financial matters. Remember that people who are ill or facing challenges are not always cordial, so they may not respond positively to discussion of their patient account balances. Make every attempt to work with each patient to develop a financial plan for settling the account balance. The healthcare facility works hard to collect every dollar, so effective financial management is essential for practice success.

Patient Education

In some cases patients may not fully appreciate all the costs involved in providing high-quality health care. The medical assistant may need to respectfully educate the patient about the basic costs associated with the services provided by the healthcare facility. Patients may not need a lengthy explanation, but they should be informed that the provider does not set his or her fees arbitrarily. The healthcare facility office is a small business, and like thousands of other small businesses, it should collect enough money to cover its operating expenses.

Legal and Ethical Issues

A patient who has filed for bankruptcy cannot be contacted or billed further. Another legal concern is that a threat to send a patient's account into collections should not be made unless this is the provider's intention. Never tell a patient that the provider intends to take action if the provider does not plan to follow through.

Because collection laws vary greatly from state to state, medical assistants should review the statutes pertaining to billing and collecting in the area of the healthcare facility's address. Develop a strong understanding of what is required of small businesses in collecting fees and billing patients for their financial responsibility. Remember that laws change often, so it is important to update the healthcare facility's policies on billing and collecting to reflect current statutes.

Professional Behaviors

The medical assistant is responsible for coordinating communication between the patient and the provider about financial issues. Some patients may act belligerently toward or try to bully the medical assistant in an effort to reduce their financial obligation. Be sure to inform the patient that the provider's decision about the patient's financial responsibility is not based on the medical assistant's discretion. Also, explain that the medical assistant represents the provider in his or her financial decision making. If the patient's behavior is out of control, politely excuse yourself and consult with the office manager. Inform the manager of all the details of the encounter, including the healthcare provider's instructions regarding the patient's account. The more information you give the office manager, the better able he or she will be to represent you in discussing the matter with the patient. During the entire encounter, remember to remain professional and treat the patient with respect, even though that respect may not be reciprocated.

SUMMARY OF SCENARIO

Brenda has learned much about the different types of bookkeeping transactions performed daily in the healthcare facility. She is never hesitant to confer with Mr. Schmidt, the CPA, whenever she has a question about how to post a transaction in the patient account record. As she gains more experience, she appreciates the important role of patient accounts collection in their practice's cash flow and their ability to cover its operating expenses.

Dr. Wilkins follows a conservative philosophy when it comes to accounts payable, which enables her to manage her finances wisely. As a result, Dr. Wilkins can provide job security to her best employees, including Brenda.

SUMMARY OF LEARNING OBJECTIVES

1. **Define, spell, and pronounce the terms listed in the vocabulary.**
   Spelling and pronouncing bookkeeping terms correctly reinforce the medical assistant's credibility. Knowing the definitions of these terms promotes confidence in communication with patients and co-workers.

2. **Define bookkeeping and all of the different transactions recorded in patient accounts.**
   Bookkeeping is the recording of financial transactions in the patient account records. Charges, payments, and adjustments can all be recorded in patient accounts.

3. **Do the following related to patient accounts records:**
   - *List the necessary data elements in patient accounts records.*
     Patient account records should include all information pertinent to collecting the account, such as the name and address of the guarantor, insurance identification, home and business telephone numbers, name of employer, any special instructions for billing, and emergency or alternative contact information.
   - *Discuss a pegboard (manual bookkeeping) system.*
     Although we live in a tech-savvy world, many providers still use a manual pegboard system. There are advantages and disadvantages in using a manual bookkeeping system.
   - *Explain when transactions are recorded in the patient account.*
     Once the provider has entered the procedures into the electronic encounter form, the medical assistant reviews the encounter form and enters the charges into the patient account record.
   - *Perform accounts receivable procedures for patient accounts, including charges, payments, and adjustments.*
     Practice management software systems automatically calculate the correct fees or charges when a CPT/HCPCS code is entered (see Procedure 18-1). All insurance payment amounts posted should also match the total amount paid on the Explanation of Benefits (EOB). The patient account record should have a column for the adjustment to be posted as a credit (Procedure 18-2).

4. **Describe special bookkeeping procedures for patient account records, including credit balances, third-party payments, and refunds; explain how to interact professionally with third-party representatives.**
   A credit balance occurs when a patient has paid in advance or an overpayment or duplicate payment is made. Third-party payments are reimbursement payments made from an insurance company that provides benefits for the patient. Refunds are made to insurance companies for overpayments made on patient accounts.
   Some tips for interacting professionally with third-party representatives include (1) before dialing provider services, have all documents readily accessible to discuss the patient account, and (2) when the health insurance representative comes on the phone, refrain from telling him or her how long the wait was; the representatives usually don't have much control over wait times.

5. **Discuss payment at the time of service, and give an example of displaying sensitivity when requesting payment for services rendered.**
   The medical assistant must believe that the provider and the facility have a right to charge for the services provided. Do not be embarrassed to ask for payment for the valuable services the clinician provides. When tact and good judgment are used in billing and collecting, patients appreciate the service they receive and the help the medical assistant provides. Give each patient individual attention and personal consideration; also, be courteous and show a sincere desire to help the patient with financial problems.

6. **Describe the impact of the Truth in Lending Act on collections policies for patient accounts.**
   If credit options are offered for patients, the healthcare facility should be in compliance with Regulation Z of the Truth in Lending Act (TILA). If an agreement exists between provider and patient that the healthcare facility will accept full payment in more than four installments, the healthcare facility must provide a Federal Truth in Lending Statement, even if no finance fees are charged, and it should be signed by the healthcare facility representative and the patient.

7. **Discuss ways to obtain credit information, and explain patient billing and payment options.**
   Credit information is confidential and should be guarded carefully. Healthcare facilities usually send patient account statements for payment in cycles, which allows a consistent flow of income to the office. A section of patient accounts is billed either weekly or biweekly, and patients send in their payments by mail, bring them in personally, or use an online payment system. Payment is usually requested at the time of service, especially if the patient uses a managed care system that requires a copayment. Medicare Advance Beneficiary Notices provide an option for patients to pay the provider's fee schedule in full to receive services that Medicare does not cover. Minors cannot be held financially responsible for a bill unless they are emancipated, and the medical profession traditionally has accepted the responsibility of providing occasional medical care for those unable to pay for services rendered. Problems can arise when a provider begins to reduce his or her fees.

8. **Review policies and procedures for collecting outstanding balances.**
   Most of today's healthcare facilities use statements from their practice management software to prompt patients to pay overdue bills. Often a message can be added to monthly statements that are increasingly more urgent, depending on the age of the account. Outstanding balances are also collected using telephone calls, e-mails, and personal discussions with the patient or guarantor. More advance collection methods must be used, under the provider's supervision, if the patient account balance goes without payment. Providers may take special circumstances into consideration (e.g., patient financial hardship) in deciding whether to assign a patient account to collection.

SUMMARY OF LEARNING OBJECTIVES—*continued*

9. **Do the following related to collection procedures:**
   - *Describe successful collection techniques for patient accounts.*
     The medical assistant can use a variety of techniques to collect patient accounts, such as collection phone calls, collection letters, and skip tracing. Often more than one technique must be used to obtain payment. Always be courteous and kind when using collection techniques.
   - *Discuss strategies for collecting outstanding balances through personal finance interviews.*
     Personal finance interviews with patients sometimes can be more effective than a whole series of collection letters. By speaking with a patient face to face, the medical assistant can come to an understanding of the problem more quickly, and an agreement about future payment plans can be reached.
   - *Describe types of adjustments made to patient accounts, including nonsufficient checks (NSF) and collection agency transactions.*
     With a check drawn on an account with insufficient funds, the bank returns the check to the healthcare facility marked "NSF" and charges the healthcare facility bank account a returned check fee. The payment posted to the patient account must be reversed. Note that the originally payment is not deleted; rather, a charge line item is added with the amount of the NSF check; the transaction description should read

   "NSF Date 02/23/20-". Many medical offices add additional line items for NSF fee charges, but this is up to the discretion of the provider. Because collection agencies charge a fee for their collection efforts, the amount credited to the patient's account might be less than the actual payment amount.

10. **Define bookkeeping terms, including *accounts receivable* and *accounts payable*.**
    Accounts receivable is money that is expected but has not yet been received. The amount charged on the encounter form becomes the account receivable for the healthcare facility. *Accounts payable* is the management of debt incurred and not yet paid. All invoices, statements, and operational expenses are included in accounts payable. Once expenses have been paid, they are no longer categorized as accounts payable.

11. **Discuss patient education, in addition to legal and ethical issues, related to patient accounts, collections, and practice management.**
    Patient accounts management and collections are critical responsibilities in the healthcare facility, and a responsible medical assistant is a great asset in this important area. The medical assistant may need to respectfully educate a patient about various things related to payment. Medical assistants should always review their state's statutes pertaining to billing and collecting.

CONNECTIONS

Study Guide Connection: Go to the Chapter 18 Study Guide. Read and complete the activities.

evolve Evolve Connection: Go to the Chapter 18 link at *evolve.elsevier.com/kinn* to complete the Chapter Review Quiz. Check out the other resources listed for this chapter to make the most of what you have learned from Patient Accounts, Collections, and Practice Management.

19

BANKING SERVICES AND PROCEDURES

SCENARIO

Laura has been working at Ambulatory Surgical Care Associates in the back office for the past 3 years. Her primary job has been preparing the daily deposits and visiting the bank every day to make the deposits. A bank representative stopped by the healthcare facility to show Laure some time efficient ways to bank with mobile depositing and online banking. Before she started her medical assisting education, Laura had worked as a part-time teller at City National Bank. She is looking forward to using online banking and managing the healthcare facility's many bank accounts.

Although Laura had some banking experience, working at Ambulatory Surgical Care Associates has helped her realize that she still has much to learn about the daily financial duties in a healthcare facility, including working with the patient account management software, making daily deposits, reconciling bank statements, and many other banking responsibilities.

Laura wants to increase the value of the healthcare facility's bank accounts by looking for bank accounts that pay a higher interest rate and by reducing the office's operational expenses. Laura also wants to encourage patients at the healthcare facility to use debit or credit cards, instead of checks, to pay for services, because she knows that returned patient checks have created problems.

While studying this chapter, think about the following questions:

- How is online banking affecting banking in healthcare facilities?
- How can an office manager determine whether an employee can be trusted with banking procedures?
- What precautions should the healthcare facility take when accepting patient payments?
- Why is making daily deposits a good idea?
- How can the office manager reconcile the bank account, and why is this important?

LEARNING OBJECTIVES

1. Define, spell, and pronounce the terms listed in the vocabulary.
2. Explain the purpose of the Federal Reserve Bank and the types of banks it manages.
3. Identify common types of bank accounts.
4. Do the following related to banking in today's business world:
   - Discuss the importance of signature cards.
   - Explain how online banking has made standard banking processes more efficient.
   - Review the benefits of customer-oriented banking.
5. Do the following related to checks:
   - Compare different types of negotiable instruments.
   - Identify precautions in accepting checks from patients.
   - Explain how checks are processed from one account to another.
   - Review the procedure followed when the healthcare facility receives a nonsufficient funds (NSF) check.
6. Identify precautions in accepting cash.
7. Discuss the use of debit and credit cards, including advantages and precautions.
8. Do the following related to banking procedures in the ambulatory care setting:
   - Describe banking procedures as related to the ambulatory care setting.
   - Explain the importance of depositing checks daily.
   - Prepare a bank deposit.
   - Compare types of check endorsements.
9. Review check-writing procedures used to pay the operational expenses of a healthcare facility.
10. Understand the purpose of bank account reconciliation for auditing purposes.
11. Discuss patient education, as well as legal and ethical issues, related to banking services and procedures.

checking account A bank account against which checks can be written and funds can be transferred to the payable party.

discretionary income Money in a bank account that is not assigned to pay for any office expenses.

embezzlement The misuse of a healthcare facility's funds for personal gain.

EMV chip technology Global technology that includes imbedded microchips that store and protect cardholder data; also called *chip and PIN* and *chip and signature.*

endorser The person who signs his or her name on the back of a check for the purpose of transferring all rights in the check to another party.

Federal Reserve Bank The central bank of the United States. The Federal Reserve system consists of a seven-member Board of Governors with headquarters in Washington, D.C., and 12 Federal Reserve banks in major cities throughout the country.

interest A payment the bank makes in exchange for using money.

negotiable instruments A document used to withdraw money from one bank account and deposit it into another.

principal A capital sum of money due as a debt or used as a fund for which interest is either charged or paid.

Financial transactions in the healthcare facility involve the accepting of funds from insurance companies and patients. Most healthcare institutions use bank accounts to deposit their reimbursements to pay their expenses. A medical assistant who works in the front office is responsible for accepting a variety of payments, endorsing and depositing checks, writing checks for office expenses, and regularly reconciling bank and credit card statements. Mobile deposit allows for healthcare facilities to deposit checks on the date payments are received because it is conveniently done in the office. The medical assistant will have to master basic math skills such as addition and subtraction for all banking functions.

BANKING IN TODAY'S BUSINESS WORLD

Banks can be used to centralize all financial transactions for a healthcare facility. The bank account details all deposits, withdrawals, and transfers so that the opening balance exactly matches the closing balance at the end of the previous month. Monthly bank account balances can help healthcare facilities establish and maintain a monthly operational budget. Banks also provide opportunities to earn **interest** and to invest for future financial gain. Overall, banks organize funds for the financial management of the healthcare facility.

Fees for banking services depend on the bank and products used (Table 19-1). The type of bank the medical practice will use is a decision made by the provider and the office manager, depending on the needs of the medical practice.

Although the **Federal Reserve Bank** manages all banks in the United States, healthcare facilities can choose from a number of different types of banks with which to do business:

- *Retail banks:* Offer basic banking services to the public; these banks have hundreds of branches to provide easy consumer access.

TABLE 19-1	Common Banking Fees		
FEE	DESCRIPTION	AVERAGE FEE	WAIVABLE?
Account maintenance fee	Fee for using the bank account	$5 to $25 per month	Some bank accounts waive monthly account maintenance fees if a specific balance is maintained in the account or if direct deposit is used.
Overdraft fee	Fee for the bank paying a check or debit when the balance is not in the account	$25 to $40 per occurrence	Not usually. To avoid the fee in the future, tie the checking account with an overdraft account just in case the balance is low.
Returned deposit fee	Fee charged when a deposited check is returned from the drawer's account	$5 to $10 per occurrence	Not usually. However, the practice can require the check drawer to cover this expense because the check did not clear his or her account.
Hard copy statement fee	Fee for the bank to send paper copies of bank statements	$5 to $10 per statement	This fee can be avoided by downloading all electronic bank statements when they are released.
Nonsufficient funds (NSF) fee	Fee charged when a check is written against an account with not enough funds and the check is returned unpaid	$25 to $40 per occurrence	Not usually. To avoid the fee in the future, tie the checking account with an overdraft account just in case the balance is low.
Transaction fee	Fee charged when too many transactions are made on a bank account	$.50 to $1.00 per transaction	Online banking is usually free, but nowadays banks are charging fees to visit bank branches and to complete transactions with customer service over the phone.

- *Commercial banks:* Offer business banking services to businesses of all sizes; they are equipped to handle large volumes of check deposits and credit card transactions.
- *Credit unions:* Nonprofit banking institutions owned by members; credit unions use the funds deposited to make loans to their members, which enables them to offer loans at lower than market rates.
- *Online banks:* Offer basic banking services at competitive rates because all banking transactions are done online; there are no branch locations to visit.

The medical assistant most likely will manage only the bank accounts set up for the income and operational expenses of the healthcare facility.

The Federal Reserve

In 1913, to provide the nation with a safer, more flexible, and stable monetary and financial system, Congress created the Federal Reserve Banking System, making it the central bank of the United States. The system consists of a seven-member Board of Governors with headquarters in Washington, D.C., and 12 Federal Reserve banks in major cities throughout the country (Figure 19-1).

The Federal Reserve Bank monitors the movement of money in the form of checks from one bank account to another. Each check has a routing number, an account number, and an American Bankers Association (ABA) number; these numbers identify which Federal Reserve Bank jurisdiction, bank location, and specific bank accounts are used in each transaction.

For additional information on the Federal Reserve System and its regional banks, visit the system's website at *www.federalreserve.gov.*

Because of the large volume bookkeeping transactions, many healthcare facilities use accounting management software and most online banking systems can download bank account data. These software systems can be complicated to use, so the medical assistant should be in regular contact with the accountant chosen by the provider who can answer questions when needed.

Common Types of Bank Accounts
Checking Accounts

By placing an amount of money on deposit in a bank, a depositor can set up a **checking account.** Simply stated, a checking account is a bank account against which checks can be written and funds can be transferred to the payable party. Banks typically charge a monthly account maintenance fee. In addition, there may be fees associated with banking services such as transferring funds to other banks or using the checking overdraft.

A provider who also owns a healthcare facility often requires at least three separate bank accounts:

- A personal checking account for depositing income and managing personal expenses
- Another checking account for depositing checks for the healthcare facility and for paying office expenses
- A savings account for monies set aside for paying insurance premiums, property taxes, and other seasonal expenses

Savings Accounts

Money that is not needed for current expenditures can be saved and deposited into a savings account. In most cases, savings accounts earn interest on the amount on deposit; that is, the bank pays the depositor a specified monthly percentage to use the money in the savings account. Interest is a payment the bank makes in exchange for using money. It usually is calculated as a percentage of the **principal**. Simple interest is computed annually. Compound interest is figured on the principal and on any previous interest that has been added to the original sum of money; in addition, compound interest can be computed using a variety of time increments (e.g., daily, monthly, quarterly, and so on). Interest-bearing checking accounts draw a small amount of interest, usually 1% or 2%, on the average daily balance. Savings accounts typically pay a higher rate of interest than checking accounts. Interest rates fluctuate with the financial market.

A standard savings account earns interest at the lowest prevailing rate and has no minimum balance requirement and no check-writing privileges. However, penalties apply for withdrawing funds from a savings account more than four times per month. The provider may deposit a certain percentage of **discretionary income** into a savings account each month to earn interest.

Money Market Savings Account

An insured money market savings account requires a minimum balance, anywhere from $500 to $5,000; it draws interest at money market rates (usually a higher percentage rate than for a regular savings account); and it allows only a specified number of checks (frequently three) to be written per month, which requires most bill payments managed through online banking. Such checks usually are written to transfer funds to a checking account. Some businesses transfer excess funds from the business checking account to a money market account over the weekend or over an extended holiday period to draw interest on the funds.

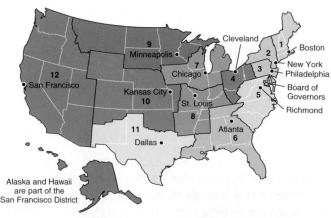

FIGURE 19-1 The 12 Federal Reserve districts.

Signature Cards

When an account is opened at a bank branch, the account signer is required to provide his or her handwritten signature on a physical or electronic card, which is kept on file with the bank. If a check comes through and some suspicion arises that the depositor's signature has been forged, bank personnel compare the signature on the check with the original on the signature card.

The provider often delegates the task of paying bills to a responsible medical assistant. In this case, any staff member who has been authorized to sign the medical facility's checks must go to the bank and add his or her handwritten signature to the signature card. Only those whose names appear on the signature card are authorized to sign checks, and the bank is responsible for verifying any questionable signatures. The provider is able to designate specific times when the secondary signer is authorized if, for example, the provider is on vacation.

Online Banking

Internet banking has changed the way financial institutions manage money. People once had to fight traffic and wait in line at crowded banks; now, they can bank from their offices any time of day. A healthcare facility's banking transactions, such as paying bills, and transferring funds between accounts, can be done online. In addition, staff members have access to supply companies online and can review costs easily from the office instead of driving to numerous companies to compare prices.

Online banking is a means of performing banking services electronically via the Internet. All banks and credit unions have this capability, and most of them offer both basic and advanced services. With basic services, a customer usually can do the following:

- Check account balances
- Transfer funds between accounts in the same bank
- Pay bills electronically and create checks
- Determine whether a check has cleared the bank
- Download account information
- View images of transactions

A major concern with online banking is fraud. Concern that unauthorized users may gain access to the healthcare facility's account balances are valid. Some experts believe that online banking involves a slightly greater risk of fraud than does conventional banking. Despite the disadvantages, studies show that Internet banking is now mainstream.

Customer-Oriented Banking

Americans want to conduct business and take care of personal concerns on laptops or cell phones on their way to and from work. In addition, the rapid pace of life requires rapid or "instant" solutions; convenience has become a basic expectation of consumers where the banking industry is concerned.

Mobile banking is a customer-oriented innovation that is emerging through the wireless technology. Using wireless devices, such as smart phones and tablets, customers can conduct a variety of financial transactions, set up alerts and notifications when bills are due, and make electronic transfers to pay these bills. Many banks offer banking software applications, which can be downloaded for free on smart phone, tablets, and computers, that allow the user to deposit checks from any location.

A healthcare facility's management personnel should consider the services available through local banks when choosing the best bank for the healthcare facility.

CHECKS

A *check* is a bank draft, or an order to pay a certain sum of money, on demand, to a specified person or entity. When a check is presented for payment, the *drawee* (the bank on which the check is drawn or written) pays the specified sum of money written on the face of the check to the *holder* (the person presenting the check for payment).

A check is considered a *negotiable* instrument. For a check to be negotiable, it must:

- Be written and signed by the drawer
- Contain a promise or order to pay a sum of money
- Be payable on demand or at a fixed future date
- Be payable to order to the drawee

To ensure that the amount is taken from the correct account number, the routing and account numbers are printed with magnetic ink on the bottom of the check. The check should have the amount written as a number and as verbiage to confirm the amount. Finally, the check must be signed and dated by the drawer of the account.

Routing and Account Numbers

A *routing transit number* (RTN) is a nine-digit code printed on the bottom left side of checks. A RTN is assigned to every banking institution under the Federal Reserve Banking System, so it identifies the bank upon which the check was drawn. RTNs also are used for direct deposits and the wiring of funds between banks. The first two digits indicate the Federal Reserve district where the bank is located. The third digit indicates the specific district office. And the rest of the digits represent the individual accounts that belong to the bank.

Bank account numbers are assigned to each individual account. No two accounts in the same financial institution can be the same, even if they belong to the same account holder. *Wire transfers* and *automated clearinghouse (ACH) transfers* use the routing and account numbers to transfer funds between exact accounts. Wire transfers are between two separate banking institutions in which both accounts are verified, so funds are available quickly. ACH transfers also involve two different banking institutions, but because both accounts are not verified, a few extra days are needed for funds to be available.

American Bankers Association Number

The *American Bankers Association number (ABA)* appears in the upper right area of a printed check. The number is used as a simple means of identifying the area location of the bank on which the check is written and the particular bank in that area. The code number is expressed as a fraction (Figure 19-2).

In the top part of the fraction, before the hyphen, the numbers 1 to 49 designate cities in which Federal Reserve banks are located or other key cities; the numbers 50 to 99 refer to states or territories. The part of the number following the hyphen is a number issued to each bank for its own identification purposes. The bottom part of the fraction includes the number of the Federal Reserve district where the bank is located and other identifying information. The ABA number is used to prepare deposit slips and to identify each check.

Types of Negotiable Instruments

The following are different types of **negotiable instruments** are documents used to withdraw money from one bank account and deposit it into another:

- Personal check
- Cashier's check
- Money order
- Business check
- Voucher check

Precautions for Accepting Checks

- Inspect the check carefully for the correct date, amount, and signature.
- Do not accept a check with corrections on it.
- Ask for a state-issued picture ID and compare the signature on the ID to the check signature.
- Do not accept an out-of-town check, government check, payroll check, starter check, unnumbered check, or a non-personalized check.
- Do not accept a third-party check. For example, Mrs. Richards, a patient, receives a check written to her by her neighbor for $30. Mrs. Richards brings the check to her visit with the provider and presents it to the clinic to pay her copayment. If the check is accepted and subsequently returned by the bank, obtaining reimbursement from the patient or the neighbor may be difficult. A check from the patient's health insurance carrier is the only exception.

- When accepting a postal money order for payment, make sure it has only one endorsement. Postal money orders with more than two endorsements will not be honored.
- Do not accept a check marked "Payment in Full" unless it does pay the account in full, up to and including the date on which it is received. If a check so marked is less than the amount due, you will be unable to collect the balance on the account once you have accepted and deposited such a check. It is illegal to cross out the words "Payment in Full."
- Do not accept a check written for more than the amount due; returning cash for the difference between the amount of the check and the amount owed is poor policy. If the check is not honored by the bank, your office suffers the loss not only of the amount of the check, but also of the amount returned in cash.

Personal Check

A personal check is drawn by a bank against funds deposited to a personal account in another bank. Patients typically write these checks for copayments and other financial responsibilities.

Cashier's Check

A cashier's check is a bank's own check, drawn on itself and signed by the bank cashier or other authorized official. A cashier's check is obtained by paying the bank the amount of the check, in cash. Many banks charge a fee for this service. Cashier's checks often are issued to accommodate a savings account customer who does not keep a checking account.

Money Order

Domestic money orders can be purchased at banks, some retail stores, and the U.S. Postal Service. Money orders often are used to pay bills by mail when a person does not have a checking account. The maximum face value varies, depending on the source. Cashier checks are preferable to money orders when larger amounts need to be paid.

Business Checks

Today, most business checks can be prepared through the online banking portal. The checkbook most widely used in the professional office is a ledger-type book with three checks per page and a

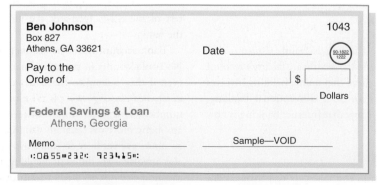

FIGURE 19-2 American Bankers Association (ABA) number.

perforated stub at the left side of the check. Checks may be bound in a soft cover or punched for a ring binder. The checks and matching stubs are numbered in sequence and preprinted with the depositor's name and account number, along with any additional information, such as address and telephone number. Business checks can also be printed through accounting management software programs when vendors submit invoices.

Voucher Check

A voucher check has a detachable voucher form or could be attached to an Explanation of Benefits (EOB). The voucher portion is used to itemize or specify the purpose for which the check was drawn. It shows the amount charged by the provider, the allowable amount, and the amount paid by the insurance company. The voucher portion of the check is removed before the check is presented for deposit; the voucher then is given to the insurance payment poster to post in the patient account record (Figure 19-3).

CRITICAL THINKING APPLICATION **19-2**

A new patient wants to pay for his services at the end of the office visit. The charge is $75. The patient writes a check for $100 and asks Laura for $25 in currency in return. How should Laura handle the situation?

How Checks Are Processed from One Bank to Another

Checks received by the drawee's bank are turned over daily to a regional banking clearinghouse, which clears each one. The identifying code numbers, printed on the face of the check with magnetic ink, enable this "clearing" process to be accomplished quickly and efficiently. Checks due from and to all banks outside a specific region are settled by electronic entries. The bank keeps the canceled checks and an electronic copy of the check is returned to the *drawer,* or the writer of the check. When the drawer needs proof of payment, a copy of the check can be requested from the bank, or the drawer can review monthly bank statements for printed copies of cleared checks. Check copies can also be obtained online through the banking portal.

Electronic Checks

In an effort to prevent check fraud, many healthcare facilities accept only electronic checks. When the patient presents a personal check to the healthcare facility, the bottom of the check, which includes the routing and account numbers, is scanned. The funds are then automatically transferred from the patient's checking account and into the healthcare facility's account. Once the transaction has been approved, the paper check is returned to the patient with "VOID" printed across it to show that it has already been used. Electronic checks reduce the time involved in transferring funds from one account to another.

Nonsufficient Funds Check (NSF)

When a check that had been deposited is returned back to the agency, it is called a *nonsufficient funds* (NSF) check ("the check

bounces"). A NSF check is not honored by the bank issuing the check, because there were not sufficient funds in the entity's bank account or the account had been closed. The medical assistant must add the amount of the check plus the NSF fee back to the patient's account balance. Some healthcare facilities will have a set amount that is billed to the patient when a check "bounces."

If the healthcare facility receives an NSF check, call the signer of the check immediately and ask him or her to stop by the office to pay the amount needed to cover the check and the additional fee. Most offices require that such payment be made by another form of payment, preferably credit card. Legal remedies are available for the provider if the check remains unpaid.

Many NSF problems can be cleared up quickly and easily with courtesy and tact, assuming the situation was simply a mistake or an oversight. Bad checks may be reported to several organizations, and once the writer is in their databases, the person will have difficulty writing a check to any business. Credit associations often are a great help when such problems arise. Turn the account over to a qualified collection agency if the practice is unable to collect on the account within a short time. To save time and resources, it may be wise to write off NSF check patient accounts with balances less than $100 if the patient has refused to pay after several requests.

CRITICAL THINKING APPLICATION **19-3**

The bank calls Laura to inform her that three of the patient checks deposited last week were NSF. What steps should Laura take to collect the NSF check amounts from the patients? Are there additional charges she can add to the patients' balances to cover the inconvenience?

CASH MANAGEMENT

Some patients may prefer to pay in cash instead of by check or by debit or credit card. Cash transactions can occur with little or no paperwork; therefore, an audit trail is harder to establish.

Patients can request a receipt when they pay cash. However, if there is no canceled check or debit/credit card slip, an employee can easily provide a receipt for payment but then pocket the money for themselves, leaving the balance on the patient's account. To prevent the mismanagement of cash, many healthcare facilities do not allow patients to pay cash for services. Healthcare facilities that have a no-cash payment policy should post a sign in the lobby to inform patients of this in advance. If a patient does not have a bank account, the medical staff can kindly refer the patient to a local money order dealer. Patients may see this as an inconvenience, but the medical assistant should explain that the policy is intended to protect the patient's account.

If the healthcare facility chooses to accept cash payments, keep in mind the following precautions:

- Make sure the cash is not counterfeit; use a marker or tool designed for this purpose to confirm its authenticity. If you suspect that the cash may be counterfeit, do not accept the payment and contact the local FBI office.
- Establish a checks and balance system in which the employee accepting cash must document cash payments on a register and in the patient's account to establish an audit trail.
- Inform patients that change cannot be made for larger bills.

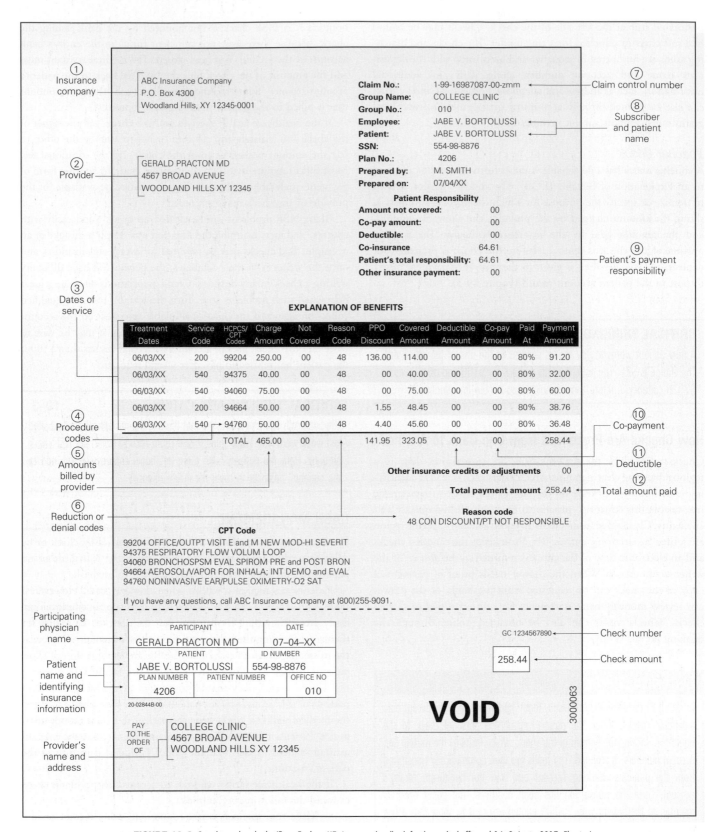

FIGURE 19-3 Sample voucher check. (From Fordney MT: *Insurance handbook for the medical office,* ed 14, St Louis, 2017, Elsevier.)

Debit Cards

The use of debit cards has vastly increased in the United States. Most debit cards are connected to a checking account. When the debit card is used, the amount of the transaction is immediately withdrawn from the available balance in the account. A personal identification number (PIN) is assigned to the card for cash withdrawal and point-of-sale (POS) purchases. The cards usually have a MasterCard or Visa logo and can be used as a credit card wherever they are accepted. The account can still be overdrawn; in most situations, when there are not enough funds in the account to make a purchase, the card is denied unless the account has some type of overdraft protection. Substantial fees may be charged if the bank elects to pay the debit when the account has insufficient funds. Currently, some banks decline debit card charges at the point of sale when an account has insufficient funds, and they do not charge an insufficient funds fee toward the attempted purchase. Stay abreast of recent banking legislation and always follow office policy when accepting debit cards as payment for medical services. The medical assistant may see various types of debit cards in the provider's office. Many states issue a debit card to individuals receiving child support payments or some types of state financial assistance.

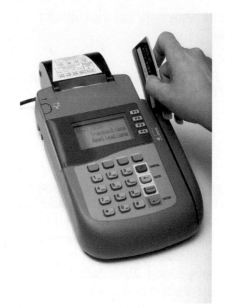

FIGURE 19-4 Example of a magnetic strip card terminal. (From Gaylor LJ: *The administrative dental assistant,* ed 3, St Louis, 2012, Saunders.)

Advantages of Using Debit Cards

Using debit cards to transfer funds has many advantages:
1. Debit cards are both safe and convenient, particularly for making payments online.
2. Transactions are completed quickly.
3. The cards can be used either as debit or credit cards. For use as a debit card, the user must have a PIN. For use as a credit card, the user often must provide identification.
4. Specific payments can be easily located online.
5. If stolen or lost, the debit card can be cancelled quickly with minimum liability.
6. Receipts and statements provide a permanent, reliable record of disbursements for tax purposes.
7. The debit card statement provides a summary of receipts.
8. The cards usually can be used anywhere that accepts MasterCard or Visa.

Credit Cards

Credit cards are one of the most common methods of payment from patients. New technology, called *contactless payment systems,* allows payment with a phone or other device that is linked to a credit or debit card. Drawbacks of credit card payments include the small processing fee that is deducted from the amount deposited into the healthcare facility's bank account. There is also an increased risk of fraud when using credit cards.

To help reduce fraud, magnetic strip cards are being replaced with cards imbedded with **EMV chip technology**. These chip cards offer advance security for in-person payments, but the EMV chip cards require a special terminal to read the chips. If a healthcare facility accepts credit or debit cards, it is important to have a terminal that processes the EMV chip cards. Businesses that cannot process the chip cards may be liable for fraud losses to their customers.

Many credit card processing terminals can accept both credit cards and debit cards (Figure 19-4), and some can also process check payments electronically. Debit card transactions use a PIN but do not need a patient's signature. Credit card transactions do not need a PIN, but patients must sign a credit card slip. Electronic check processing requires patients to submit a signed check in which the routing number and account number are scanned by the credit card terminal. Once these numbers have been scanned, a transfer of funds into the healthcare facility's bank account is initiated. All three types of accounting transactions will transfer the amount charged directly into the healthcare facility's bank account.

Although using the credit card processing terminal incurs per-transaction charges, valuable time is saved because an office employee does not need to visit the bank branch to make the daily deposit. Credit card transactions also can reduce the chances of money mismanagement in the office, such as **embezzlement**.

Precautions for Accepting Credit and Debit Cards

Just as the medical assistant must take precautions when accepting checks, care must be taken when accepting a credit or debit card as payment for medical services. The first precaution should be to make certain the person presenting the card is the person to whom it was issued. Always ask for a state-issued ID, and compare the name and signature to the ones on the credit card. Follow the healthcare facility's policy on verifying identity if the name on the state-issued ID does not match the name on the credit card. Sometimes, a married couple may use each other's cards, but if the office is strict about the card acceptance policy, then the spouse may need to be present in the office for the medical assistant to accept the card. Some patients may use a prepaid credit card, which is purchased with cash and does not have the patient's name printed on it, to make payments on their accounts. These cards, if allowed by office policy, pay just like a normal credit card. If a patient becomes belligerent if his or her credit card is denied, refer him or her to the office manager.

BANKING PROCEDURES IN THE AMBULATORY CARE SETTING

Healthcare facilities use bank accounts to deposit (as cash, checks, or debit or credit card transactions) and to pay their operational expenses by check or credit card (Box 19-4).

BOX 19-4 Accounting Management Software

Accounting management software can simplify the banking transactions of healthcare facilities. This type of software is compatible with many online banking portals; therefore, daily transactions can be downloaded directly into the accounting program. Diligent medical assistants who download daily can manage all account balances on a regular basis. Office expenses and invoices can be entered into the accounting management software as accounts payable, and payments can be scheduled for entered invoices. Checks to vendors can be printed at any time from the accounting software, documenting the transaction—and documented transactions make bank reconciliation a snap!

Making Bank Deposits

The medical assistant should make daily bank deposits, which minimizes the risks of keeping large sums of money on hand, and it also makes the money available for paying expenses. Depositing checks daily is important for these reasons:

- Checks may have a restricted time payment or may be lost, misplaced, or stolen over time.
- A stop-payment order may be placed, or it may be returned for insufficient funds.
- Prompt processing is a courtesy to the payer.

Preparing the Deposit

The medical assistant must prepare a deposit slip (ticket) that accompanies the funds being deposited. The deposit slip can be paper or electronic and itemizes the cash or checks being deposited. It provides the bank account information into which the funds need to be deposited (Figure 19-5). All details of the daily deposit should be recorded in the accounting software program; each check should be entered separately. The check number, payer, and check amount should also be recorded in the accounting software program so that the deposit amount from the software matches the bank deposit record. Many banks require that deposits be made before 3 PM if the deposit is to be credited that business day (Procedure 19-1).

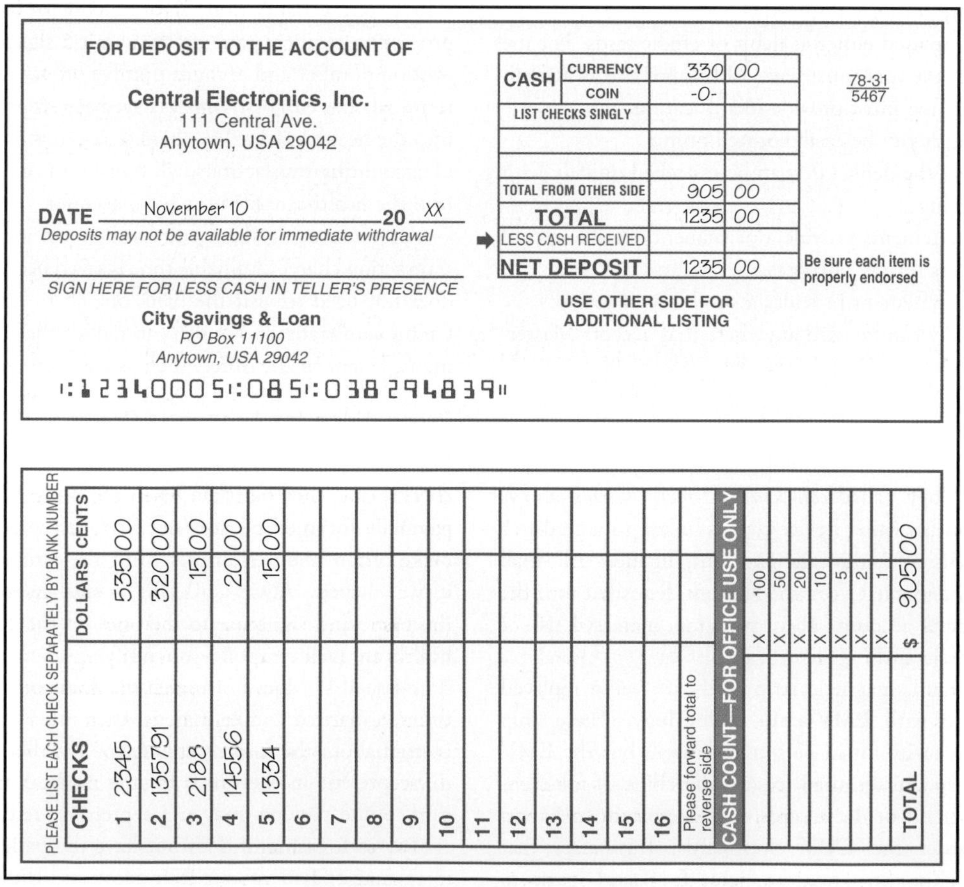

FOR DEPOSIT TO THE ACCOUNT OF

Central Electronics, Inc.
111 Central Ave.
Anytown, USA 29042

DATE November 10 20 XX
Deposits may not be available for immediate withdrawal

SIGN HERE FOR LESS CASH IN TELLER'S PRESENCE

City Savings & Loan
PO Box 11100
Anytown, USA 29042

⑆1234000 5⑆:085⑆:038 294839⑈

CASH	CURRENCY	330	00
	COIN	-0-	
LIST CHECKS SINGLY			
TOTAL FROM OTHER SIDE		905	00
TOTAL		1235	00
LESS CASH RECEIVED			
NET DEPOSIT		1235	00

78-31 / 5467

Be sure each item is properly endorsed

USE OTHER SIDE FOR ADDITIONAL LISTING

PLEASE LIST EACH CHECK SEPARATELY BY BANK NUMBER

CHECKS		DOLLARS	CENTS
1	2345	535	00
2	135791	320	00
3	2188	15	00
4	14556	20	00
5	1334	15	00
6			
7			
8			
9			
10			
11			
12			
13			
14			
15			
16			
Please forward total to reverse side			
TOTAL		$ 905	00

CASH COUNT—FOR OFFICE USE ONLY: X 100, X 50, X 20, X 10, X 5, X 2, X 1

FIGURE 19-5 Front and back of a deposit slip.

Other options to deposit checks include using a credit card terminal that processes checks electronically at the time of payment. Small healthcare facilities can snap a picture of the check and use the bank's app to do a mobile deposit. For facilities receiving a high volume of checks, a mobile check scanner can be used (Figure 19-6). Checks are scanned individually and are documented as a bank transaction on the monthly statement. Mobile deposits can save staff time and do not require a deposit slip since the software (app) is linked to the bank account being used. When using mobile deposits, the daily deposit amount must match the exact daily deposit amount in the accounting management software.

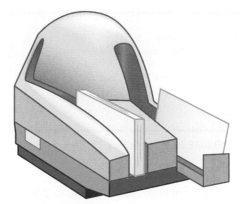

FIGURE 19-6 Mobile check scanner.

PROCEDURE 19-1 | Prepare a Bank Deposit

Goal: *To prepare a bank deposit for currency, coins, and checks.*

Scenario: *The following checks need to be deposited: #3456 for $89; #6954 for $136; #9854-10 for $1366.65; #8546 for $653.36; and #9865 for $890.22. The following currency and coins need to be deposited: (19) $20 bills; (10) $10 bills; (46) $5; (73) $1; (43) quarters; and (155) nickels. The healthcare facility's name is Walden-Martin Family Medicine Clinic, account number 123-456-78910, and the bank is Clear Water Bank, Anytown, Anystate.*

EQUIPMENT and SUPPLIES

- Checks, currency, and coins for deposit (see scenario)
- Check for endorsement
- Calculator
- Paper method: bank deposit slip
- Electronic method: SimChart for the Medical Office (SCMO)

PROCEDURAL STEPS

1. Gather the documents to be used. For the electronic method, enter into the Simulation Playground in SCMO. Click on the Form Repository icon. On the INFO PANEL, click on Office Forms and then select Bank Deposit Slip.
2. Add the date on the deposit slip.
3. Using the calculator, calculate the amount of currency to be deposited. Enter the amount in the CURRENCY line, completing the dollar and cent boxes.

4. Calculate the amount of coins to be deposited. Enter the amount in the COIN line, completing the dollar and cent boxes.
5. Add the currency and coins and enter the total amount in the TOTAL CASH line.
6. For each check to be deposited, enter the check number, the dollars, and cents. List each check on a separate line.
   PURPOSE: The bank requires that each check be listed separately, and it also helps when verifying the checks before the deposit.
7. Calculate the total to be deposited and enter the number in the TOTAL FROM ATTACHED LIST box.
8. Enter the number of items deposited in the TOTAL ITEMS box.
9. Before completing the deposit slip, verify the check amounts listed and recalculate the totals. For the electronic method, click on SAVE.
   PURPOSE: It is crucial to verify the accuracy of check amounts and totals.
10. Place a restrictive endorsement on the check(s).
    PURPOSE: To protect checks from loss or theft.

Check Endorsements

An endorsement is a signature plus any other writing on the back of a check by which the **endorser** transfers all rights in the check to another party. Endorsements are made with either a pen or rubber ink stamp. The medical assistant needs to endorse the back of the check in the box indicated. Regardless of how checks are deposited, they all need to be endorsed.

Types of Endorsements

Four principal kinds of endorsements can be used: blank, restrictive, special, and qualified. Blank and restrictive endorsements are most commonly used.

Blank Endorsement. In a blank endorsement, the payee signs only his or her name. This makes the check payable to the bearer. It is the simplest and most common type of endorsement on personal checks but should be used only when the check is to be cashed or deposited immediately.

Restrictive Endorsement. A restrictive endorsement specifies the purpose of the endorsement (Figure 19-7). It is used in preparing checks for deposit to the provider's checking account.

Special Endorsement. A special endorsement includes words specifying the person to whom the endorser makes the check payable. For instance, a check written to Helen Barker as the payee may be endorsed to the provider by writing on the back of the check as follows:

Pay to the order of
Theodore F. Wilson, M.D.
Helen Barker

```
Pay to the Order of
Midwest National Bank
Main Branch
For Deposit Only
ROBERT SPALDING
301-012697
```

FIGURE 19-7 Example of a restrictive endorsement.

The check is still negotiable but requires Dr. Wilson's signature or endorsement.

Qualified Endorsement. With a qualified endorsement, the effect of the endorsement is qualified by disclaiming or destroying any future liability of the endorser. Usually the words "without recourse" are written above by an attorney who accepts a check on behalf of a client but who has no personal claim in the transaction.

Methods of Endorsement

Any endorsement should match exactly with the name on the pay to line of the check. If the name of the payee is misspelled, the payee usually must endorse the check the way the name is spelled on the face, followed by the correctly spelled signature.

Stamp. As checks from patients and other sources arrive, they should be recorded in the ledger and immediately stamped with the restrictive endorsement "For Deposit Only." This is a safeguard against lost or stolen checks. Most banks accept routine stamp endorsements that are restricted to For Deposit Only if the customer is well known and maintains an established account.

Signature. Some insurance checks or drafts require a personal signature endorsement; a stamped endorsement is not acceptable. This is stated on the back of the check. In such cases ask the payee to endorse the check, then stamp immediately below the signature the restrictive endorsement "For Deposit Only."

USING CHECKS FOR HEALTHCARE FACILITY EXPENSES

How to Write a Check

Checks are written in ink or produced using software. Write or key the check by the following steps:
- Date the check using one of these formats: May 23, 20XX; 05/23/XX; or 5/23/XX.
- On the "Pay to the Order of" line, correctly write or key the person's name or the company's name.
- On the line with the dollar sign, write out the exact amount of the check starting next to the dollar sign (e.g., $135.00, not $135).
- On the line below the recipient's name, write out the amount, making sure to start at the left edge. The cents are written in a fraction. Draw a single line through the rest of the line to prevent any additions (e.g., One hundred thirty-five and 50/100_____).
- On the Memo line, indicate the purpose of the payment (optional).

- The check needs to be signed to be valid. If the provider is signing the check, clip the invoice to the check and place it on the provider's desk for a signature. If you are responsible for signing checks, your name must be on the signature card on file at the bank. For checks over a certain amount, two signatures will be needed.
- If you make a mistake when writing the check, it cannot be altered by crossing out or changing anything that was written. You will need to void the check and rewrite another check. Write "VOID" on the stub and on the check. File the voided check with other accounting documents for auditing purposes. If using accounting software, indicate the check number has been voided in the software.

Preventing Check Fraud in the Healthcare Facility

The National Check Fraud Center suggests the following steps to minimize the chance of check fraud in the healthcare facility:
- Check bank statements immediately after receiving them. If check fraud is not reported within 30 days of receipt of a monthly statement, the bank usualy does not have to reimburse the loss.
- Make sure all extra checks, deposit slips, bank statements, and records are stored securely (e.g., locked file cabinet or secure electronic folder).
- Bank statements and records should be maintained for up to 7 years and then shredded before disposal.

For more information on how to prevent check fraud or what to do if fraud occurs, consult the National Check Fraud Center's website at *ckfraud.org*.

Writing Cash Checks

A check is made payable to Cash and is completely negotiable. Because these checks are easily cashed, it is poor policy to write cash checks until a person is physically at the bank. These checks most often are used to replenish petty cash funds. Some bank personnel may require that the person receiving the cash endorse the check. Many experts in the banking business advise their customers not to endorse a check written for cash often; if a problem arises, the person who endorses the check is liable. To avoid being accused of embezzlement, a medical assistant should never endorse a check written from the facility's account that is written for cash.

Mailing Checks

When checks are sent through the mail, the check should not be visible through the envelope. Either place the check within a letter or fold it into a plain sheet of paper. Checks may be folded at the right end to conceal the amount of money written. Make sure the envelope is sealed before mailing. The medical assistant should personally mail all checks as soon as possible.

Overdraft

When a depositor draws a check for more than the amount on deposit in the account, the account is overdrawn. Issuing a check for more than the amount on deposit in the bank is illegal. Such a check is said to "bounce." Should this happen through error or oversight and a check is written by an established depositor, the bank may honor the check and notify the depositor that the account is overdrawn. If the bank thus pays or covers the check, it issues an overdraft on the depositor's account. Considerable fees ($10 to $35) normally are charged for an overdraft.

Stop-Payments

A depositor or check writer who wants to rescind the check has the right to request that the bank stop payment on it. Stop-payment orders should be used only when absolutely necessary; as with overdrafts, most banks charge a fee for this service. Reasons for stop-payment requests include:

- Loss of a check
- Disagreement about a purchase
- Disagreement about a payment

PAYING BILLS TO MAXIMIZE CASH FLOW

Establish a systematic plan for paying bills. Some offices have incorporated an online bill paying system and pay bills as soon as they are received. In establishing the procedure for accounts payable, a medical assistant should keep in mind that most vendors allow 30 days to pay. When each invoice is received, check the "terms," which usually are located at the top of the document. Sometimes occasions arise when a bill can be discounted if a bill is paid within a specified time, such as 10 days. A few vendors offer a discount (normally 1% to 2%) if bills are paid within a shorter time; such discounts usually are indicated at the bottom of invoices or billing statements. If the terms say "Net 30," this means the total amount of the bill is due within 30 days.

Remember to allow a certain number of days for mailing (2 to 5, depending on where the payment is sent). If the business checking account is an interest-bearing one, do not pay bills before their due date. In this way, the funds in the account continue to draw interest until it is time to write the check. Also, if the practice has a weekly service (e.g., a laundry or cleaning service) that bills several times a month, accumulate the invoices and issue only one check per month.

Online Bill Pay

Online banking is a common practice for personal and business accounts. The bank pays bills by automatically debiting the customer's account and crediting the merchant's account. Many bills can be scheduled through the online banking portal (Figure 19-8). However, not all vendors accept electronic transfers in payment of bills. It will take longer for vendors to receive payment, so schedule payments accordingly. Some routine bills that are due monthly or on a regular billing cycle, such as insurance premiums, rent payments, and utility bills, can be set up to be automatically withdrawn on the online banking portal. All banking transactions can be downloaded into an accounting management program for efficient money management. Online banking also is an excellent way to research the checks that have cleared the bank and to compute accurate bank balances.

Direct Deposit

Direct deposit, also known as *electronic funds transfers* (EFT), is the electronic payment of payroll, money owed to vendors or business establishments, and payments from government agencies. Direct deposit payments are safe, secure, efficient, and less expensive than paper checks. Their greatest advantage is the cost savings: the U.S.

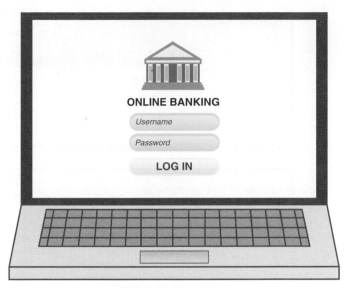

FIGURE 19-8 Online banking portal.

government pays $1.03 to issue each check payment, but only 10.5¢ to issue a direct deposit. Electronic processing becomes more prevalent each day, and business transactions are processed faster and more efficiently through electronic means.

Reward Credit Cards

More and more vendors are accepting credit cards for payment. Many different credit cards offer rewards, such as airline points, hotel rewards, reward points for products, or cash back rewards. If one of these credit cards is used for monthly expenses instead of a checking account, the provider can earn a variety of rewards. To get the greatest advantage from the credit card, be prepared to pay the credit card balance in full at the end of each billing statement to avoid interest charges.

BANK STATEMENTS AND RECONCILIATION

The bank creates a statement at the end of each monthly period, and the medical assistant can download the bank statement directly into the accounting management software, which has a *reconciliation* feature. The purpose of reconciliation is to start with the beginning balance and then add all deposits and subtract all checks and other debit transactions, leaving the ending statement balance. It is extremely important to make sure at the end of reconciliation that the ending balance is achieved. The bank statement reconciliation is used as an audit, or to ensure that the bank is managing the funds in the account accurately. Any errors on the bank statement should be reported to the bank immediately. Bank statements typically contain the following elements (Figures 19-9 and 19-10):

- Beginning balance
- Deposits made
- Checks paid (including images of all cleared checks)
- Transfer transactions
- Online payment transactions
- Bank charges
- Ending balance

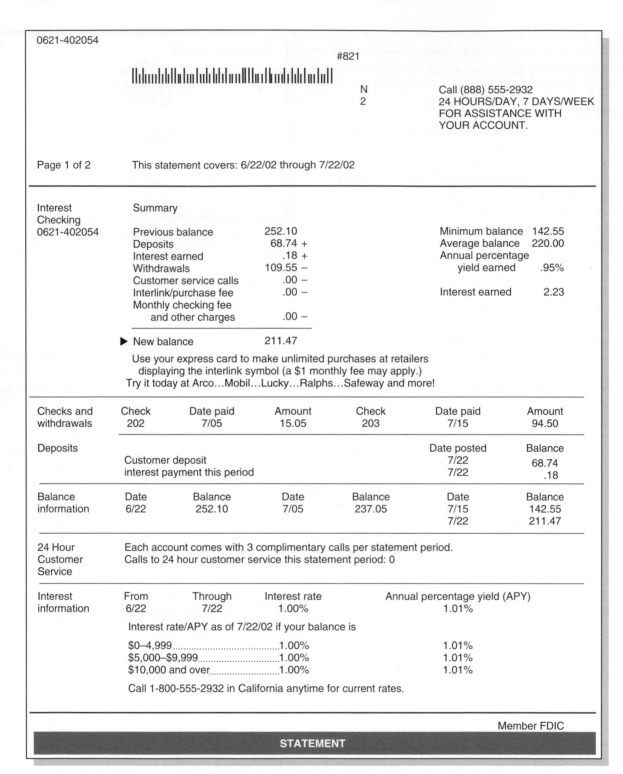

0621-402054

#821

llıılıdllılıılıılılıllıllıılIllıılıllllıllıllıılıılll

N
2

Call (888) 555-2932
24 HOURS/DAY, 7 DAYS/WEEK
FOR ASSISTANCE WITH
YOUR ACCOUNT.

Page 1 of 2   This statement covers: 6/22/02 through 7/22/02

Interest
Checking
0621-402054

Summary

Previous balance	252.10		Minimum balance	142.55
Deposits	68.74 +		Average balance	220.00
Interest earned	.18 +		Annual percentage	
Withdrawals	109.55 −		yield earned	.95%
Customer service calls	.00 −			
Interlink/purchase fee	.00 −		Interest earned	2.23
Monthly checking fee				
and other charges	.00 −			
▶ New balance	211.47			

Use your express card to make unlimited purchases at retailers
  displaying the interlink symbol (a $1 monthly fee may apply.)
Try it today at Arco…Mobil…Lucky…Ralphs…Safeway and more!

Checks and withdrawals	Check	Date paid	Amount	Check	Date paid	Amount
	202	7/05	15.05	203	7/15	94.50

Deposits			Date posted	Balance
Customer deposit			7/22	68.74
interest payment this period			7/22	.18

Balance information	Date	Balance	Date	Balance	Date	Balance
	6/22	252.10	7/05	237.05	7/15	142.55
					7/22	211.47

24 Hour Customer Service

Each account comes with 3 complimentary calls per statement period.
Calls to 24 hour customer service this statement period: 0

Interest information

From	Through	Interest rate	Annual percentage yield (APY)
6/22	7/22	1.00%	1.01%

Interest rate/APY as of 7/22/02 if your balance is

$0–4,999.....................................1.00%		1.01%
$5,000–$9,999.............................1.00%		1.01%
$10,000 and over.........................1.00%		1.01%

Call 1-800-555-2932 in California anytime for current rates.

Member FDIC

STATEMENT

FIGURE 19-9 Example of a regular checking account statement.

This worksheet is provided to help you balance your account

1. Go through your register and mark each check, withdrawal, Express ATM transaction, payment, deposit or other credit listed on this statement. Be sure that your register shows any interest paid into your account, and any service charges, automatic payments, or Express Transfers withdrawn from your account during this statement period.

2. Using the chart below, list any outstanding checks, Express ATM withdrawals, payments or any other withdrawals (including any from previous months) that are listed in your register but are not shown on this statement.

3. Balance your account by filling in the spaces below.

ITEMS OUTSTANDING		
NUMBER	AMOUNT	
TOTAL	$	

Enter

The new balance shown on
this statement .... $_____

Add

Any deposits listed in your register $_____
or transfers into your account which $_____
are not shown on this statement. $_____
                                                           +$_____
                                        _____
                                        Total................+ $_____

Calculate the subtotal.. $_____

Subtract

The total outstanding checks and
withdrawals from the chart at left ....– $_____

Calculate the ending balance

This amount should be the same
as the current balance shown in
your check register.. $_____

If you suspect errors or have questions about electronic transfers

If you believe there is an error on your statement or Express ATM receipt, or if you need more information about a transaction listed on this statement or an Express ATM receipt, please contact us immediately. We are available 24 hours a day, seven days a week to assist you. Please call the telephone number printed on the front of this statement. Or, you may write to us at United Trust Company, P.O. Box 327, Anytown, USA.

1. Tell us your name and account number or Express card number.

2. As clearly as you can, describe the error or the transfer you are unsure about, and explain why you believe there is an error or why you need more information.

3. Tell us the dollar amount of the suspected error.

You must report the suspected error to us no later than 60 days after we sent you the first statement on which the problem appeared. We will investigate your question and will correct any error promptly. If our investigation takes longer than 10 business days (or 20 days in the case of electronic purchases), we will temporarily credit your account for the amount you believe is in error, so that you may have use of the money until the investigation is completed.

FIGURE 19-10 Reverse side of a bank statement, which is used for reconciling a checking account.

What to Do When the Balances Do Not Match

When a medical assistant manages a large number of transactions from check deposits and bill payment activities, it can be challenging to match the closing balance of the bank statement with the closing balance indicated in the accounting management software. Keeping accurate records of deposits and bill payment activities makes the bank reconciliation much smoother. All deposit copies should be maintained with a copy of the calculator tape totaling the day's deposit. Every online bill pay transaction should be recorded accurately in the accounting management system.

If you have diligently recorded every transaction and the balances still do not match, ask yourself the following questions:

- Is your arithmetic correct? Could a deposit, check, or online bill pay amount be transposed?
- Did you forget to include one of the outstanding checks?
- Did you fail to record a deposit or did you record one twice?

Most banks ask to be notified within a reasonable time (e.g., 10 days) of any error found in the statement. The bank statement should be reconciled as soon as it is received. Most banks provide a form for reconciliation on the last page of the bank statement.

Bank Statement Reconciliation Formula

Bank statement balance	$ _____
Minus outstanding checks	$ _____
Plus deposits not shown	$ _____
Corrected bank statement balance	$ _____
Checkbook balance	$ _____
Minus any bank charges	$ _____
Corrected checkbook balance	$ _____

If the two corrected balances agree, stop there. If they do not agree, subtract the lesser figure from the greater figure; the difference usually provides a clue to the error. For instance, if the shortage is $35, examine all the transactions for $35 on the statement and checkbook register and determine whether one of them has a posting error. Check the math and make sure all figures were added and subtracted correctly. Look at each figure and make sure none has been transposed. These tips usually catch the mistake.

CLOSING COMMENTS

Patient Education

It should be emphasized that patients are financially responsible for balances on their accounts; patients should be informed of the healthcare facility's payment policy at the very first appointment. If a patient submits an NSF check, the medical assistant should immediately call the patient and explain the problem, requesting that he or she correct the matter as soon as possible. It is important to remember, however, that most overdrafts are simply the result of mathematic errors or a delay in deposited funds being available for withdrawal. Therefore, the medical assistant should be patient and courteous when discussing NSF issues with patients. However, patients need to know that overdrafts are costly not only to them but also to the medical facility.

Legal and Ethical Issues

If a mistake is made in preparing a check, do not destroy the check. Rather, write "VOID" across the face of the check, make a note on the check stub, and file the check with other important accounting documents available for auditing purposes.

A stop-payment order may be placed with the bank in an emergency, such as when a check is lost or a disagreement occurs with regard to a purchase or payment.

Do not accept a check made payable to another party without the endorsement of the person who gives the check to you. If the check is returned by the bank for any reason, the check will be charged to the last endorser, not the last person to receive the money.

Professional Behaviors

Despite the advances in online banking, the healthcare facility will need a responsible employee to handle money to be deposited or withdrawn from the bank. The healthcare facility manager should be diligent in ensuring that the individual handling the bank deposits or transactions is trustworthy. An employee in this position should undergo a background check, including a credit check, and drug screening. It also is wise for the practice to take out a *fidelity bond*, which is a financial protection against any fraudulent behavior by the bonded employee. Detailed money management policies prevent the misuse of the healthcare facility's funds and/or embezzlement. An effective healthcare facility manager recognizes the power of unaccounted money and protects employees by establishing strict money management rules.

SUMMARY OF SCENARIO

After the visit by the bank representative, Laura has implemented a few changes in bank account management, which has increased productivity in the office. For one, Laura requested that the bank send a mobile deposit machine so this could be done in-house; this has saved Laura a lot of time.

Laura has also set up online bill pay and manages all invoice payments through the banking portal online. She sits down once a month and sets up all payments for the month. In this way she can budget the office expenses for the month and can transfer unused funds to a money market account that pays a higher interest rate.

Laura is working closely with the providers at Ambulatory Surgical Care Associates to make some financial policy changes in the office to streamline banking processes. As of January 1 of the new year, the sign at the healthcare facility's lobby window will explain that cash will no longer be accepted for services and that a $0.25 fee will be charged for the use of a credit or debit card. Laura believes that handling fewer checks will eliminate returned patient checks.

SUMMARY OF LEARNING OBJECTIVES

1. **Define, spell, and pronounce the terms listed in the vocabulary.**
Spelling and pronouncing terms correctly reinforce the medical assistant's credibility. Knowing the definitions of these terms promotes confidence in communication with patients and co-workers.

2. **Explain the purpose of the Federal Reserve Bank and the types of banks it manages.**
The Federal Reserve Bank manages all banks in the United States. Healthcare facilities have a choice among different types of banks with which to do business, such as retail and commercial banks, credit unions, and online-only banks.

3. **Identify common types of bank accounts.**
The bank accounts most commonly used by healthcare facilities are checking, savings, and money market accounts.

4. **Do the following related to banking in today's business world:**
   - *Discuss the importance of signature cards.*
   When an account is opened at a bank branch, the depositor is required to provide a handwritten signature on a physical or electronic card, which is kept on file with the bank. If a check comes through and some suspicion arises that the depositor's signature has been forged, bank personnel compare the signature on the check with the original on the signature card.
   - *Explain how online banking has made standard banking processes more efficient.*
   Online banking allows healthcare facilities to perform mobile deposits, thereby reducing the number of times a staff member visits the bank branch. Online banking also provides up-to-the-minute account balances, online bill pay, and easy account balance transfers so that the healthcare facility's manager can spend less time managing the bank account.
   - *Review the benefits of customer-oriented banking.*
   Customer-oriented banking opens opportunities for customers to perform banking tasks from their office instead of going to the bank regularly. The Federal Reserve Banks are located across the United States. Local branches operate under the assigned Federal Reserve Bank.

5. **Do the following related to checks:**
   - *Compare different types of negotiable instruments.*
   The different types of negotiable instruments used to transfer funds from one bank account and deposit them in another are the personal check, cashier's check, money order, business check, and voucher check.
   - *Identify precautions in accepting checks from patients.*
   When accepting a check, compare the name and address on the check to the name and address in the patient's health record. Scan the check carefully for the correct date, amount, and signature. Do not accept a check with corrections on it. If you do not know the person presenting a personal check, ask for identification and compare signatures.
   - *Explain how checks are processed from one account to another.*
   Local branches are assigned a routing number, which is printed on the bottom left side of the check. The check also has the specific account

number assigned by the branch, which specifies the account from which funds are taken. When a check is presented to the bank, the check is sent to a regional banking clearinghouse, which requests funds from the check-sponsoring financial institution. Then the funds are moved from the payer's account to the payee's account. The endorsement on the back of the check includes the number of the account into which the funds are to be deposited.
   - *Review the procedure followed when the healthcare facility receives a nonsufficient funds (NSF) check.*
   When the healthcare facility is informed that a patient's check has been returned for nonsufficient funds, the patient should be contacted immediately. Inform the patient that the balance plus the overdraft fee is payable by money order or debit or credit card immediately. The patient should also be informed that he or she can no longer pay by check for any future services.

6. **Identify precautions in accepting cash.**
Many healthcare facilities refuse to accept cash from patients to prevent employees being tempted to embezzle. In addition, cash cannot be deposited by mobile deposit, and maintaining records for accepting cash can be difficult.

7. **Discuss the use of debit and credit cards, including advantages and precautions.**
The advantages of debit cards include their safety and convenience, in addition to the availability of receipts and statements. The most important precaution in accepting credit cards is to verify the patient's identity by asking to see the person's state-issued ID. Patients must know the debit card's PIN, so this is considered a verification of identity.

8. **Do the following related to banking procedures in the ambulatory care setting:**
   - *Describe banking procedures as related to the ambulatory care setting.*
   Banking procedures include withdrawals, deposits, writing checks, reconciling bank statements, paying bills, and other transactions, most of which can be done conveniently in the healthcare facility through online banking or through accounting management software.
   - *Explain the importance of depositing checks daily.*
   Deposits should be made daily for these reasons: a stop-payment order may be placed; the check may be lost, misplaced, or stolen; delay may cause the check to be returned because of insufficient funds; the check may have a restricted time for cashing; prompt processing is a courtesy to the payer; and the accounts receivable may be inflated because payments have not been deposited daily.
   - *Prepare a bank deposit.*
   Bank deposits should be made daily. The process for preparing a bank deposit is outlined in Procedure 19-1.
   - *Compare types of check endorsements.*
   Endorsements include (1) a blank endorsement, in which the payee simply signs his or her name on the back of the check; (2) a restrictive endorsement, which specifies in which bank and which specific account the funds are to be deposited; (3) a special endorsement,

Continued

SUMMARY OF LEARNING OBJECTIVES—*continued*

which names a specific person on the back of the check as payee; and (4) a qualified endorsement, which disclaims future liability. This type of endorsement is used when the person who accepts the check has no personal claim in the transaction.

9. **Review check-writing procedures used to pay the operational expenses of a healthcare facility.**
   Writing checks is a routine and basically simple function; however, certain guidelines should be followed to prevent potential problems. The bank account should have a check signer that is on file with the bank, and correction fluid for errors should not be used on checks.

10. **Understand the purpose of bank account reconciliation for auditing purposes.**
    The procedure for reconciliation starts with the beginning balance; then, all deposits are added, and all checks and other debit transactions are

subtracted—the ending statement balance should be left. It is extremely important to make sure that the ending balance is achieved at the end of reconciliation. The bank statement reconciliation is used to audit the account; that is, to ensure that the bank is managing the funds in the account accurately. Any errors on the bank statement should be reported to the bank immediately.

11. **Discuss patient education, in addition to legal and ethical issues, related to banking services and procedures.**
    Patients are financially responsible for the balance on their accounts, and they should be informed of the healthcare facility's payment policy at the very first appointment. Do not accept a check made payable to another party without the endorsement of the person who gives you the check.

CONNECTIONS

Study Guide Connection: Go to the Chapter 19 Study Guide. Read and complete the activities.

evolve Evolve Connection: Go to the Chapter 19 link at *evolve.elsevier.com/ kinn* to complete the Chapter Review Quiz. Check out the other resources listed for this chapter to make the most of what you have learned from Banking Services and Procedures.

SUPERVISION AND HUMAN RESOURCE MANAGEMENT

20

SCENARIO

Katherine Martinson is the office manager for Fair Oaks Pediatrics, a pediatric group practice in a metropolitan area. The office manages a full appointment schedule each day. Katherine encourages the medical office staff to communicate and work as a cohesive team to meet the goal of providing exceptional care to the practice's young patients. Katherine knows that positive motivation will encourage the office team to meet this goal. At weekly staff meetings, employees are free to offer their suggestions on office procedures. Katherine regularly consults her team members and always asks for their thoughts on how the office can function more effectively. She recognizes that employees need to feel that they are part of the team, and by implementing some of the procedures her team members suggest, she creates a forward-thinking and empowered work environment for the office staff.

Katherine has been praised by the pediatricians as a transformational manager because she has implemented new and efficient health information systems and technologies in the pediatrics practice. In addition, when an office position becomes vacant, Katherine is careful about whom she hires. She always checks at least three references per applicant and verifies each previous place of employment. She also always requests a background check, a credit check,

a drug test, and a bond if the applicant will be assigned to manage office money matters.

Katherine trains each new employee herself, using the office's policies and procedures manual. She makes sure the employee knows that this manual also contains a detailed job description, so the employee knows the duties expected of his or her job. Katherine regularly reviews employee performance and keeps checklists that reflect that new employees are trained accurately. All new employees are probationary until they have been evaluated by Katherine at 90 days after hire. She works hard to improve the types of benefits offered to her team, to improve employee satisfaction and retention.

Katherine makes sure each employee has the tools needed to do his or her job effectively. She also trains the team in ways to reduce expenses and waste in the medical office. Major office changes are presented to the entire staff, and although the pediatricians make the final decision, Katherine seeks the suggestions of the employees. The cooperative attitude between the management and employees of the healthcare facility provides a great atmosphere for teamwork, and Katherine and the pediatricians are pleased with the team-building atmosphere they have implemented.

While studying this chapter, think about the following questions:

- How friendly should office managers become with the staff members?
- Why are checking references and a background check important when considering a new staff member?
- How should negative employee evaluations be handled?
- How can the office manager promote a teamwork atmosphere in the medical office?

LEARNING OBJECTIVES

1. Define, spell, and pronounce the terms listed in the vocabulary.
2. Define the qualities and responsibilities of a successful office manager in a healthcare facility.
3. Explain the chain of command in the medical office.
4. Do the following related to the power of motivation:
   - Identify several ways in which employees are motivated.
   - Explain how the abuse of power and authority can negatively affect productivity in a healthcare facility.
5. Do the following related to creating a team atmosphere:
   - Discuss strategies to create a team environment in the healthcare facility.
   - Recognize and overcome communication barriers.
   - Demonstrate respect for individual diversity, including gender, race, religion, age, economic status, and appearance.

6. Summarize strategies to introduce a new office manager.
7. List several ways to prevent burnout.
8. Do the following related to finding the right employee for the job:
   - Identify the need to find the right employee for an opening in the medical office.
   - Review a general job description for medical assistants.
   - Explain how to search through résumés and applications for potential candidates.
   - List and discuss legal and illegal interview questions.
   - Explain how to select the most qualified candidates.
   - Identify follow-up activities the office manager should perform after an interview.

VOCABULARY

diversity The inclusion of every individual, despite age, religion, race, disability, and/or gender, in the medical practice.

affable Pleasant and at ease in talking to others; characterized by ease and friendliness.

blatant Completely obvious, conspicuous, or obtrusive, especially in a crass or offensive manner; brazen.

chain of command A series of executive positions in order of authority.

cohesive Sticking together tightly; exhibiting or producing cohesion.

compliance Ensuring that the healthcare facility meets standards and regulations according to the office's established policies and procedures.

disparaging Slighting; having a negative or degrading tone.

empower To delegate more responsibilities to employees (a management theory).

extern A student working in an ambulatory care environment, who is learning the job and not earning a wage.

Human Resources File (HR File) Contains all documents related to an individual's employment.

incentives Things that incite or spur to action; rewards or reasons for performing a task.

mentor A steady employee whom a new staff member can approach with questions and concerns.

retention A term referring to actions taken by management to keep good employees.

subordinate Submissive to or controlled by authority; placed in or occupying a lower class, rank, or position.

The management of a professional healthcare facility can greatly influence the success of the business. Good management allows the provider to see and treat patients in a functional environment with the confidence that the business side of the facility is operating as it should be. A well-managed office is not something that just happens. Great effort and teamwork are necessary to ensure that the day-to-day activities are carried out efficiently and that the many details needing attention are handled urgently.

Although most medical assistants do not enter medical office management right after graduation, they can look forward to advancing their careers as they gain experience. The information in this chapter can help the medical assistant understand what it takes to become a good manager. Many of these traits can be developed as a new employee after graduation, such as punctuality, respect, and responsibility. Additionally, the medical assistant will learn the employment process from the office manager's point of view. This information also is valuable to a new medical assistant who is applying for a position. By studying office management, the medical assistant prepares for future management positions, but also learns to see both the employee side and the manager side of the operating healthcare facility.

TODAY'S OFFICE MANAGER

The office manager in today's medical facilities must be able to perform many different tasks successfully. The more duties the office manager can perform, the more valuable he or she is to the facility. This is why many medical office managers seek opportunities for continuing education. Office managers should always be

open to learning more management responsibilities because taking on management positions usually results in an increase in salary and benefits. A capable medical assistant who is ready to learn will advance quickly and find a variety of opportunities in the healthcare industry.

Qualities of an Effective Manager

- Uses good judgment
- Organized and manages time well
- Enjoys pursuing continuing education
- Creative and problem solving
- Has leadership ability
- Fair with all employees
- Takes a personal interest in employees
- Remains calm under stress
- Sees the potential of fellow employees
- Can communicate with staff, patients, providers, insurance companies, and upper management
- A good listener
- Approachable
- Comfortable using the computer

Responsibilities of the Medical Office Manager

The responsibilities of medical office managers vary from practice to practice. Some providers take a much more active role in office management than others. The best management plan for the provider is to hire a trustworthy, reliable office manager and then allow the manager to run the daily business aspects of the office. This frees the provider to concentrate on taking care of patients (Figure 20-1).

Some of the tasks performed by the medical office manager include:

- Preparing and updating the policies and procedures manual
- Training and evaluating employees to ensure they follow the healthcare facility's policies and procedures
- Establishing job descriptions for each position in the medical office
- Recruiting future employees
- Conducting performance and salary reviews
- Terminating employees
- Planning staff meetings
- Building strong teams in the office
- Establishing workflow guidelines
- Ensuring human resource compliance with all federal and state regulations
- Improving the office's operational efficiency
- Supervising the purchase and care of equipment
- Educating patients on aftercare, insurance benefits, and their financial responsibility
- Marketing for the practice

Office management is most successful when an office policies and procedures manual is developed and followed.

Variables Affecting Responsibilities in an Ambulatory Healthcare Setting

- Office size
- Number of providers
- Whether medical billing is done in-house or outsourced
- Number of employees
- Amount of provider/owner involvement in daily activities

CHAIN OF COMMAND IN THE MEDICAL OFFICE

If the office has only one medical assistant, that individual must be able to assume many management responsibilities, with co-operation from the provider. When the office has two medical assistants, one administrative and one clinical, the administrative medical assistant often is expected to assume management duties.

A facility with three or more employees should designate one person as supervisor or office manager. This individual needs management skills and experience in personnel supervision. Employees answer to the office manager, and the office manager answers to the provider. A **chain of command** allows the office staff to consult with the provider about administrative or clinical problems, complaints, or grievances; this allows the individuals whom the provider has placed in charge to have the first opportunity to solve problems. It also allows the provider to check on the operation of the office, disseminate information on policy changes, and correct errors or grievances by dealing with one person instead of all employees.

Office management problems often can be prevented by clearly defining areas of authority and the responsibilities of each employee. Many office managers claim that friction among workers is their most common personnel problem. The importance of the chain of command cannot be overemphasized, and the provider must not undermine the office manager's authority by circumvention. When employees know what is expected of them, they can plan both their daily and long-term work more effectively.

THE POWER OF MOTIVATION

Managers have a great deal of influence over the staff they supervise. Successful managers must be interested in people they work with on a daily basis. It is said that if one helps others get what they want in life, the individual usually also gets what he or she wants.

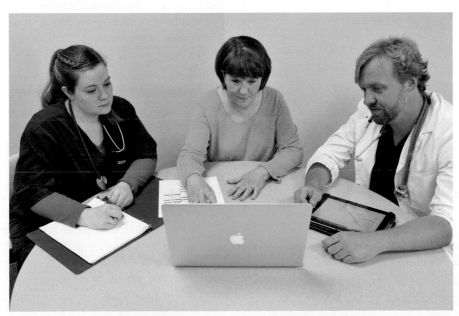

FIGURE 20-1 Staff training is a regular part of an office manager's job.

Successful managers learn that their employees should be encouraged to perform at optimum levels, and managers should be confident enough in their own skills to give credit to employees who develop ideas and concepts for the team. These managers know how to let their employees help them "look good." A manager with a group of outstanding employees usually is looked on as an effective leader.

Frederick Herzberg, known as the Father of Job Enrichment, stated, "Quality work that fosters job satisfaction and health enjoys top priority in industry all over the world." In his book, *The Motivation to Work,* Herzberg stated three points:

1. Jobs must be satisfying and must motivate employees to grow and reach their full capabilities.
2. Employees who show greater ability should be given more responsibility.
3. If the job does not allow the employee to use his or her full ability, a different employee who can grow and find motivation in the work should be placed in that position.

Effective medical office managers, or office team leaders, recognize that employees are more than static workers. Therefore, motivation is a key component to developing successful employees.

The Power of Motivation

A number of factors can motivate a person to reach a goal, including:
- Challenging work
- Money
- Recognition
- Satisfaction
- Freedom
- Fear
- Family
- Insecurity
- Competition
- Fulfillment
- Integrity
- Honor
- Reputation
- Responsibility
- Prestige
- Needs
- Love

Any of these motivators can prompt an employee to action. There are two general types of motivation. *Intrinsic motivation* is internal, or originates within a person. Intrinsic motivation is long term and can be focused toward a lifelong goal. *Extrinsic motivation* is external and more material in nature. Generally, extrinsic motivation is short-lived and less satisfying than intrinsic motivation.

CRITICAL THINKING APPLICATION   20-1
The staff is nervous about the implementation of a new EHR system, and morale has been low because training has been taking a long time. How can Katherine reassure her team of her confidence in their potential?

Keeping the Management Relationship Professional

When people work together for an extended period, they often become **affable**, and sometimes relationships develop into close friendships. This is a normal occurrence, but the office manager must be careful about becoming too close to his or her employees. When the relationship is friendly, reprimanding an employee when needed sometimes is difficult. Some employees take advantage of a good relationship with the office manager and may begin to arrive late or call in sick more than usual. A healthy respect for each other must be maintained. The manager can have a good rapport with employees without becoming overly friendly, and this is the best policy. Some facilities have strict rules about fraternization with subordinates outside the work facility. It is advisable to keep the relationship on a professional level at all times.

Use of Incentives and Employee Recognition

The staff of the provider's office should feel satisfaction with the working conditions and atmosphere in the facility. The office manager plays a part in ensuring that this happens.

CRITICAL THINKING APPLICATION   20-2
The clinical medical assistants at the Fair Oaks Pediatrics office usually celebrate payday by going out to eat after work every other Friday. After about 6 months on the job, they invite Katherine to join them. Should she go with the employees? Why or why not?

Most offices plan parties for Christmas or at other times during the year. Are these good for employee morale, or should they be avoided?

Incentives give employees reasons to perform over and above the level expected of them. An important element to incentive success is that management established clear and attainable goals. If the staff meets or exceeds a goal that has been set, the provider may elect to provide tickets to a sports or entertainment event for the entire staff. Some providers have an incentive program for outstanding patient account collection for a given period. These ideas provide a goal for the employees to work toward and an opportunity to expand their efforts as a team.

Incentives and Employee Recognition

Incentives and employee recognition should reward employees for a job well done; also, they will motivate staff members to keep up the great work! Here are some sensible incentives and employee recognition opportunities:
- After an office accomplishment, take the office out to lunch, order lunch into the office, or schedule a potluck lunch.
- Recognize an employee for his or her exceptional work during a team meeting with a personalized certificate and modest award.
- Set aside a specific time to play office games, trivia, or bingo for modest prizes at the end of a workweek.
- Schedule a weekend activity, such as a company picnic, to which employees can invite their families.

Recognition is a strong method of improving employee morale and encouraging outstanding performance. Certificates for peak performance are a great way to motivate employees. For instance, the office manager may decide to award a certificate each month to the employee who provides the highest rated customer service. Patients could even be involved by allowing them to nominate employees for this honor. When an award is at stake, most employees enjoy participating and striving to accomplish the goals that have been set.

CRITICAL THINKING APPLICATION   **20-3**

Katherine has noticed that the medical coding department has been running behind, more than usual. As a result, health insurance reimbursements have been lagging. What can Katherine do to motivate her employees?

Abuse of Power and Authority

Unfortunately, managers may abuse the power they have. As a result, the patients, the staff, and the overall morale of the office suffer. A manager who puts up barriers and erects emotional walls with employees has difficulty building effective office teams. Some managers use other people as tools to get what they want, and other managers cling to upper management, relating only to the inner circle of decision makers in the facility.

When an organization has no checks and balances, power can be abused. Working with a manager who cannot look inside himself or herself and see mistakes is difficult. Some managers stress rules and conformity, leaving no gray areas where a **subordinate** is concerned. Some show a false humility and pretend to care, but most employees can see right through this half-effort at a relationship. Others only hire "yes" people, who agree with everything the manager says. All these are abuses of power and indications of a poor manager.

These types of managers cannot be successful for an extended time. Eventually their conduct negatively affects the quality of care given to patients. It doesn't take long before upper management grows tired of unresolved office issues, such as high employee turnover and dissatisfied patients. Future candidates for jobs in medical office management should focus on developing the qualities of an effective manager, so that they are ready when ineffective managers must be replaced.

CREATING A TEAM ATMOSPHERE

Teamwork is critical in the medical profession. Communication improves when staff members collaborate as a team in the healthcare workplace, and improved communication can reduce medical errors and increase patient satisfaction. Therefore, the manager must promote an atmosphere in which employees are willing to work together toward common goals. Morale in the office may be low because of recent changes in policies or procedures, changes in staff or management, recent terminations of employees, lack of business, or for any number of other reasons. Some managers try to shield employees from negative information, but this practice can cause rumors to circulate and worsen morale.

One of the most effective ways to improve employee morale is to communicate openly and honestly. Regular staff meetings, e-mails, and memos are critical for good communication and the smooth operation of a medical facility (Figure 20-2). Communicating changes and developments that affect employees helps to improve morale. Morale can also be improved by scheduling activities that involve the families of employees.

Recognize and Overcome Barriers to Communication

Effective communication is important to increase efficiency and improved teamwork. Recognizing barriers to communication in the workplace is critical to the health of the team. The following are five barriers that can occur in a healthcare agency. It is important for the

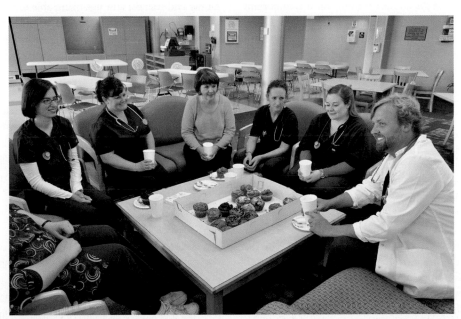

FIGURE 20-2 Communication is vital when building a team. Employees appreciate good communication with management. Sharing good and bad news openly with employees leads to fewer rumors and eases workers' concerns.

medical assistant to recognize the barriers and help the team overcome them.

- **Physical separation barriers** In large healthcare facilities, employees can be separated by departments or even by distance, if they are in different buildings. Communicating via email can be difficult and communication cues can be missed, leading to misinterpretation of the message. Using technology (e.g., videoconferencing and webcams) can help employees interact and strengthen communication.
- **Language barriers** Our workplaces are becoming more diverse. Employees live and train in different areas, learning different communication styles and different words for the same thing. For instance, a surgical instrument may be known by several names, as a result of providers training in different parts of the world. Supervisors who encourage awareness and acceptance of everyone's language and culture differences will strengthen the team's communication.
- **Status barriers** People may perceive that only those in higher ranking positions in a healthcare organization are important. This can lead to communication barriers and malfunctioning teams. It is important for the supervisor to promote awareness and acceptance that everyone counts and every position on the team is important.
- **Gender difference barriers** Males and females communicate differently, with females typically preferring a closer, more personal communication style than males. In some situations, the minority gender in an organization may not be as comfortable in communicating with peers. It is important for the supervisor to ensure that all employees, regardless of gender, feel empowered to communicate openly with others.
- **Cultural diversity barriers** Behaviors, words, and gestures have different meanings from one cultural group to another. How persons of different cultural groups communicate can also be different. For instance, some cultural groups do not believe in eye contact, whereas other groups may perceive a person to be lying or uncomfortable if eye contact is minimal. It is important for the supervisor to help the team embrace the cultural differences among the members, and educating the team on the differences can help promote understanding and cohesion.

INTRODUCING A NEW OFFICE MANAGER

The medical assistant will encounter various reactions when entering a facility as the new office manager. Often, he or she will face negative reactions from employees. They may have felt an intense loyalty to the previous manager and may resent that that person left for another job or was terminated, or they may have settled into a routine with an office manager they had worked with easily for many years. Most individuals resist change, and getting accustomed to a new supervisor can be extremely stressful. A new office manager wants to create a positive work environment; therefore, he or she must find ways to win the support of current employees.

The first thing a new office manager can do to begin gaining support is nothing. Never storm into an office and begin making radical changes in the first few days. Always observe for at least a few weeks and make notes about problem areas. Then, meet with the provider and share the information observed and present a plan

for changes. Ask for the provider's suggestions because he or she may know the history of difficult situations and can provide guidance in moving forward with plans for change.

After discussing these plans with the provider, use strategy to try to move employees toward achieving office goals. Schedule individual meetings with employees and allow them to tell you three things they like about their jobs, three things they dislike, and three things they need to do their jobs more effectively. This information provides a preliminary road map for management because the employees' responses give the new manager an excellent idea about what is important to them and where the problem areas are in the office. Hold staff meetings and move toward eliminating negative aspects and increase positive aspects of employees' jobs. These strategies will help employees realize that the new manager can get things done and that their opinions matter.

Realize that some employees still will resist, which may make the new office manager feel frustrated. At some point staffing changes may be necessary, and this might include terminating employees who do not get on board with the office moving in a positive direction. Although any terminations are stressful for the entire office, realize that this is a common situation when new managers begin their positions. This process is the first step in building a functional team.

PREVENTING BURNOUT

Burnout is defined as exhaustion of physical or emotional strength or motivation, usually as a result of prolonged stress or frustration. Medical professionals are particularly susceptible to burnout because of the intensity of their jobs, in which even small decisions can affect a patient's life.

Some of the causes of burnout include a stressful, disorganized home or work environment; poor human relations skills; a feeling of being out of control of one's life; excessive expectations from supervisors or family members; long work hours or time away from family and friends; and not being able to relax either at home or in the work environment. Management may make efforts to prevent employee burnout, but ultimately the employee must take steps to prevent it.

Personal Tips for Preventing Burnout

- Ask for help.
- Devote specific times to introspection or meditation.
- Understand what can be changed and what cannot be changed.
- Get some exercise.
- Organize and prioritize tasks.
- Understand your personal limitations.
- Take short vacations at least twice a year.
- Identify goals and try to perform only tasks that lead to reaching them.
- Consider options, including changing jobs.
- Personalize your work space with pictures and comforting items.
- Get a good understanding of a position and the stress involved before accepting it.

FINDING THE RIGHT EMPLOYEE FOR THE JOB

The most important asset of any healthcare facility is a staff that genuinely cares for patients. From providers to the receptionist, all play a vital role in the quality of the healthcare delivered. Hiring staff members who can be molded into a **cohesive** team is not an easy task. Care should be taken to choose employees who have the necessary skills and the right personality for the ambulatory care facility.

When the need for a new employee arises, the office manager should discuss with the providers the type of employee needed and the job description for that individual. Ask what qualities the providers desire for the position and the tasks for which the person will be responsible. Once the need has been established and the duties confirmed, the office manager can begin the recruiting process.

One of the most effective methods of finding new employees is allowing medical assistant students to complete their practicum at the healthcare facility. This provides the student the opportunity to learn about the facility and the staff, providers, and supervisor to see how the student interacts with others. Even if no openings exist, supervisors can ask the students for a resume to keep on file until a position opens up. Another effective method for finding new employees is advertising on local job boards. Larger facilities will post the job on their employment website page and link to other job boards. Smaller agencies will usually advertise on local free or low-cost job boards and advertise in local newspapers.

When creating an online ad or a job posting on an employment website, list the basic responsibilities and expectations for the position. Briefly describe the office, location, and the qualifications needed. Some offices also list a few of the benefits offered to attract applicants and also may disclose a salary range.

Job Description for a Medical Assistant

Medical assistants are qualified for a variety of tasks in the ambulatory care site. To fill any open medical assisting positions, the manager must determine which specific experience meets the facility's needs. With experience, professional skills can develop in specific aspects in the medical assisting profession. The website *monster.com* provides the following general job description for medical assistants.

Medical Assistant's Job Responsibilities
Helping patients through information, services, and assistance.

Medical Assistant's Job Duties
- Interviews patient to collect health data; records medical history and confirms purpose of the visit.
- Collects vital patient data by taking blood pressure, weight, and temperature; reports patient history summary.
- Secures patient's private information and preserves patient confidentiality according to HIPAA standards.
- Performs diagnostic and procedural coding, medical billing, and collection procedures for all patient accounts.
- Schedules patient appointments in the medical office and for surgery. Prepares the health record, pre-admit paperwork, and all required consent forms.
- Counsels patients on following provider's orders and answers patients' questions about follow-up care.
- Manages biohazardous waste and infection control to protect patients and medical office staff.
- Works with the medical care team to create a safe, secure, and healthy work environment by following office policies and procedures.
- Maintains inventory for medical supplies in the office by taking stock, placing orders, and verifying receipts.
- Supports healthcare facility equipment maintenance by following operating instructions, troubleshooting equipment failure, conducting preventive maintenance, and calling for repairs.
- Displays exceptional customer service to all patients, regardless of age, race, gender, religion, or socioeconomic background.

Medical Assistant's Skills and Qualifications
Customer service, clinical skills, written and verbal communication, infection control management, time management, scheduling, professionalism, confidentiality, working on a team.

Job Description

The job description is a tool designed to inform job candidates about the duties they would be expected to perform. Well-written and detailed job descriptions list the essential functions of the job and reveal the chain of command the employee should follow when questions or concerns arise. These documents provide a good guideline for potential employees so that they will understand exactly what is expected of them and their responsibilities at work.

Job descriptions are essential in the search for the perfect candidate. They highlight the specific educational background and skill set needed to be successful in the position. A clear job description in the hiring process increases the chance that an applicant with the required skills will apply for the open position. If a job description is too vague, many unqualified applicants may apply, and sorting through all the applications to find the right person for the position will be difficult.

The job description should include a statement that says the employee must perform any additional duties as assigned by the supervisor. With this statement in place, the employee cannot say, "That's not my job." All employees should be willing to pull together and assist with any tasks, but this statement gives added weight to assignments that are not specified in the written job description.

An effective manager understands the phrase "inspect what you expect." When duties are assigned, the manager should ensure that the tasks were completed correctly and in a timely manner. New employees should be monitored to make sure their delegated tasks are being done and done right. Without inspection, the manager cannot know whether the new employee is meeting expectations. Once employees have earned a degree of trust, inspecting their work is not as necessary as in the beginning. Some managers practice a skill called "management by walking around." By strolling through the areas where subordinates work, managers can observe and hear about issues that might be brewing, and at the same time improve morale by offering encouragement and praise.

Reviewing Applications

Depending on the situation, the manager may look at the applications as they come in or at the closing date. With today's technology, many agencies are having applicants submit cover letters, resumes, and applications online, although some still use paper documents. The first step in reviewing resumes includes separating out those that meet the minimal qualifications and those that do not. Typically, the minimal qualification includes successful completion of a medical assistant program and/or a medical assistant credential.

From those that meet the minimal qualifications, divide those into three stacks: those to call for an interview, possible candidates but not the strongest, and those that will not be called for an interview. Usually, the manager makes these decisions after reviewing the resume. Those with related experience, strong related skill sets (e.g., customer service), no unexplained employment gaps, and customized, error-free resumes and cover letters are more apt to be moved to the top of the pile.

Online Job Applications

Many healthcare facilities request job applicants to complete their employment application online. The online job application portal is beneficial for the job applicant and the health facility. The health facility can provide specific details about the open medical assisting positions, including the job responsibilities, a brief description of the benefits package, and a description of the company, including its mission statement. For the healthcare facility employer, online medical assisting applicants can be filtered by each individual professional experience, skills, certifications, and educational background. These portals allow employers to ask for more information specific to the job description; they can reduce the pool of applicants to just a few skilled candidates.

Once the original stack of applications has been reviewed, the office manager can return to the qualifying applications to determine which candidates to interview. Careful judgment and objectivity must be used in the search for an employee suitable for the healthcare facility. The manager should review the final applications with the following questions in mind:

- Does the applicant's grammar meet the office's standards? Can the applicant write a business letter?
- Does the applicant have basic computer skills?
- Has the applicant been employed previously in an ambulatory care facility? What were some of his or her responsibilities? Is this experience in line with the job description of the open position?
- If the applicant was previously employed, how long was he or she in the last position? Why did the applicant leave?
- Does the applicant seem to accept and enjoy responsibility? Does he or she have any professional goals that the medical office can train the individual to achieve?
- What is the applicant's formal education? Is he or she registered or certified?
- Is the applicant a member of a professional organization? Does he or she attend meetings?

Arranging the Personal Interview

In many of the larger healthcare facilities, a human resources representative will conduct a prescreening interview either over the phone or using technology like Skype. At this time, basic questions can be asked by the representative to gauge the interest of the applicant. That information is then forwarded to the office manager. In other agencies, the office manager may conduct the prescreening interview, to evaluate the person's telephone voice, attitude, and communication skills. In addition, the manager may want to ask several questions about the person's education, skills, and professional experience. Because the employee probably will speak with patients on the telephone, a qualified candidate should speak with ease. Those who perform well during the prescreening phone call should be scheduled for an interview.

CRITICAL THINKING APPLICATION 20-4

Katherine was impressed with Carol Limpken's résumé and application, but when scheduling an interview on the telephone, she noticed that Carol's grammar was not as professional as Katherine would like. Should this influence Katherine's decision whether to hire Carol?

Why is speech such an important issue in a healthcare facility?

Should Katherine be concerned about a candidate's grammar and spelling errors on the résumé or application? Why or why not?

Set a time for the personal interview when the applicant can be given undivided attention. An applicant who is being considered for employment should have an opportunity to see the facility during a period of fairly normal activity. The candidate who is interviewed in a peaceful, quiet office may not be prepared for the activity on a normal working day.

Before interviewing any applicant, become thoroughly familiar with the federal, state, and local fair employment practice laws affecting hiring practices. The Equal Employment Opportunity Act of 1972 prohibits inquiries into an applicant's race, color, gender, religion, and national origin. Inquiries about medical history, arrest records, or previous drug use also are illegal. Office managers must research the laws that pertain to employment in their own states or work with the human resources team, who are more familiar with these laws. It is important to develop a list of questions that will be asked to all interviewees. Creating a question list before the interviews helps to ensure no illegal questions are asked and that all interviewees are fairly evaluated (Table 20-1).

Laws Affecting Employment

Numerous laws affect the way employees are treated, from the interview through the end of employment. The office manager should be familiar with these laws and how they affect the practice.

Fair Labor Standards Act

- State standards for minimum wage and overtime pay; employees must be paid minimum wage and time and a half for overtime hours, as they apply
- Prohibits those under age 18 from performing certain kinds of work and restricts the hours of workers under age 16

Occupational Safety and Health Act
- Regulates conditions affecting employees' safety and health in the workplace

Workers' Compensation
- Regulates the benefits of employees who have been injured on the job
- Determines pay for employees who are not working because of an on-the-job injury

Family and Medical Leave Act
- Requires employers of 50 or more employees to offer up to 12 weeks of unpaid, job-protected leave to eligible employees for the birth of a child, an adoption, or a personal or family illness

Pregnancy Discrimination Act
- Forbids employers to refuse to hire a woman based on pregnancy, childbirth, or related medical conditions
- Requires employers to hold open a job for a pregnancy-related absence the same length of time that a job would be held open for employees on sick or disability leave

Americans with Disabilities Act
- Prohibits discrimination against individuals with disabilities

Age Discrimination Act
- Prevents discrimination in hiring on the basis of age
- Prevents discrimination in promoting, discharging, and compensating employees

The Interview

The interview is usually conducted by the office manager or with a panel of employees. If a panel is being used, they should meet before the interview to create a list of interview questions and discuss the flow of the interview. Each interviewee needs to be asked the same questions.

The interview typically starts with an introduction of the interviewers and a review of the job description. Usually, the first question (e.g., "Tell us about yourself") is meant to put the person at ease and get a summary of the person's professional and educational background. As the interview progresses, different types of questions will be asked to explore the person's past experiences and personality. Straightforward questions relate to the position duties. Behavioral questions are given to explore how the person behaved during a difficult past situation to anticipate how he or she might handle

future issues. Situational questions help the interviewers understand how the person would handle a hypothetical situation. The interviewers use the questions to explore the person's personality and past experiences and to judge how the person might fit into the existing team.

After the questions are completed, the manager should give the interviewee an opportunity to ask questions. Some interviews conclude with a discussion of the benefits and pay, but many times this occurs when the job is being offered to the applicant, since the human resources representative is the best resource for this information. Lastly, the office manager should give the interviewee an idea of the next steps in the process and when the decision will be made. If the person hasn't completed an application form, it is important to have that completed before the person leaves. References should also be collected from the interviewee.

Once the applicant leaves, the interviewers should rate or summarize their impressions of the applicant, listing the strengths and weaknesses on the interview question form. Be objective and professional and do not write **disparaging** information. The form will be kept on file in case of discrimination claims in hiring practices.

Usually, discussions of the candidate among the interview team are not encouraged until after all the interviews are completed. After all the interviews are conducted, the interviewers as a group should rank the candidates and finalize the top choices.

Bonding of Employees

To protect their business establishments from embezzlement or other financial loss caused by employees who handle large sums of money, providers often purchase fidelity bonds. Fidelity bonds reimburse the medical practice for any monetary loss caused by employees. Bonding normally requires a personal background investigation. The three types of bonding are:
- *Position-schedule bonding,* which covers a specific position rather than an individual, such as a bookkeeper or receptionist
- *Blanket-position bonding,* which covers all employees
- *Personal bonding,* which covers specific individuals

Follow-Up Activities

Always carefully check all references and follow through on any leads for information. Contact all listed references. When speaking with a candidate's former employer, be sure to "listen between the lines." Note the tone of the replies to the questions. Do not ask questions

TABLE 20-1 Legal and Illegal Interview Questions	
LEGAL QUESTIONS	**ILLEGAL QUESTIONS**
• Why did you leave your last job?	• How long have you been working?
• What are your strengths and weaknesses?	• When was the last time you used drugs?
• What motivates you to succeed?	• Do you have any children?
• What are some of your hobbies?	• What religion do you practice?
• Are you willing to work more than 40 hours a week?	• Are you married?

that might incriminate the person answering them. The following questions are effective as an introduction:

- When did (the applicant) work for you? For how long?
- What were his or her duties and responsibilities? Did the employee assume responsibility well?
- Did the employee work well in a team environment? Did any conflicts arise that we should know about?

Some employers provide information only on the date of hire, job title, and date of termination of the employment. However, if the employer states, "She worked in our office from May, 2011, to July, 2012, and is not eligible for rehire," the reasonable assumption is that the employee did not perform well. The tone of voice and emphasis on the word "not" should be clues that this person is probably not right for the job. Still, if all other references are glowing, call and ask the applicant about the facility that gave the negative response. There could be a reasonable explanation for what might have been a bad experience. Respect the company's policy and do not press for further information.

After the applicant list has been narrowed to two or three candidates whose references have been checked thoroughly, a second interview may be arranged. The providers may want to participate in these interviews.

Selecting the Right Applicant

Once the final interviews have been conducted, it is time to choose the best candidate. Never rely strictly on a "gut instinct" about a potential employee. Base hiring decisions on logical conclusions drawn from all contacts with the applicant, including:

- Grammar and enunciation
- Office manners and customer service skills
- Professional appearance
- Work history
- Match to required job skills
- Friendly, personable attitude

When a decision has been reached to hire someone, either a human resource representative or the office manager will contact the person. This is the most common time to discuss wages and benefits. The applicant may request 2 to 3 days to think over the offer. Make sure you have a firm date when the applicant will make his or her decision.

When the position is filled, the human resources representative or the office manager needs to contact all the applicants and explain the job has been filled. This notification can occur through email, a letter, or a phone call. Be courteous in the notification and thank the individual for applying.

PAPERWORK FOR NEW EMPLOYEES

The office manager should develop a checklist of the paperwork needed for newly hired staff members and all the information that should be covered with the new employee at the start of the job. Basic new employee paperwork often includes:

- HIPAA confidentiality statement
- Computer passwords and agreement statement
- Job application
- Form I-9 (Employment Eligibility Verification)
- W-4 Form (Employee's Withholding Allowance Certificate)

- Notice of Workers' Compensation coverage
- Consent for background check, drug testing, and search (if applicable)
- Acknowledgment of receipt of company handbook or policy manual
- Agreements regarding pay, wage deductions, benefits, schedule, work location, and so on
- Notices of at-will employment status
- Direct deposit application
- Occupational Safety and Health Administration (OSHA) compliance acknowledgement or checklist

All of these forms, once completed and signed, should be kept in the employee's personnel file. Other forms and paperwork may be necessary that vary from state to state and company to company. The Form I-9 (Employment Eligibility Verification) is required by the federal government (Figure 20-3). This form must be completed for all newly hired employees to verify their identification and authorization to work in the United States. The most current form is available at http://www.uscis.gov along with training materials. The newly hired employee should complete the first section of the form and provide it to the human resource representative or office manager on the first day of work. The remaining information is completed by the representative or manager. Specific documents need to be shown to prove the person's identification and authorization to work in this country. A person who cannot provide the required documentation should not be allowed to remain as an employee.

Employees should also understand the *at-will employment* status. Under the at-will employment principle, the employer can terminate the employment at any time, for any reason/cause and without notice. Unless the employer violated labor laws or the employee rights, the employee has little recourse. Only a few states protect employees from termination without good cause. At-will employment also means that the employee can leave the employment at any time, but professionally it is important to give the employer the required notice.

ORIENTATION AND TRAINING: CRITICAL FACTORS FOR SUCCESSFUL EMPLOYEES

The hiring process does not end with hiring a new employee. Orientation and training help new employees understand what is expected and develop to their full potential (Figure 20-4). A critical error made when bringing new staff members aboard is failing to provide them with a fair orientation and training period.

Some managers assign a **mentor** to assist the new employee during the initial probationary period. This type of "buddy" system is a good practice because the new person does not feel isolated and alone during the first few weeks on the job.

Acquaint the new employee with the following:

- Staff members and their names
- Physical environment and layout of the office
- Nature of the practice and specialty
- Types of patients seen in the office
- Office policies and procedures
- Employee benefits
- Short- and long-range expectations
- HIPAA and computer training

Department of Homeland Security
U.S. Citizenship and Immigration Services

**Form I-9, Employment
Eligibility Verification**

Read instructions carefully before completing this form. The instructions must be available during completion of this form.

ANTI-DISCRIMINATION NOTICE: It is illegal to discriminate against work-authorized individuals. Employers CANNOT specify which document(s) they will accept from an employee. The refusal to hire an individual because the documents have a future expiration date may also constitute illegal discrimination.

Section 1. Employee Information and Verification *(To be completed and signed by employee at the time employment begins.)*

Print Name: Last   First   Middle Initial   Maiden Name

Address *(Street Name and Number)*   Apt. #   Date of Birth *(month/day/year)*

City   State   Zip Code   Social Security #

I am aware that federal law provides for imprisonment and/or fines for false statements or use of false documents in connection with the completion of this form.

I attest, under penalty of perjury, that I am (check one of the following):

- [ ] A citizen of the United States
- [ ] A noncitizen national of the United States (see instructions)
- [ ] A lawful permanent resident (Alien #) _____
- [ ] An alien authorized to work (Alien # or Admission #) _____
  until (expiration date, if applicable - *month/day/year*) _____

Employee's Signature   Date *(month/day/year)*

Preparer and/or Translator Certification *(To be completed and signed if Section 1 is prepared by a person other than the employee.) I attest, under penalty of perjury, that I have assisted in the completion of this form and that to the best of my knowledge the information is true and correct.*

Preparer's/Translator's Signature   Print Name

Address *(Street Name and Number, City, State, Zip Code)*   Date *(month/day/year)*

Section 2. Employer Review and Verification *(To be completed and signed by employer. Examine one document from List A OR examine one document from List B and one from List C, as listed on the reverse of this form, and record the title, number, and expiration date, if any, of the document(s).)*

List A	**OR**	**List B**	**AND**	**List C**

Document title: _____   _____   _____

Issuing authority: _____   _____   _____

Document #: _____   _____   _____

Expiration Date *(if any)*: _____   _____   _____

Document #: _____

Expiration Date *(if any)*: _____

CERTIFICATION: I attest, under penalty of perjury, that I have examined the document(s) presented by the above-named employee, that the above-listed document(s) appear to be genuine and to relate to the employee named, that the employee began employment on *(month/day/year)* _____ **and that to the best of my knowledge the employee is authorized to work in the United States.   (State employment agencies may omit the date the employee began employment.)**

Signature of Employer or Authorized Representative   Print Name   Title

Business or Organization Name and Address *(Street Name and Number, City, State, Zip Code)*   Date *(month/day/year)*

Section 3. Updating and Reverification *(To be completed and signed by employer.)*

A. New Name *(if applicable)*   B. Date of Rehire *(month/day/year) (if applicable)*

C. If employee's previous grant of work authorization has expired, provide the information below for the document that establishes current employment authorization.

Document Title: _____   Document #: _____   Expiration Date *(if any)*: _____

I attest, under penalty of perjury, that to the best of my knowledge, this employee is authorized to work in the United States, and if the employee presented document(s), the document(s) I have examined appear to be genuine and to relate to the individual.

Signature of Employer or Authorized Representative   Date *(month/day/year)*

Form I-9 (Rev.) Y Page 4

FIGURE 20-3 The I-9 Form (Employment Eligibility Verification) is designed to help the employer gather the documents necessary to prove that an employee is eligible to work in the United States.

Continued

LISTS OF ACCEPTABLE DOCUMENTS
All documents must be unexpired

LIST A	LIST B	LIST C
Documents that Establish Both Identity and Employment Authorization	**Documents that Establish Identity**	**Documents that Establish Employment Authorization**
	OR	AND
1. U.S. Passport or U.S. Passport Card	1. Driver's license or ID card issued by a State or outlying possession of the United States provided it contains a photograph or information such as name, date of birth, gender, height, eye color, and address	1. Social Security Account Number card other than one that specifies on the face that the issuance of the card does not authorize employment in the United States
2. Permanent Resident Card or Alien Registration Receipt Card (Form I-551)		2. Certification of Birth Abroad issued by the Department of State (Form FS-545)
3. Foreign passport that contains a temporary I-551 stamp or temporary I-551 printed notation on a machine-readable immigrant visa	2. ID card issued by federal, state or local government agencies or entities, provided it contains a photograph or information such as name, date of birth, gender, height, eye color, and address	3. Certification of Report of Birth issued by the Department of State (Form DS-1350)
4. Employment Authorization Document that contains a photograph (Form I-766)	3. School ID card with a photograph	4. Original or certified copy of birth certificate issued by a State, county, municipal authority, or territory of the United States bearing an official seal
	4. Voter's registration card	
5. In the case of a nonimmigrant alien authorized to work for a specific employer incident to status, a foreign passport with Form I-94 or Form I-94A bearing the same name as the passport and containing an endorsement of the alien's nonimmigrant status, as long as the period of endorsement has not yet expired and the proposed employment is not in conflict with any restrictions or limitations identified on the form	5. U.S. Military card or draft record	
	6. Military dependent's ID card	5. Native American tribal document
	7. U.S. Coast Guard Merchant Mariner Card	
	8. Native American tribal document	6. U.S. Citizen ID Card (Form I-197)
	9. Driver's license issued by a Canadian government authority	
	For persons under age 18 who are unable to present a document listed above:	7. Identification Card for Use of Resident Citizen in the United States (Form I-179)
6. Passport from the Federated States of Micronesia (FSM) or the Republic of the Marshall Islands (RMI) with Form I-94 or Form I-94A indicating nonimmigrant admission under the Compact of Free Association Between the United States and the FSM or RMI	10. School record or report card	8. Employment authorization document issued by the Department of Homeland Security
	11. Clinic, doctor, or hospital record	
	12. Day-care or nursery school record	

Illustrations of many of these documents appear in Part 8 of the Handbook for Employers (M-274)

Form I-9 (Rev.) Y Page 5

FIGURE 20-3, cont'd

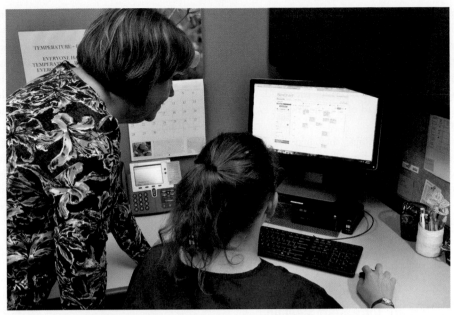

FIGURE 20-4 The training of successful employees begins with the job orientation.

Types of Employee Benefits

- *Employer-sponsored health insurance:* The employer pays a percentage of the employee's health insurance premium.
- *Dental and vision benefits:* The employer may offer dental and vision benefits for employees but may choose not to sponsor any of the premium.
- *Cafeteria plan:* A tax-free account in which employees can invest some of their paycheck and from which they can withdraw amounts for qualified health and/or child day care expenses.
- *401k retirement account matching:* The employer matches the exact amount or a percentage of the investment the employee makes every pay period (2% to 3%), up to a specific amount ($1,500).
- *Life insurance:* The employer pays for a small life insurance policy (usually up to $15,000) for minimal after-death expenses.
- *Disability insurance:* A benefit employees pay for that pays them if they are disabled and unable to work.

All new employees should be required to familiarize themselves with important office policies and procedures by reviewing the manual. It is advisable for the manager to require the employee to sign a statement verifying that the manual has been read.

Make sure the employee's file is complete before allowing the person to work even 1 hour. Also, make sure all federal and state regulations that apply to new employees have been met.

CRITICAL THINKING APPLICATION   **20-5**

Katherine is hiring a new employee who must begin work on the following Monday because the staff has been short one person for approximately 2 weeks. However, Katherine will be going on vacation the same day. How can she ensure that the new employee is trained properly?

Staff Development and Training

Continuous training and staff development are vital aspects of any medical facility. Technology is always advancing, so all employees must be kept up to date. Meetings should be held at least quarterly to ensure **compliance** in the use of health information technologies and the safety of patient health information. The staff should be trained to use the latest techniques and current regulations when dealing with issues that confront the medical facility. Keep an eye out for e-mails for seminar opportunities that will allow employees to earn continuing education units (CEUs) and develop more skills that will benefit the office. Ask employees to suggest topics about which they'd like to learn more and look for those opportunities. Professional organizations, such as the American Association of Medical Assistants (AAMA) and the American Medical Technologists (AMT), offer CEUs on a regular basis; encourage all staff members to become certified and to join professional organizations. Most hospitals have numerous continuing education classes that they allow employees of affiliated healthcare offices to attend.

Staff Meetings

As discussed, staff meetings are a formal channel used to keep the office manager and other team members current and communicating on a regular basis. One of the most common complaints from office personnel is that they are unable to discuss problems with the providers. The solution to this issue may be to hold regular staff meetings, which may be scheduled as frequently as weekly but should be held no less often than quarterly. Some of the best ideas on improvement come from the office staff; the expression and exchange of good ideas should be encouraged.

Set aside a specific time for regular meetings at an hour when most people can attend with the least disruption (Procedure 20-1). The meetings need not be long or overly formal, but to be effective, they must be planned and organized. There must be a leader, and someone should be appointed to take notes. The effectiveness of the leader, a person who can balance firmness with fairness, is an important aspect of the meeting. This usually is either the provider or the office manager or supervisor. All members of the staff should be encouraged to submit ideas for discussion.

Draw up a simple agenda listing the issues to be discussed and prepare any supporting data needed for the meeting. The agenda can be distributed to the team members ahead of the meeting so everyone can prepare and participate.

There are many kinds of staff meetings; they may be purely informational, problem-solving, or brainstorming meetings. They may be work sessions for updating manuals, training seminars, or whatever is necessary to the individual practice. Meetings also may be scheduled to discuss new ideas and any changes in office procedures. Some meetings are held simply to resolve specific problems. The staff meeting must not be allowed to deteriorate into a gripe session. Individual complaints should be handled privately.

The meeting agenda might be similar to that of any business meeting:

1. Reading of the last meeting's minutes
2. Discussion of any unfinished business
3. Discussion of any problems in the clinical area
4. Discussion of any problems in the administrative area
5. Discussion of any problems in common areas
6. Adjournment

Some providers like to combine the staff meeting with breakfast or lunch. The time or place is not important as long as it meets the needs of the practice. Meetings should be conducted democratically, and without interruption. Meetings should be kept as brief as possible. Always follow up on the items discussed; otherwise, the only result will be frustration and a reluctance to discuss problems at future meetings. The status of action items from the staff meeting should be introduced in the next staff meeting as *minutes*.

PROCEDURE 20-1   Prepare for a Staff Meeting

Goal: *Prepare for the meeting by creating an agenda and notifying the staff.*

Scenario: *You are a medical assistant team leader in a family practice department. Over the last 2 months there has been an increase in patient complaints related to long wait times in the reception area. Your supervisor asks you to prepare for a staff meeting to discuss these complaints and find ways to increase patient satisfaction.*

EQUIPMENT and SUPPLIES

- Computer with word processing software and email
- Paper and pen

PROCEDURAL STEPS

1. Using word processing software, create an agenda. Start by stating the attendees, start and end time, and location of the meeting.
2. Add the purpose and goal of the meeting.
3. Add a list of items to be discussed. The list needs to support or relate to the purpose of the meeting.
   PURPOSE: A well-written agenda provides the reader all the necessary information regarding the meeting.
4. Identify any supplies or materials the attendees should bring to the meeting.
5. Create a professional email to the attendees informing them of the meeting. The email should have an appropriate topic on the subject line. It should include a greeting, appropriate message, and a closing.

NOTE: In some facilities, the email can be sent as an invitation through the scheduling software. When the person accepts the invitation, a notation is then made on the person's schedule.

6. Use correct grammar, spelling, capitalization, and sentence structure in both the agenda and email.
   PURPOSE: Mistakes in the agenda and/or email can impact the reader's understanding of the information.
7. Proofread both the email and the agenda. Attach the agenda to the email and send it.
8. Create a list of items and equipment need for the meeting (e.g., whiteboard, easel pad and easel, projector, and computer).
9. Create a list of activities needed to prepare for the meeting and prepare the room for the meeting (e.g., appoint a person to take notes and order food).

Delegation of Duties

Delegating duties to subordinates allows managers to concentrate on the most critical aspects of their own jobs. Delegation also provides an opportunity to **empower** employees to develop their skills and experiences. Some managers are hesitant to assign duties to employees because they believe the tasks are too important not to be performed by staff employees. This hesitation suggests either a refusal to release control or mistrust of the employees. However, these manager types are typically overrun with tasks and unable to complete them. Managers should place trust in employees who have earned it and allow them to prove their abilities. Mistrust is a symptom of a poor hire. Discover the strengths of individual employees and then assign them tasks that will allow them to use those strengths. For example, if a medical assistant was hired to do administrative duties but is good with phlebotomy, empower the employee to assist with venipunctures whenever needed.

USING PERFORMANCE REVIEWS EFFECTIVELY

A new employee should be granted a probationary period. The traditional period is 60 to 90 days, but many employers believe that 2 weeks is sufficient to determine whether the employee will be able to learn and adapt to the position. Set a specific date for a performance review covering the probationary period when the new employee is hired. This review should not be squeezed in between patient visits or be given a token few minutes at the end of a day. Schedule a time that provides the opportunity to relax and talk. Tell the new employee how well expectations have been met and whether there are any deficiencies; then give the employee an opportunity to ask questions. Sometimes an employee fails to perform because he or she was never told what was expected. Although the probationary period does not always allow time to train an individual fully for a specific position, it is fair to assume that the potential for being a satisfactory employee can be judged at this time. Now is the time to talk about any problems and make suggestions for improvement. Sometimes the employee is released after an unsuccessful probationary period.

The formal performance appraisal usually occurs at the end of the probationary period and then at the hiring date anniversary. A typical appraisal includes feedback on teamwork, punctuality and attendance, motivation, accuracy with skills, customer service, professionalism, and potential continuing education and future goals. In many facilities, the appraisal relates to the pay increase the person will receive. Agencies do performance appraisals differently, yet one of the more common methods is for the supervisor to gather input from peers that work with the employee. The 360-degree evaluation is a process in which the supervisor, peers, and those who interact with the employee outside of the department provide feedback for the performance appraisal. If an employee works well with peers in the department, yet is rude and unprofessional to employees in other areas of the facility, the 360-degree evaluation will provide that information. This evaluation process holds the employee accountable for all his or her interactions in the facility.

When negative information is to be relayed to the employee during a performance appraisal, sandwich the negative comment between two positive ones whenever possible. For instance, tell the employee, "Jewel, you are a pro at greeting patients and making them feel at home. I would like to see you improve your time management skills, however, because I feel you are spending too much time with individual patients. I must confess that they feel a part of the clinic family. Let's work on some time management issues, and keep making them feel so welcome!"

Managers also may use the "feel, felt, found" approach when talking with employees about their performance. For example, "Jewel, I feel the same way you do about patients taking up a lot of our time. I know there are some that want to talk with us for hours, and I have felt the pressure of wanting to make them feel comfortable but having so much to do, too. I have found that if I explain that I have a meeting or another patient to assist, they are very understanding and not offended. Perhaps you can try that approach, too."

No supervisor enjoys giving an evaluation (Figure 20-5) that is not a positive one. It is difficult to know exactly where to begin when the employee has not performed as expected or hoped. Perhaps the best way to open the conversation is to say, "Rebecca, your review today is not going to be a positive one. It seems that we do not have a meeting of the minds about your duties and our expectations of you. Let's talk about your performance and discuss whether this position is a good match for you." Having detailed documentation of performance issues leaves little room for argument and places the manager on the offensive. The employee may be apprehensive or even defensive at this point, but the phrasing will certainly get his or her attention, and the discussion should produce either the motivation to improve or the clarity that termination is in order.

Problem Employees

Occasionally, employees do not perform at the expected level or demonstrate unprofessional behaviors. Counseling these employees

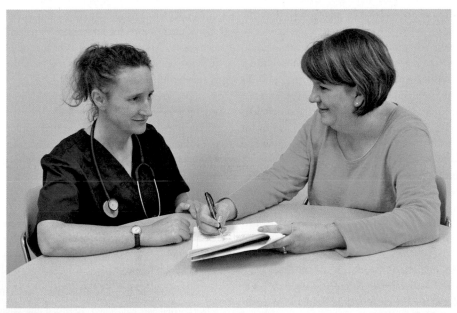

FIGURE 20-5 Performance evaluation and development plan. Performance evaluations should be considered tools that help employees reach their personal goals and the goals of the organization.

to determine the source of their difficulties is the first step toward resolution. Many employees can be redirected to become productive staff members with a little patience and understanding on the manager's part. Employees who display a willingness to improve their attitude are worth the investment the office manager makes to help them succeed.

Many offices allow one verbal warning before written reprimands go into the employee's file. It is important that the manager document the specific times, dates, and descriptions of incidents, even issues like tardiness. If the manager does not make a habit of writing a *formal warning* in the employee's **human resources file (HR file)**, there may be insufficient documentation of problems. The manager should never be in a position in which the termination of an employee cannot be justified through documentation.

CRITICAL THINKING APPLICATION   **20-6**

Katherine has two employees who have never seemed to get along. One of the employees has a history of being vindictive and manipulative, but never in an obvious enough way for Katherine to have sufficient proof to reprimand her in writing. One day, one of the employees comes to Katherine's office to report that she saw the other employee, who has an exemplary record, taking drugs from the supply cabinet. How does Katherine handle this situation? What steps should Katherine take from here?

Terminating Employees

Terminating an employee is unpleasant at best, but if the ground rules are decided in advance, written into the office policies and procedures manual, and explained to all employees, the problem is partially solved. The policies must be applied equally and impartially to all employees. The providers of the healthcare facility will most probably make the final decision on dismissal, but it may be based on the recommendation of the office manager. Unless there are mitigating factors that suggest otherwise, the person who does the hiring should do the firing.

A probationary employee who does not prove satisfactory should be dismissed at the end of the probationary period, with tact and a full explanation of the reasons for dismissal. In all fairness, an individual should be told why the employment is being ended and not be given weak excuses or untruths that do not help correct deficiencies. If the manager is not straightforward in giving the reason for dismissal, the employee will not have the opportunity to grow and improve his or her performance.

An employee who has been in service for some time and is not performing satisfactorily should be warned and given an explanation of the specific improvements expected. If a second chance does not produce improvement in performance or attitude, dismissal must follow. It should be done privately, with tact and consideration.

Most practice consultants believe that firing should come close to the end of the day and end of the workweek, after all other employees have left, and that the break should be clean and immediate. If the office policy provides for 2 weeks' notice when an employee resigns, the provider may want to offer 2 weeks' pay unless the circumstances that led to the dismissal were extremely **blatant**. A dismissed employee should never be allowed to train or influence a replacement.

The exit meeting should be planned just as carefully as the employment interview. Be honest with the employee. Discuss both the employee's assets and liabilities and give the reasons for the termination. There is no need to dwell on the employee's deficiencies. These should have been thoroughly discussed at the warning interview, and the employee need only be told that the necessary improvements have not been made. Listen to the employee's feedback, unless it becomes lengthy or abusive. This may reveal some important administrative problems that need correction.

After dismissing an employee, do not leave that person in the office unattended. Request the office keys and any other equipment in the employee's possession immediately, before the dismissed employee leaves the building, and block all access to the healthcare facility's electronic health records (EHRs). Most states have strict payday laws that do not allow holding the final paycheck for any reason. Do not offer to give the employee a good reference unless it can be done sincerely. If there is any indication that an employee may become abusive or violent once told about the termination, the supervisor should bring a representative from the human resources department or security to the final interview. It is possible that an employee can "snap" and suddenly become violent; however, more often it is the warning flags raised by an employee's behavior before termination that justify care in the termination interview. This is why supervisors should always document any strange or suspicious employee behavior and any breach of office policy or procedures in the employee's personnel file, according to office policy. Documenting everything creates a clear picture of the employee's actions throughout the time of employment. Of course, the supervisor must be willing to confront an employee about his or her negative actions in the workplace.

Some specific employee behaviors in the workplace, such as embezzlement, insubordination, and violation of patient confidentiality, are grounds for immediate dismissal without warning. These behaviors display a lack of respect for the healthcare facility and can lead to the mistreatment or endangerment of patients if the employee is not terminated immediately.

Occasionally an employee voluntarily leaves a position without giving a valid reason. The provider or office manager may want to follow up with a letter to the former employee to determine whether a problem prompted the resignation. The employee may reveal serious issues with other personnel or with the office that need to be addressed and corrected.

CRITICAL THINKING APPLICATION   **20-7**

While Katherine is explaining to a particularly poor employee why she plans to terminate her, the employee begins screaming and accusing Katherine of discrimination and harassment. How should Katherine handle this situation? What are Katherine's options if the employee does not stop the inappropriate behavior?

Fair Salaries and Raises

Medical office managers should recruit employees who want to remain with the office for a long time. There are always such situations as a part-time worker returning to college, or a summer worker going back to school. However, good employee **retention** is the goal.

To retain good employees, the practice must pay them a fair salary with regular raises if they perform as expected. The office manager can find information about salary comparisons on the Internet. Periodically review job descriptions and salary analyses online to see whether the salary the medical facility offers is comparable to that for similar jobs in the area.

Merit raises are increases based on an employee's commendable performance. Cost of living increases are given when earned, usually after specific periods or annually, and are based on national statistics and trends. An employee who is promoted should also be awarded a salary increase. When the office pays a fair salary for work done, the facility retains happy employees.

CLOSING COMMENTS

Medical assistants are not likely to go into office management immediately after graduation. The goal of this chapter is to introduce and discuss further professional opportunities in office management and the supervision of the healthcare facility staff. Successful office managers care about their employees and the vision for the healthcare facility. The areas of authority and responsibility must be clearly defined to prevent management problems. A detailed office policies and procedures manual helps the healthcare manager run an efficient facility.

Legal and Ethical Issues

Office managers must stay abreast of current employment laws and regulations for all the different agencies that govern the medical office. Joining a local office managers' association can help the manager keep the office up to date and in compliance. Periodic online checks of the websites of various organizations (e.g., OSHA) are a good way for the office manager to keep up with the most recent changes in policies and rules.

HIPAA compliance training should be required for all healthcare facilities. The facility's office manager should be knowledgable not only about all HIPAA provisions, including those affecting the privacy and security of patient health information, but also about the penalties associated with information breaches.

Professional Behaviors

Managers that encourage their staff create a strong team in the healthcare facility. By focusing on team building, office managers can accomplish more tasks efficiently, delegate some of their workload, and promote high-quality patient care. Office managers can become immersed in their daily office responsibilities; however, they must keep in mind that slacking off on staff training and team development meetings results in lower office productivity. Staff meetings should be scheduled in advance and their attendance should be mandatory for all staff members.

SUMMARY OF SCENARIO

Katherine has had a positive effect on her team at the Fair Oaks Pediatrics office. She treats her employees well and is fair about administering office policies and procedures. Her staff appreciates her flexibility and professionalism as she manages the day-to-day operations of the facility. Katherine treats her employees as team members, never speaking to them as if she were superior to them. She shares vital information with the staff so that they feel a part of the whole team, and she believes that even negative information should be relayed to the staff so that everyone is aware of the challenges the office faces. She makes strong hiring decisions and firmly believes in a good orientation and training program. Dr. Elaine Collins, the senior member of the pediatrician staff, has placed a great deal of trust in Katherine, and she has performed well, proving to be a reliable office manager.

Katherine knows that she should display a friendly attitude toward her staff members when it is appropriate to do so. She is kind and considerate and treats the staff as individuals. She does not fraternize with them but is open to having lunch with the staff at various times and participates in all casual office activities. She maintains a healthy distance so that she can be an effective manager, but she listens to those who are experiencing difficulty and is compassionate about helping whenever possible.

Katherine knows that when hiring for a vacant position, she must be diligent in checking references so that she brings reliable, qualified individuals on board as staff members. Unless she receives acceptable references, she will not hire a medical assistant to become a part of her team. Once she hires someone, she conducts a thorough training program and takes special care to share the experience and skills of the new staff member with the rest of the team.

When Katherine must give a negative employee evaluation, she states that fact at the beginning of the meeting. Although she is compassionate, she is able to point out a staff member's shortcomings in a detailed, fair way. She usually is willing to give an employee time to improve, but if he or she fails to perform, Katherine does not hesitate to end the employment.

Katherine leads a group of cooperative team members who function well together every day, and this results in an efficient office and a pleasant work environment.

SUMMARY OF LEARNING OBJECTIVES

1. **Define, spell, and pronounce the terms listed in the vocabulary.**
   Spelling and pronouncing medical terms correctly reinforce the medical assistant's credibility. Knowing the definitions of these terms promotes confidence in communication with patients and co-workers.

2. **Define the qualities and responsibilities of a successful office manager for a healthcare facility.**
   The provider counts on the office manager to run the business aspects of the office so that he or she can focus on providing good patient care. A high degree of trust is placed in the office manager. A good office manager is fair and flexible. Good communication skills are necessary, as is attention to detail. The manager should care about the employees and have a sense of fairness. The ability to remain calm in a crisis is important, as are the use of good judgment and the ability to multitask. Successful medical office managers work to promote a positive team environment to facilitate cohesion.

3. **Explain the chain of command in the medical office.**
   The provider/owner is ultimately responsible for all activities in the medical office. The provider and the medical office manager work together to handle the day-to-day activities. The provider trusts the medical office manager to handle employee issues. The medical office manager also defines job descriptions so that each member of the team is aware of his or her responsibilities.

4. **Do the following related to the power of motivation:**
   - *Identify several ways in which employees are motivated.*
     Employees are motivated by various factors, including money, praise, insecurity, honor, prestige, needs, love, fear, satisfaction, and many others. An effective manager attempts to discover what motivates an employee to do a good job. Employees can also be motivated by incentives and recognition.
   - *Explain how the abuse of power and authority can negatively affect productivity in a healthcare facility.*
     A manager who berates and insults the staff members because he or she feels superior to them creates a distrusting, stressful, and nonproductive environment. Eventually the conduct of these types of managers negatively affects the quality of the care given to patients.

5. **Do the following related to creating a team atmosphere:**
   - *Discuss strategies to create a team environment in the medical office.*
     Teamwork is critical in the medical profession. In the healthcare facility, the manager must promote an atmosphere in which employees are willing to work together toward common goals. Morale in the facility may be low because of recent changes in policies or procedures, changes in staff or management, recent terminations of employees, lack of business, or any number of other reasons. The wise manager takes steps to improve employee morale continuously, including scheduling frequent meetings and keeping employees abreast of changes and developments that affect them.
   - *Recognize and overcome barriers to communication.*
     It is important for the medical assistant to recognize the barriers and help the team overcome them. Physical separation barriers can be

   reduced by using technology (e.g., video-conferencing and webcams). Language barriers can be addressed by encouraging awareness and acceptance of everyone's language and cultural differences. Status barriers can be reduced by promoting awareness and acceptance that everyone counts and every position on the team is important. Gender difference barriers can be addressed by helping all employees feel empowered to communicate openly with others. Cultural diversity barriers can be reduced by helping the team embrace the cultural differences among the members and educating the team on the differences.
   - *Demonstrate respect for individual diversity including gender, race, religion, age, economic status, and appearance.*
     Encouraging workplace diversity is part of the method of encouraging strong teams in the healthcare facility. Management should focus on the strengths that each staff member brings to the team. Staff members should be trained to provide the best medical care they can for all patients, without discrimination.

6. **Summarize strategies to introduce a new office manager.**
   As a new office manager, the first thing you can do to begin gaining support is nothing. Never storm into an office and begin making radical changes in the first few days. Work with the providers to determine the office goals. Then, schedule individual meetings with employees; allow them to tell you three things they like about their jobs, three things they dislike, and three things they need to do their jobs more effectively. After discussing your findings with the providers, use strategy to put the helpful suggestions into practice and attempt to move employees toward achieving the office goals.

7. **List several ways to prevent burnout.**
   Some of the causes of burnout include a stressful, disorganized home or work environment; poor human relations skills; a feeling of being out of control of one's life; excessive expectations from supervisors or family members; long work hours or time away from family and friends; and not being able to relax either at home or in the work environment. Although management may make efforts to prevent employee burnout, the employee ultimately must take steps to prevent it.

8. **Do the following related to finding the right employee for the job:**
   - *Identify the need to find the right employee for a job opening in the medical office.*
     From the providers to the receptionist, all play a vital role in the quality of healthcare delivered to patients. Hiring staff members who can be molded into a cohesive team is not an easy task. Care should be taken to choose employees who have the necessary skills and the right personality for the ambulatory care facility. When the need for a new employee arises, the office manager should discuss with the providers the type of employee required and the job description for that individual.
   - *Review a general job description for medical assistants.*
     Medical assistants are qualified for a variety of tasks in the healthcare facility. To fill an open medical assisting position, the manager must

SUMMARY OF LEARNING OBJECTIVES—*continued*

determine the specific experience that meets the facility's needs. Management should summarize the educational and skills sets needed to be successful at the position in the job description.

- *Explain how to search through résumés and applications for potential candidates.*

  Résumés and applications should be reviewed for accuracy and completeness. Gaps in employment dates should be explained fully, and the office manager should verify any references. Documents should be legible, and the information should be consistent and without oversights.

- *List and discuss legal and illegal interview questions.*

  The interviewer should be aware of various federal and state laws protecting the interviewee. Title VII of the Civil Rights Act of 1964, as amended by the Equal Employment Opportunity Act of 1972, prohibits inquiries into an applicant's race, color, gender, religion, and national origin. Inquiries about a person's medical history, arrest record, or previous drug use also are illegal. Most states have laws designed to protect the rights of job applicants, and these laws may impose additional restrictions. Office managers must research the laws that pertain to employment in their own states.

- *Explain how to select the most qualified candidates.*

  The first step in reviewing resumes includes separating out those that meet the minimal qualifications and those that do not. From those that meet the minimal qualifications, divide those into three stacks: those to call for an interview, possible candidates but not the strongest, and those that will not be called for an interview. Those with related experience, strong related skill sets (e.g., customer service), no unexplained employment gaps, and customized, error-free resumes and cover letters are more apt to be moved to the top of the pile.

- *Identify follow-up activities the office manager should perform after the interview.*

  When the interview is over, the office manager or interview team should immediately take a few moments to rate or summarize the applicant's strength and weaknesses. After all the interviews have been conducted, the team then rates the interviewees and identifies the top candidates. References are checked and a second interview may occur before the final person has been selected.

9. **Review new employee orientation, including paperwork, training, and development; also, explain how to conduct a staff meeting with an agenda.**

The office manager should develop a checklist of the paperwork needed for newly hired staff and all the information that should be covered with the new employee at the start of the job. Basic new employee paperwork often includes a job application; Form I-9 (Employment Eligibility Verification); W-4 Form (Employee's Withholding Allowance Certificate); Notice of Workers' Compensation coverage; consent for a background check and drug testing; acknowledgement of receipt of the company handbook or policy manual; agreements regarding pay, wage deductions, benefits, schedule, work location, and so on; notices of at-will employment status; acknowledgement of ethics statement; direct deposit application; and the OSHA compliance acknowledgement or checklist. Orientation and training help new employees to understand what is expected and to develop to their full potential.

The process for arranging a staff meeting is outlined in Procedure 20-1.

10. **Discuss strategies for addressing a problem employee, giving an employee a poor evaluation, terminating an employee, and determining fair salaries and raises.**

When negative information is to be relayed to an employee during a performance appraisal, the office manager should sandwich the negative comment between two positive ones whenever possible. Counseling these employees to find the source of their difficulties is the first step toward resolution. Many employees can be redirected to become productive staff members with a little patience and understanding on the manager's part. The manager should have good documentation of the problems that led to the poor evaluation. An employee who has been in service for some time and is offering unsatisfactory performance should be warned and given an explanation of the specific improvements expected. If a second chance does not produce improvement in performance or attitude, dismissal must follow. It should be done privately, with tact and consideration.

To keep good employees, the practice must pay a fair salary with regular raises if the staff member performs as expected. The office manager can find information about salary comparisons on the Internet. The manager should periodically review job descriptions and salary analyses online to see whether the salary the medical facility offers is comparable to those for similar jobs in the area.

CONNECTIONS

Study Guide Connection: Go to the Chapter 20 Study Guide. Read and complete the activities.

evolve Evolve Connection: Go to the Chapter 20 link at *evolve.elsevier.com/kinn* to complete the Chapter Review Quiz. Check out the other resources listed for this chapter to make the most of what you have learned from Supervision and Human Resource Management.

21

MEDICAL PRACTICE MARKETING AND CUSTOMER SERVICE

SCENARIO

Medical assistant Monica Raymond was hired by the Clear Skin Dermatology practice 2 years ago, after she had graduated from a medical assisting program. Dr. Julie Huang regularly praises Monica for her customer service skills. Dr. Huang is aware that effective marketing is essential to grow the practice, so she has asked Monica if she would be willing to assume some marketing responsibilities for the practice. Dr. Huang knows that Monica is comfortable using the Internet and is social media–savvy. Monica is excited about this opportunity. She realizes that she first must determine the type of patients the practice usually serves.

Dr. Huang has suggested a small budget and a few marketing tools that Monica may want to implement. In turn, Monica has suggested some updates to staff members' training, to improve their customer service skills and thus patient retention.

Monica has started designing the practice's website. She plans to incorporate a few features she found on other medical practice websites, including online appointment scheduling, an "ask the provider" e-mail exchange, and uploading of new patient intake forms. Knowing the importance of social networking, Monica intends to establish the dermatology practice on several social media platforms, such as Facebook and YouTube.

While studying this chapter, think about the following questions:

- Why is it important to identify the target market?
- What are some cost-effective marketing tools that a healthcare practice can use?
- Can social media help a healthcare practice stay in closer communication with its patients? If so, how?
- Why is customer service so important when delivering patient care?
- What type of resources can the healthcare practice provide to meet the needs of its patients?

LEARNING OBJECTIVES

1. Define, spell, and pronounce the terms listed in the vocabulary.
2. Do the following related to the marketing needs of a healthcare practice:
   - Explain the need for marketing for a healthcare facility.
   - Identify the target market.
   - Discuss why a SWOT analysis is important to identify the target market.
3. Do the following related to marketing tools:
   - Review ways a healthcare practice or facility can promote their practice through community involvement.
   - Define and discuss automated call distribution.
   - Explain how newsletters and blogs can be effective marketing tools.
   - Discuss marketing through print ads in magazines and newspapers.
   - Determine the value of Internet marketing for a healthcare practice or facility.
4. Distinguish between advertising and public relations.
5. Discuss the value of marketing through social media.
6. Develop website content, organization, and design to attract new patients; also, review strategies to increase website traffic.
7. Explain how to successfully deliver high-quality customer service, including how to identify with patients, and the value of patient surveys.
8. Identify strategies to manage problem patients.
9. Review the importance of the new patient information packet, and develop a current list of community resources related to patients' healthcare needs.
10. In the role of patient navigator, facilitate referrals to community resources.
11. Define a patient-centered medical home (PCMH).
12. Discuss applications of electronic technology (e.g., telemedicine) in professional communication.

VOCABULARY

advocate An individual who represents the patient when healthcare decisions are made.

blog An online journal that providers can use to share their experiences in caring for patients.

cost benefit analysis An assessment that weighs the benefit of attracting patients against the cost required.

liaison An individual assigned to communicate between multiple parties when the financial responsibilities of a deceased patient's estate are settled.

patient-centered medical home (PCMH) A model philosophy intended to improve the effectiveness of primary care. This approach is promoted by the National Committee for Quality Assurance (NCQA).

patient navigator A person who identifies patients' needs and barriers and assists by coordinating care and identifying community and healthcare resources to meet the needs.

site map A list of all Web page links on a website.

social media Internet-sponsored, two-way communication between individuals, individuals and businesses, or between businesses.

target market The groups of people most likely to need the medical services the practice offers.

telemedicine Video-conferencing technology that enables the delivery of quality healthcare at a distance.

A medical practice is a business; therefore, success lies in bringing in new patients and retaining current patients to maintain cash flow. Marketing and customer service are both essential for a healthcare facility to grow. *Marketing* is the process of informing the local community of the medical procedures and services the healthcare practice provides. Once customers visit the healthcare facility and become patients, customer service can enhance their experience so they want to return.

Marketing can be expensive and ineffective at increasing patient traffic if it is not planned out well. Some healthcare facilities work hard to find patients in the community, but then lose the patients' business through the lack of customer service. Customer loyalty ensures the longevity of a healthcare business. Therefore, following a well-thought-out marketing plan and building loyalty through customer service can ensure the healthcare practice's long-term financial success.

TABLE 21-1   Marketing Strategies for the Medical Office

STRATEGY	COST
Maintain a professional website	$$$
Manage an active Facebook, Twitter, Instagram, and/or other social media handle	No cost
Actively participate in community health fairs and events	$
Mail yearly checkup reminders	$$
Purchase billboard or magazine advertisements promoting the medical office	$$$$
Invite the public to an open house	$

MARKETING NEEDS OF THE HEALTHCARE FACILITY

All healthcare practices must have some sort of marketing plan to attract new patients. There are many ways to market a healthcare practice. A billboard near a freeway is a great way to promote the practice because of the number of potential patients it can reach; however, this type of marketing can be very expensive. A healthcare practice can print business cards for about $20 and then have someone leave a card at all the stores in a retail center. Although relatively inexpensive, this method doesn't ensure that the right patients are being reached (Table 21-1). The most important element of the marketing plan is to identify the right target market.

Identifying the Target Market

Identifying the **target market** is the key to successful marketing. Reaching the target market means that the targeted groups are made aware of the healthcare practice and what it has to offer.

The first step in identifying the target market is to determine who will need the medical procedures and services the healthcare facility offers. For example, the elderly population would most benefit from a long-term care facility. Women who are or who want

to become pregnant would benefit from an obstetrician's office and so on.

To bring more focus to the target market, the healthcare practice can review the demographics of its current patients. It may find, for example, that most of the patients for the long-term care facility come from the 78253 ZIP code. A gynecologist's office may find that most of its patients are between the ages of 20 and 25. In established medical offices, the medical assistant should keep a spreadsheet file for all patients with the following fields:

- Reason for visit
- Patient's age
- ZIP code
- Gender
- Marital status
- Ages of children
- How the patient found out about the healthcare facility

These demographics provide the details of the healthcare facility's specific target market. To identify the target market further, a SWOT analysis should be performed.

SWOT Analysis

The acronym SWOT stands for:

S – Strengths
W – Weaknesses
O – Opportunities
T – Threats

The SWOT analysis provides an evaluation of the business environment (Figure 21-1). This tool evaluates how economic forces affect the healthcare facility internally and externally. The Strengths and Weaknesses categories evaluate internal economic forces, and the Opportunities and Threats categories evaluate external economic forces.

Strengths and Weaknesses. The strengths of a healthcare practice are the advantages it has over its competitors, such as in the following categories:

- Reduced patient wait times
- Advanced medical technique and health information technology
- Flexible appointment hours
- Patient information Web portals
- E-prescribing

Weaknesses are the exact opposite of strengths. In other words, the weaknesses tool evaluates whether the healthcare practice's competitors are better in any of these categories.

No healthcare practice has only strengths. It would be too expensive for the practice to offer every benefit for their patients, but not be able to gain all the patients in their target market. Therefore, the healthcare practice should perform a **cost benefit analysis**, which is an assessment that weighs the benefit of attracting patients against the cost required. For example, a healthcare practice could invest in an in-house magnetic resonance imaging (MRI) machine, which would cost millions of dollars in lease payments over the next 5 years. But how many patients will use the machine in their healthcare facility? How much revenue will having the equipment generate for the medical office? Are there more significant advantages compared to referring patients go to a laboratory facility for an MRI?

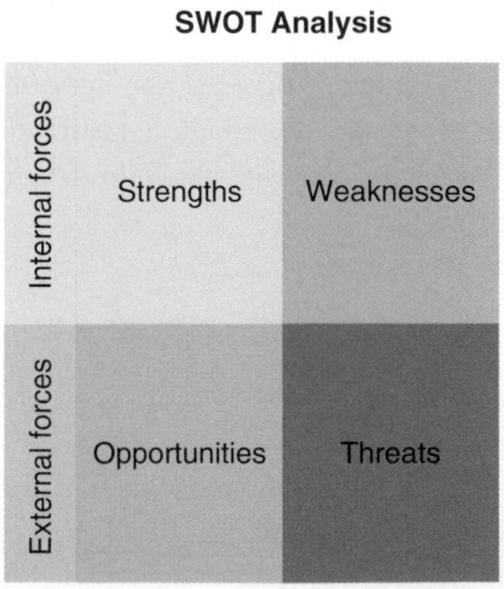

Opportunities and Threats. Opportunities review the prospect of increased business due to external forces. Healthcare practices have little or no control over the external market environment; however, a practice that recognizes opportunities can improve its internal strengths. Likewise, disregarding changes in the market can worsen a practice's weaknesses.

Some examples of opportunities include:

- Medical technology that reduces the cost of healthcare and hospital stays
- The increased number of Americans with health insurance because of the Affordable Care Act
- Electronic management of patient information, which reduces the time needed to care for each patient
- Public health campaigns, which highlight the importance of seeing the provider for specialized care

Threats can damage the long-term viability of a healthcare practice. A key threat is resisting the integration of electronic health record (EHR) systems into the practice. EHR systems facilitate the delivery of quality healthcare to patients and can support the continuity of patient care through collaboration among different healthcare providers. Although the implementation of electronic systems in healthcare facilities can be expensive at first, the long-term market outlook for them is good.

CRITICAL THINKING APPLICATION   **21-1**

Monica reviews the clinic's spreadsheet file of dermatology patients and finds that 40% of the patients come in for treatment of their acne. Would it be a good idea for the dermatology practice to expand its treatments for acne patients?

MARKETING TOOLS

As mentioned, some marketing strategies can be very expensive and also ineffective. Once the target market has been clearly identified, a number of marketing tools can effectively increase patient volume.

Promoting the Practice Through Community Involvement

Patients trust medical offices that participate in the local community. Some healthcare practices have participated in local health fairs offering free screenings, have partnered with farmer's markets to promote healthier eating, or even sponsored a local 5K run/walk to encourage exercise. To increase the healthcare practice's involvement in the community, some staff members can attend public community events and distribute brochures and pamphlets about conditions such as diabetes, heart disease, and hypertension. The practice may also sponsor specific charities annually. Some healthcare practices have volunteer programs in which staff members are recognized for their participation in community activities. Screenings for cholesterol and blood pressure checks are good ways to market a practice and gain new patients. The more the public views the healthcare practice actively participating in the community, the more likely it is that this will increase the number of appointments made at the medical office.

SWOT Analysis

FIGURE 21-1 A SWOT analysis can be done to define the target market.

Automated Phone Calls

Automated appointment reminders are a popular means of communicating with a large number of patients. A computer dials multiple phone numbers at the same time and plays a recorded message. Similar systems can send out text messages because most patients use their cell phones as their primary phone line. For instance, if a healthcare practice is planning to move to another part of the city, a program could be initiated to notify all patients that the office will be moving after a certain date. The message could include the address of the new location and even prompt patients to "Press 1" if they need to schedule an appointment. The same principle could be applied to news about an upcoming health fair or a special seminar about a certain illness.

Newsletters and Blogs

Many providers refer their patients to medical research about a variety of health topics, including ways to be treated. Some providers communicate this medical information as an e-newsletter, which is sent periodically, typically every month. However, providers are careful not to offer medical advice electronically; the intention of the e-newsletter should be to inform patients about health conditions that the provider typically sees in the medical office. For example, as an introduction to outdoor summer activities, an e-newsletter may promote healthy sun habits, such as wearing hats, sunglasses, and sunscreen. Or, in the fall, the provider can publish an e-newsletter to discuss ways to avoid catching the flu and may include a short video on how to properly wash hands to prevent the spread of disease.

A **blog** is an online journal that providers can use to share their experiences in caring for patients. Usually, providers do not follow a schedule for blog posts; they post when they have an experience to share for prevention, for care, and to inform. For example, a provider may document a patient who came in with a second-degree sunburn. To protect the patient's identity, the provider must uphold all privacy and confidentiality rules established by the Health Insurance Portability and Accountability Act (HIPAA), but he or she can post how the patient suffered through an unfortunate incident that could have been prevented. Sometimes blogs can include a v-log, or video log; at times providers post surgery videos online to inform patients of the services they provide.

Print Ads in Magazines and Newspapers

Advertising in magazines, newspapers, or mailers can inform the public of the healthcare practice and the services it offers. However, it is important to ensure that the target market can be reached by advertising this way because it is significantly more expensive and reaches a wider audience. Advertising in local magazines and/or newspapers is a more effective marketing strategy and can establish a business in the community. Magazine and newspaper ads can be effective tools, but finding free sources to promote the practice is less of a strain on the budget and allows expansion in other areas. The effectiveness of a newspaper and magazine marketing strategy can be evaluated by asking new patients how they learned about the practice. If a significant percentage mention the magazine or newspaper ad, the target market was reached.

Mailers are postcards or flyers that are mailed directly to hundreds of homes in a geographic area (Figure 21-2). This practice can be costly, and the target market may be wider than the area covered in the mailing, so the strategy may not be as effective. The more specialized the service the healthcare practice offers, the less likely it is that a mailer campaign could reach the target market and thus would be successful in increasing patient traffic.

Internet Marketing

Nowadays it is common to read many customer reviews on websites before patronizing a business. Businesses with more and better reviews tend to attract new customers. A healthcare practice has many opportunities to build a strong reputation through Internet marketing because patients can post reviews of their experiences on many different popular websites. The key is to ask every patient before he or she leaves to post a review of the services the person received; as the number of reviewers grows, the potential for new patients also will grow. A medical assistant can take responsibility for monitoring customer reviews on websites to confirm that the reviews are mostly positive. Some websites allow businesses to address negative comments, so the medical assistant should be ready to post a reply, such as, "We're sorry that you feel you did not receive the care that you deserve. Please feel free to call our office manager, Grace Townsend, to discuss how we could have improved your experience. Thank you for your feedback."

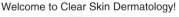

Welcome to Clear Skin Dermatology!

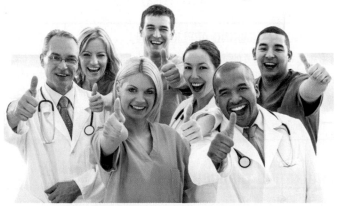

FIGURE 21-2 A mailer promoting the healthcare facility.

ADVERTISING VERSUS PUBLIC RELATIONS

There is a difference between advertising and public relations. Advertising involves creating or changing attitudes, beliefs, and perceptions by influencing people with purchased broadcast time, print space, or other forms of written and visual media. Broadcast time could take the form of television commercials, radio broadcasts, or audiovisual aids. Print could be a newspaper, magazine, or trade journal, and written and visual media may include a flier, brochure, or billboard.

Public relations is a similar field but relies more on news broadcasts or reports, magazine or newspaper articles, and blogs and radio reports to reach the audience. Most public relations efforts are free, but often it is difficult to get others interested enough in the activities the medical practice is planning to warrant coverage.

Addressing Bad Press

Occasionally a healthcare facility will face some cases of medical error, poor healthcare delivery, the leaking of personal health information, and/or mitigating circumstances that have found their way into the national headlines. Because healthcare is a personal issue, negative health news stories can destroy the trust the community has in the provider and the medical office. The first defense is to establish a high standard of customer service in the medical practice. Many patients will overlook small mistakes if the medical staff is apologetic and humble about the error.

If a medical error has been published in any type of media, it is wise for the medical practice to post an official apology statement on its website. This statement should not defend the actions of the provider and/or the medical practice, but rather express concern for any that were negatively affected in any way. The statement should also inform the public of the practice's rededication to delivering quality healthcare to all its current patients. A copy of the statement can also be displayed in the reception area of the medical office.

After the error has been published, the medical practice and the provider must work to overcome the stigma. Greater participation in the local community can help win back patients' trust, but patience and diligence may be needed to rebuild a thriving medical practice. It may be wise for a medical practice to hire a public relations consultant to help it improve its image in the community.

CRITICAL THINKING APPLICATION   21-4

A few weeks ago a patient posted on a public review website that she had had a bad reaction to a chemical peel she received at the clinic; she also complained that the medical office staff had done nothing to rectify the problem. This is the most recent review. What can Monica do to address the negative customer review?

MARKETING THROUGH SOCIAL MEDIA

Social media (e.g., Facebook, Twitter, YouTube) allow for two-way communication between a business and the consumer. Social media

outlets promote the business, and customers can respond positively or negatively about the service they received. Traditional media outlets, such as newspapers and magazines, allow only limited ability to respond; a person can write a letter to the editor of a newspaper, but the letter is not an immediate two-way exchange. Social media are considered a blending of technology and social interaction that creates an effective marketing tool.

Many websites now have icons that link to Facebook, Instagram, Twitter, YouTube, Pinterest, and other types of social media to promote interaction, in the hope of creating loyal patient relationships.

Medical offices are taking advantage of social media to promote the services they offer. Just like the "About Us" Web page, social media allow patients to gain insight into the care delivered. Providers can post nutritional counseling videos on YouTube, announce a community event on Twitter, and post the event pictures on Instagram. Patients can use Facebook to refer their friends and family to the medical practice. At-home remedies for some conditions, such as migraines, can be posted on Pinterest. Social media can bring the provider-patient relationship closer without the provider spending more time with the patient.

It is easy to understand how an aggressive, well-planned social media approach can positively affect the financial health of a practice. These outlets put individuals "into" the Web, making the experience more interactive and responsive. A medical assistant who can promote the healthcare practice on social media in a professional way is a valuable asset to the practice.

BUILDING A MEDICAL PRACTICE WEBSITE

One of the most popular and beneficial marketing tools for the healthcare facility is a professional website. An essential part of the marketing budget is the cost of having a Web developer create a website and maintain it on a monthly basis (Figure 21-3).

Five basic steps are involved in building a website for a medical practice:

1. Choosing a website name
2. Creating a site map
3. Designing the pages, including graphics and written content
4. Increasing traffic to the website
5. Using social media to increase public awareness of the website

Choosing a Website Name

Choosing a website name should be part of the healthcare facility's marketing strategy. Patients should commonly associate the website name with the medical office. The ideal website name typically is 7 to 15 letters and is related to the practice's name. The Internet has been around for some time, so many website names have already been taken; therefore, an Internet search should be done to check the availability of the preferred name before it is given to the Web page designer. Most websites begin with *www.*, followed by the name with no spaces, and usually end with *.org*, *.com* or *.net*. Some other website endings (e.g., *.gov* for government sites and *.edu* for educational institutions) would not be appropriate for a healthcare facility.

There is no requirement that the website name reflect the provider's name or the name of the medical office. Some practices identify themselves as the local specialist, as in *www.riversidegastroenterologists.com*.

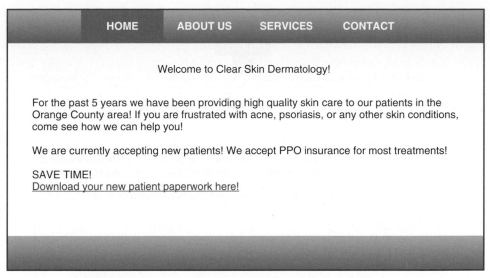

FIGURE 21-3 Common website format, with an introduction to the healthcare facility and site map.

Creating a Site Map

A successful website will attract many patients. An organized **site map** makes the website user friendly. When the website is designed, it is important to identify which informational pages should be included. A standard basic website has a Home page, an About Us page, a Testimonials or Information page, a Specials page, and a Contact Us page.

Home Page

The Home page is the introduction to the entire website. It is the first page viewed when the patient types the website into the address bar. The purpose of the Home page is to introduce the medical practice to the patient. Design is a key element of this page; colors should be appealing to the eye, and there should be a balance of images and content.

The Home page should contain the practice's name, the address, phone number, and any social media handles. The links to other pages, or the navigational menu, on the website should also be presented vertically or horizontally along the Web page. Most medical practices have a link to a patient portal, which provides access to personal health records; the user name and password are assigned by the practice. Typically the link to new patient paperwork also is found on the Home page.

About Us Page

The About Us page offers a unique opportunity to introduce all the healthcare providers in the medical office. Many healthcare facilities include photos of their providers, medical professionals, and/or support staff. These profiles are a marketing tool in that they inform possible patients about the services the medical practice offers. Each profile should include a friendly photograph of the medical practitioner, biographic information about his or her background, the number of years in practice, and a personal note. The personal note should focus on the type of care the patient can expect to receive.

Testimonials or Information Page

The Testimonials or Information page is an opportunity for the practice to customize the website. Some healthcare facilities prefer to include positive patient reviews about the practice; the page could have a link to a public reviewer website with more reviews. Other medical offices use the page for more informational purposes by publishing monthly e-newsletters here. The page can also be used to present any research papers a provider in the practice has published. The content of this page is up to the discretion of the medical staff.

Specials Page

Healthcare facility management decides the content of the Specials page. There may be times in the year when a practice, in an effort to attract more patients, can offer specials for various services. Many patients who still do not have health insurance look for specials for more affordable healthcare. For example, the practice can offer a special for flu vaccination for $20, no appointment necessary. Offering specials shows that the medical practice is invested in the good health of the community in general, not just in those with health insurance.

Contact Us Page

The Contact Us page contains a form that patients can fill out to be contacted for more information. This page also can be used as an "Ask the Provider" e-mail service (Figure 21-4). The patient can send an e-mail to the provider and expect a response within the next 24 hours. This type of provider-patient communication is popular and can increase patient retention.

Once the form has been filled out, the data collected are sent to the medical office e-mail address associated with the Web page. A medical assistant should be assigned to monitor this e-mail to respond to the patient in a timely manner.

Designing Pages

Once the site map has been created, the Web designer can begin brainstorming ideas about what the site will look like on the computer screen. Graphics, color choices, animation, and fonts enhance a website's look, and those four elements should be kept in balance. For example, smaller fonts make the text difficult to read for patients

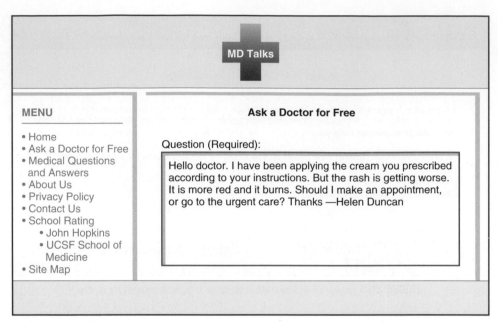

FIGURE 21-4 *"Ask the Provider" e-mail feature in the patient portal.*

with poor vision. Too many graphics crowd out the content of the website. The navigational menus should be designed so that viewers can move easily through the site. Most users appreciate a means to go back to the page previously viewed, and they become frustrated with sites that have an excessive number of pop-up boxes. Consistency is important, so it is a good idea to keep the same design theme on each page of the website.

Photographs, graphics, and video can add fun to the website, but be careful not to overdo them. Larger graphic files can take time to download. Most people will not wait longer than about 10 seconds for a Web page to load before clicking elsewhere. When you design Web page graphics, remember that smaller is better. Graphics can be found by searching for "index of GIF files" or "GIF library." Always respect any copyrights that are designated on any graphic file used. Many websites offer these file for free or charge a small fee.

The most important part of the website is the script, which should be developed by the office manager and the provider. It has been said that every word in a book must add to the story, and this is a good way to look at the text in a website. Avoid too much repetition, and remain clear about what is being communicated on the site. Headings and titles help clarify the theme of each page. Use a spell-checker before uploading the message and making it available for public viewing.

Hyperlinks are words or graphics on a Web page that, when clicked, take the viewer to another page or another website. To add a hyperlink, simply highlight the text field or graphic, select the hyperlink icon, and specify the destination address, or the *uniform resource locator* (URL). Always specify the full URL to ensure that the link directs the user to the desired page.

Increasing Website Traffic

A well-organized website has no value if patients are not aware that it exists. When patients search medical offices in their geographic area on a search engine website, the website should pop up. In order for the search engine to pick up the website, the Web designer includes appropriate key words into the website developer code. All healthcare facility websites should include keywords such as city, state, medical specialty, types of insurances accepted, and so on. These keywords are not viewable on the website but are included in the design code.

Website traffic should be monitored on a regular basis by healthcare facility management. Counters often can be added to the website that indicate how many people have viewed it. This helpful tool allows the medical practice to track how many people are viewing which pages. A sharp decline in website traffic may indicate a technical problem with the website, so it is important to monitor website traffic regularly and ensure that all Web pages are working properly.

HIGH-QUALITY CUSTOMER SERVICE

Once a patient comes to a medical practice, the key is to retain the patient for his or her future care needs. High-quality customer service not only can retain loyal patients, but also prompts them to refer their friends and family to the healthcare facilty. The delivery of high-quality customer service, therefore, is also considered an effective marketing tool.

Loyal Patients

The most effective way to increase the number of patients is word of mouth. When patients are satisfied with the treatment they receive, they refer other patients to the provider. However, if they are dissatisfied, they will tell everyone they know about their negative experience, which may affect the facility's future business.

Because patients often have a choice about who provides their healthcare services, it is important that the healthcare facility become the patient's first choice. Some patients are so loyal to a certain provider that even if their healthcare coverage no longer pays for visits, they continue to see that provider.

A Helpful Attitude

The provider and staff members should project a helpful attitude in every contact with the patient. They should sincerely ask, "How may I help you?" and then take steps to assist the patient in whatever way possible (Figure 21-5). Instead of pointing in the general direction of the radiology department, a staff member should take the patient there and introduce him or her to the receptionist. Instead of telling a patient on the telephone, "Ann handles the insurance billing. I'll transfer you to her," say, "One moment, Mrs. Brown, let me see if Ann is at her desk." Place Mrs. Brown on hold, call Ann, and let her know that she has a call. Then return to Mrs. Brown, tell her that Ann is at her desk, and transfer the call at that time. Be courteous and kind to every patient and visitor to the office. Good customer relations must be one of the primary goals of the medical facility. Patients count on staff members to be reliable and available to help them to the best of their abilities.

Office management should emphasize to all staff members the importance of delivering quality customer service. Staff meetings should be scheduled regularly to discuss customer service failures, review how those situations should have been handled, and recognize staff members who display high-quality customer service.

Identifying with Patients

Patients appreciate staff members who can be empathetic with the problems patients are facing. This is especially effective when a patient is upset or angry. For example, if a patient comes to the office complaining that charges were placed on his account for procedures that were not performed, the medical assistant may respond with a phrase such as, "Mr. Roberts, I understand that you are upset about these additional charges. Let me do some research on your account and let you know what I find. Let me help you by doing this ..."

Identifying with the patient shows understanding on the part of the staff member, no matter how upset the patient may be. Always acknowledge and restate the patient's concern. It proves that the medical assistant was listening and is interested in resolving the problem.

Remember, it costs much more to find new customers than to keep existing customers happy. Providing helpful, personal service impresses even the most difficult patient. To patients and visitors to the clinic, the employees to whom they speak represent the whole practice. Perceptions and opinions likely will be formed based on experiences with only one person. Each individual employee must be aware that to the patient, each employee is the healthcare practice.

CRITICAL THINKING APPLICATION   21-5

Monica thinks it would be beneficial for staff members to receive some of the dermatologic treatments so that they can recommend them to patients. Monica takes her idea to the providers as a marketing tool. Could this be a strong marketing tool? Might the staff members relate to patients better after experiencing the same medical treatments?

What Do Patients Expect?

First, patients expect to be treated according to the Golden Rule. They expect their concerns to be met with responsiveness, which means that the medical assistant should have a caring attitude (Figure 21-6). They also expect the professionals in the medical office to be knowledgeable about their field or specialty. An insurance biller should know more than just the basics of insurance filing. The office manager should have a certain degree of authority to handle problems and complaints. Patients also expect confidentiality and trust from the staff of the medical office. They expect an organized office that runs on schedule. They also expect that if a staff member promises to do something, it is as good as done.

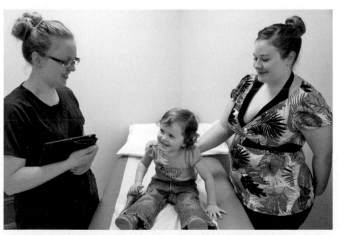

FIGURE 21-5 Helpful staff members provide the best customer service.

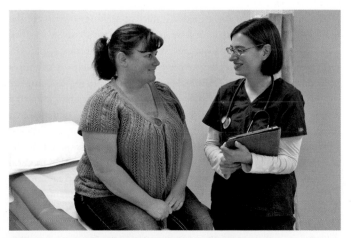

FIGURE 21-6 Friendly staff members are the best marketing tool. A smile is an excellent way to make patients feel welcome in the medical facility.

Thank you so much for visiting Clear Skin Dermatology! We want to ensure your experience with us was excellent! Your experience is important to us, so please share your thoughts by completing this survey. All surveys are confidential and are used to improve our service only. Thank you so much for your time and we look forward to caring for you soon!

	YES	NO
1. Is the location of our office convenient?	☐	☐
2. Do you find our reception area comfortable?	☐	☐
3. Do you feel relaxed in the reception area?	☐	☐
4. Do you find our front office personnel (Receptionist, etc.)	☐	☐
Friendly?	☐	☐
Courteous?	☐	☐
Rude or indifferent?	☐	☐
5. Do you find our business personnel (practice manager, billing specialist, etc.)	☐	☐
Friendly?	☐	☐
Courteous?	☐	☐
Rude or indifferent?	☐	☐
6. Are phone calls handled in a prompt, courteous, competent manner?	☐	☐
7. Do we provide adequate help with your insurance?	☐	☐
8. Have you received a copy of our financial policies?	☐	☐
9. Have our payment and billing policies been explained to your satisfaction?	☐	☐
10. Do you find our nurses and other clinical allied health workers:	☐	☐
Friendly?	☐	☐
Courteous?	☐	☐
Rude or indifferent?	☐	☐

Comments/complaints: _____
_____
_____
_____

FIGURE 21-7 Sample patient survey.

Patient Surveys

There is no better way to understand the quality of the care delivered than by asking the patients themselves! A patient survey (Figure 21-7) is vital for a medical practice seeking to evaluate the level of quality provided to their patient. Surveys can be mailed, e-mailed, or posted in the patient Web portal. Realistically, patients unhappy with the care they received are more likely to submit a patient survey. Sending friendly reminders for patients to complete the survey would be appropriate. Some medical offices have offered a small reward for completing the survey, such as a $10 gift card to a local coffee shop.

Successful medical practices take these surveys seriously by addressing patients' commendations and concerns. The medical office manager should review some of the responses during monthly staff meetings to discuss any changes that can be implemented to improve customer service. For the most part, surveys are anonymous. However, if a patient identifies himself or herself and addresses a specific concern, the office manager should contact the patient immediately to offer a possible remedy.

Phrases and Body Language That Undermine Successful Customer Service

The following are examples of phrases and body language that should never be used when speaking with patients or visitors.

- "I don't know."
  Say instead: "I'm not exactly sure, but I will find out." Medical assistants will not know the answer to every question, but they must be willing to find out the information.
- "I don't care."
  Say instead: "We care about your concerns and want to help." If the medical assistant cannot honestly make this statement, he or she should consider another profession.
- Body language that implies the staff member can't be bothered with the patient's concern.
  Instead: Look at the patient directly and say, "I truly want to give this matter my full attention. How can I contact you once I have looked into it?"

Some people may expect immediate attention and service, but they may have to be patient and wait their turn to receive assistance.

- "Ask someone else."
  Say instead: "I will be happy to find out who handles that for you." The medical assistant should never project the attitude that the patient's concerns are unimportant.
- "It's not my job."
  Say instead: "I am not one of the employees who files insurance, but I will be happy to ask Amanda, our insurance supervisor, to contact you and answer your questions." Do not ever tell the patient or a supervisor that a certain duty is not your responsibility. Find the right person to help the patient.
- "It's not my fault."
  Say instead: "I was not involved with that decision, but I know that our office manager would be happy to speak with you about it." Although blame should never be placed on another employee, any touchy issue should be referred to the office manager, especially if the medical assistant is not the final decision-making authority.
- "I didn't do it."
  Say instead: "I will see if I can get to the root of this issue." Be willing to assist the patient even if you are not involved in the situation at hand.
- "I know that."
  Say instead: "Yes, I understand. Let me try to help you." Do not use sarcasm, and never make snippy remarks.
- "I'm right, you're wrong."
  Say instead: "Our policy is clear about this matter, but let's see if we can come up with a compromise." Accusatory remarks should never be made to a patient.

All of the preceding alternate phrases give the patient a more positive view of both the office and those who work in it.

PROBLEM PATIENTS

Patients can sometimes be quite challenging for the provider's staff and office manager. Most patients are genuinely concerned about their health and are very cooperative. However, a few patients require extra understanding, which may lead to intervention by the office manager. Types of problem patients may include those who are:

- Complainers
- Angry
- Needy
- Demanding
- Violent
- Nonpaying
- Noncompliant
- Drug seeking
- Reschedulers

The office manager may act as a **liaison** between the patient and the providers when issues arise that are somewhat complicated. Some patients may feel ignored or mistreated by office staff. Others may have a general lack of trust that makes complying with the provider's orders difficult for them. Cultural differences, social issues, and financial problems all can affect a patient's compliance and attitude.

Both the medical assistant and the office manager should serve as patient **advocates**, but they can never hold back information the provider needs to know. For instance, if a patient tells the medical assistant or office manager that he has been smoking, although he told the provider he quit, the information must be presented to the provider. Information that is shared with the medical assistant must be shared with the provider, even if the patient objects. Medical assistants should inform the patient respectfully that they are ethically obligated to share all information collected with the provider.

"WELCOME TO OUR OFFICE" PACKET

Only a very small percentage of practices have a Welcome to Our Office packet that explains the operational and service aspects of the practice. Yet, the provider and staff can easily compile a patient information booklet cooperatively during a staff meeting. Experience has shown that if such a packet is given to every new patient, the number of patient calls to the office can be reduced by an average of 20% to 30%. It also can reduce misunderstandings and forgotten instructions. The packet should be custom tailored to the specific practice.

Introduction to the Medical Office

The welcome packet should begin with an introduction letter to the practice. The information should be the same or similar to what would be found in the "About Us" Web page on the website. The healthcare facility letterhead should be used, which includes the address, contact numbers, website, and/or any social media user names.

A statement of philosophy frequently is included in the introduction, followed by a description of the practice. Consider this example:

> The doctors and staff would like to welcome you to our office. We work as a team with the goal of providing prompt and thorough care to improve your health. We are always working to improve our care and service in any way possible. Our practice is limited exclusively to dermatology and related disorders. Therefore, it is important for each patient to have a primary care provider, such as a pediatrician, a family provider, or an internist, to oversee the patient's primary medical care. Our role is most effective as a consultant to your primary care provider.

List all providers in the practice; state their educational backgrounds, training, and board certifications; and define their specialties. List the names of key clinical and administrative staff members, such as registered nurses and nurse practitioners, medical assistants, the office manager, and the business manager. Provide the practice address, a map of how to get there, and information about the parking facilities.

Missed Appointments and Cancellation Policy

The office policy regarding missed appointments and cancellations, telephone calls, and the function of the answering service should also be mentioned in the welcome packet. For example:

> We always strive to answer telephone calls quickly, but at times you may be asked to wait as we finish handling prior patient calls. Your call is important to us, and we appreciate your patience. If you wish to speak to the provider, the receptionist will take your information and the provider will contact you during the next available break or at the end of the office day. Our triage nurse and the provider's medical assistant also would be happy to help you.

> If you want to speak to a doctor, your call usually will be returned during the next available break period or at the end of the office day. Therefore, the receptionist usually will take a message, and your call will be returned as soon as possible. Please inform the receptionist if your problem is urgent, and he or she will inform the doctor. Patients can also use the "Ask the Provider" e-mail service located on the "Contact Us" page on the website.

> **In case of emergency, call 911**. If you have a nonemergency concern, one of the doctors in the group is always on call. You may reach him or her by calling our office telephone number (714) 555-2323; the answering service will put you in touch with the doctor on call at that time. Our doctors are on staff at St. Joseph Hospital (714) 555-3333, and for children, Children's Hospital of Orange County (714) 555-4444.

Medical Office's Financial Policy

Spell out the practice's policies on billing and collection procedures, and make it clear that patients are responsible for their financial portion of the fees. If payment is expected at the time of service, add this in the welcome folder. Keep the language simple and straightforward so that the message is clear:

> We ask that our services be paid for at the time they are rendered. There is usually a greater charge for the initial visit because this involves more time and evaluation than follow-up visits. If you are referred to an outside office for laboratory testing or special x-ray procedures, you will be billed separately by that office. We will bill your insurance on your behalf; thank you for accepting financial responsibility for the amount the health insurance assigns as your co-insurance and/or deductible.

Patient Information Web Portal

Patients should be granted access to their patient portal through the healthcare facility website. The username and password are assigned at the patient's first office visit. Patients can gain access to laboratory reports, test results, consultation reports, and any other medical encounter records in their personal Web portal.

Patients can also request pharmaceutical refills, update health insurance information, and request an appointment through the patient portal. However, patients should be aware that the patient Web portal manages records from this specific medical office, not from any other specialists, laboratories, or hospitals.

Patient Instruction Sheets

In most medical offices, some patient procedures are performed over and over again. Instead of attempting to instruct a patient orally each time, the practice can develop instruction sheets (Figure 21-8) that can be reviewed with the patient and then uploaded to the patient portal. The following are some suggested topics for patient instruction sheets:

- Preparation for an x-ray procedure or laboratory tests
- Preoperative and postoperative instructions
- Dietary guidelines
- Performing an enema
- Dressing a wound
- Taking medications
- Using a cane, crutches, walker, or wheelchair
- Care of casts
- Exercise therapy

List of Community Resources

Community organizations can collaborate with the healthcare provider to meet the patient's health needs. As a participant in the health of the local community, the practice should generate a list of community resources to assist patients in their efforts to improve their health (Procedure 21-1). These resources can represent a wide variety of services, such as:

- Meals assistance and food banks
- Adult day care services and centers
- Grief support groups
- Chronic disease support groups
- Medical equipment suppliers
- Home healthcare centers
- Long-term healthcare facilities (e.g., convalescent care, skilled nursing facilities, rehabilitation centers, and psychiatric hospitals)
- Assisted-living information
- Hospice services
- Immunization clinics
- Smoking cessation programs
- Local board of health
- Alcoholics and Narcotics Anonymous meetings

Local communities have many outreach programs with which the healthcare practice should network. For example, the American Cancer Society provides support to cancer patients in the community by providing rides to treatment, lodging near treatment centers, and hair loss and mastectomy products. The healthcare facility should maintain and update the list of resources on a regular basis, but it is not responsible if the services are no longer available.

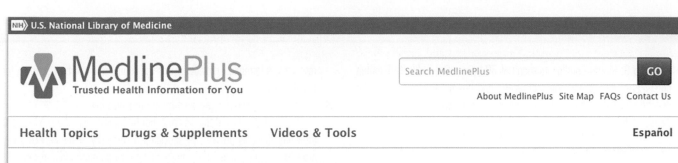

MedlinePlus
Trusted Health Information for You

Search MedlinePlus [GO]

About MedlinePlus Site Map FAQs Contact Us

Health Topics   **Drugs & Supplements**   **Videos & Tools**   **Español**

Home → Drugs, Herbs and Supplements → Clindamycin and Benzoyl Peroxide Topical

Clindamycin and Benzoyl Peroxide Topical
pronounced as (klin da mye' sin) (ben' zoe ill) (per ox' ide)

Why is this medication prescribed?

The combination of clindamycin and benzoyl peroxide is used to treat acne. Clindamycin and benzoyl peroxide are in a class of medications called topical antibiotics. The combination of clindamycin and benzoyl peroxide works by killing the bacteria that cause acne.

How should this medicine be used?

The combination of clindamycin and benzoyl peroxide comes as a gel to apply to the skin. It is usually applied twice a day, in the morning and evening. To help you remember to use clindamycin and benzoyl peroxide gel, apply it at around the same times every day. Follow the directions on your prescription label carefully, and ask your doctor or pharmacist to explain any part you do not understand. Use clindamycin and benzoyl peroxide gel exactly as directed. Do not use more or less of it or use it more often than prescribed by your doctor.

To use the gel, follow these steps:

1. Wash the affected area with warm water and gently pat dry with a clean towel.

2. Use you fingertips to spread a thin layer of gel evenly over the affected area. Avoid getting the gel in your eyes, nose, mouth, or other body openings. If you do get the gel in your eyes, wash with warm water.

3. Look in the mirror. If you see a white film on your skin, you have used too much medication.

4. Wash your hands.

Other uses for this medicine

This medication may be prescribed for other uses; ask your doctor or pharmacist for more information.

FIGURE 21-8 Sample patient instruction sheet.

PROCEDURE 21-1	Develop a Current List of Community Resources Related to Patients' Healthcare Needs and Facilitate Referrals

Goal: *Identify community resources related to patients' healthcare needs and to facilitate referrals to community resources in the role of a patient navigator.*

EQUIPMENT and SUPPLIES

- Computer with Internet and/or a telephone book
- Paper and pen
- Community Resource Referral Form or referral form

- **Scenario 1:** Herman Miller is a 72-year-old male who was just diagnosed with dementia. He currently lives with his daughter, Ruby, who works full-time. Ruby is feeling overwhelmed with being his only caregiver and realizes that she needs to find someone to provide care to her father while she is working.

- **Scenario 2:** Leslie Green just tested positive for pregnancy. She is still a teenager and doesn't feel that she has a support system to help her make decisions.

PROCEDURE 21-1   —continued

- **Scenario 3:** Marcia Carrillo's husband of 30 years, died suddenly 1 month ago. Marcia stated that she feels alone and has no one to talk to. Her daughter feels that she needs the support of others who have gone through the same thing.

PROCEDURAL STEPS

1. Identify the possible types of community resources that would assist the patient and/or family.
   PURPOSE: A variety of community resources are available for patients and families dealing with chronic illnesses and death. The resources range from daycare, meals, transportation, medical equipment, assistive living, support groups, and reduced costs for medications.
2. Using the Internet and/or the phone book, identify local resources for the patient. Make a list of resources for the patient and/or family member. Include the name of the organization, the addresses, and the contact information.
   PURPOSE: As an advocate and patient navigator, it is important to provide patients and families with the contact information for various community

resources. Information provided helps the family find the best solution for the situation.

3. Summarize the services provided by the organization.
   PURPOSE: Patients and families may not be familiar with the services that local organizations provide. By providing a summary of the services, you are educating the patient and family, and it may promote them to seek out these services.
4. (Role-play) Provide the patient and/or family member with the list of resources and identify which service(s) they would be interested in.
5. Use professional, tactful verbal and nonverbal communication as you work with the patient and family.
   PURPOSE: Patients and family members are more apt to respond positively to assistance if the medical assistant's communication is professional, empathic, and tactful. Talking down to patients or acting superior are unprofessional behaviors that negatively impact the working relationship with patients.
6. Complete the referral form to help facilitate the referral to community resource(s).

THE PATIENT NAVIGATOR

The **patient navigator** program was established at the Harlem Hospital Center in 1990 to assist cancer patients in accessing quality healthcare. With the assistance of the 2005 Patient Navigator, Outreach and Chronic Disease Prevent Act, many patient navigator positions were funded throughout the U.S. Today, patient navigator positions are found in clinics and hospitals around the country, helping patients find emotional, financial, administrative, or cultural resources within the healthcare community and the local community.

There are many models for patient navigator programs, but the goal is the same—to help patients find the resources they need. Patient navigators are responsible for, but not limited to, the following:

- Interview patients to identify their needs and barriers to wellness and healthcare.
- Provide patients resources based on their needs and barriers.
- Coordinate appointments and care for patients.
- Assist with reducing language barriers, by identifying bilingual providers and translators.
- Discuss special needs patients have with their healthcare team.
- Identify community resources, which may include transportation, medical equipment, adult daycare and assistive living, support groups, low cost medication programs, low-cost preventative screening and immunizations, and adoption services.

A medical assistant can work in the patient navigator role and assist the healthcare team by identifying patients' needs and barriers to wellness and healthcare. The medical assistant then matches the patient to appropriate community resources (e.g., support groups, low cost/free meals, and transportation) and provides the patient with information on the resources (see Procedure 21-1). For healthcare related resources (e.g., medical equipment, hospice), the medical assistant works with the provider and completes the required insurance and referral forms.

PATIENT-CENTERED MEDICAL HOME

The **patient-centered medical home (PCMH)** is a model philosophy intended to improve the effectiveness of primary care. This approach is promoted by the National Committee for Quality Assurance (NCQA). The PCMH model sets the following standards in the delivery of primary health care:

- Providers and patient care teams should work together to bring care to the patient.
- Patients should be treated with respect, dignity, and compassion by the medical care team.
- Medical care should be coordinated with the patient's needs and wants.
- The use of health information technology should be maximized in the delivery of patient care.
- A chain of command that creates a forum for decision making for the entire patient care team should be established; this helps organize and unify network practices.

The intent of the PCMH model is to improve healthcare in America by transforming how primary care is organized and delivered. The model has five key domains (Table 21-2):

- Comprehensive Care
- Patient-Centered Care
- Coordinated Care
- Accessible Services
- Quality and Safety

TABLE 21-2   Key Domains of the Patient-Centered Medical Home (PCMH)

DOMAIN	DESCRIPTION
Comprehensive Care	The PCMH is designed to meet a majority of a patient's physical and mental health care needs through a team-based approach to care.
Patient-Centered Care	The delivery of primary care oriented toward the whole person. This can be achieved by partnering with patients and families through an understanding of and respect for culture, unique needs, preferences, and values.
Coordinated Care	The PCMH coordinates patient care across all elements of the healthcare system, such as specialty care, hospitals, home healthcare, and community services, with an emphasis on efficient care transitions.
Accessible Services	The PCMH seeks to make primary care accessible through minimizing wait times, enhanced office hours, and after-hours access to providers through alternative methods, such as telephone or e-mail.
Quality and Safety	The PCMH model is committed to providing safe, high-quality care through clinical decision-support tools, evidence-based care, shared decision making, performance measurement, and population health management. Sharing quality data and improvement activities also contribute to a systems-level commitment to quality.

From the Agency for Healthcare Research and Quality: pcmh.ahrq.gov.

Health Internet Technology (IT), the workforce, and finance support these key domains. Health IT supports PCMH by collecting and storing relevant data to improve process outcomes. The workforce, which includes the team of providers and other healthcare personnel, provides care based on PCMH principles. Finance calls for the reform of health insurance reimbursement for primary care services.

ELECTRONIC TECHNOLOGY IN PROFESSIONAL COMMUNICATION

Telemedicine

More and more, providers are using technology to improve the care delivered to their patients. Advances in video conferencing technology have enabled providers to evaluate and treat patients who live hundreds of miles away. Telemedicine opens health care access to many patients in rural areas where access is limited. Patients in rural areas must drive farther to receive care; because of this inconvenience, many of these patients go without regular medical care. Case studies have shown that providers who use telemedicine improve not only the quality of the patient's health, but also customer service.

Video conferencing through a secured Web portal in which the provider can view the patient for evaluation. Some telemedicine organizations provide 24-hour support for patients all over the country. Providers can allow patients to keep the recording of the consultation so they can remember the provider's recommendations. Telemedicine also has greatly reduced the number of unnecessary emergency and urgent care visits.

CLOSING COMMENTS

Marketing is essential to the future financial success of a medical practice. Once a target market has been identified, many different marketing tools can be used to assist the practice in attracting new patients. A well-organized website is useful for reaching new patients and creating a loyal relationship with current patients. The most inexpensive marketing strategy is delivering exceptional customer service. Providing good customer service is a commitment that must be made by every employee of the healthcare practice, every single day. There will be times when the customer does not act respectfully, but he or she should be treated with dignity and respect at all times. In addition, a skilled customer service provider has a knack for making the customer think he or she was right all along! For medical practices, providing good service results in an excellent reputation for the clinic, built by those who matter most—the patients.

Patient Education

A practice's marketing efforts provide endless opportunities for patient education. Most providers agree that part of the obligation of the medical profession is to educate patients about healthcare issues specific to their needs. Medical assistants should listen carefully to the patient's needs and then make referrals to community resources if these can help the patient meet his or her health needs. For patients who are more private about their personal health struggles, it may be beneficial to post links to different online resources, such as Alcoholics Anonymous meetings and stop smoking seminars.

Legal and Ethical Issues

The provider must take care that patients do not use the information in brochures or on the practice website as medical advice or as a substitute for the provider's medical advice. Before attaching a link to another website, the medical assistant must be sure the site is reputable; government websites are always recommended. The patient may consider information on the practice's website to be an extension of the provider's advice, so make sure everything on the website is accurate.

The provider should carefully review all printed information used to promote the medical facility. Make sure there are no misleading statements. A stated disclaimer should be included to remind patients that the information given in brochures and on websites is for general use only. Patients should be advised to discuss specific issues with the provider or to use the "Ask the Doctor" feature.

Professional Behaviors

Building a successful medical practice starts with effective marketing tools and strong customer service standards. As mentioned, customer service is the key to building a loyal patient base and growing the practice through referrals. Medical assistants, whether just out of school already established in their career must strive to provide patients with good customer service. Patients do not hesitate to tell the provider if the medical assistant is not cordial and helpful. Providing excellent customer service is mandatory for every employee of the practice.

SUMMARY OF SCENARIO

Monica is confident that a simple marketing plan will enable the practice to experience steady, continuous expansion. She has performed a SWOT analysis and reviewed the spreadsheet of patient demographics and determined a specific target market.

A monthly newsletter and the practice's website are some of the marketing tools Monica plans to use to reach the target market. One of her first steps is to develop an annual calendar of special events and community outreach. The newsletter, which will provide health information and details about upcoming events, will be available both in print and online. The patients in the office database who have e-mail addresses will automatically receive a computer-generated e-mail message with a link that takes them directly to the online newsletter. Monica also has planned one special community event for each month of the upcoming year.

Monica plans to track the responses to each event promoted on the healthcare facility website to determine what marketing tools were most effective in promoting the clinic. The website allows her to count the number of visits and to determine which pages are the most popular. She will keep Dr. Huang informed, and be open to their suggestions. Monica also has found that using social media for marketing has increased traffic to the practice's website, which offers patients several options to increase their knowledge about health-related subjects and find opportunities to participate in events that promote good health.

The clinic's staff members understand that no matter what efforts are used to promote the practice and obtain new patients, it is their responsibility to provide exceptional customer service so that patients are happy with their experience. People have choices as to who provides their healthcare, so they must be treated cordially and fairly by medical professionals who truly want to serve their needs.

SUMMARY OF LEARNING OBJECTIVES

1. **Define, spell, and pronounce the terms listed in the vocabulary.**
   Spelling and pronouncing medical terms correctly reinforce the medical assistant's credibility. Knowing the definitions of these terms promotes confidence in communication with patients and co-workers.

2. **Do the following related to the marketing needs of the healthcare practice:**
   - *Explain the need for marketing for a healthcare practice or facility.*
     All healthcare practices and facilities must have a marketing plan in order to attract new patients. There are many ways to market a healthcare practice/facility.
   - *Identify the target market.*
     Identifying the *target market* (i.e., the groups of people most likely to need the medical service provided by the practice) is the key to successful marketing. Reaching the target market means that the targeted groups are made aware of the practice and what it has to offer.
   - *Discuss why a SWOT analysis is important to identify the target market.*
     A SWOT analysis provides an evaluation of the business environment. This tool evaluates how economic forces affect the healthcare practice internally and externally. The strengths and weaknesses categories evaluate internal economic forces, and the opportunities and threats categories evaluate the external economic forces.

3. **Do the following related to marketing tools:**
   - *Review ways a healthcare practice or facility can promote itself through community involvement.*

   Patients trust medical practices that participate in the local community. Some practices participate in local health fairs to provide free screenings and farmers' markets to promote healthier eating. Some even sponsor a local 5K run/walk to encourage vigorous exercise. The more the public views the practice as active in the community, the more likely it is that this will increase the number of appointments made at the medical office.
   - *Define and discuss automated call distribution.*
     Automated call distribution is a popular means of communicating with large numbers of people. A computer dials multiple numbers at the same time and plays a recorded message, which can be the actual provider with news about a new procedure or a new associate joining the practice.
   - *Explain how newsletters and blogs can be effective marketing tools.*
     Many providers refer their patients to the same medical research about a variety of health topics, including ways to be treated. Some providers communicate this medical information as an e-newsletter, which is sent periodically, typically every month. However, providers must be careful not to offer medical advice electronically; the intention of the e-newsletter should be to inform patients about health conditions that the provider typically sees in the medical office.
   - *Discuss marketing through print ads in magazines and newspapers.*
     If the marketing budget allows, advertising in magazines and newspapers or through mailers can inform the public about the practice and the services it offers. However, it is important to ensure that the

target market can be reached by advertising this way because it is significantly more expensive and reaches a wider audience. Advertising in local magazines and/or newspapers is a more effective marketing strategy and can establish the practice in the community.

- *Determine the value of Internet marketing for a healthcare practice or facility.*

On the Internet, businesses that have a greater number of and more favorable reviews tend to attract new business. There are many opportunities for a healthcare practice to build a strong reputation through Internet marketing because there are many different popular websites in which people post reviews of their experiences. The key is to ask every patient before he or she leaves to post a review of the services the person received; as the number of reviewers grows, the potential for new patients also will grow.

4. **Distinguish between advertising and public relations.**

Advertising is a medium that attempts to create or change attitudes, beliefs, and perceptions through printed material, the Internet, or other forms of communication. Public relations is a similar field but relies more on news broadcasts or reports, magazine or newspaper articles, and radio reports to reach the audience.

5. **Discuss the value of marketing through social media.**

A social media outlet promotes a business, and customers can respond positively or negatively about the service they received. Traditional media outlets, such as newspapers and magazines, allow only limited ability to respond; a person can write a letter to the editor of a newspaper, but the letter does not generate an immediate two-way response. Social media is considered a blending of technology and social interaction that creates an effective marketing tool.

6. **Develop website content, organization, and design to attract new patients; also, review strategies to increase website traffic.**

A successful website will be able to attract many patients. An organized site map makes a site user friendly. In the design of a website, it is important to identify which informational pages should be included. A standard basic website has a Home page, an About Us page, testimonials or an informational page, specials, and a Contact Us page.

A well-organized website has no value if patients are not aware that it exists. When patients search for medical offices in their geographic area on a search engine website (e.g., Google), the practice's website should pop up. To enable the search engine to pick up the website, the Web designer must include appropriate key words in the website developer code. All medical office websites should include keywords such as city, state, medical specialty, types of insurances accepted, and so on. These keywords are not viewable on the website but are included in the design code.

7. **Explain how to successfully deliver high-quality customer service, including how to identify with patients, and the value of patient surveys.**

High-quality customer service not only can create a loyal patient, it can prompt that patient to refer his or her friends and family so that they can receive the same quality of care. Therefore, delivering high-quality customer service is considered an effective marketing tool.

For staff members, identifying with the patient means showing understanding, no matter how upset the person may be. Always acknowledge and restate the patient's concerns. This proves that the medical assistant was listening and is interested in resolving the problem.

For a medical practice seeking to evaluate the quality of its customer service, periodic evaluation is vital. Patients' perspectives can provide insight into areas needing improvement that staff members may not be able to perceive from inside the office. Evaluations can be mailed, e-mailed, or posted on the patient Web portal.

8. **Identify strategies to manage problem patients.**

Cultural differences, social issues, and financial problems all can affect a patient's compliance and attitude. The rare patient may have a personality disorder or psychological problem that staff members find frustrating as they provide medical treatment. Some patients may have a general lack of trust that makes complying with the provider's orders difficult for them.

9. **Review the importance of the new-patient information packet.**

Experience has shown that if an information packet is given to every new patient, the number of patient calls to the office can be reduced by an average of 20% to 30%. This also can reduce misunderstandings and instances of forgotten instructions. The packet should be custom tailored to the specific practice.

10. **In the role of patient navigator, facilitate referrals to community resources.**

Patient navigators help identify patients' barriers and needs to wellness and healthcare. The patient navigators then provide patients with referrals or information about community resources. For healthcare related needs, the patient navigator works closely with the patient's healthcare team to resolve the issues.

11. **Define a patient-centered medical home (PCMH).**

The patient-centered medical home (PCMH) is a model philosophy intended to improve the effectiveness of primary care. This approach is promoted by the National Committee for Quality Assurance (NCQA).

12. **Discuss applications of electronic technology (e.g., telemedicine) in professional communication.**

Video conferencing takes place through a secure Web portal in which the provider can view the patient for evaluation. Some telemedicine organizations provide 24-hour support for patients all over the country.

CONNECTIONS

Study Guide Connection: Go to the Chapter 21 Study Guide. Read and complete the activities.

evolve Evolve Connection: Go to the Chapter 21 link at *evolve.elsevier.com/kinn* to complete the Chapter Review Quiz. Check out the other resources listed for this chapter to make the most of what you have learned from Medical Practice Marketing and Customer Service.

22 SAFETY AND EMERGENCY PRACTICES

SCENARIO

Cheryl Skurka, CMA (AAMA), has been working for Dr. Peter Bendt for approximately 6 months. During that time, a number of patient emergencies have occurred in the office, and even more potentially serious problems have been managed by the telephone screening staff. Cheryl is concerned that she is not prepared to assist with emergencies in an ambulatory care practice. She decides to ask Dr. Bendt for assistance, and he suggests that she work with the experienced screening staff to learn how to manage phone calls from patients calling for assistance.

Dr. Bendt is participating in a community-wide preparedness effort focused on both natural and human-made disasters, and he expects his practice and employees to be ready to respond if needed. This includes creating plans both to maintain the safety of patients and employees in the facility and to provide assistance as needed in a community emergency.

While studying this chapter, think about the following questions:

- What should Cheryl learn about the medical assistant's responsibilities in an emergency situation?
- What are some of the general rules for managing a medical emergency in an ambulatory care practice?
- What types of questions does the telephone screening staff ask if a patient calls with a medical emergency?
- What information from these phone calls should be documented?
- Is it important for Cheryl to be able to recognize life-threatening emergencies and to be prepared to respond to them? Why?
- What are some of the typical patient emergencies that occur in a healthcare facility?
- How should Cheryl instruct a patient to control bleeding from a hemorrhaging wound?
- What safety practices should be followed in the healthcare facility to protect patients and employees from potential harm?
- What is the medical office's responsibility in preparing for community emergencies?
- Are there common health emergency topics for patient education that Cheryl should be prepared to present?
- What legal factors should Cheryl keep in mind when handling ambulatory care emergencies?

LEARNING OBJECTIVES

1. Define, spell, and pronounce the terms listed in the vocabulary.
2. Describe patient safety factors in the medical office environment.
3. Interpret and comply with safety signs, labels, and symbols and evaluate the work environment to identify safe and unsafe working conditions for the employee.
4. Do the following when it comes to environmental safety in the healthcare setting:
   - Identify environmental safety issues in the healthcare setting
   - Discuss fire safety issues in a healthcare environment
   - Demonstrate the proper use of a fire extinguisher
5. Describe the fundamental principles for evacuation of a healthcare facility and role-play a mock environmental exposure event and evacuation of a provider's office.
6. Discuss the requirements for proper disposal of hazardous materials.
7. Identify critical elements of an emergency plan for response to a natural disaster or other emergency.
8. Maintain an up-to-date list of community resources for emergency preparedness.
9. Describe the medical assistant's role in emergency response.
10. Summarize typical emergency supplies and equipment.
11. Demonstrate the use of an automated external defibrillator.
12. Summarize the general rules for managing emergencies.
13. Demonstrate telephone screening techniques and documentation guidelines for ambulatory care emergencies.
14. Recognize and respond to life-threatening emergencies in an ambulatory care practice.
15. Describe how to handle an unresponsive patient and perform provider/professional-level CPR.
16. Discuss cardiac emergencies and administer oxygen through a nasal cannula to a patient in respiratory distress.
17. Identify and assist a patient with an obstructed airway.
18. Discuss cerebrovascular accidents and assist a patient who is in shock.
19. Determine the appropriate action and documentation procedures for common office emergencies, such as fainting, poisoning, animal bites, insect bites and stings, and asthma attacks.

VOCABULARY

arrhythmia (uh-rith′-me-uh) An abnormality or irregularity in the heart rhythm.

asystole (ay-sis′-toh-le) The absence of a heartbeat.

cyanosis (si-an-oh′-sis) A blue coloration of the mucous membranes and body extremities caused by lack of oxygen.

diaphoresis (di-uh-fuh-re′-sis) The profuse excretion of sweat.

ecchymosis (eH-kih-moh′-sis) A hemorrhagic skin discoloration commonly called bruising.

emetic (eh-met′-ik) A substance that causes vomiting.

fibrillation Rapid, random, ineffective contractions of the heart.

hematuria (he-muh-tuhr′-e-uh) Blood in the urine.

idiopathic (ih-dee-oh-path-ik) Pertaining to a condition or a disease that has no known cause.

mediastinum (me-de-ast′-in-um) The space in the center of the chest under the sternum.

myocardium (my-oh-kar′-de-um) The muscular lining of the heart.

necrosis (neh-kroh′-sis) The death of cells or tissues.

photophobia An abnormal sensitivity to light.

polydipsia Excessive thirst.

Safety Data Sheets (SDSs) Documents that accompany hazardous chemicals and substances and outline the dangers, composition, safe handling, and disposal of these items. Safety Data Sheets must be formatted to conform to the Globally Harmonized System (GHS), which mandates that SDS have 16 standardized sections arranged in a strict order.

thrombolytics Agents that dissolve blood clots.

transient ischemic attack (TIA) Temporary neurologic symptoms caused by gradual or partial occlusion of a cerebral blood vessel.

The medical assistant typically is responsible for making the healthcare facility as accident proof as possible. This requires attention to a number of factors. For example, cupboard doors and drawers must be kept closed; spills must be wiped up immediately; and dropped objects must be picked up. The medical assistant also should make sure that all medications are kept out of sight and away from busy patient areas. If children are in the office, all sharp objects and potentially toxic substances must be kept out of reach. In addition, the medical assistant should never leave a seriously ill patient or a restless, depressed, or unconscious patient unattended.

SAFETY IN THE HEALTHCARE FACILITY

Patient Safety

Patient safety is a critical component of the quality of care provided in a healthcare facility. The U.S. Department of Health and Human Services (DHHS) has conducted extensive research on the features of safe patient environments in providers' offices. The DHHS has found the following factors to be crucial to patient safety.

- Open lines of communication must be established among all employees about possible safety issues, and employees must work together to solve these problems before a patient is injured.
- If an injury occurs (e.g., a medication is administered to the wrong patient), policies and procedures must be in place so that all employees recognize the potential for an error and protocols are established for preventing a similar problem in the future.
- Procedures must be standardized in the facility's policies and procedures manual so that all employees can refer to specific guidelines on how procedures should be performed. For example,

in the case of a blood spill, the policies and procedures manual must outline a specific, step-by-step procedure for cleaning up the spill that safeguards both patients and staff members.
- The facility must provide ongoing staff training in patient safety factors.
- Staff members must work as a team to maintain a safe environment for patients. For example, all staff members must follow Standard Precautions to prevent the spread of disease in the facility.

Throughout this text, you have learned about situations that could result in serious harm to your patients. You must constantly be on guard to protect patients from possible injury. For example, studies have shown that healthcare workers frequently confuse drug names, which results in administration of the wrong medication; they also fail to identify a patient correctly before performing a procedure and neglect to perform hand sanitization consistently, thus promoting the spread of infectious diseases. The medical assistant is an important link in the delivery of quality and *safe* care. Can you think of anything you have learned thus far in your studies that could help keep patients safe in the provider's office?

Employee Safety

The healthcare facility should safeguard patients as well as staff members from the possibility of accidental injury. This includes making sure the facility has appropriate safety signs throughout the building as well as appropriate symbols and labels that identify potentially dangerous items (Figure 22-1). Data compiled by the Occupational Safety and Health Administration (OSHA) reveal that the leading causes of accidents in an office are slips, trips, and falls. You must think and work safely to prevent accidents. The following

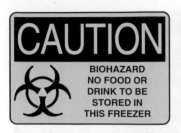

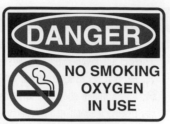

Fire extinguisher

Manual Station
Pull Station/
Fire Alarm Box

Fire hose
or standpoint

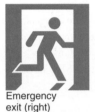
Emergency
exit (right)

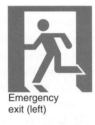
Emergency
exit (left)

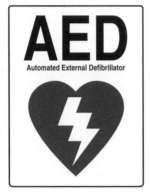
Automated External Defibrillator (AED)

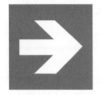

Emergency exit directional arrows
(Can be rotated in increments of 45 degrees)

FIGURE 22-1 Safety signs, symbols, and labels.

are some suggestions from OSHA for vigilant accident prevention methods (Procedure 22-1).

1. Use proper body mechanics in all situations. For example, bend your knees and bring a heavy item close to you before lifting rather than bending from your back; push heavy items rather than pulling them; and use a gait belt or ask for assistance when transferring patients.
2. Constantly check the floors and hallways for obstructions and possible tripping hazards, such as telephone and computer cables or boxes.
3. Store supplies inside cabinets rather than on top, where they can fall off and injure someone; store heavier items on lower shelves so they do not have to be lifted any higher than necessary.
4. Clean up spills immediately; slippery floors are a danger to everyone.
5. Use a step stool to reach for things, not a chair or a box that could collapse or move.
6. Have handrails and grab bars available as needed in the facility; use them, and encourage patients to use them.
7. Do not overload electrical outlets.
8. Perform a safety check of the facility routinely; look for unsafe or defective equipment, torn carpeting that could catch heels, adequate lighting both inside and outside the facility, and so on.

A primary concern for personnel and patient safety is infection control. Standard Precautions protocols require employers to provide appropriate and adequate personal protective equipment (PPE). The goal is to protect staff members from occupational exposure to blood-borne pathogens while at the same time safeguarding patients in the facility. OSHA's guidelines include managing sharps and providing current safety-engineered sharps devices; providing hepatitis B immunization free of charge to all employees at risk of exposure to blood and body fluids; using latex-free supplies as much as possible to prevent allergic reactions in both staff members and patients; identifying all chemicals in the facility with **Safety Data Sheets (SDSs)** and adequately storing potentially dangerous substances; and performing proper hand hygiene consistently throughout the workday.

Another serious concern that faces all of us today is the prevention of workplace violence. Unfortunately, rarely does a week go by without reports of violence in a public place. Employees in a healthcare facility are no exception. We started the text with information about and exercises in communication techniques in the workplace: problem solving, therapeutic communication, and assertive behavior. All of these are helpful in dealing with a difficult patient. Employers should provide training on how to identify potentially violent patients and should discuss safe methods for managing difficult patients. Many employers offer training on how to manage assaultive behaviors. Procedure 22-2 presents a scenario that deals with employee safety. Follow the steps of this procedure to learn how to handle such a situation.

OSHA Updates for Signs, Symbols, and Labels

In September, 2013, the Occupational Safety and Health Administration (OSHA) updated standard formats for safety signs, symbols, and labels. This is the first standard change since 1971. The revised standards regulate the color, shape, symbols, and wording that can be used on safety signs and labels. Figure 22-1 shows some examples of the types of signs, symbols, and labels that should be used in an ambulatory care office. The four major types of signs are:

- *Danger signs* (identify the most severe and immediate hazards)
- *Caution signs* (warn of possible hazards that require added precautions)
- *Safety instruction signs* (communicate directions for safety actions)
- *Biologic hazard signs* (identify an actual or potential biohazard)

OSHA specifies the format of each type of sign, the information that must appear, and where each type of sign must be used. Tags or labels must contain a signal word ("Danger," "Caution," "Biologic Hazard," "BIOHAZARD," or the biologic hazard symbol) and a major message, which states a specific hazard or safety instruction. Employers are required to train workers about the information conveyed on safety signs and labels. The signs and labels use graphic symbols and specific colors to explain the sign's warning or message so that the problem of language barriers is minimized (see Procedure 22-1).

PROCEDURE 22-1	Evaluate the Work Environment to Identify Unsafe Working Conditions and Comply With Safety Signs and Symbols

Goal: *To assess the healthcare facility for possible safety issues and develop a safety plan.*

Scenario: *Work with a partner to evaluate environmental safety in the laboratory at your school. Record your results and discuss them with the class. After all members of the class have shared their observations, develop a safety plan for your laboratory.*

EQUIPMENT and SUPPLIES

- Pen and paper
- Document or manual on policies and procedures for environmental safety issues in the facility

PROCEDURAL STEPS

1. Check the floors and hallways for obstructions and possible tripping hazards, including torn carpets, possible spills, protruding electrical cords, and so on.
   PURPOSE: To prevent accidental falls.
2. Check storage areas to make sure the tops of cabinets are clear and heavier items have been stored closer to the floor.
   PURPOSE: To prevent injuries from items falling off shelves and to limit the lifting of heavy items.
3. Assess the location and security of handrails and grab bars placed around the facility. They should be placed at all stairs, in restrooms, and in any other areas where staff members or patients may need assistance.
   PURPOSE: Handrails and grab bars help safeguard staff members and patients and provide assistance where needed.
4. Examine all electrical plugs and outlets to prevent electrical overload.
   PURPOSE: Overloading electrical outlets could cause a fire.
5. Check all equipment to make sure it is in safe working condition.
6. Make sure all lights are working (both inside and outside the facility), that lighting is adequate, and that light fixtures are in good condition.
   PURPOSE: Adequate lighting both inside and outside the facility helps prevent accidents, and faulty fixtures can be a fire hazard.
7. Check the working condition of smoke alarms, and examine all fire extinguishers.
   PURPOSE: To monitor the function of smoke detectors and make sure fire extinguishers are charged.
8. Make sure evacuation routes are posted throughout the facility, along with floor plans with clearly marked exit routes.
   PURPOSE: Every room in the facility must have a map with exit routes marked on it to make sure that even those who are unfamiliar with the facility's floor plan can safely reach an exit in case of an emergency.
9. Assess the laboratory's compliance with the safety signs, symbols, and labels required by the Occupational Safety and Health Administration (OSHA). Are all signs, symbols, labels in place and posted properly?
10. Record your observations and share them with the class.
    PURPOSE: To compile a comprehensive list of problem areas.
11. Based on group discussion, develop a plan of action for improving the safety of the laboratory.
    PURPOSE: The student-generated safety plan can be incorporated into the laboratory's policies and procedures manual.

PROCEDURE 22-2   Manage a Difficult Patient

Goal: *To communicate with an angry patient in a safe, therapeutic manner. The following procedure is part of an overall employee safety plan.*

Scenario: *You are working at the admissions desk when an extremely angry patient comes storming into the office, screaming about a mistake on his bill. Although the facility uses an outside billing center, you recognize that you should attempt to help the patient and try to defuse the situation. Remember: Call 911 immediately and alert any available security if you or one of your co-workers is threatened with violence.*

EQUIPMENT and SUPPLIES

- Patient's record
- Telephone
- Facility's policies and procedures manual

PROCEDURAL STEPS

1. Although it is important to safeguard patients' privacy, do not ask an angry patient into an isolated room; do not close the door.
   PURPOSE: To protect yourself, remain in an open area. If you are in a room with an angry patient, keep the door open and stand close to the door so that you can leave the room quickly if necessary.

2. Alert other staff members to the situation, if possible.
   PURPOSE: To have assistance nearby; call 911 immediately if you feel physically threatened.

3. If you do not feel physically threatened, allow the patient to blow off steam.
   PURPOSE: Attempting to interrupt the patient to give a logical reason for the problem will only make him angrier. Allowing him to continue to yell helps him release the anger so that you can work on a reasonable solution to the problem. Call 911 if at any time you feel threatened.

4. When the patient begins to slow down, offer supportive statements, such as, "I understand it is frustrating to receive a bill you think is unfair." Continue to make supportive statements until the patient is calmer (think of it as the patient screaming his way up a mountain; sooner or later, he is going to run out of steam; when he begins to slow down, you can then start offering supportive statements).

PURPOSE: Providing verbal support helps defuse the situation and gives the patient the opportunity to become calmer and reach a rational level where you can discuss the problem.

5. Once you can discuss the situation, ask the patient for the details of the problem. Gather as much information as possible so you can work together on a possible solution.

6. After determining the problem, suggest a possible solution to the patient. For example, tell him that you will contact the billing office with the information and will make sure they get back to the patient as soon as possible.
   PURPOSE: Use therapeutic techniques, including restatement, reflection, and clarification, to gather details and work on a possible solution with the patient. Make sure you follow up with the action to prevent future outbursts.

7. Report the incident to your supervisor and document the patient's problem and the agreed-upon action in the patient's health record, taking care not to use judgmental statements.
   PURPOSE: Documenting the patient's problem and the agreed-upon solution allows for continuity of care if follow-up is needed. The patient's medical record is a legal document, and all judgmental statements must be avoided.

8. Discuss your approach to managing the difficult patient at the next staff meeting. With your supervisor's permission, summarize your approach and include it as part of the facility's Employee Safety Plan.
   PURPOSE: The safety plan should be reviewed frequently, and revisions should be made as needed.

Environmental Safety

Environmental safety guidelines include numerous work safety practices, such as office security, management of smoke detectors and fire extinguishers, posting of designated fire exit routes, and securing certain items (e.g., narcotics, dangerous chemicals) in locked storage areas in the facility. In addition to these concerns, staff members should constantly be on the alert for possible safety hazards in and around the building, such as improper lighting, unlimited access to the facility, and inadequate use of security systems.

The medical assistant must be prepared to use a fire extinguisher to prevent injury to patients and to protect the medical facility (Procedure 22-3). An ABC fire extinguisher is effective against the most common causes of fire, including cloth, paper, plastics, rubber, flammable liquids, and electrical fires. Most small extinguishers empty within 15 seconds, so it is important to call 911 immediately if the facility fire is not small and confined. If the fire is small, no heavy smoke is present, and you have easy access to an exit route, use the closest fire extinguisher. However, do not hesitate to evacuate the facility if you believe any danger exists to yourself or others.

Methods of Fire Prevention and Response

- Store potentially flammable chemicals and supplies according to the manufacturers' guidelines.
- Inspect electrical equipment and cords throughout the facility; take care not to overload outlets.
- If a fire is suspected, immediately disconnect oxygen supplies or turn off oxygen tanks to prevent an explosion.
- Smoke alarms should be located throughout the facility, checked periodically, and replaced as needed.
- Fire safety equipment should be available and current. Fire extinguishers must be inspected at least annually. If an extinguisher is discharged, it must be replaced immediately.
- Fire extinguishers should be located in multiple sites throughout the facility and mounted on the wall for easy access.
- If you smell smoke or suspect a fire, immediately notify the fire department (or call 911) and evacuate the facility. Do not use elevators if a fire is suspected.

CRITICAL THINKING APPLICATION 22-1

Cheryl is in the middle of a busy day; patients are in all of the examination rooms, and the waiting room is full. She walks past the patient bathroom and smells smoke. She opens the door and sees smoke and flames coming from the wastebasket. What should she do? Write down your response to this scenario and share it with your classmates.

PROCEDURE 22-3 Demonstrate the Proper Use of a Fire Extinguisher

Goal: *To role-play the safe and proper use of a fire extinguisher.*

EQUIPMENT and SUPPLIES

- Portable, office-size ABC fire extinguisher that has been discharged

PROCEDURAL STEPS

Role-play the following with a discharged ABC fire extinguisher.
1. Pull the pin from the handle of the extinguisher.
2. Aim the discharge from the extinguisher toward the bottom of the flames. PURPOSE: Aiming the fire extinguisher directly onto the fire may spread the flames.
3. Squeeze the handle of the extinguisher so that it begins to discharge.
4. Sweep the extinguisher from side to side toward the base of the fire until it is out or until fire officials arrive.
5. Check on the safety of all patients and other personnel.

Each facility should have a policy and procedure in place for evacuating the building. According to OSHA, the facility's plan first should identify the situations that might require evacuation, such as a natural disaster or a fire. The following provisions should be included in the facility's evacuation plan.
- An emergency action coordinator must be designated, and all employees must know who this individual is. This person (usually the office manager) is in charge if an emergency occurs.
- The coordinator is responsible for managing the emergency at the facility and for notifying and working with community emergency services.
- Evacuation routes with clearly marked exits must be posted in multiple locations throughout the facility. Maps of floor diagrams with arrows pointing to the closest exits are an easy means of

finding the closest door out, even for individuals unfamiliar with the facility.
- Exit doors must be clearly marked, well lit, and wide enough for everyone to evacuate.
- Hazardous areas in the facility that should be avoided during an emergency evacuation must be identified, such as areas where chemicals and oxygen tanks are stored.
- A meeting place outside the facility must be designated for all those evacuating to make sure everyone got out of the facility safely.
- Employees should be trained to assist any co-worker or patient with special needs.
- A designated individual must check the entire facility, including restrooms, before exiting. He or she must make sure to close all doors (especially designated fire doors) when leaving to try to contain the fire or other disaster (Procedure 22-4).

Evacuation Levels

Four levels of evacuation are possible, depending on the severity of the need for evacuation:

Shelter in place: Staff stops all routine activities in preparation for possible evacuation of the facility; close doors/windows for initial protection from fire and smoke.

Horizontal evacuation: Patients and staff move away from immediate danger, but if the facility is located in a multifloor structure, everyone remains on that floor until it is determined that the entire building should be evacuated.

Vertical evacuation: A specific floor in a building is evacuated vertically (i.e., toward the ground level) to prepare for evacuation outside.

Total or full evacuation: The facility is completely evacuated (this is used only as a last resort).

PROCEDURE 22-4   Participate in a Mock Environmental Exposure Event: Evacuate a Provider's Office

Goal: *To role-play an environmental disaster and implement an evacuation plan.*

Scenario: *Role-play the following scenario with your lab group: The building next door to the provider's office where you work is on fire. One member of the group is the designated emergency action coordinator, two individuals are responsible for helping patients with special needs out of the facility, and one person is designated to be the last to leave after the building is clear. In a community emergency situation, certain staff members may be designated to provide immediate assistance to survivors. Two medical assistants are sent to help with fire victims. How could medical assistants help in this situation? After the evacuation is complete, meet in a designated spot to discuss the process and see whether any aspects of the evacuation plan could be improved. Document the steps taken throughout the mock environmental event.*

EQUIPMENT and SUPPLIES

- Pen and paper
- Document or manual on policies and procedures for evacuation of the facility and response to an environmental disaster

PROCEDURAL STEPS

1. In an actual emergency, an emergency action coordinator is in charge.
   PURPOSE: All employees must know who this individual is (usually it is the office manager) and must follow his or her lead in safely responding to the emergency situation.
2. The student who is role-playing the emergency action coordinator is responsible for managing the emergency at the facility and for notifying and working with community emergency services.
   PURPOSE: The coordinator or someone designated by the coordinator must notify community emergency services of the fire; the coordinator works with emergency services to provide care at the scene.
3. Fire victims are being cared for across the street, where a triage and treatment center has been set up by the police, fire, and emergency responder units in the city. Two students role-play staff members who are sent to assist with the victims:
   - Use therapeutic communication techniques to calm and care for victims
   - Implement appropriate Standard Precautions
   - Monitor and record vital signs
   - Gather pertinent health histories
   - Observe victims for possible complications, such as breathing problems, shock, angina, and so on
   - Immediately report to emergency responders any life-threatening changes in a patient's status
   - Use first aid skills as needed

4. The coordinator designates an employee to shut down immediately any combustibles (e.g., oxygen tanks).
   PURPOSE: To prevent an explosion if the fire spreads.
5. Using the posted evacuation routes, role-play staff members following floor plan diagrams to the closest safe exit. Identify any hazardous areas in the facility that should be avoided during the emergency evacuation. Role-play staff members assisting patients, especially those with special needs (e.g., individuals in wheelchairs) during the building evacuation.
   PURPOSE: Evacuation routes must be posted throughout the facility, and exit doors must be clearly marked, well lit, and wide enough for everyone to evacuate. The doors facing the building on fire should not be used because this could be a hazard.
6. Role-play the staff member delegated to check that everyone has left the facility and that fire doors have been closed before he or she leaves the building.
   PURPOSE: To make sure the building is clear and that any fire is contained. This person should leave immediately if there is danger.
7. Role-play evacuated personnel and patients meeting in a designated area to count heads and make sure everyone exited the facility safely.
   PURPOSE: To make sure everyone safely evacuated the facility.
8. After everyone has been accounted for and the patients are secure, role-play staff members reporting to the emergency triage area to provide assistance to rescue workers and victims.
9. Discuss with the class the evacuation exercise and response to a community disaster.
10. Document the specific steps taken during the facility evacuation and your role in the exercise. What were the strengths and weaknesses of the group's response to an environmental emergency?
    PURPOSE: To reflect on the learning activity.

DISPOSAL OF HAZARDOUS WASTE

The chapter on Infection Control explained the management of biohazardous waste; the use of PPE when the potential exists for exposure to blood and body fluids; the importance of flushing the eyes with an eye wash unit if they are exposed to potentially infectious or toxic material; and the consistent use of sharps containers. Regardless of individual responsibilities in the facility, all employees must be aware of potentially dangerous situations and must comply with all safety measures to protect themselves and their patients.

OSHA defines regulated waste as any contaminated item that might release blood or other potentially infectious material; contaminated supplies with dried blood or other potentially infectious material on their surfaces; contaminated sharps; and waste products that contain blood or other potentially infectious material. Healthcare facilities must make special arrangements for the disposal of regulated waste, which often costs as much as 10 times more than regular garbage disposal. It therefore is important to put only supplies contaminated with blood or body fluids into red bag collection systems and sharps containers. The following measures should be used for proper disposal of hazardous materials in the provider's office.

- Place signs on or near the biohazard container to identify its purpose and the materials that should be deposited in it. All biohazardous waste containers should display a biohazard label.
- Make sure all biohazardous waste containers are covered and have a foot pedal for opening and closing the container. This prevents the spread of infectious material and reduces the likelihood that noninfectious material will be tossed inside. Biohazard containers should be kept only in treatment areas where contaminated materials are likely to be produced.
- Place a regular garbage container next to a biohazard container to encourage staff members to use the biohazard bags only as needed.
- Place only sharps in sharps containers; gauze, bandages, and so on belong in a contaminated waste container. Noninfectious items, such as patient gowns that are not contaminated with body fluids, and packaging material, belong in the regular trash.

EMERGENCY PREPAREDNESS

Ambulatory care centers and hospitals may be the first to recognize and initiate a response to a community emergency. If an infectious outbreak is suspected, Standard Precautions should be implemented immediately to control the spread of infection. If the problem has the potential to affect a large number of individuals in the community (e.g., suspected food contamination), a communications network should be established to notify local and state health departments and perhaps federal officials. Your employer may participate in an annual community disaster preparedness drill designed to help facilities improve their response to natural disasters and other emergencies.

Community preparation and response to emergencies are managed by several agencies, including the Office of Civil Defense,

Local Emergency Management Agency (LEMA), Emergency Services, or Homeland Security. Local governments are responsible for creating a system that coordinates police, fire, emergency medical services, public health, and area healthcare response to community-wide emergencies. These agencies develop an all-hazards response plan that would be appropriate for any community emergency. Local officials can turn to state, regional, or federal officials for assistance as needed.

Every healthcare facility should have a policy that includes specific procedures for the management of emergencies on site. When a new employee starts on the job, part of the orientation process is to review the site's policies and procedures manual. As a new employee, be sure to get answers to any questions you have about emergency management in that particular facility.

Staff members should discuss emergencies that may occur and should have an emergency action plan for rapid, systematic intervention. For instance, local industries may present unique problems that call for very specialized care. Plan for these, and ask the provider's advice on the procedures to follow and the supplies to have on hand. If the facility has several employees, each should be assigned specific duties in the event of an emergency. Organization and planning make the difference between systematic care for patients and complete chaos.

Emergency Plan for a Natural Disaster or Other Emergency in an Ambulatory Care Facility

- Evacuate the facility as needed.
- Include procedures for the protection of patients' health records. If the facility uses electronic health records (EHRs), make sure this information is backed up on offsite systems.
- In the case of a community emergency, provide care to the extent possible within the facility.
- Coordinate services between the ambulatory facility and other local healthcare systems, including hospitals and public health departments.
- Provide staff and supplies as needed to help in a community emergency.
- Maintain up-to-date phone trees to notify staff members of an emergency.
- Educate patients in emergency preparedness.

CRITICAL THINKING APPLICATION 22-2

A chemical plant is located about three blocks from Dr. Bendt's office. The office staff is brainstorming ideas about what should be done if an accident occurs at the plant. Based on what you have learned so far about emergency preparedness, what do you think should be included in the office's emergency plan?

Community Resources for Emergency Preparedness

Most communities have an emergency medical services (EMS) system. This system includes an efficient communications network (e.g., the emergency telephone number 911), well-trained rescue personnel, properly equipped ambulances, an emergency facility that is open 24 hours a day to provide advanced life support, and a hospital intensive care unit for victims.

More than 100 poison control centers in the United States are ready to provide emergency information for the treatment of victims of poisoning. Every healthcare facility is required to post a list of local emergency numbers. This list should be kept in plain sight and should be known to all office personnel. A good place to post this vital information is next to all the phones in the facility. Include on the list the numbers for the local EMS system, poison control center, ambulance and rescue squad, fire department, and police department (Procedure 22-5).

Contact Information for Emergency Preparedness

Keep the following telephone numbers readily available in the facility:
- Local hospital numbers, including the emergency department, infection control officer, administration contacts, and public affairs office
- Local and state health department numbers
- Centers for Disease Control and Prevention (CDC) Emergency Response Office
  - Telephone: 800-232-4636
  - Website: www.cdc.gov/phpr/index.htm

The Centers for Disease Control and Prevention (CDC) recommends that all healthcare facilities be aware of possible agents of bioterrorism, including anthrax, botulism, plague, and smallpox. The provider is responsible for diagnosing and reporting any suspected cases, but the medical assistant may be involved in patient care and certainly will participate in preventing the spread of infection in the facility. As with any suspected infectious disease, Standard Precautions should be used to control disease transmission. These precautions should be implemented with all patients, regardless of their diagnosis or possible infection status.

Infection control procedures for bioterrorism threats include the following:
- Sanitize your hands routinely.
- Wear disposable gloves when contamination with blood and body fluids is possible.
- Use masks/eye protection or face shields if you may be splashed by secretions or blood and body fluids.
- Wear impermeable gowns to protect your skin and clothes as needed; remove them promptly and wash your hands to prevent transmission of infectious material.
- Sanitize, disinfect, and sterilize equipment, supplies, and environmental surfaces.
- Dispose of contaminated waste in appropriate biohazard containers.

Another resource that can aid with community emergency preparedness is the Laboratory Response Network (LRN), which coordinates with the DHHS, the CDC, the Federal Bureau of Investigation (FBI), and the Association of Public Health Laboratories

(APHL) to ensure an effective laboratory response to bioterrorism threats. The LRN links state and local public health laboratories, and veterinary, agriculture, military, and water- and food-testing laboratories to protect U.S. citizens from bioterrorism, chemical terrorism, and other public health threats.

Community emergency preparedness plans are required by the federal government so that a coordinated response is in place if a natural disaster occurs. The federal government requires all healthcare facilities, including private providers' offices, to be prepared to provide medical services and to contribute medical supplies if a natural disaster or other emergency occurs in the area.

Emergency preparedness plans are designed to coordinate the care provided by all healthcare facilities and agencies in the community, including local emergency management agencies, EMS, fire departments, law enforcement agencies, the American Red Cross, and the National Guard. Each of these groups can provide crucial services during a community emergency.

Medical assistants also can contribute to rescue and emergency efforts. Services that might be performed by trained medical assistants include providing emergency first aid at the site of a disaster; conducting patient interviews in an empathetic manner while using therapeutic communication to help calm victims and gather important health-related information; helping with mass vaccination efforts or antibiotic distribution; performing documentation and electronic health record management; ensuring compliance with the procedures required by Standard Precautions; assisting with patient education efforts; and performing phlebotomy and laboratory procedures according to their skill level.

Psychological Aspects of an Emergency Situation

Everyone involved in an emergency situation experiences a certain amount of anxiety and stress. The Centers for Disease Control and Prevention (CDC) recommends that the following actions be included in a facility's emergency preparedness plan to minimize these negative psychological effects on both healthcare workers and patients:

- Provide fact sheets for employees and patients to help them understand the dangers of certain emergencies, and encourage employee participation in disaster drills.
- Plan in advance for effective communication and action in response to an emergency; the plan should include methods for coordinating a response with local and state agencies and media sources.
- Put into place a method for clearly explaining emergency situations to patients and healthcare workers; offer immediate evaluation and treatment of an infectious outbreak.
- Treat acute anxiety with reassurance and explanation; provide follow-up counseling for employees as needed.

Further information on emergency preparedness can be found at the following CDC websites:
- Emergency preparedness planning: www.bt.cdc.gov/planning
- Coordinating Office for Terrorism Preparedness and Emergency Response (COTPER): www.bt.cdc.gov

PROCEDURE 22-5 | Maintain an Up-to-Date List of Community Resources for Emergency Preparedness

Goal: To develop and maintain a list of community agencies that would respond to a natural disaster or other emergency.

Scenario: Your employer asks you to develop a list of groups in your community that are part of the community-wide emergency preparedness plan that has been mandated by the state and federal governments. Using multiple resources, develop a comprehensive list of emergency services for your area.

EQUIPMENT and SUPPLIES

- Telephone
- Internet access
- Pen and paper
- Electronic record

PROCEDURAL STEPS

1. Start with an online search for the area office of the Local Emergency Management Agency (LEMA), which is sponsored by the Department of Homeland Security. If available, investigate the LEMA website for information about the emergency preparedness plan in your community. You can begin the search at the website *www.ready.gov*; the Federal Emergency Management Agency (FEMA) website is *www.fema.gov*.
   PURPOSE: To develop emergency preparedness plans by starting with the federal and state governments.

2. Gather contact information for local police, fire, and emergency medical services (EMS); post this information next to all telephones in the facility.
   PURPOSE: To ensure that emergency services contact information is immediately available in case of an emergency in the facility.

3. Investigate services provided by your local Public Health office and the American Red Cross.
   PURPOSE: To coordinate services available to potential victims in the community.

4. Organize the information gathered about community resources for emergency preparedness. With your supervisor's approval, post a copy of this information in all appropriate locations in the facility. Prepare a database in the computer that can be updated as the information changes.

ASSISTING WITH MEDICAL EMERGENCIES

First aid is the immediate care given to a person who has been injured or has suddenly taken ill. Knowledge of first aid and related skills often can mean the difference between life and death, temporary and permanent disability, or rapid recovery and long-term hospitalization. The medical assistant may be responsible for initiating first aid in the office and continuing to administer first aid until the provider or the trained medical team arrives. Every medical assistant should successfully complete a course for the professional in cardiopulmonary resuscitation (CPR) and should continue to hold a current CPR card as long as he or she is employed.

Basic knowledge of CPR and life support skills needs to be updated regularly, because procedures change as new techniques are developed. For example, both the American Red Cross and the American Heart Association (AHA) now recommend training on automated external defibrillators (AEDs) for all healthcare workers.

Medical assistants need up-to-date training in current emergency practices. They should encourage their local professional chapters to offer workshops on the management of emergencies in an ambulatory care practice, in addition to community-wide emergency preparedness. Being prepared for both types of emergencies is important. The facility's employees must be ready to respond both to emergencies on site and to natural disasters or other emergencies that affect the community.

Medical assistants are not responsible for diagnosing emergencies, especially over the telephone, but they are expected to make decisions about emergency situations on the basis of their medical knowledge and training. If any doubt exists about how to manage a particular situation or emergency phone call, the medical assistant should not hesitate to consult the provider, the office manager, or some other, more experienced member of the healthcare team.

The Medical Assistant's Role in Performing Emergency Procedures

- Perform only the emergency procedures for which you have been trained.
- If an emergency occurs in the facility, notify the provider.
- If a provider cannot be located, immediately contact the local emergency medical services team (EMS or 911).

Emergency Supplies

Emergency supplies consist of a properly equipped "crash cart" or box of items needed for a variety of emergencies (Figure 22-2). The contents vary to some degree, depending on the types of emergencies the particular office might expect to encounter and whether pediatric patients are seen in the practice. Emergency supplies should be kept in an easily accessible place that is known to all personnel in the office, and the supplies should be inventoried regularly. Expiration dates of medications and sterile supplies must be checked weekly or monthly, along with the status of available oxygen tanks and related

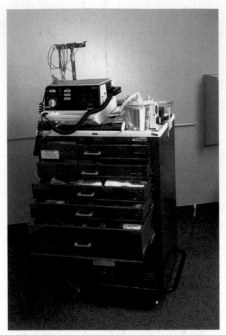

FIGURE 22-2 Office emergency cart with defibrillator. Drawers are marked for easy retrieval of emergency supplies.

materials. The cart should be replenished with fresh supplies after every use. Each time crash cart supplies are checked, a log must be completed and signed for legal purposes.

Emergency pharmaceutical supplies should include certain basic drugs, such as epinephrine, which has multiple uses in emergency situations. As a vasoconstrictor, it controls hemorrhage, relaxes the bronchioles to relieve acute asthma attacks, is administered for an acute anaphylactic reaction, and is an emergency heart stimulant used to treat shock. Epinephrine should be available in a ready-to-use cartridge syringe and needle unit. These units are supplied in 1-mL cartridges.

Other drugs used include atropine, digoxin (Lanoxin), nitroglycerin (Nitrostat), lidocaine (Xylocaine), and sodium bicarbonate. Atropine reduces secretions, increases the respiratory rate and heart rate, and is a smooth muscle relaxant. It is administered in a cardiac emergency for **asystole**, or it can be used to treat bradycardia. Digoxin is a cardiac drug used to treat **arrhythmia** and congestive heart failure (CHF); it is good for emergency use because it has a relatively rapid action. Nitroglycerin is a vasodilator that is given to relieve angina; it acts by dilating the coronary arteries so that an increased volume of oxygenated blood can reach the **myocardium**. Lidocaine is used intravenously to treat a cardiac arrhythmia and locally as an anesthetic, and sodium bicarbonate corrects metabolic acidosis, which typically occurs after cardiac arrest. Many of the medications administered during a medical emergency are given intravenously (IV), which is outside of the medical assistant's scope of practice.

Emergency medical supplies also should include an **emetic**, such as syrup of ipecac, which causes vomiting soon after the syrup is swallowed, and activated charcoal, an antidote that is swallowed to absorb ingested poisons. Narcan, an antidote given intravenously for narcotic drug overdoses, is administered when indicated to raise blood pressure and increase the respiratory rate. Antihistamines for

the treatment of allergic reactions and for anaphylaxis need to be available to treat any allergic responses to medications administered in the facility. Such antihistamines include Benadryl for minor reactions and Solu-Medrol, a corticosteroid, for severe anaphylactic reactions.

Other medications also may be found in a crash cart. For example, isoproterenol (e.g., Isuprel, Medihaler-Iso, Norisodrine), an antispasmodic used to treat bronchospasms (e.g., as in an asthma attack), also is effective as a cardiac stimulant. Phenobarbital and diazepam (Valium) are used for convulsions and/or sedative effects. Furosemide (Lasix) is used for CHF. Glucagon is used primarily to counteract severe hypoglycemic reactions (low blood glucose) in patients with diabetes who are taking insulin.

Basic Emergency Supplies

Equipment
- Adhesive tape in 1- and 2-inch widths
- Airways (variety of types and sizes)
- Alcohol wipes
- Ambu bag with assorted sizes of facial masks
- Antimicrobial skin ointment
- Bandage scissors
- Cotton balls and cotton swabs
- Cardiopulmonary resuscitation (CPR) masks (adult and pediatric)
- Defibrillator
- Elastic bandages in 2- and 3-inch widths
- Filter needles
- Flashlight with batteries
- Gauze pads, 2 × 2- and 4 × 4-inch widths, and roller bandage (sterile and nonsterile)
- Gloves (sterile and nonsterile) in multiple sizes
- Hot and cold packs (instant type)
- Intravenous catheters, tubing, solutions (variety of types, including D_5W and Ringer's lactate), and tourniquet
- Laryngoscope with blades
- Lubricant
- Endotracheal tubes (variety of sizes with stylets)
- Personal protective equipment (PPE), including impervious gowns, splash guards or goggles, and booties
- Portable oxygen tank with regulator, mask, and nasal cannula
- Roller gauze (Ace bandages and gauze dressing) in various sizes
- Sharps container
- Sphygmomanometer (pediatric and adult regular and large sizes)
- Splints (various sizes)
- Sterile dressings (miscellaneous sizes, including two abdominal pads)
- Steri-Strips, dermal glue, or suturing material
- Suction machine and catheters
- Syringes and needles (assorted sizes and gauges)
- Tongue blades
- Tubex cartridge system
- Venipuncture supplies and butterfly units

Medications

- Activated charcoal (bottle of 29 to 50 g)
- Antihistamine (injectable and oral)
- Atropine
- Dextrose
- Diazepam (Valium)
- Digoxin (Lanoxin), injectable
- Diphenhydramine (Benadryl)
- Epinephrine (Adrenalin), injectable
- Furosemide (Lasix)
- Glucagon and/or glucose tablets
- Ipecac syrup
- Isoproterenol (Isuprel), injectable
- Lidocaine (Xylocaine), injectable and spray
- Naloxone (Narcan), injectable
- Nitroglycerin tablets
- Phenobarbital, injectable
- Sodium bicarbonate, injectable
- Methylprednisolone (Solu-Medrol), injectable
- Sterile water and saline for injection

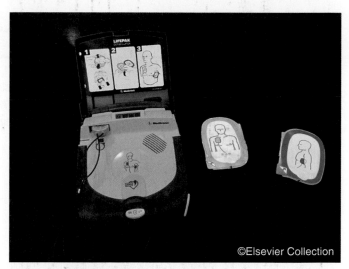

©Elsevier Collection

FIGURE 22-3 Fully automated external defibrillator (AED).

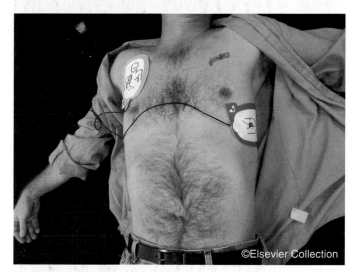

©Elsevier Collection

FIGURE 22-4 Connect the adhesive pads to the automated external defibrillator (AED) cables; apply the pads to the patient's chest at the upper right sternal border and at the lower left ribs over the cardiac apex.

Defibrillators

The medical assistant may be required to assist the healthcare team with defibrillation of emergency patients. Defibrillation is indicated when a patient is in ventricular **fibrillation** (VF). VF is a severe cardiac arrhythmia that is caused by uncoordinated, rapid firing of the electrical system of the heart, which makes it impossible for the ventricles to empty. In the absence of ventricular emptying, the patient has no pulse, blood pressure drops to zero, and the patient could die within 4 minutes unless help is given immediately.

Defibrillators are devices that send an electrical current through the myocardium by means of handheld paddles (in a healthcare facility) or self-adhesive pads applied to the chest. This electrical shock causes momentary asystole, giving the heart's natural pacemaker an opportunity to resume the heart rate at a normal rhythm.

An automated external defibrillator has a computerized system that analyzes a cardiac rhythm and delivers voice-prompt instructions on how to operate the device (Figure 22-3 and Procedure 22-6). AEDs use self-adhesive pads that record and monitor the cardiac rhythm, and the device instructs the rescuer when to deliver the electrical charge. The apex-anterior position is the most commonly used pad position, with the anterior (sternum) pad placed to the right of the upper sternum, and the apex pad placed under the individual's left nipple at the left middle axillary line (Figure 22-4). To defibrillate a female individual, the apex pad is placed next to or underneath the left breast. The AED self-adhesive pads are packaged with expiration dates so these should be checked periodically.

Precautions for Automated External Defibrillators

- Neither the individual nor the rescuer should be in contact with any metal during defibrillation. Do not place the AED pad over jewelry, and remove the patient's glasses to prevent injuries.

- When available, a pediatric-dose AED system should be used for children 1 to 8 years of age (it should not be used on infants younger than 1 year old). These systems deliver a reduced shock dose for victims up to about 8 years old or weighing 55 pounds.
- All clothing (including bras) must be removed; pads must be applied directly to the skin. If the individual has a great deal of hair on the chest, try to push the hair aside before applying the pads; or, apply the pads and quickly remove them to remove hair from the area, then reapply new pads. The machine will prompt you by stating "Check electrode" if the connection is poor.
- To prevent burns, make sure the individual is lying on a dry surface and the chest is dry before applying the pads.
- If the patient has an implanted defibrillator or pacemaker, it will be obvious from the bulged area under the surface of the skin on the chest. Apply the AED pads at least 1 inch away from implants to prevent interference.

PROCEDURE 22-6	Maintain Provider/Professional-Level CPR Certification: Use an Automated External Defibrillator (AED)

Goal: *To defibrillate adult victims with cardiac arrest. Most adult victims in sudden cardiac arrest are in ventricular fibrillation. The survival rate for victims with ventricular fibrillation is as high as 90% when defibrillation occurs within the first minute of collapse; however, the survival rate declines 7% to 10% with every minute defibrillation does not occur.*

EQUIPMENT and SUPPLIES

- Automated external defibrillator (AED) for practice
- Approved mannequin

PROCEDURAL STEPS

These steps are to be performed only on an approved mannequin.

If the healthcare worker witnesses a cardiac arrest, an automated external defibrillator (AED) should be used as soon as possible. If cardiopulmonary resuscitation (CPR) has already been started, continue performing CPR until the AED machine is turned on, pads are applied, and the machine is ready.

1. Place the AED near the victim's left ear. Turn on the AED.
2. Attach electrode pads to the victim's bare dry chest as pictured on the AED. Place the electrodes at the sternum and apex of the heart. Make sure the pads are in complete contact with the victim's chest and that they do not overlap (see Figure 22-4).
3. All rescuers must clear away from the victim. Press the ANALYZE button. The AED analyzes the victim's coronary status, announces whether the victim is going to be shocked, and automatically charges the electrodes (Figure 1).

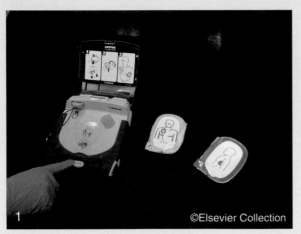
1   ©Elsevier Collection

4. All rescuers must clear away from the victim. Press the SHOCK button if the machine is not automated. You may repeat 3 analyze-shock cycles.
5. Deliver 1 shock, leaving the AED attached, and immediately perform cardiopulmonary resuscitation (CPR), starting with chest compressions.
6. After 5 cycles (about 2 minutes) of CPR, repeat the AED analysis and deliver another shock, if indicated. If a nonshockable rhythm is detected, the AED should instruct the rescuer to resume CPR immediately, beginning with chest compressions.
7. If the machine gives the No Shock Indicated signal, assess the victim. Check the carotid pulse and breathing status and keep the AED attached until emergency medical services (EMS) arrives.
   <u>PURPOSE:</u> Continue to monitor breathing and circulation because these can stop at any time. Keep the AED pads in place to diagnose ventricular fibrillation quickly if it occurs.

GENERAL RULES FOR EMERGENCIES

A medical assistant will face two types of emergencies in an ambulatory care practice: office emergencies and home emergencies. Common office emergencies and their management are discussed later in this chapter. Besides dealing with actual emergency situations on site, a medical assistant frequently is the first person to interact with patients facing potential emergencies at home. It is estimated that one third of the telephone calls received in a provider's office involve some type of problem that requires attention. An immediate decision must be made on how to manage that problem: by giving home care advice, scheduling an appointment, or, in life-threatening cases, notifying EMS. Many facilities, under the direction and approval of the provider, create a reference list of appropriate questions for specific patient complaints.

Regardless of how emergency phone calls are managed in the facility where you work, consider the following general rules when faced with an emergency:

- It is most important to stay calm. Reassure the patient and make him or her as comfortable as possible.

- Assess the situation to determine the nature of the emergency. Decide whether the need is immediate. This decision requires calm judgment and medical knowledge.
- Obtain as much information as possible to determine the appropriate action.
- Immediately refer any concerns to the office supervisor or provider.

Telephone Screening

Each time the phone rings in a healthcare facility, a person with a possible life-or-death situation may be on the other end of the line. One of the most important tasks performed by medical assistants every day is answering the phones and managing patients' needs efficiently and appropriately. The following emergency action principles serve as a guide for managing emergency phone calls in an ambulatory care practice.

- If the patient's situation is life-threatening, activate EMS/911.
- *Never put a caller with a life-threatening emergency on hold, and always be the last to hang up.*
- Remain on the line until help arrives and you have talked to EMS personnel.
- Immediately record the names of the caller and the patient, the location, and the phone number in case the connection is lost.
- If you are unsure how to manage the emergency situation, contact the provider.
- If the patient is referred to an emergency department (ED), call the ED to notify the staff of the patient's arrival, and make a follow-up call to determine the patient's condition.
- Gather as much information as possible about what is wrong with the patient and when the problem started. Obtain details about the patient's condition, including the following:

- What is the patient's level of consciousness? Alert, responsive, lethargic, or confused? Did the patient lose consciousness at any time? If so, for how long?
- What is the character of the patient's respirations (and pulse, if the caller is able to determine this): normal, rapid, shallow, or difficult?
- Is there bleeding? If so, how much and from where?
- Is there a suspected head or neck injury? If so, has the patient been moved? Is there a suspected fracture? Where?
- Does the patient have a history of this problem?
- Any there other symptoms, such as fever, vomiting, diarrhea, or pain?
- Obtain details about what has been done for the patient. For example:
  - Medication—What, when? Dose, effectiveness? Current allergies?
- Thoroughly document the information gathered and any actions taken, including notification of EMS, whether the patient was sent to the ED or an appointment was scheduled, all home care recommendations, and whether the provider was notified and when.

Based on the outcome of the telephone interaction, a decision is made on when the provider will see the patient (Procedure 22-7). Emergency calls require activation of EMS or immediate attention as soon as the patient arrives. Urgent calls require a same-day appointment if the patient has an acute condition or is in severe discomfort. Such cases would include a young child with a high fever or a patient who complains of moderate to severe abdominal pain. A new patient will have to be worked into the day's schedule, which may cause a delay in currently scheduled appointments. Patients with other, less urgent problems can be scheduled for appointments within the next 3 to 4 days.

PROCEDURE 22-7	Perform Patient Screening Using Established Protocols: Telephone Screening and Appropriate Documentation

Goal: *To assess the direction of emergency care and to document information appropriately in the patient's record.*

Scenario: *Cheryl is working with the telephone screening staff members when they receive a call from the mother of a 5-year-old patient. The mother reports that her son fell and cut his arm. What type of information should Cheryl gather about the injury? What action should be taken? How should the incident be documented?*

EQUIPMENT and SUPPLIES

- Patient record
- Notepad and pen or pencil
- Facility's emergency procedures manual
- Computer scheduling program
- Area emergency numbers

PROCEDURAL STEPS

1. Stay calm and reassure the caller.
   <u>PURPOSE</u>: To enable you to gather accurate details about the patient's condition.

2. Verify the identity of the caller and the injured patient.
3. Immediately record the name of the caller and the patient, their location, and the phone number.
   <u>PURPOSE</u>: To be able to contact the caller if the connection is lost.
4. Determine whether the patient's condition is life-threatening. Quantify the amount of blood loss, whether the patient is alert and responsive, and whether breathing is normal. Notify emergency medical services (EMS) if necessary.
   <u>PURPOSE</u>: Notify emergency services immediately if the patient is in danger.

PROCEDURE 22-7 —*continued*

5. If EMS is notified, stay on the line with the caller until EMS personnel arrive at the scene.
   PURPOSE: Never break a phone connection in the case of a life-threatening emergency.

6. If EMS is not needed, gather details about the injury to determine whether the patient can be seen in the office or should be referred to an emergency department (ED). Consider the following questions:
   - Is there a suspected head or neck injury? Has the patient been moved?
   - Is there a possible fracture? If so, where?
   - Is bleeding present? Can it be easily controlled?
   - Are there any other symptoms?
   - Is there anything pertinent in the patient's health history that would complicate the situation?
   - Has the caller administered any first aid? If so, what was done?

7. Based on the information gathered, determine when the patient should be seen in the office if he or she has not been referred to an ED.

PURPOSE: Most emergencies are scheduled for an immediate office visit. This may require altering the current appointment schedule.

8. At any point in this process, do not hesitate to consult the provider or experienced staff or refer to the facility's emergency procedures manual to determine how to manage the patient's problem.

9. Always allow the caller to hang up first, just in case more information or assistance is needed.

10. Document the information gathered, the actions taken or recommended, any home care recommendations, and whether the provider was notified.
    PURPOSE: To have a legal record of the management of the emergency and a comprehensive description of the patient's condition and the recommended management.

7/13/20– 1:25 PM: Pt's mother reports child fell against a window and lacerated his arm. Bleeding is moderate but controlled. No reported signs of dyspnea or altered consciousness. Mother will bring child to office immediately for provider assessment. Cheryl Skurka, CMA (AAMA)

Management of On-Site Emergencies

An emergency can occur at any time to anyone. Always follow Standard Precautions when you are at risk for coming into contact with blood or body fluids. When an emergency occurs, it is impossible to determine the level of infection. All body fluids must be considered infectious, and appropriate precautions must be taken to prevent cross-contamination. If the situation is life-threatening, notify EMS and stay with the patient until you are relieved by the EMS provider or the provider in your office. It is important to document all details of the incident in the patient's health record.

Documentation of an On-Site Emergency

1. Patient's name, address, age, and health insurance information
2. Allergies, current medications, and pertinent health history
3. Name and relationship of any person with the patient
4. Vital signs and chief complaint
5. Sequence of events, beginning with how the problem occurred, any changes in the patient's overall condition, and any observations made about the patient's condition
6. Details about procedures or treatments performed on the patient

CRITICAL THINKING APPLICATION 22-3

Cheryl is working the front desk when a patient comes into the office limping. She tells Cheryl that she fell in the parking lot and hurt her ankle. Cheryl helps the patient into an exam room and begins to interview her. Role-play the situation with a classmate and make a list of at least 10 questions Cheryl should ask the patient.

Life-Threatening Emergencies

If a patient in the facility shows any signs of unresponsiveness, the provider must be brought to the patient immediately. If no provider is available in the facility, EMS must be activated. Even when a provider is present, the provider may order you to call 911 for immediate emergency care. Put on gloves before you begin to assess the patient, because any emergency situation may involve exposure to blood or body fluids.

Unresponsive Patient

If a patient is able to talk to you, he or she has an open airway. If the patient does not respond to a simple question (e.g., "Are you OK?"), gently shake the person's shoulder to check responsiveness. If the patient does not respond, you must assume that the patient is unconscious. Immediately call for help and activate EMS if that is office policy.

To care for an unresponsive patient, first assess the patient's respirations to determine whether the person is breathing. When the patient collapsed, the tongue may have gone limp and occluded the trachea. Just by changing the individual's position and opening the airway, you may provide all the assistance the patient needs to breathe independently.

If the patient is face down, roll the victim onto his or her back while supporting the head, neck, and back. Apply the head tilt–chin lift movement to open the airway. The tongue is attached to the lower jaw, so moving the jaw forward automatically opens the patient's airway. If a head or neck injury is suspected, the neck should be manipulated as little as possible; therefore, the airway should be open with the jaw-thrust maneuver. Both of these actions relieve possible obstruction of the trachea by the tongue.

Check for breathing or only gasping for breath while checking the carotid pulse at the same time for 10 seconds. Look for a rise in the chest while listening or feeling for air exchange (Figure 22-5). Breathing may stop suddenly for a variety of reasons, including shock, disease, and trauma. If no breaths are detected but there is a pulse, artificial ventilation must be started immediately because death can occur within 4 to 6 minutes. Barrier devices should be kept on hand for artificial respiration (Figure 22-6), and these should be used if rescue breaths are required (Procedure 22-8).

Administer one breath every 5 to 6 seconds (about 10 to 12 breaths per minute). Check the carotid pulse about every 2 minutes. If there is no pulse, begin chest compressions immediately at a ratio of 30 compressions to 2 breaths with about 100 to 120 compressions per minute.

The AHA uses the acronym CAB (*c*ompressions, *a*irway, *b*reathing) to help people remember the order for performing the steps of CPR (see Procedure 22-8).

When both breathing and pulse stop, the victim has suffered sudden death. Sudden death has many causes, including heart disease, choking, drowning, poisoning, suffocation, electrocution, and smoke inhalation. CPR must be started immediately to attempt to revive the patient and to prevent permanent damage to body organs, especially the brain. Continue CPR until the victim begins to move, an AED is available and ready to use, professional help arrives, or you are too exhausted to continue. If the patient has a pulse but is not breathing, continue rescue breathing and occasionally monitor the pulse until help arrives.

For specific procedures and precautions in the management of respiratory and cardiac emergencies, refer to the *Standard First Aid Manual* of the American Red Cross or the *American Heart Association CPR Manual*, or those organizations' websites. As stated earlier, all healthcare workers should have a current Certification for the Professional in CPR.

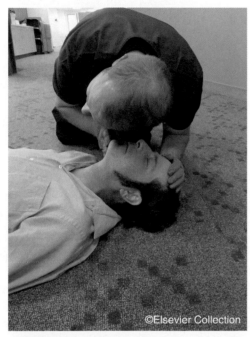

FIGURE 22-5 Checking for breathing in an unconscious patient.

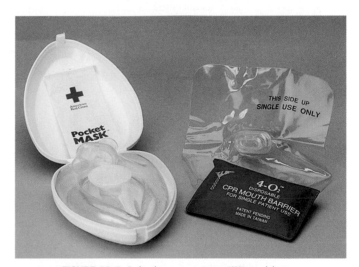

FIGURE 22-6 Cardiopulmonary resuscitation (CPR) mouth barriers.

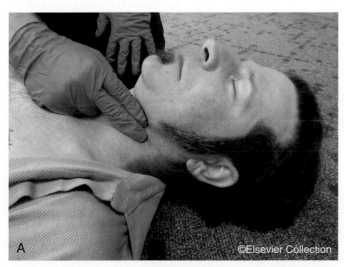

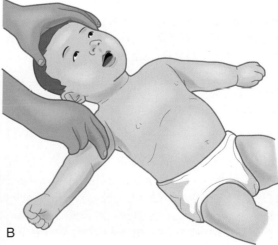

FIGURE 22-7 A, In an adult, check for a carotid pulse. **B,** In an infant, check for a brachial pulse.

PROCEDURE 22-8 | Maintain Provider/Professional-Level CPR Certification: Perform Adult Rescue Breathing and One-Rescuer CPR; Perform Pediatric and Infant CPR

Goal: *To restore breathing and blood circulation when respiration or the pulse (or both) has stopped.*

EQUIPMENT and SUPPLIES

- Disposable gloves
- Cardiopulmonary resuscitation (CPR) ventilator masks for adults, children, and infants
- Approved mannequins

PROCEDURAL STEPS

These steps are to be performed only on approved mannequins.

CPR on an Adult

1. Establish unresponsiveness. Tap the victim and ask, "Are you OK?"
   PURPOSE: To determine whether the victim is conscious.
2. If unresponsive, shout for help. Activate the emergency response system. Put on gloves and get a ventilator mask.
   PURPOSE: As soon as it is determined that an adult victim requires emergency care, activate emergency medical services (EMS). Most adults with sudden, nontraumatic cardiac arrest are in ventricular fibrillation. The time from collapse to defibrillation is the single most important predictor of survival.
3. Put the person on his or her back on a firm surface.
4. If an AED is immediately available, deliver 1 shock if instructed by the device, then begin CPR.
5. If an AED is not available, check for breathing or only gasping to breathe while at the same time checking the carotid pulse for 10 seconds.
6. If there is no pulse, start chest compressions. Kneel at the victim's neck and shoulders a couple of inches away from the chest. Place the heel of the hand over the lower part of the sternum, between the nipples but above the xiphoid process.
7. Place your other hand on top of the first and interlace or lift your fingers upward off the chest (Figure 1).
   PURPOSE: This position gives you the most control, allowing you to avoid injuring the victim's ribs as you compress the chest.

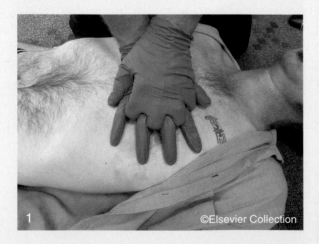

©Elsevier Collection

8. Bring your shoulders directly over the victim's sternum as you compress downward, keeping your elbows locked (Figure 2).

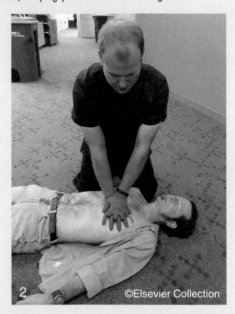

©Elsevier Collection

9. Use your upper body weight (not just your arms) as you push straight down on the sternum at least 2 inches but no more than 2.4 inches in an adult victim. Relax the pressure on the sternum after each compression, but do not remove your hands from the sternum.
   PURPOSE: The depth of compression is needed to circulate blood through the heart. Movement of the hands may injure the victim. Relieving the pressure on the chest between contractions allows the heart to completely fill with blood before the next compression.
10. After performing 30 compressions (at a rate of about 100-120 compressions per minute), perform the head tilt–chin lift maneuver to open the airway. Tilt the victim's head by placing one hand on the forehead and applying enough pressure to push the head back; with the fingers of the other hand under the chin, lift up and pull the jaw forward. Look, listen, and feel for signs of breathing. Place your ear over the mouth and listen for breathing. Watch the rising and falling of the chest for evidence of breathing. If breathing is absent or inadequate, open the airway and place the ventilator mask over the victim's mouth and nose (Figure 3).
    PURPOSE: To open the airway and determine whether the victim is breathing. Give 2 breaths, each breath delivered over 1 second, holding the ventilator mask tightly against the face while tilting the victim's chin up to keep the airway open. Remove your mouth from the mouthpiece between breaths to allow time for the patient to exhale between breaths.

PROCEDURE 22-8   —continued

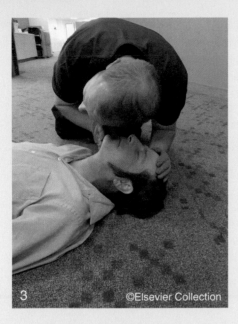

3   ©Elsevier Collection

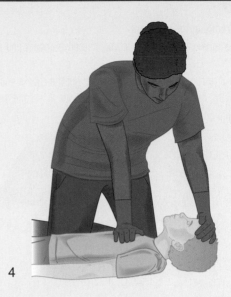

4

11. Check the patient's pulse (at the carotid artery for an adult or older child; at the brachial artery for an infant). If a pulse is present, continue rescue breathing (1 breath every 6 seconds—about 10 breaths per minute). If no signs of circulation are present, begin cycles of 30 chest compressions (at a rate of about 100-120 compressions) followed by 2 breaths.

12. If the person is still not responding after 5 cycles (about 2 minutes) and an AED is now available, apply it and follow the prompts. Administer 1 shock, then resume CPR, starting with chest compressions, for 2 more minutes before administering a second shock. Continue 30 : 2 cycles of compressions and ventilations. If an AED is not available, continue CPR until the person shows signs of movement or EMS personnel take over.

CPR on a Child

The procedure for giving CPR to a child ages 1 through 8 is essentially the same as that for an adult. The differences are as follows:

- Perform 5 cycles of compressions and breaths on the child (30 : 2 ratio, about 2 minutes) before calling 911 or the local emergency number or using an AED. If another person is available, have that person activate EMS while you care for the child.
  PURPOSE: It is important to provide immediate circulation of oxygenated blood to a child to prevent brain damage. Most pediatric cardiac arrests occur because of a secondary problem, such as airway occlusion, rather than a cardiac problem. If you know there is an airway obstruction, clear the obstruction and then proceed with CPR (Figure 4).

- Use only one hand to perform chest compressions.
  PURPOSE: The pediatric sternum requires less force to achieve the needed depression.
- Breathe more gently.
- Use the same compression-to-breath ratio as used for adults (30 compressions followed by 2 breaths per cycle); after 2 breaths, immediately begin the next cycle of compressions and breaths.
- After 5 cycles (about 2 minutes) of CPR without response, apply an AED if available. Use pediatric pads for children ages 1 through 8; if pediatric pads are not available, use adult pads. Do not use an AED on children younger than age 1. Administer 1 shock, if instructed to do so, then resume CPR, starting with chest compressions, for 2 more minutes before administering a second shock.
- Continue until the child responds or help arrives.

Infant Cardiac Arrest

Infant cardiac arrest typically is caused by lack of oxygen from drowning or choking. If you know the infant has an airway obstruction, clear the obstruction; if you do not know why the infant is unresponsive, perform CPR for 2 minutes (about 5 cycles) before calling 911 or the local emergency number. If another person is available, have that person call for help immediately while you attend to the baby.

CPR on an Infant

- Draw an imaginary line between the infant's nipples. Place two fingers on the sternum just below this intermammary line.
- Gently compress the chest at a rate of 100 to 120 per minute.
- Administer 2 breaths after every 30 compressions.
- After about 5 cycles of a 30 : 2 ratio, activate EMS.
- Continue CPR until the infant responds or help arrives.

PROCEDURE 22-8   —*continued*

Rescue Breathing for an Infant

Use an infant ventilator mask or cover the baby's mouth and nose with your mouth.

13. Give 2 rescue breaths by gently puffing out the cheeks and slowly breathing into the infant's mouth, taking about 1 second for each breath (Figure 5).

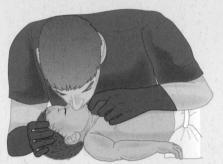

5

14. Remove your gloves and the ventilator mask valve, and discard them in the biohazard container. Disinfect the ventilator mask per the manufacturer's recommendations. Sanitize your hands.

15. Document the procedure and the patient's condition.

Cardiac Emergencies

Chest pain or angina can be associated with heart and lung disease, in addition to a few other conditions. It can be quite serious; a patient with chest pain is treated as a cardiac emergency until a provider has ruled this out. A heart attack, or *myocardial infarction,* usually is caused by blockage of the coronary arteries, which reduces the amount of blood delivered to the myocardium. The most common signal of a heart attack is an uncomfortable pressure, squeezing, fullness, or pain in the center of the chest (symptoms in women, which may be different, are presented in the following box). This may spread to the shoulder, neck, jaw, or arms. The pain may not be severe. The lips and fingernails may turn blue, which is a sign of **cyanosis** (Figure 22-8), or the patient may have a gray, ashen appearance. Frequently the patient clutches the chest in pain. This pain may radiate from the **mediastinum** down the left arm and up the left side of the neck. The pulse may be rapid and weak, and the patient often complains of nausea. Other symptoms include sweating (**diaphoresis**); indigestion; shortness of breath (SOB); cold, clammy skin; and a feeling of weakness (*general malaise*). Unfortunately, most people deny that the problem is serious until they require immediate medical attention.

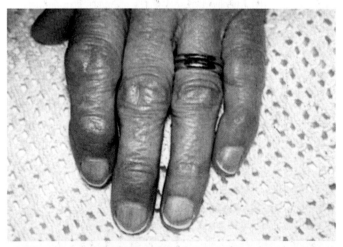

FIGURE 22-8 Cyanosis of the nail beds. (Kamal A, Brockelhurst JC: *Color atlas of geriatric medicine,* ed 2, St Louis, 1991, Mosby.)

Signs and Symptoms of Myocardial Infarction in Women

Women may experience symptoms that are different from those traditionally associated with a heart attack. Women's symptoms include a combination of the following:

- Back pain or aching and throbbing in the biceps or forearms
- Shortness of breath (SOB)
- Clammy perspiration
- Dizziness (vertigo): Unexplained lightheadedness or syncopal episodes
- Edema, especially of the ankles and/or lower legs
- Fluttering heartbeat or tachycardia
- Gastric upset
- Feeling of heaviness or fullness in the mediastinum

Immediately report any of these signs or symptoms to the provider. If the provider is not available, activate EMS. Use a wheelchair to move the patient to an examination room. Breathing will be easier if the patient's head is slightly elevated or if the patient is in a Fowler's or semi-Fowler's position. Keep the patient quiet and warm. Loosen all tight clothing. Take vital signs, including both apical and radial pulses. The provider may order oxygen started on the patient to relieve dyspnea (Procedure 22-9). Bring the emergency cart into the room and open the medication drawer so that the provider can quickly prepare the medications needed. These may include epinephrine (adrenaline), atropine, digitalis, calcium chloride, or morphine.

If the patient is conscious, ask about any medication that he or she has recently taken or is carrying. If the patient has an established heart disorder, the person may be carrying nitroglycerin tablets; these tablets are administered sublingually and may be given with the patient's consent (Figure 22-9). If the provider is in the office or is on the way, connect the patient to the electrocardiograph machine and record a few tracings. If the patient becomes unresponsive before the provider or EMS arrives, it may be necessary to start rescue breathing if no evidence of respirations is noted. If chest pain progresses to cardiac arrest and loss of circulation, CPR must be performed until help arrives.

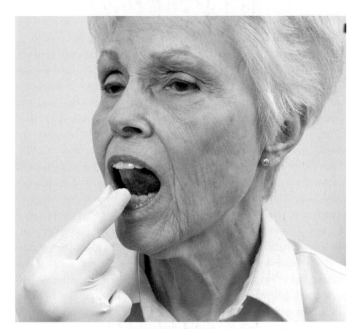

FIGURE 22-9 Nitroglycerin is administered beneath the patient's tongue.

PROCEDURE 22-9   Perform First Aid Procedures: Administer Oxygen

Goal: *To provide oxygen for a patient in respiratory distress.*

EQUIPMENT and SUPPLIES

- Provider's order
- Patient's health record
- Portable oxygen tank
- Pressure regulator
- Flow meter
- Nasal cannula with connecting tubing

PROCEDURAL STEPS

1. Gather equipment and sanitize your hands.
2. Greet and identify the patient, introduce yourself, and explain the procedure.
   PURPOSE: A nasal cannula is applied with a nasal prong in each nostril and the tab resting above the upper lip. Patients who will be using oxygen at home need to be taught how to open an oxygen tank or to use an oxygen compressor. It is vital that patients and their families understand the dangers of oxygen use in the home. They must avoid open flames and must not smoke when oxygen is in use because it is combustible. The provider typically writes an order for the number of liters of oxygen to be delivered and for home healthcare services to set up the equipment in the patient's home.
3. Check the pressure gauge on the tank to determine the amount of oxygen in the tank.
4. If necessary, open the cylinder on the tank one full counterclockwise turn, then attach the cannula tubing to the flow meter.
5. Adjust the administration of the oxygen according to the provider's order. Usually the flow meter is set at 1 to 4 liters per minute (LPM). Check to make sure oxygen is flowing through the cannula.

6. Insert the tips of the cannula into the nostrils and adjust the tubing around the back of the patient's ears (Figure 1).

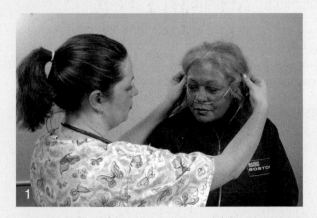

7. Encourage the patient to breathe through the nose with the mouth closed.
8. Make sure the patient is comfortable, and answer any questions he or she may have.
9. Sanitize your hands.
10. Document the procedure, including the number of liters of oxygen being administered and the patient's condition. Continue to monitor the patient throughout the procedure and document any changes in condition.

7/24/20– 3:05 PM: R 28 and labored. Oxygen initiated at 4 LPM via nasal cannula per provider order. Pt observed for signs of dyspnea and tachypnea. Cheryl Skurka, CMA (AAMA)

Choking

Choking is usually caused by a foreign object, often a bolus of food, lodged in the upper airway. The victim may clutch the neck between the thumb and the index finger (Figure 22-10); this universal distress signal should be viewed as a sign the victim needs help. If the victim has good air exchange or only partial airway obstruction and can speak, cough, or breathe, do not interfere, but encourage the patient to continue coughing until the object is expelled. Monitor the patient for signs of respiratory distress, such as pallor and cyanosis. If the patient has a pronounced wheeze or a very weak cough, he or she has a partial airway obstruction with poor air exchange and may need help. If the patient is unable to speak, breathe, or cough, a complete airway obstruction exists, and quick action must be taken to clear the airway. With complete obstruction, the patient eventually loses consciousness from lack of oxygen to the brain. This condition may lead to respiratory and cardiac arrest. If the object is not removed, the victim may die within 4 to 6 minutes. Procedure 22-10 presents the steps involved in clearing an obstructed airway in an adult. The procedure for removal of a foreign airway obstruction is exactly the same for a child older than 1 year of age.

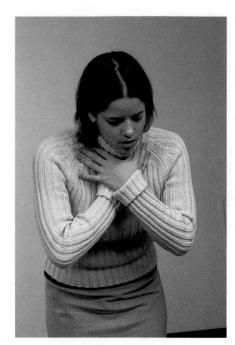

FIGURE 22-10 Universal sign of choking.

| PROCEDURE 22-10 | Perform First Aid Procedures: Respond to an Airway Obstruction in an Adult |

Goal: *To remove an airway obstruction and restore ventilation.*

EQUIPMENT and SUPPLIES

- Disposable gloves
- Ventilation mask (for unconscious victim)
- Approved mannequin for practicing removal of a foreign body airway obstruction (FBAO) in an unconscious person

PROCEDURAL STEPS

Responsive Adult

1. Ask, "Are you choking?" If the victim indicates yes, ask, "Can you speak?" If the victim is unable to speak, tell the victim you are going to help.
   <u>PURPOSE</u>: If the victim is unable to speak, is coughing weakly, and/or is wheezing, he or she has an obstructed airway with poor air exchange, and the obstruction must be removed before respiratory arrest occurs.
2. Stand behind the victim with your feet slightly apart.
   <u>PURPOSE</u>: With an obstructed airway, the victim may lose consciousness at any time. The rescuer must be prepared to lower the unconscious victim to the floor safely.
3. Reach around the victim's abdomen and place an index finger into the victim's navel or at the level of the belt buckle (Figure 1). Make a fist of the opposite hand (do not tuck the thumb into the fist) and place the thumb side of the fist against the victim's abdomen above the navel. If the victim is pregnant, place the fist above the enlarged uterus. If the victim is obese, it may be necessary to place the fist higher in the abdomen. It may be necessary to perform chest thrusts on a victim who is pregnant or obese.
   <u>PURPOSE</u>: The fist should be placed in the soft tissue of the abdomen to avoid injury to the sternum or rib cage.

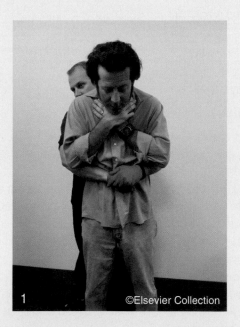

1   ©Elsevier Collection

4. Place the opposite hand over the fist and give abdominal thrusts in a quick inward and upward movement.
   <u>PURPOSE</u>: Abdominal contents pushing against the diaphragm force trapped air out of the lungs, and with it the obstruction.
5. Repeat the abdominal thrusts until the object is expelled or the victim becomes unresponsive.

Unresponsive Adult Victim

The technique for an unresponsive victim is to be practiced only on an approved mannequin.

1. Carefully lower the patient to the ground, activate the emergency response system, and put on disposable gloves.
2. Immediately begin cardiopulmonary resuscitation (CPR) at cycles of 30:2 (compressions to breaths) using the ventilator mask.
   PURPOSE: Higher airway pressures are maintained with chest compressions than with abdominal thrusts.
3. Each time the airway is opened to deliver a rescue breath during CPR, look for an object in the victim's mouth and remove it if visible. If no object is found, immediately return to the cycle of 30 chest compressions.
4. A finger sweep should be used only if the rescuer can see the obstruction.
5. Continue cycles of 30 compressions to 2 rescue breaths until the obstruction is removed or emergency medical services (EMS) arrives.

6. If the obstruction is removed, assess the victim for breathing and circulation. If a pulse is present but the patient is not breathing, begin rescue breathing.
7. Once the patient has been stabilized or EMS has taken over care, remove your gloves and the ventilator mask valve and discard them in the biohazard container. Disinfect the ventilator mask per the manufacturer's recommendations. Sanitize your hands.
8. Document the procedure and the patient's condition.

7/22/20– 8:35 AM: Pt in waiting room, clutching throat and coughing weakly. After confirming pt choking, abdominal thrusts performed until foreign body expelled. Pt breathing without difficulty; R 18 and regular. Incident reported to provider. Cheryl Skurka, CMA (AAMA)

To dislodge a foreign object from the airway of an infant up to 1 year of age, place the baby face down over your forearm and across your thigh. The head should be lower than the trunk, and you should support the baby's head and neck with one hand. Using the heel of your other hand, deliver 5 blows to the back, between the infant's shoulder blades (Figure 22-11, *A*). Holding the baby between your arms, turn the infant face up, keeping the head lower than the trunk. Using two fingers, deliver 5 thrusts to the midsternal area at the infant's nipple line (Figure 22-11, *B*). Examine the infant's mouth, and if the object is visible, pluck it out with your fingertips. *Never perform a finger sweep on an infant.* A baby's oral cavity is too small for a finger sweep, and such an action may only push the obstruction farther into the airway. If the obstruction is not visible, administer 2 rescue breaths by covering the baby's nose and mouth with your mouth, or use a pediatric ventilator mask if available. Repeat the sequence until the foreign body is expelled or help arrives.

If a choking victim is in the late stages of pregnancy, chest compressions should be delivered by placing your cupped hands above

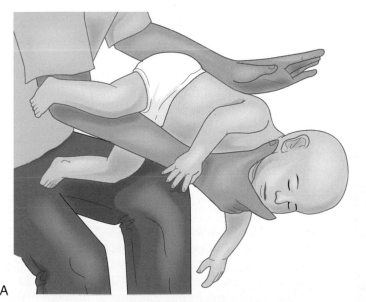

A

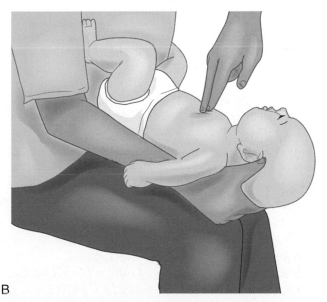

B

FIGURE 22-11 A, Back blows are administered to an infant supported on the arm and thigh. **B,** Chest thrusts are administered in the same position as for cardiac compressions.

the uterus to prevent possible trauma to the infant. If the patient is obese and you are unable to wrap your arms around the abdomen, perform chest compressions as you would for a pregnant woman.

The abdominal thrust maneuver also can be performed on yourself if you are choking and no one is nearby to help you. Press your fist into your upper abdomen with quick, upward thrusts, or lean forward and press the abdomen quickly against a firm object, such as the back of a chair.

Cerebrovascular Accident (Stroke)

A cerebrovascular accident (CVA), or stroke, is a disorder of the cerebral blood vessels that results in impairment of the blood supply to part of the brain. This interruption in normal circulation of blood through the brain leads to some degree of neurologic damage, temporary or permanent, depending on the severity of oxygen deprivation to the brain cells.

A minor stroke, or **transient ischemic attack (TIA)**, usually does not cause unconsciousness, and symptoms depend on the location of the circulatory problem in the brain and the amount of brain damage. TIA symptoms are temporary and may include headache, confusion, vertigo, ringing in the ears *(tinnitus)*, temporary paralysis or weakness of one side of the body, transient limb weakness, slurred speech, and vision problems. TIA episodes indicate that the patient is at risk for a major stroke.

Symptoms of a major stroke include unconsciousness, paralysis on one side of the body, difficulty breathing and swallowing, loss of bladder and bowel control, unequal pupil size, and slurring of speech.

Home recommendations for a patient who has suffered a major stroke should begin with notifying the provider and/or activating EMS. Keep the patient lying down and lightly covered. Maintain an open airway. To prevent choking, position the head so that any secretions drain from the side of the mouth. If the patient is lying on the floor, did not fall, and shows no indications of a head or neck injury, he or she can be placed in the recovery position as follows (Figure 22-12):

1. Place the patient's arm that is farthest from you alongside and above the head; place the other arm across the chest.
2. Bend the leg that is closest to you, and after placing one arm under the patient's head and shoulder and the other hand on

the flexed knee, roll the patient away from you while you stabilize the head and neck. The patient's head should be resting on the extended arm.

The recovery position uses gravity to drain fluids from the mouth and keep the trachea clear. Keep the patient in this position until the person is alert or help arrives. Do not give the patient anything to eat or drink. Vital signs should be measured at regular intervals and recorded for the provider.

Advances in early treatment of strokes show great promise in preventing long-term neurologic deficits. However, to prevent permanent brain damage, **thrombolytics** must be administered intravenously within 3 hours of the onset of symptoms. If a patient does not know when the symptoms began (e.g., the person woke up with the symptoms) or cannot accurately tell the provider when the symptoms started, the time allotted for administration begins from the point at which the patient last was known to be asymptomatic. Intracranial hemorrhage must be ruled out before treatment begins. The earlier the treatment starts, the better the neurologic outcomes. The best possible outcomes are seen in patients who receive thrombolytic therapy within 90 minutes of the onset of symptoms.

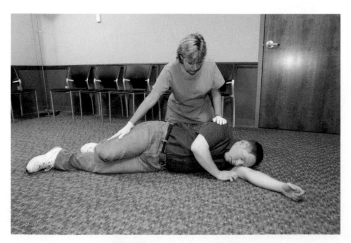

FIGURE 22-12 Recovery position.

Warning Signs of Stroke: *FAST*

The American Stroke Association developed the mnemonic FAST to help people spot the signs of a sudden stroke. If any of these are present, 911 should be called immediately.

Face drooping	• Does one side of the face droop or is it numb?
	• Ask the person to smile. Is the person's smile uneven?
Arm weakness	• Is one arm weak or numb?
	• Ask the person to raise both arms. Does one arm drift downward?
Speech difficulty	• Is speech slurred? Is the person unable to speak or hard to understand?
	• Ask the person to repeat a simple sentence, such as, "The sky is blue." Is the sentence repeated correctly?
Time to call 911	• If someone shows any of these symptoms, even if the symptoms go away, call 911 and get the person to the hospital immediately. Note the time the first symptoms appeared.

Source: American Heart Association and The American Stroke Association.

CRITICAL THINKING APPLICATION   22-4

Thomas Antonio, a 67-year-old patient, calls to report that when he woke up this morning, the left side of his face was drooping and he had difficulty seeing out of his left eye. The symptoms went away in about 2 hours, and he is feeling fine now. The schedule does not show any openings for 2 days. When should Cheryl make an appointment for Mr. Antonio? What questions should Cheryl ask him?

Shock

Shock is a state of collapse caused by failure of the circulatory system to deliver enough oxygenated blood to the body's vital organs. Injury, hemorrhage, infection, anesthesia, drug overdose, burns, pain, fear, or emotional stress can cause this physiologic reaction. Shock can be immediate or delayed, and it is potentially fatal. Many different types of shock can occur, but the signs and symptoms are universal. The most common indicators are a pale, gray, or cyanotic appearance; moist but cool skin; dilated pupils; a weak, rapid pulse; marked hypotension; shallow, rapid respirations; lethargy or restlessness; nausea and vomiting; and extreme thirst.

If a patient shows signs of shock, maintain an open airway and check for breathing and circulation. Place the patient supine with the legs elevated approximately 1 foot to return the blood from the legs to vital organs. Loosen all tight clothing and cover the patient with a blanket for warmth (Procedure 22-11). Do not move the patient unnecessarily. Fluids may be given by mouth if the patient is alert. Because shock can evolve into a life-threatening situation, only basic first aid should be administered, and the patient should be transported to the hospital as soon as possible.

Types and Causes of Shock

Anaphylactic: A severe allergic reaction

Insulin: Severe hypoglycemia caused by an overdose of insulin

Psychogenic or *mental:* Excessive fear, joy, anger, or emotional stress

Hypovolemic or *hemorrhagic:* Excessive loss of blood

Cardiogenic: Myocardial infarction, pulmonary embolism, or severe congestive heart failure

Neurogenic: Dilation of blood vessels as a result of brain or spinal cord injury

Septic: Systemic infection

PROCEDURE 22-11 | Perform First Aid Procedures: Care for a Patient Who Has Fainted or Is in Shock

Goal: *To assess and provide emergency care for a patient who has fainted.*

EQUIPMENT and SUPPLIES

- Patient's record
- Sphygmomanometer
- Stethoscope
- Watch with second hand
- Blanket
- Footstool or box
- Pillows
- Oxygen equipment, if ordered by provider:
  - Portable oxygen tank
  - Pressure regulator
  - Flow meter
  - Nasal cannula with connecting tubing

PROCEDURAL STEPS

1. If warning is given that the patient feels faint, have the patient lower the head to the knees to increase the blood supply to the brain (Figure 1). If this does not stop the episode, have the patient lie down on the examination table or lower the patient to the floor. If the patient collapses to the floor when fainting, treat with caution because of possible head or neck injuries.

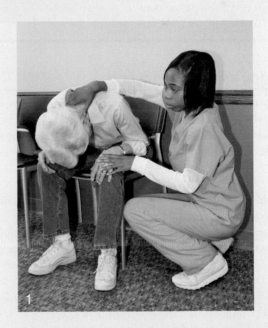

2. Immediately notify the provider of the patient's condition and assess the patient for life-threatening emergencies, such as respiratory or cardiac arrest. If the patient is breathing and has a pulse, monitor the patient's vital signs.

3. If the patient has fainted and vital signs are unstable or the patient does not respond quickly, activate emergency medical services (EMS).
   PURPOSE: Fainting may be a sign of a life-threatening problem.

4. Activate EMS if the patient shows signs of shock—pale, gray, or cyanotic appearance; moist but cool skin; dilated pupils; a weak, rapid pulse; marked hypotension; shallow, rapid respirations; or lethargy or restlessness.

PROCEDURE 22-11 —continued

5. Look, listen, and feel for breathing and check the pulse. Maintain an open airway and continue to monitor vital signs.
6. Loosen any tight clothing and keep the patient warm, applying a blanket if needed.
7. If a head or neck injury is not a factor, elevate the patient's legs above the level of the heart using a footstool with pillow support if available (Figure 2).
   PURPOSE: Elevating the legs assists with venous blood return to the heart. This may relieve symptoms of fainting or shock by elevating the blood pressure and increasing blood flow to vital organs.

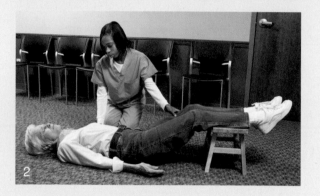

8. Continue to monitor vital signs, and apply oxygen by nasal cannula if ordered by the provider until the patient recovers or EMS arrives.
9. If the patient vomits, roll the patient onto his or her side to prevent aspiration of vomitus into the lungs.
10. If the patient completely recovers, assist the patient into a sitting position. Do not leave the patient unattended on the examination table.
11. Document the incident, including a description of the episode, the patient's symptoms and vital signs, the duration of the episode, and any complaints. If oxygen was administered, document the number of liters and how long oxygen was administered.

7/29/20— 4:18 PM: Pt in waiting room states she feels faint. Pt lowered to floor, clothing loosened, legs elevated. Provider notified. P 88 and regular, R 22, BP 112/60. Syncopal episode persisted for 90 sec, feeling of vertigo lasted 10 min post syncope. Pt transferred to exam room via wheelchair after recovery. Cheryl Skurka, CMA (AAMA)

COMMON OFFICE EMERGENCIES

The remainder of this chapter highlights typical emergencies seen in an ambulatory care practice or in telephone triage situations. Table 22-1 summarizes common emergencies, the questions that should be asked, and possible actions for home care.

Fainting (Syncope)

Fainting, or *syncope*, is a common emergency. It usually is caused by a transient loss of blood flow to the brain (e.g., a sudden drop in blood pressure), which results in a temporary loss of consciousness. It can occur without warning, or the patient may appear pale; may feel cold, weak, dizzy, or nauseated; and may have numbness of the extremities before the incident. The greatest danger to the patient is an injury from falling during the attack. Therefore, if a patient has syncopal symptoms, immediately place the individual in a supine position. Loosen all tight clothing and maintain an open airway. Apply a cold washcloth to the forehead. Measure and record the patient's pulse, respiratory rate, and blood pressure, and report the findings to the provider. Keep the patient in a supine position for at least 10 minutes after the person regains consciousness. A complete patient history can help determine the possible causes of the attack (e.g., a history of heart disease or diabetes). Document the details of the episode and how long it took the patient to recover completely (see Procedure 22-11).

If the patient does not recover quickly, the provider may activate EMS for transport to the hospital. Syncope might be a brief episode in the development of a serious underlying illness, such as an abnormal heart rhythm or shock, that could lead to sudden cardiac death.

Poisoning

Poisonings are considered medical emergencies and are the sixth leading cause of accidental pediatric death in the United States. Poisoning can occur by oral intake, absorption, inhalation, or injection. Over-the-counter (OTC) medications (e.g., acetaminophen); detergents and bleach; plants; cough and cold medicines; and vitamins cause most cases of poisoning seen in young children. Other typical household poisons include drain cleaner, turpentine, kerosene, furniture polish, and paint (Figure 22-13). Signs and

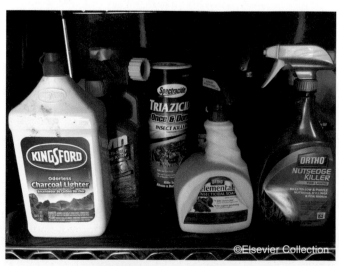

FIGURE 22-13 Hazardous household materials.

TABLE 22-1   Telephone Screening of Possible Emergency Situations

EMERGENCY SITUATION	SCREENING QUESTIONS	HOME CARE ADVICE
Syncope	• Was the patient injured? • Does the patient have a history of heart disease, seizures, or diabetes?	• Syncope does not necessarily indicate a serious disease. If injured by a fall, the patient may need to be evaluated and treated. • The patient should get up very slowly to prevent a recurrence; he or she should then take it easy and drink plenty of fluids. • If the patient is to be seen, someone should accompany him or her to the provider's office.
Animal bites	• What kind of animal (pet or wild)? • How severe is the injury? • Where are the bites? • When did the bites occur?	• The health department or police should be notified. Every effort must be made to locate the animal and monitor its health. • If the skin is not broken, wash the area well and observe for signs of infection.
Insect bites and stings	• Does the patient have a history of an anaphylactic reaction to insect stings? • Does the patient have any of these: difficulty breathing, a widespread rash, or trouble swallowing?	• If the patient has a history of anaphylaxis and has an EpiPen, the EpiPen should be used immediately and emergency medical services (EMS) notified. • Activate EMS if the patient is having systemic symptoms. • An antihistamine (Benadryl) relieves local pruritus.
Asthma	• Does the patient show signs of cyanosis? • Has the patient used prescribed inhalers?	• If a patient with asthma is unable to speak in sentences, has poor color, and is struggling to breathe even after using an inhaler, he or she should be seen immediately or EMS should be activated.

Burns	• Where are the burns located, and what caused them?
	• Are signs of shock present—moist, clammy skin; altered consciousness; and rapid breathing and pulse?
	• If the burn is more than 2 days old, are signs of infection present—foul odor, cloudy drainage?
		• Activate EMS for the following:
		  • Burns on the face, hands, feet, or perineum
		  • Burns caused by electricity or a chemical
		  • Burns associated with inhalation
		  • Signs of shock are present
		• The patient must receive a tetanus shot if he or she has not had one in more than 10 years.
		• Schedule an urgent appointment if signs of infection are reported.

Wounds	• Is the bleeding steady or pulsating? • How and when did the injury occur? • Does the patient have any bleeding disorders, or is the patient taking anticoagulant drugs? • Is the wound open and deep?	• Pulsating bleeding usually indicates arterial damage; activate EMS. • If the injury was caused by a powerful force, other injuries also may have resulted. • Patients taking anticoagulants or who have diabetes or anemia require an urgent appointment. • A gaping, deep wound requires sutures.
Head injury	• Did the patient pass out or have a seizure? Is the patient confused or vomiting? Is a clear fluid draining from the nose or ears?	• If the answer is yes to any of these questions; activate EMS.

symptoms of poisoning, which vary greatly, include burns on the hands and mouth, stains on the victim's clothing, open bottles of medicines or chemicals, changes in skin color, nausea or stomach cramps, shallow breathing, convulsions, heavy perspiration, dizziness or drowsiness, and unconsciousness.

If you receive a phone call about a suspected poisoning, tell the caller not to hang up and not to leave the victim unattended. Call the local poison control center and forward all directions to the caller. Syrup of ipecac has been recommended in the past for home use when a child ingests a poisonous substance, but the

American Academy of Pediatrics now recommends that syrup of ipecac not be kept in the home. There are several reasons for this decision:

- Ipecac should not be given if the child swallowed chemicals that cause burns on contact because the substance can burn the gastrointestinal tract again when it is vomited.
- People with eating disorders often use ipecac to make themselves throw up.
- Ipecac may make it difficult to keep down other drugs that are needed to treat the poison.

If parents believe a child has ingested a poisonous substance, they should call the national poison control center at 1-800-222-1222, or call 911. (Always remember, though, that the best treatment is prevention; parents should be reminded to keep poisonous substances out of sight and out of reach of children). If the patient is to be seen by the provider or sent to the hospital, tell the caller to bring the container of poison or a sample of the vomitus so that the chemical contents of the substance can be verified.

What to Ask When a Poisoning Is Reported

- Victim's name, weight, and age
- Name of the poison taken and any information on the label
- How much was taken
- How long ago the poison was ingested
- Whether vomiting has occurred
- Whether the person has any pertinent symptoms, such as difficulty breathing or an altered state of consciousness
- Whether any first aid has been given, and if so, what

CRITICAL THINKING APPLICATION   22-5
A young mother calls in a panic to report that her 18-month-old daughter swallowed at least half a bottle of cough syrup. The child is fussy and very sleepy, and the mother wants to give her ipecac immediately. What should Cheryl do?

Animal Bites

Possible complications from animal bites include rabies, tetanus, and local skin infection. Any animal bite that is extensive or deep should be seen by a provider. Human infection with rabies is rare; however, if the bite is made by a domestic animal, the animal should be kept quarantined and under observation for 10 days to be monitored for signs of the disease. The animal should not be killed, because a positive finding of rabies is almost impossible to make if the animal has been dead for an extended time. If the bite is made by a bat, raccoon, or any other wild animal, the animal is assumed to be rabid, and the patient must undergo a series of rabies vaccine injections. Local skin infection can be prevented by immediately cleansing the area with antimicrobial soap and water. If the bite breaks the skin (including human bites), the patient's tetanus immunization status must be checked and, if needed, a booster or the entire four-dose tetanus series must be administered as indicated.

Insect Bites and Stings

The bite or sting of an insect can be irritating and painful because of the chemical toxin injected by the insect, but it usually is not serious. Typical symptoms—inflammation, itching (pruritus), and edema—are local and are confined to the area of the bite. In rare cases, a severe allergic reaction may occur; this is a potentially dangerous situation that can lead to anaphylaxis. Signs and symptoms of a systemic allergic reaction include a dry cough, a feeling of tightening in the throat or chest, swelling or itching around the eyes, widespread hives (urticaria), wheezing, dyspnea, and hypotension. Difficulty talking is a sign of urticaria or edema in the throat and may indicate the onset of complete airway obstruction. This is a sign of a true emergency. Epinephrine and oxygen should be ready for immediate administration on the provider's orders. Antihistamines and corticosteroids may be used, but these agents act considerably slower than epinephrine. If acute anaphylactic shock develops, death may occur within 1 hour without medical intervention.

If the stinger is still lodged in the skin, scrape it off with a dull knife, a credit card, or a fingernail. Be careful not to squeeze the stinger, because this injects more venom into the skin. Apply an ice bag to the site to relieve pain and slow absorption of venom. Calamine lotion or hydrocortisone cream may be applied to relieve itching. If the patient has a history of allergies, especially to insect venom, he or she should have access to an EpiPen injection system; this should be used immediately after the sting. In this case, the patient should be transported to the nearest hospital for immediate care.

Removal of a Tick

Ticks can cause a number of diseases, including Rocky Mountain spotted fever and Lyme disease. The tick embeds its head into the skin to obtain blood, and it should be removed intact by the following method:
1. Do not handle ticks with uncovered fingers; use tweezers to prevent personal contamination.
2. Place the tips of the tweezers as close as possible to the area where the tick has entered the skin.
3. With a slow, steady motion, pull the tick away from the skin. Try not to squeeze or crush the tick. If the tick's entire body is not removed, make an appointment with a provider to have the site evaluated.
4. After removal, place the tick directly into a sealable container. Disinfect the area around the bite site using standard procedures.
5. If the tick is removed at home, the provider may suggest that it be brought to the office to be tested for disease.

Asthma Attacks

Asthma is characterized by expiratory wheezing, coughing, a feeling of tightness in the chest, and shortness of breath. During an asthma attack, two different physiologic responses occur. The lining of the respiratory tract becomes inflamed and edematous and produces mucus, which results in narrowing of the air passages. At the same time, bronchospasms occur, which also constrict the airways. The quality and severity of attacks vary greatly among patients, and treatment must be individualized to minimize or eliminate chronic symptoms. If the patient is prescribed a bronchodilator inhaler, it should be used at the first indication of symptoms. Depending on the severity of the attack, give the patient an appointment for the same day as the call, or consult the provider. The provider may recommend that the patient go directly to the ED for emergency respiratory care.

Seizures

Seizures may be **idiopathic**, or they may result from trauma, injury, or metabolic alterations, such as hypoglycemia or hypocalcemia. A *febrile* seizure is transient and occurs with a rapid rise in body temperature over 101.8°F (38.8°C). Febrile seizures typically occur in children between 6 months and 5 years of age. Many different types of seizures occur, but all are caused by a disruption in the electrical activity of the brain.

If a patient suffers a grand mal seizure, which involves uncontrolled muscular contractions, the most important point is to protect the patient from possible injury. Clear everything away from the patient that could cause accidental injury, and observe him or her until the seizure ends. Do not place anything into the person's mouth, because it may damage the teeth or tongue and force the tongue back over the trachea. Do not hold the patient down, because this may result in muscle injuries or fractures. If unconsciousness persists after the seizure has subsided, place the patient in the recovery position to maintain an open airway and allow drainage of excess saliva. After the seizure is over, let the patient rest or sleep, but never leave the person alone. If the provider is not in the office, check the office policies and procedures manual to determine how to manage the situation (Procedure 22-12).

Call 911 for emergency assistance in any of the following situations:

- The patient does not regain consciousness within 10 to 15 minutes.
- The seizure does not stop within a few minutes.
- The patient begins a second seizure immediately after the first one.
- The patient is pregnant.
- Signs of head trauma are present.
- The patient is known to have diabetes.
- The seizure was triggered by a high fever in a child.

PROCEDURE 22-12   Perform First Aid Procedures: Care for a Patient With Seizure Activity

Goal: *To assess and provide emergency care for a patient who has a grand mal seizure.*

EQUIPMENT and SUPPLIES

- Patient's record
- Sphygmomanometer
- Stethoscope
- Watch with second hand
- Blanket
- Pillows

PROCEDURAL STEPS

1. If warning is given that the patient might have a seizure, help lower the patient to the floor. If the patient collapses with a seizure, clear everything away from the patient that could cause accidental injury. If you cannot remove all hard items (e.g., the examination table), pad the hard edges with a blanket or pillow.
   PURPOSE: The patient could be injured when uncontrollable muscular contractions occur with the seizure.

2. Immediately check the time on your watch and call for help.
   PURPOSE: To time the length of the seizure and alert the provider of the patient's seizure activity.

3. Observe the patient throughout the seizure but do not restrain or confine the patient's movements.
   PURPOSE: Stay with the patient for the entire seizure, but do not restrain movement. Restraining the patient may cause musculoskeletal injury.

4. Do not place anything in the patient's mouth during the seizure.
   PURPOSE: The patient's jaw is typically clamped tight during the seizure and trying to force something between the teeth can cause injury.

5. After the muscular contractions have ended, roll the patient into the recovery position on his or her side, with the top knee bent and the head resting on the extended arm closest to the floor.
   PURPOSE: This position helps maintain an open airway.

6. Loosen any tight clothing and keep the patient warm, using a blanket if needed. Let the patient rest, but never leave the patient alone.
   PURPOSE: To maintain patient safety and comfort.

7. If the provider is not in the facility, check the policies and procedures manual to determine how to follow up with the patient.

8. Activate emergency medical services (EMS) if any of the following conditions are present:
   - The patient does not regain consciousness within 10 to 15 minutes.
   - The seizure does not stop within a few minutes.
   - The patient begins a second seizure immediately after the first one.
   - The patient is pregnant.
   - Signs of head trauma are present.
   - The patient is known to have diabetes.
   - The seizure was triggered by a high fever in a child.

9. If the patient completely recovers, assist him or her into a sitting position, check vital signs, and make sure there is someone to accompany the person home.

10. Document the incident, including a description of the episode, the patient's symptoms and vital signs, the duration of the seizure activity, and any complaints.

Abdominal Pain

Abdominal pain is a symptom caused by many different problems, which can range from acute discomfort to life-threatening complications. The clinician should see every patient who reports abdominal pain; the question is how soon the patient should be seen. A patient with acute onset of severe, persistent abdominal pain, especially when this is accompanied by fever, should receive medical attention as soon as possible. Abdominal pain has a variety of causes, including intestinal infection, appendicitis, ectopic pregnancy, inflammation, hemorrhage, obstruction, and tumor.

Treatment in the ambulatory care office depends on the cause of the pain; however, the medical assistant should follow these general guidelines:

- Keep the patient warm and quiet.
- Have an emesis basin available.
- Administer nothing by mouth (NPO).
- Do not apply heat to the abdomen unless so instructed by the provider.
- Administer analgesics as ordered.
- Check and record the patient's vital signs and follow the provider's orders.

Screening Guidelines for Assessing Abdominal Pain

- Assess for shock-related signs and symptoms: diaphoresis; cold, clammy skin; cyanosis or gray pallor; rapid respirations; altered state of consciousness.
- Is the pain severe and constant, or does it come in waves?
- Has the patient had any bloody or tarry stools?
- Is the patient's temperature higher than 101° F (38.3° C)?
- Could the patient be pregnant or has she missed a menstrual period?
- Has the patient experienced continuous vomiting or severe constipation?
- Are any urinary symptoms present, such as frequency, **hematuria**, or flank pain?

- Does the patient have chest pain, shortness of breath, or a continuous cough?
- Does the patient have a history of serious illness, such as diabetes, heart disease, or cancer?

Sprains and Strains

Sprains are tears of the ligaments that support a joint; *strains* are injuries to a muscle and its tendons. Both types of injury may damage surrounding soft tissues and blood vessels and nearby nerves. With a sprain, the victim develops edema and **ecchymosis** around the injury, and any movement of the joint, especially a twisting one, produces pain. Usually no swelling or discoloration is seen with a strain, and only mild tenderness is noted unless the injured muscle or tendon is used.

Tendon strains and ligament sprains take several weeks to heal, whereas muscle tears usually heal in 1 to 2 weeks because muscle has such a rich blood supply. These injuries are treated by elevating the affected area and applying mild compression and ice. Swelling is reduced if ice is applied within 20 to 29 minutes of the injury. After 24 to 36 hours, alternating applications of mild heat and ice usually are indicated. The patient may be advised to immobilize the part.

Fractures

A fracture is a break or crack in a bone, which can result from trauma or disease. Fractures are very painful and affect the patient's ability to freely move the injured part. When a patient with a fracture is brought into the office, the medical assistant should make the patient as comfortable as possible. Place the patient in a position that supports the affected area at the joints above and below the suspected fracture and does not place strain on the injury. Notify the provider immediately and proceed according to the orders given. Emergency treatment for fractures includes preventing movement of the injured part through splinting, elevation of the affected extremity, application of ice, and control of any bleeding (Procedure 22-13). If a patient with an open fracture (i.e., the bone is protruding through the skin) is seen in an ambulatory care office, he or she should be transported to the ED.

PROCEDURE 22-13   Perform First Aid Procedures: Care for a Patient With a Suspected Fracture of the Wrist by Applying a Splint

Goal: *To provide emergency care for and assessment of a patient with a suspected fracture of the wrist.*

EQUIPMENT and SUPPLIES

- Patient record
- Sphygmomanometer
- Stethoscope
- Watch with second hand
- Splint with padding
- Ace or roller bandage material
- Gloves and sterile dressing (if any open areas on the skin)

PROCEDURAL STEPS

1. Gather equipment and sanitize your hands.
2. Greet and identify the patient, introduce yourself, and explain the procedure.
   <u>PURPOSE</u>: To relieve the patient's anxiety and earn his or her cooperation with the procedure.
3. Obtain vital signs.

PROCEDURE 22-13 *—continued*

4. Assess the area of the suspected fracture for swelling, bleeding, bruising, or protruding bones.

5. If the skin is broken, put on gloves and cover the area with a sterile dressing.
   PURPOSE: Infection control and compliance with Standard Precautions procedures.

6. Moving the limb as little as possible, place the padded splint under the lower arm and wrist.
   PURPOSE: Avoid moving the limb any more than necessary to prevent movement of the fracture and further pain.

7. The area must be immobilized by the splint above and below the suspected fracture.
   PURPOSE: Immobilizing the joint above and below the injury keeps the joint in place, preventing further injury and pain.

8. Secure the splint in place by rolling an Ace bandage or roller bandage around the splint and arm, starting at the arm and rolling down to the wrist and hand.

9. Check the pulse in the affected arm. Note the color and temperature of the skin and the color of the nails.
   PURPOSE: To make sure the splint and bandage have not been applied too tightly.

10. Make sure the patient is comfortable, and answer any questions he or she may have.

11. Sanitize your hands.

12. Document the procedure, including the condition of the patient, the reported pain level, and application of the splint.

7/24/20– 1:05 PM: Temporary splint applied to Ⓛ wrist per provider order. Pt reports some relief of discomfort, with pain at 6 on a 1-10 scale. Hand warm and normal color, nail beds pink, and radial pulse easily palpated. BP 132/80, P 88 and regular, R 22. Cheryl Skurka, CMA (AAMA)

Burns

Burns are among the most common causes of injury in the United States. Burn injuries can result from flame, heat, scalds, electricity, chemicals, or radiation. The skin surface may be reddened, blistered, or charred. The depth and extent of a burn are the major determinants in classifying its severity. The extent of the pain is directly proportional to the extent of the surface area burned and the depth and nature of the burn.

To screen a burn injury, the medical assistant must know what caused the burn, its location and approximate size, the depth of the burn, and whether any additional injuries occurred. If the patient reports a chemical burn, it is important to have the person immediately remove all clothing that may have come into contact with the chemical and flood the affected area with running water to flush the irritant off the skin. If the chemical is not quickly flushed away or remains in the patient's clothing, the agent will continue to burn the skin and may do very serious damage.

The percentage of the body surface area burned can be estimated using the Rule of Nines (Figure 22-14). With this assessment tool, the amount of burned tissue can be quickly calculated. The Rule of Nines divides the body into areas approximately equal to 9% of the total body surface area. When a burn victim is assessed, the affected regions are combined to yield an estimate of the total percentage of burned tissue. Partial-thickness burns over 15% of the total body surface and full-thickness burns of less than 2% can be treated in the ambulatory care office if the patient can be seen immediately. Patients with larger body surface area involvement or other complications should be transported immediately to a hospital, preferably one with a burn unit.

Tissue Injuries

Patients may report any of several different types of wounds. A *contusion* is a closed wound with no evidence of injury to the skin; it typically is caused by blunt trauma, appears swollen and discolored,

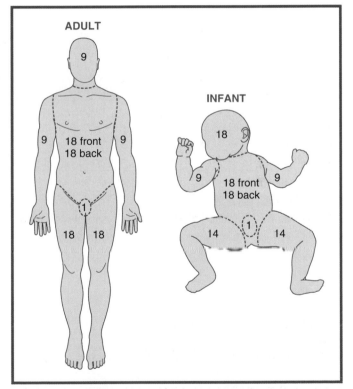

FIGURE 22-14 Rule of Nines classification of burns.

and is painful. A contusion results in a painful bruise, but the skin remains intact. A scrape on the surface of the skin (e.g., a skinned knee, rug burn) is called an *abrasion*. A deeper, jagged wound is called a *laceration*. Additional tissue damage may occur around a laceration; depending on its depth, the wound may need to be repaired surgically. A *puncture* wound occurs when an object is forced into the body (e.g., stepping on a nail). If an object is lodged in body tissues, the best course is to leave it there, stabilize it as much as possible with rolled-up material, and transport the individual to a clinic or ED. The puncture may have severed blood vessels, and if the object is removed, considerable bleeding may occur. An injury in which tissue is torn away (e.g., complete or partial removal of a finger) is known as an *avulsion*.

Lacerations are common presentations in a primary care provider's office. A lacerated wound shows jagged or irregular tearing of the tissues. The severity depends on the cause of the laceration, the site and extent of the injury, and whether the area is contaminated. The injury that caused the laceration also may have damaged blood vessels, nerves, bones, joints, and organs in the body cavities.

When the patient arrives at the facility, put on gloves and notify the provider immediately. Have the patient lie down, and cover the injured area with a sterile dressing (use a dressing that is thick enough to absorb the bleeding) (Procedure 22-14). Reassure the patient and explain your actions as much as possible. Ask the patient when he or she last received a tetanus inoculation, and record the date in the patient's record. If it has been longer than 10 years, the provider probably will want a booster injection given.

Wounds that are not bleeding severely and that do not involve deep tissue damage should be cleaned with antimicrobial soap and water to remove bacteria and other foreign matter. If the laceration is extremely dirty, the provider may want the area irrigated with sterile normal saline solution.

A butterfly closure strip may be used over small lacerations to hold the edges together. If the wound is superficial and has straight edges, it may be closed with a microporous tape (e.g., Steri-Strips)

(Figure 22-15), which eliminates the discomfort of suturing and suture removal. Another wound closure option is a tissue adhesive product (e.g., Dermabond fluid or LiquiBand), which forms a strong, flexible closure similar in strength to nylon suture material. Tissue adhesive products are very useful for closing simple lacerations in children; they provide an antimicrobial and waterproof coating to the wound site that lasts several days, even with repeated washing.

After the clinician closes the wound, the medical assistant typically applies a sterile dressing to the site. The size and thickness of the dressing depend on the type of wound.

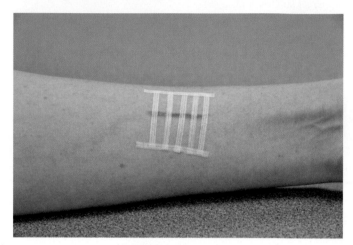

FIGURE 22-15 Steri-Strips.

PROCEDURE 22-14 Perform First Aid Procedures: Control Bleeding

Goal: *To stop hemorrhaging from an open wound.*

EQUIPMENT and SUPPLIES

- Patient's record
- Gloves (sterile if available)
- Appropriate personal protective equipment (PPE) as specified by Occupational Safety and Health Administration (OSHA) guidelines, including:
  - Impermeable gown
  - Goggles or face shield
  - Impermeable mask
  - Impermeable foot covers, if indicated
- Sterile dressings
- Bandaging material
- Biohazard waste container

PROCEDURAL STEPS

1. Sanitize your hands and put on appropriate PPE.
   PURPOSE: To follow Standard Precautions.
2. Assemble equipment and supplies.
3. Apply several layers of sterile dressing material directly to the wound and exert pressure.
   PURPOSE: Direct pressure to a wound slows or stops the bleeding. Sterile supplies are needed to prevent wound infection.

4. Wrap the wound with bandage material. Add more dressing and bandaging material if the bleeding continues.
5. If bleeding persists and the wound is on an extremity, elevate the extremity above the level of the heart. Notify the provider immediately if the bleeding cannot be controlled.
6. If the bleeding still continues, maintain direct pressure and elevation; also apply pressure to the appropriate artery. If the bleeding is in the arm, apply pressure to the brachial artery by squeezing the inner aspect of the middle upper arm. If the bleeding is in the leg, apply pressure to the femoral artery on the affected side by pushing with the heel of the hand into the femoral crease at the groin. If the bleeding cannot be controlled, activate emergency medical services.
7. Once the bleeding has been brought under control and the patient has been stabilized, discard contaminated materials in an appropriate biohazard waste container.
8. Disinfect the area, then remove your gloves and discard them in a biohazard waste container.
9. Sanitize your hands.
10. Document the incident, including details of the wound, when and how it occurred, the patient's symptoms and vital signs, treatment provided by the provider, and the patient's current condition.

Nosebleeds (Epistaxis)

A nosebleed, or *epistaxis*, is a hemorrhage that usually results from the rupture of small vessels in the nose. Nosebleeds can be caused by injury, disease, hypertension, strenuous activity, high altitudes, exposure to cold, overuse of anticoagulant medications (e.g., aspirin), and nasal recreational drug use. Bleeding from the anterior nostril area usually is venous, whereas bleeding from the posterior region usually is arterial and is more difficult to stop. Treatment of epistaxis varies according to the amount of bleeding and the presence of other conditions, and whether the patient is taking anticoagulant medications.

If the bleeding is mild to moderate and from one side of the nose, the patient should sit up, lean slightly forward, and apply direct pressure to the affected nostril by pinching the nose. Constant pressure should be continued for 10 to 15 minutes to allow clotting to take place. If the bleeding cannot be controlled, insert a clean gauze pad into the nostril, and notify the provider. If the provider is not available, proceed with standard EMS protocols. Bleeding should be considered a medical emergency if it is bilateral and continuous or if it occurs in a patient who has a bleeding disorder or has been prescribed anticoagulants.

Head Injuries

The severity of head injuries can vary greatly. The history of the injury (i.e., details about what it is and how it happened) is crucial for determining appropriate management. With a head injury, the patient may appear normal; may experience dizziness, severe headache, mental confusion, or memory loss; or may even be unconscious. Loss of consciousness may be brief or prolonged; it may appear immediately or may be delayed. The victim may experience vomiting; loss of bladder and bowel control; and bleeding from the nose, mouth, or ears. The pupils of the eyes may be unequal and nonreactive to light.

All head injuries must be considered serious. Notify the provider or contact EMS immediately. If evidence of a neck injury is seen, stabilize the neck and do not attempt to move the victim. Do not administer anything by mouth. Keep the patient warm and quiet. Watch the pupils of the eyes and record any changes. Measure vital signs and record the extent and duration of any unconsciousness. If the patient is at home or is sent home after the provider's assessment, he or she should be watched closely for 24 hours after the injury for any change in mental status.

Foreign Bodies in the Eye

The eye is a delicate organ with a unique structure that demands special handling. This kind of emergency is uncomfortable, and it often is extremely difficult to keep the patient from rubbing the eye. Tell the patient not to touch the eye in any way. The provider may order ophthalmic topical anesthetic drops to relieve pain. The patient should be placed in a darkened room to wait for the provider because **photophobia** is common with eye irritations. If a contusion and swelling are present, cold, wet compresses can help. Ask the patient to close both eyes and cover them with eye pads until the provider arrives. The provider may order an eye irrigation to remove the object. The medical assistant should not attempt to search for or remove an object in the eyes.

Heat and Cold Injuries

Exposure to extremes in temperature can cause minor to severe injuries. Heat injuries occur most often on hot, humid days and result in cramps, heat exhaustion, or heatstroke. Heat-related muscle cramps may be the first sign of *heat exhaustion,* which is a serious heat-related condition. Patients with heat exhaustion appear flushed and report headaches, nausea, vertigo, and weakness. *Heatstroke,* the most dangerous form of heat-related injury, results in a shutdown of body systems. Patients with heatstroke have red, hot, dry skin; altered levels of consciousness; tachycardia; and rapid, shallow breathing. This is a true medical emergency. If heat-related problems are recognized in the early stages and are adequately treated, the patient does not usually develop heatstroke. Management of heat-related conditions includes getting the person out of the heat; loosening clothing or removing perspiration-soaked clothing; and giving the person cool electrolyte drinks if he or she is alert. An effective way to lower the victim's temperature is to apply cool, wet cloths and then fan the moist skin so that heat is released from the body by evaporation.

The two types of cold-related injuries are frostbite and hypothermia. *Frostbite,* which is the actual freezing of tissue, occurs when the skin temperature falls to a range of 14° to 25° F (−10° to −3.9° C). Prolonged exposure of the skin to cold causes damage similar to a burn. The tissue may appear gray or white, may be swollen, and may have clear blisters; in full-thickness frostbite, the skin may show signs of tissue **necrosis**, including blackened areas and severe deformity. The more advanced the frostbite, the more serious the tissue damage and the more likely the body part will be lost. Frozen tissue has no feeling, but as thawing occurs, the patient reports itching, tingling, and burning pain. Mild frostbite can be managed by applying constant warmth to the affected areas; this can be done by immersing the area in warm water (no warmer than 105° F [40.6° C]) or by wrapping it in warm, dry clothing. Friction should never be used because this could increase tissue damage. If blisters have formed or if evidence of full-thickness frostbite is seen, the patient should be transported to the nearest ED.

Hypothermia is a medical emergency that may result in death unless the patient receives immediate assistance. Systemic hypothermia occurs when the core body temperature drops below 95° F (35° C). Signs and symptoms of hypothermia include shivering, numbness, apathy, and loss of consciousness. If hypothermia is suspected, activate EMS and provide care for any life-threatening conditions until help arrives. Remove the victim's wet clothing and wrap the victim in blankets while moving him or her to a warm place. If the victim is alert, give warm liquids and apply heating pads (using a barrier to prevent burns) or chemical hot packs to help slowly raise the core body temperature.

Dehydration

A person dehydrates when more water is excreted than is taken in. Dehydration can be a very serious health emergency, leading to convulsions, coma, and even death. Infants, young children, and older adult patients are at greatest risk of developing serious complications from dehydration. Severe dehydration may be caused by excessive heat loss, vomiting, diarrhea, or lack of fluid intake. Symptoms include vertigo; dark yellow urine or no urine output for 8 to

10 hours; extreme thirst; lethargy or confusion; and abdominal or muscle cramps. If the patient shows any of these symptoms and is unable to retain fluids, schedule an urgent appointment or recommend that the patient be taken to the ED. Replacement of lost fluids is vital, so the patient should be encouraged to drink water, tea, sports drinks, fruit juice, or Pedialyte.

Diabetic Emergencies

Diabetes mellitus is caused by a malfunction in the production of insulin in the pancreas or by an inability of the cells to use insulin. Insulin is required on the cellular level so that glucose can be used for energy. Two different diabetic emergencies can occur, one caused by *hyperglycemia* (high blood glucose levels) and the other by *hypoglycemia* (low blood glucose levels).

Insulin shock is caused by severe hypoglycemia, which results when a patient with diabetes takes too much insulin, does not eat enough food, or exercises an unusual amount. Signs and symptoms, which have a rapid onset, include tachycardia, profuse sweating (diaphoresis), headache, irritability, vertigo, fatigue, hunger, seizures, and coma. It is important to provide glucose immediately, preferably

in the form of glucose tablets, which have a known, concentrated quantity of glucose.

Diabetic coma results from severe hyperglycemia, which develops because the body is not producing enough insulin; the patient eats too much food or is very stressed; or the patient has an infection. The symptoms of impending diabetic coma, which develop more slowly than those of insulin shock, include general malaise, dry mouth, polyuria, **polydipsia**, nausea, vomiting, SOB, and breath with an acetone (or "fruity") smell. If the patient or caregiver calling for an appointment reports these symptoms, notify the provider immediately because the patient typically would be admitted to the hospital.

In an emergency situation, if a patient diagnosed with diabetes mellitus shows signs and symptoms of a diabetic emergency, the patient should be given glucose. If the problem is caused by insulin shock (hypoglycemia), the patient will improve quickly after receiving glucose; if it is caused by diabetic coma (hyperglycemia), a small amount of added glucose will not affect the patient's condition, and he or she must be transported to the hospital regardless (Procedure 22-15).

PROCEDURE 22-15   Perform First Aid Procedures: Care for a Patient With a Diabetic Emergency

Goal: *To provide emergency care for and assessment of a patient with insulin shock or a pending diabetic coma.*

EQUIPMENT and SUPPLIES

- Patient record
- Sphygmomanometer
- Stethoscope
- Watch with second hand
- Disposable gloves
- Glucometer
- Disposable lancet
- Glucose tablets
- Insulin
- Insulin syringe unit
- Alcohol swabs
- Sharps container

PROCEDURAL STEPS

1. Gather equipment and sanitize your hands.
2. Greet and identify the patient and introduce yourself.
   PURPOSE: To relieve patient anxiety and earn patient cooperation.
3. Obtain vital signs.
4. If the patient is known to have diabetes, observe for signs and symptoms that indicate a diabetic emergency.
   - Signs and symptoms of insulin shock or hypoglycemia: Rapid onset of vertigo, fatigue, hunger, tachycardia, profuse sweating, headache, irritability, seizures, and coma.
   - Signs and symptoms of impending diabetic coma or hyperglycemia: Symptoms develop more slowly than those of insulin shock; these include general malaise, dry mouth, polyuria, polydipsia, nausea,

vomiting, shortness of breath (SOB), and breath with an acetone (or "fruity") smell.

5. Immediately report patient's condition to the provider and follow his or her orders.
   PURPOSE: A diabetic emergency can be life-threatening.
6. In an emergency situation, if a patient diagnosed with diabetes mellitus shows signs and symptoms of a diabetic emergency, the patient should be given glucose.
   PURPOSE: If the problem is caused by insulin shock (hypoglycemia), the patient will improve quickly after receiving glucose; if it is caused by diabetic coma (hyperglycemia), a small amount of added glucose will not affect the patient's condition, and he or she must be transported to the hospital regardless.
7. Follow the provider's orders and administer 15 g of carbohydrate immediately, preferably in the form of glucose tablets because they have a known concentrated quantity of glucose. If glucose tablets are not available give the patient $\frac{1}{2}$ cup of fruit juice or 5 or 6 pieces of hard candy.
   PURPOSE: To quickly stabilize the patient's blood glucose level.
8. Check the patient's blood glucose levels with a glucometer and monitor vital signs.
   PURPOSE: To monitor the patient's current blood glucose level and the patient's condition so the provider can determine appropriate treatment.
   - If the blood glucose level is below 80 mg/dL (insulin shock), administer another 15 g of carbohydrate. Wait 15 minutes and check the glucometer reading again. If the level is still low, repeat steps 7 and 8.

PROCEDURE 22-15 —*continued*

- If the patient's blood glucose levels are elevated (diabetic coma) administer insulin as ordered by the provider

  <u>PURPOSE</u>: To lower blood glucose levels to within a normal range.

9. Continue to monitor the patient and follow the provider's orders for continued care.
   - A patient with insulin shock can be stabilized by continued monitoring of the blood glucose level and administration of glucose every 15 minutes until levels reach normal.
   - A patient with pending diabetic coma may need to be transported to the hospital.

10. Dispose of used supplies and gloves in the appropriate biohazard containers (sharps containers for used lancets and injection unit).

11. Sanitize your hands.

12. Document the actions taken and the patient's condition, including vital signs, glucometer readings, administration of glucose and/or insulin, and whether the patient was stabilized and discharged or emergency medical services (EMS) were activated and the patient was transported to the hospital.

CLOSING COMMENTS

Patient Education

Emergencies can occur anywhere. Patients need to learn how to handle emergency situations both by the example of healthcare workers and through instruction. The medical assistant must remain calm, screen the situation, call for help, and be prepared to administer appropriate first aid. Brochures on home safety can be used to help teach patients methods for preventing accidents in the home.

All patients, even children, should understand how to contact EMS. This is especially important for families with members who have chronic diseases that can be life-threatening, such as heart conditions, severe allergic reactions, diabetes, and asthma. Patients should be encouraged to post important numbers next to the telephone; these include emergency numbers (local EMS and poison control center) and the primary care provider's number. Families with young children must childproof their homes, taking special care to keep potentially poisonous substances stored where children cannot get into them. Placing "Mr. Yuk" stickers on containers of poisonous substances can be an excellent educational tool for young children.

Medical assistants must remember to keep their American Red Cross or AHA certifications current, and they should take advantage of community workshops to maintain and extend their skills. Also, a list of community safety workshops should be posted in an area where patients can see it, and they should be encouraged to attend. Your participation in emergency care workshops, in addition to encouraging others to participate, may help to save lives.

Legal and Ethical Issues

The medical assistant works in the healthcare environment as the provider's agent. Although you are responsible for your own actions, the provider is legally responsible for the care you administer to patients while working in the healthcare facility. You are responsible for knowing the limitations placed on medical assistants in your state and for adhering strictly to your employer's emergency care policies and procedures. Medical assistants are not qualified to diagnose a patient's problem, but they are responsible for acting appropriately in a medical emergency.

Most states have enacted Good Samaritan laws to encourage healthcare professionals to provide medical assistance at the scene of an accident without fear of being sued for negligence. These statutes vary greatly, but all have the intent of protecting the caregiver. A provider or other healthcare professional is not legally obligated to provide emergency care at the site of an accident, regardless of the ethical and moral considerations. Legal liability is limited to gross neglect of the victim or willfully causing further injury to the victim. As a caregiver, you are required to act as a reasonable person and cannot be held liable for personal injury resulting from an act of omission. Good Samaritan statutes provide for evaluation of the caregiver's judgment but are in effect only at the site of an emergency, not at your place of employment.

If you have not been trained in CPR, you cannot be expected to perform the procedure at the emergency site. However, in many states, a healthcare provider with CPR training and skills who is present at the scene can be declared negligent if cardiac arrest occurs and he or she does not administer CPR to the victim.

If the victim is conscious or if a member of his or her immediate family is present, obtain verbal consent to perform emergency care. Consent is implied if the patient is unconscious and no family member is present.

Medical assistants also can play a key role in the community response to natural or human-caused disasters. The medical assistant is cross-trained to perform multiple administrative and clinical duties that would prove very useful in an emergency. These include management of medical records, interacting professionally with patients, performing diagnostic tests, performing phlebotomy and administering medications, assisting with procedures, and administering first aid and CPR as needed. Because of their wide range of skills, medical assistants serve as useful volunteers on local emergency response teams. Investigate agencies and organizations that are committed to emergency preparedness in your community and see how a medical assistant could help these organizations if an emergency arises.

Professional Behaviors

In addition to legal responsibilities, you have an ethical responsibility to your patients to provide the highest standard of care. Always act in the best interest of the patient, and never hesitate to ask the provider and/or the office manager for immediate assistance when faced with a medical emergency. Many types of emergencies can be handled in the provider's office. In an emergency situation, decisions that must be made quickly can determine whether the patient lives. A medical assistant must be prepared to act calmly and efficiently in all emergency situations.

Critical thinking is a crucial part of managing medical emergencies. The ability to ask pertinent questions, consider all available information, and distinguish between relevant and irrelevant patient feedback can make the difference in the immediate management of an emergency situation. Both the provider and the patient rely on the professional medical assistant when he or she is managing potentially serious phone calls and/or caring for a patient with a medical emergency in the healthcare setting.

SUMMARY OF SCENARIO

Cheryl has learned through her work with the telephone screening team and involvement with emergencies in the office how important it is to gather complete information about emergency situations and to act calmly and knowledgeably when managing patient problems. She knows she needs to maintain her certification in CPR for the Professional and to continue to participate in workshops on emergency care so she is prepared for the wide variety of patient problems seen in the ambulatory care practice. Working with the screening staff has reinforced the importance of documenting all interactions on the telephone and all information gathered during patient visits.

Cheryl recognizes that medical assistants in the office must follow the facility's policies and procedures manual for handling emergencies. They must plan ahead and complete their designated duties if an emergency occurs; use community emergency services as needed; and keep emergency supplies and equipment well stocked and ready for any possible emergency. She recognizes that understanding first aid practices for common patient emergencies allows her to assist patients by providing instruction on the phone or by performing specific skills when emergencies occur in the facility.

Cheryl has investigated her legal standing as a medical assistant in her home state and recognizes her responsibilities when a patient calls or shows up at the office with a medical emergency. She will continue to refer to the more experienced screening staff members or to Dr. Bendt when she has questions, but she now feels more confident in managing emergency situations at work. She also recognizes her role as part of the healthcare team if an emergency situation arises in her community.

SUMMARY OF LEARNING OBJECTIVES

1. **Define, spell, and pronounce the terms listed in the vocabulary.**
   Spelling and pronouncing medical terms correctly reinforces the medical assistant's credibility. Knowing the definitions of these terms promotes confidence in communication with patients and co-workers.

2. **Describe patient safety factors in the medical office environment.**
   The medical assistant must be constantly on guard to protect patients from possible injury. Methods for achieving this goal include communicating openly about patient safety issues, following standard procedures when delivering patient care, and working as part of a team to ensure patients' safety.

3. **Interpret and comply with safety signs, labels, and symbols and evaluate the work environment to identify safe and unsafe working conditions for the employee.**
   The four major types of signs are danger signs (identify the most severe and immediate hazards); caution signs (possible hazards that require added precautions); safety instruction signs (designed to communicate directions for safety actions); and biologic hazard signs (identify an actual or potential biohazard). OSHA specifies the format of each type of sign, the information that must appear, and where each type of sign must be used (see Figure 22-1 and Procedures 22-1 and 22-2).

4. **Do the following when it comes to environmental safety in the healthcare setting:**
   - Identify environmental safety issues in the healthcare setting
   - Discuss fire safety issues in a healthcare environment
   - Demonstrate the proper use of a fire extinguisher

   Medical assistants must be constantly on the alert for potentially unsafe conditions; must consistently follow the guidelines established by OSHA for infection control; and must follow safety procedures to prevent workplace violence. Combustibles should be stored properly; electrical equipment must be monitored for safety; smoke detectors and fire extinguishers should be checked routinely; and the facility should be evacuated if a fire breaks out. Procedure 22-3 details the proper use of a fire extinguisher.

5. **Describe the fundamental principles for evacuation of a healthcare facility and role-play a mock environmental exposure event and evacuation of a provider's office.**
   An emergency action coordinator should be designated. This person is in charge of delegating duties to staff members. Exit maps should be posted in multiple areas around the facility. Patients and staff members should be evacuated safely and should meet in a designated

SUMMARY OF LEARNING OBJECTIVES—*continued*

spot to make sure all staff members and patients have escaped (see Procedure 22-4).

6. **Discuss the requirements for proper disposal of hazardous materials.**

OSHA has established specific rules about biohazard waste disposal, including the use of sharps containers and red bag collection systems, which must be used properly to avoid disease transmission.

7. **Identify critical elements of an emergency plan for response to a natural disaster or other emergency.**

Ambulatory care centers may be the first to recognize and initiate a response to a community emergency. Standard Precautions should be implemented immediately to control the spread of an infection. A communication network should be established to notify local and state health departments and perhaps federal officials. Every healthcare facility should have a standard policy with specific procedures for the management of emergencies on site. The CDC recommends that a facility's safety plan include multiple steps to minimize the negative psychological effects of an emergency situation.

8. **Maintain an up-to-date list of community resources for emergency preparedness.**

See Procedure 22-5.

9. **Describe the medical assistant's role in emergency response.**

Medical assistants can provide considerable help in a community emergency. They can use therapeutic communication to gather patient data; monitor injured victims; perform first aid and monitor vital signs; and help with any medically related service.

10. **Summarize typical emergency supplies and equipment.**

A provider's office must have a centrally located crash cart or emergency bag stocked with all emergency supplies, equipment, and medication. This material must be inventoried consistently and maintained. This chapter provides a detailed list of materials that should be readily available for an on-site emergency, including a defibrillator if indicated by the provider's practice.

11. **Demonstrate the use of an automated external defibrillator.**

See Procedure 22-6.

12. **Summarize the general rules for managing emergencies.**

Management of emergencies requires a calm, efficient approach. The medical assistant should assess the nature of the emergency and determine whether EMS should be activated, or whether the patient requires an immediate or urgent appointment. As many details about the situation as possible should be gathered, and the provider should be consulted when the medical assistant is in doubt.

13. **Demonstrate telephone screening techniques and documentation guidelines for ambulatory care emergencies.**

Telephone screening is one of the medical assistant's most important tasks. Emergency action principles should be used to determine the level of a patient's emergency. These include determining whether the situation is life-threatening and obtaining the patient's contact information, in addition to all pertinent information about the injury and the patient's signs and symptoms. This information must be shared with the

provider, and all details must be documented in the patient's record (see Procedure 22-7).

14. **Recognize and respond to life-threatening emergencies in the ambulatory care practice.**

Life-threatening emergencies require immediate assessment, referral to the provider or, if the provider is not present, activation of EMS. While waiting for assistance, the medical assistant should check for breathing and circulation. Rescue breaths or CPR is administered if indicated. Depending on the patient's signs and symptoms, the person should be monitored for signs of a heart attack; the Heimlich maneuver is performed for an airway obstruction; the patient is evaluated for signs of a CVA and is assessed for shock. The medical assistant should ask for help when indicated and should perform appropriate procedures based on the patient's presenting condition.

15. **Describe how to handle an unresponsive patient and perform provider/professional-level CPR.**

See Procedure 22-8 for instructions on performing adult, pediatric, and infant rescue breathing and CPR.

16. **Discuss cardiac emergencies and administer oxygen through a nasal cannula to a patient in respiratory distress.**

See Procedure 22-9.

17. **Identify and assist a patient with an obstructed airway.**

Procedure 22-10 presents instructions for assisting an adult with an obstructed airway. Infants with an obstructed airway should receive alternating back blows and chest thrusts with attempted rescue breaths until the item is dislodged or help arrives.

18. **Discuss cerebrovascular accidents and assist a patient who is in shock.**

A stroke is a disorder of the cerebral blood vessels that results in impairment of the blood supply to part of the brain. Symptoms of a major stroke include paralysis on one side of the body, difficulty swallowing, loss of bladder and bowel control, and slurring of speech. Procedure 22-11 explains how to assist a patient in shock.

19. **Determine the appropriate action and documentation procedures for common office emergencies, such as fainting, poisoning, animal bites, insect bites and stings, and asthma attacks.**

The medical assistant should always follow Standard Precautions when caring for a patient with a medical emergency. Documentation of emergency treatment should include information about the patient; vital signs; allergies, current medications, and pertinent health history; the patient's chief complaint; the sequence of events, including any changes in the patient's condition since the incident; and any provider's orders and procedures performed (see Table 22-1).

20. **Discuss seizures and perform first aid procedures for a patient having a seizure.**

See Procedure 22-12.

21. **Discuss abdominal pain, sprains and strains, and fractures, and perform first aid procedures for a patient with a fracture of the wrist.**

See Procedure 22-13.

Continued

SUMMARY OF LEARNING OBJECTIVES—*continued*

22. Discuss burns and tissue injuries, and control of a hemorrhagic wound.
    See Procedure 22-14.

23. Discuss nosebleeds, head injuries, foreign bodies in the eye, heat and cold injuries, dehydration, and diabetic emergencies; also, perform first aid procedures for a patient with a diabetic emergency.
    See Procedure 22-15.

24. Apply patient education concepts to medical emergencies.
    Patients should know how to contact emergency personnel, and families with young children should have telephone numbers for poison control posted. Educating patients in how to care for minor emergencies at home is an important part of telephone triage in the ambulatory care practice. Encouraging patients to participate in community safety workshops and to become certified in CPR may help prevent emergencies and save lives.

25. Discuss the legal and ethical concerns arising from medical emergencies.
    Good Samaritan laws, which vary from state to state, are designed to protect any individual from liability, whether a healthcare professional or a layperson, if he or she provides assistance at the site of an emergency. The law does not require a medically trained person to act, but if emergency care is given in a reasonable and responsible manner, the healthcare worker is protected from being sued for negligence. This protection, however, does not extend to the workplace.

CONNECTIONS

Study Guide Connection: Go to the Chapter 22 Study Guide. Read and complete the activities.

evolve Evolve Connection: Go to the Chapter 22 link at *evolve.elsevier.com/ kinn* to complete the Chapter Review Quiz. Check out the other resources listed for this chapter to make the most of what you have learned from Safety and Emergency Practices.

CAREER DEVELOPMENT AND LIFE SKILLS

23

SCENARIO

Michelle, Krysia, and Zacarias (or Zac to his friends) met during their first semester of college and have developed a great friendship over the last few months. They will be graduating from the medical assistant program in less than 6 weeks. Michelle just graduated from high school a year ago. Krysia entered the military just after her high school graduation and spent 10 years in the Marines. Zac has been out of high school for several years and worked in a factory. He started as a line worker and gradually advanced to supervisory positions, but because of downsizing, his position was eliminated and he went back to school. These friends are looking forward to graduation and getting jobs as medical assistants.

As these three friends discuss finding a job, Michelle is hesitant about the job search experience. Her only work experience is 2 years as a waitress at a local restaurant. She has never created a résumé or a cover letter. She only had a very informal interview with the restaurant owner before she was given the job. Krysia is concerned about her military career. The positions she held were not related to healthcare. She managed inventory, supervised others, and was also deployed to many hot spots around the world. Zac has a lot of experience in the factory setting, but he feels that world is so different from healthcare. As they talk with each other, it is clear that each person has a unique situation and they all must take a closer look at their past experiences as they prepare for their job search adventure.

While studying this chapter, think about the following questions:

- What experience from a medical assistant's background can be utilized in a healthcare position?
- How can a résumé market a medical assistant's characteristics and experiences to potential employers?

- How can the medical assistant organize the job search experience?
- What is considered professional dress for an interview?
- How should a medical assistant prepare for an interview?
- What are appropriate follow-up activities after the interview?

LEARNING OBJECTIVES

1. Define, spell, and pronounce the terms listed in the vocabulary.
2. Describe the four personality traits that are most important to employers.
3. Explain the three areas that need to be examined to determine one's strengths and skills.
4. Discuss career objectives and describe how personal needs affect the job search.
5. Do the following related to finding a job:
   - Explain the two best job search methods.
   - Discuss traditional job search methods.
   - Describe various ways to improve your opportunities.
   - Discuss the importance of being organized in your job search.
6. Discuss the three types of résumé formats, describe how to prepare a chronologic résumé and cover letter, and discuss the importance and format of both the résumé and cover letter.
7. Discuss how to complete an online portfolio and job application.

8. Describe how to create a career portfolio.
9. Do the following related to the job interview:
   - List and describe the four phases of the interview process.
   - List and discuss legal and illegal interview questions.
   - Practice interview skills for a mock interview.
   - Create a thank-you note for an interview.
10. Do the following related to getting a job:
    - Discuss the importance of the probationary period for a new employee.
    - List some common early mistakes of which a new employee should be aware.
    - Discuss how to be a good employee and how to deal with supervisors.
    - Explain why a performance appraisal rating is usually not perfect.
    - Discuss how to pursue a raise and how to leave a job.
11. Discuss various life skills needed in the workplace.

counteroffer Return offer made by one who has rejected an offer or a job.

dignity Being worthy of honor and respect from others.

interpersonal skills Ability to communicate and interact with others; sometimes referred to as "soft skills."

job boards Web site that posts jobs submitted by employers and can be used by job seekers to identify open positions.

mock Simulated; intended for imitation or practice.

networking Exchange of information or services among individuals, groups, or institutions; also, meeting and getting to know individuals in the same or similar career fields and sharing information about available opportunities.

proofread To read and mark corrections.

rectify (rek'-tih-fi) To correct by removing errors.

skill set A person's abilities or skills.

vocation The work in which a person is regularly employed.

Each day a person exists is a small portion of a whole—a part of a person's entire lifetime. The events that happen during a day, no matter how small, shape the future. In the same way, the events that happen in the life of a medical assistant play a role in shaping his or her career. Every day, the medical assistant "writes a résumé"—through actions that reveal strengths, highlight skills, and summarize accomplishments—that builds on his or her **vocation**. Each duty performed becomes a part of the medical assistant's sum of experience and is important in the overall growth of the individual. Each action taken can have an effect on the future for the medical assistant. If the actions are professional, accurate, and performed to the individual's utmost ability, the résumé the medical assistant is writing will be one that leads to greater opportunities. If the medical assistant performs poorly, the résumé will be one that does not reflect trustworthiness and dependability. The small decisions made each day greatly affect the overall impression the medical assistant makes in the workplace.

Most people seeking employment have never had any type of formal training in the job search process. A graduating medical assistant student should take advantage of job search training for three reasons:

- It will reduce the amount of time spent searching for a job.
- It will increase the chances of receiving better wages through negotiation.
- It will help reduce the fears of looking for work and interviewing.

MOVING ON TO THE NEXT PHASE OF LIFE

As you move toward graduation, you may be experiencing many emotions. You might be excited about finishing your medical assistant program. You might be scared of the changes that will be occurring over the next months. The thought of finding a job might be overwhelming. These are common feelings of graduates regardless of the career path they have chosen. The important step before graduation is to prepare for the next phase: getting a job.

Preparing for the job-seeking phase is very important. By understanding the characteristics that employers want; identifying your strengths, experiences, and skills; and developing your career objectives, you are ready to market yourself to potential employers through your résumé and interview experiences. Early preparation and marketing yourself to employers, even before graduation, can be the key to landing a job soon after graduation.

UNDERSTANDING PERSONALITY TRAITS IMPORTANT TO EMPLOYERS

As you start with your job search, it is important to understand what employers are looking for in an employee. With the cost and time invested in training new employees, it is crucial employers find the right new employee. Many employers will agree that they can help refine employees' technical skill proficiencies, but it is more difficult to help evolve or change personality traits. The four personality traits that are most important to employers are: collaboration and **interpersonal skills**, professionalism, compassion, and sincere interest in the job.

Collaboration and interpersonal skills are crucial to productivity in today's fast-paced, ever-changing healthcare environment. Employers look for people who can blend well with the current staff. It is important that the new employee is flexible, dependable, supportive of peers, and remains calm under pressure. Employers also look for people who will provide excellent customer service by having outstanding interpersonal skills, which include communication skills and good manners (Figure 23-1). Effective verbal communication involves clear, thoughtful communication. Being focused, calm, polite, and interested in the other person are traits of effective verbal communication. In addition, appropriate nonverbal communication is crucial in the healthcare setting. Your body language relays more to your patients and peers than any words you could use. Eye contact, posture, voice, and gestures provide insights into a person's attitude (Figure 23-2). Listening is also critical when working with peers and patients. For effective communication to occur, listening must occur. Appropriate questions can draw others into the conversation and show others you are listening and care. Using communication techniques such as rephrasing, reflecting, paraphrasing, and asking for clarification are also excellent ways of demonstrating active listening skills. Good manners and a basic understanding of the diversity of other cultures also help facilitate communication.

Professionalism is a trait that employers evaluate from their first contact with interested potential employees. From the application and résumé to the interview, employers are building their perceptions of the candidates' professionalism. Being professional not only encompasses your dress and grooming habits but also your flexibility, punctuality, honesty, attention to detail, and abilities to follow directions, prioritize, and manage time. Employers are looking for loyal employees who provide a professional image

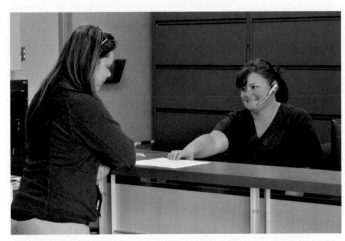

FIGURE 23-1 Having good communication skills and good manners are necessary to provide excellent customer service.

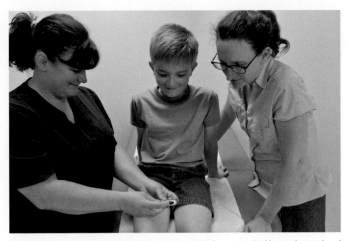

FIGURE 23-3 Enjoyment of the job is paramount. Medical assistants should enjoy their work and give compassionate, friendly care to all patients.

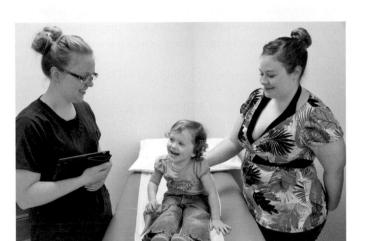

FIGURE 23-2 It is important that medical assistants working in a family practice or pediatric setting have a positive attitude and enjoy working with children.

CRITICAL THINKING APPLICATION   **23-1**

Think of the three friends. Michelle just graduated from high school and has 2 years of waitressing experience. Krysia has ten years in the military, where she managed inventory, supervised others, and was deployed to many hot spots around the world. Zac has been working in a factory, advancing to supervisory positions. Now think about the personality traits that employers want. What personality traits might each friend possess? Explain your answer.

- Create your own list of the personality traits that employers want and you possess.

to patients, families, and other customers of the healthcare organization.

Having compassion and providing **dignity** and respect to others is the third trait that is important to employers. Many people go into healthcare to help others, but lack the compassion and respect that is needed when caring for others. Not only do healthcare employees provide technical skills during patient care, they also need to help support and maintain the dignity of the patient. Compassion and respect help healthcare employees connect to patients and their families. Acts of kindness and thoughtfulness that alleviate stress are welcomed by patients.

The last personality trait that employers are looking for is genuine interest in the job. This trait can be seen during the interview when the candidate asks thoughtful questions regarding the position and the agency. Genuine interest in the job extends beyond the hiring phase into the day-to-day operations. Being interested in one's job and looking for ways to improve procedures and provide better patient care are important behaviors to demonstrate to the employer. This genuine interest is reflected in your attitude and performance in the workplace (Figure 23-3). It helps ease your transition into a new job and promotes your success.

Assessing Your Strengths and Skills

As you prepare to market yourself to potential employers, you need to examine your strengths and skills in three different areas. You need to identify the personality traits, technical skills, and transferable job skills that you possess.

As you contemplate the personality traits that employers want, try to honestly identify which of those skills and strengths you have. Many people will tell potential employers what they think the employer wants to hear. They claim to be a "team player," "communicate well," be "dependable," and so on, but employers need more. Words in your résumé or cover letter or voicing these statements in the interview is not enough to convince the potential employer that you truly have those characteristics. Early on in the preparation phase, make a list of the qualities that you believe you possess. Then for each characteristic, provide one or two pieces of "evidence" to support your claims. Your "evidence" may be a past job review or practicum evaluation where the author indicates your strengths and characteristics. These are excellent documents to include in your portfolio, which will be discussed later in the chapter. Using stories of situations where you portrayed those characteristics is another way to illustrate you have the qualities, and you can share these during the interview if pertinent to the questions asked.

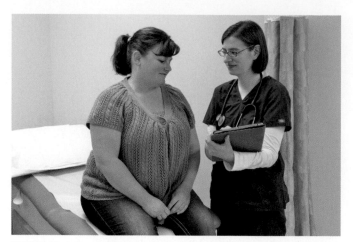

FIGURE 23-4 The potential employer needs to know about the technical skills you have practiced in the classroom and practicum setting.

Employers also need to know about your technical skills. Technical skills for medical assistants can be skills related to clinical procedures, such as phlebotomy, injections, electrocardiograms (ECGs), and obtaining vital signs (Figure 23-4). Technical skills can also be related to administrative procedures and may include software proficiency, keyboard speed, reception duties, and coding procedures. You may be able to provide supporting documentation of your technical skills through the use of practicum skill checklists or through a portfolio. Technical skills might also include skills that you obtained outside of the medical assistant program but still relate to your chosen career. For instance, you worked as a phlebotomist at a local hospital. Many of the technical skills you perform as a phlebotomist may relate to a clinic position.

The last area that needs to be examined during the preparation phase of job seeking is your transferable job skills. These are skills that a person develops in one job or experience that can be transferred to another job. Potential transferable skills include: customer service, compassion and empathy, strong communication and listening, computer skills, teamwork, time management and prioritizing, creativity, leadership, organization, problem solving, and grace under pressure. Many of these skills may sound familiar; they also are characteristics employers are looking for and were discussed in an earlier section.

Identifying transferable job skills can be difficult for many people. Job descriptions for past experiences can be very useful, but many times these are not available. To start, make a list of your past jobs, military experience, and volunteer opportunities. Then ask yourself which of the potential transferable skills you developed and used during that experience. For instance, you have waited on customers in a restaurant. Most wait staff need strong communication and listening skills. Prioritizing and customer service skills are also required. If you worked in a factory setting, communications skills, teamwork, and problem solving might be traits you developed. If you had military experience, strong communication skills, grace under pressure, and prioritizing might be just a few of the skills you developed during your time serving the country. This list of transferable job skills will be utilized as you create your résumé and prepare for your interview.

CRITICAL THINKING APPLICATION   **23-2**
What might be some transferable skills that the three friends, Michelle, Krysia, and Zac, possess? Explain your answer.
- Using the list you have already started, add on the personality traits, technical skills, and transferable job skills that you possess. Also, indicate why you believe you have these skills (e.g., which job or experience helped you develop the skill).

DEVELOPING CAREER OBJECTIVES

Each medical assistant has a reason for entering the healthcare field. This basic desire should influence decisions concerning his or her career choices. Because medical assisting is such a versatile profession, a medical assistant has numerous options after graduation.

Medical assistant students should take some time to think about what they want from their careers. While attending school and subsequently completing the practicum, ideas may surface about the area of healthcare or a specific agency in which the medical assistant most wants to work.

When developing career objectives, the medical assistant should start by asking several questions:
- What areas and skills did I enjoy in practicum?
- Where do I want to be in 5 years?
- Where do I want to be in 10 years?
- What additional skills do I need to get where I want to go?

Write down the questions and answers and go into specific detail. Set realistic goals and develop a plan as to how and when they will be reached. Remember career objectives are reached over time. It is important to know where you want to be, so you can start down the right path to reach your goals. Keep your list of goals available and visible so you can revisit them frequently.

CRITICAL THINKING APPLICATION   **23-3**
For the following four questions, write down your answers and explain them. These answers will help you as you start the job search process.
- What areas and skills did I enjoy in practicum?
- Where do I want to be in 5 years?
- Where do I want to be in 10 years?
- What additional skills do I need to get where I want to go?

KNOWING PERSONAL NEEDS

After evaluating your skills and strengths and developing your career objectives, you need to evaluate your needs. Potential jobs for medical assistants can include different wages, benefits, hours, and locations. Most people have a salary minimum and specific benefits they require to meet their needs and living expenses. Some people have specific hours that work better for them. People with children may need a job that allows them to be home with their children after school. For medical assistants who do not drive or have a reliable mode of transportation, the location of a job will be important to consider. Evaluating your personal needs will help you find a job that matches your requirements.

FINDING A JOB

Many people have misconceptions about the job market that exists today. Fortunately, the medical field is not an industry that sees high levels of unemployment. Usually healthcare employment remains high even in a poor economy. However, graduation from a medical assisting program does not guarantee that the student will obtain employment. Completion of the program gives the medical assistant the job skills needed to work, but a good attitude and positive outlook are essential for success in the job search. In addition, the medical assistant should always be open to new and better opportunities.

Some job seekers assume that potential employers will not interact with students until they graduate and passed a credential examination (i.e., Certified Medical Assistant [CMA] through the American Association of Medical Assistants [AAMA], Registered Medical Assistant [RMA] through the American Medical Technologists [AMT]). However, prospecting before graduation is a smart idea. Some employers do not require credential examinations and others may hire a medical assistant with an understanding that within a period of time the employee needs to obtain the credential. Many employers are interested in hiring new graduates. They consider new graduates "teachable," meaning they can train and "mold" them into the employee they require. Employers recognize that new graduates have more current knowledge and skills in certain healthcare areas including coding and electronic health records (EHRs).

Two Best Job Search Methods

Although there are many ways to find employment, two methods have proved to be the best and most effective: networking and checking job boards.

Networking is the exchange of information or services among individuals, groups, or institutions. When related to a job search, networking involves meeting and getting to know individuals in the same or similar career fields and sharing information about available opportunities. A medical assistant should begin to form a network of friends, business associates, co-workers, and acquaintances early in training, and he or she should stay in contact with these people throughout the job search and beyond (Figure 23-5). E-mail, LinkedIn, Facebook, Twitter, and other electronic advances make staying in touch with former classmates and instructors very easy.

A medical assistant can network through family, friends, and other healthcare professionals. The practicum is the best networking experience. During a practicum, the student meets and works alongside many healthcare professionals. These professionals continually evaluate the student's performance. It is not uncommon that when healthcare professionals find a student who portrays the qualities of a professional medical assistant, they want to assist that student in finding a job. They may offer to provide a future job reference. They may provide the student with insight on potential openings. It is crucial that the medical assistant student looks at the practicum as a constant job interview and strives to do his or her best. As the

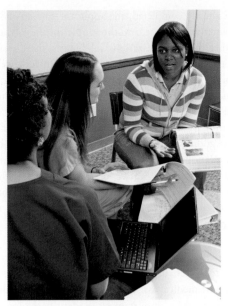

FIGURE 23-5 Stay in touch with classmates. They are excellent networking contacts and may be able to provide job leads.

practicum progresses, students can inquire about potential job openings, either through their mentor, supervisor, or the agency's human resource department. Toward the end of the practicum, the student may want to ask the mentor if he or she would be willing to provide a reference or a letter of recommendation. When the practicum experience concludes, the medical assistant student should formally thank the supervisor, the mentor, and the department with a note and also provide the supervisor with a résumé and cover letter.

Another way to network with professional medical assistants is to join a medical assistant organization. The members who attend regular meetings often know about job leads in the area. Friends and family members can be on the lookout for potential opportunities and may help by asking their friends and personal physicians/providers if they are aware of positions that will open for applications soon.

Checking **job boards** is the other most common method of identifying job opportunities. Large healthcare organizations usually have their own Web sites and many include an employment or career section that lists available jobs. Some of these larger organizations allow job seekers to register, complete an online application, and upload a résumé and cover letter. These sites will then generate e-mails to job seekers when jobs are posted. By having the online application already completed, the applicant can upload a customized cover letter and résumé, and thus apply for the job very quickly.

Besides healthcare organizations' job boards, there are local, state, and national job boards. Local job boards may include websites from your school or your community's media (i.e., newspaper, television, radio) agencies. Smaller healthcare organizations tend to advertise using these boards because the cost is less than national sites and they are aiming for a local audience. The Department of Workforce in each state addresses unemployment and provides a job board for job seekers. National job boards, like Monster and Indeed, provide job seekers the ability to search for openings across the country. Medical assistant jobs available in the federal government can be found at www.usajobs.gov. National organizations, like the American Association of Medical Assistants (AAMA) or their local chapters, also post jobs.

When looking for a medical assistant position, it is important for job seekers to search beyond "medical assistant" jobs. Many job boards will post medical assistant types of positions under different job titles. It may take a bit of research to identify the local titles used for medical assistants in different regions or with specific employers. A good search method to utilize if unsure of the job title is to look in the allied health positions and review the educational requirements for different positions. Some agencies will use terms such as "technicians" or "coordinator" for medical assistant jobs. Make a list of job titles related to medical assisting and search by those as you identify potential openings.

CRITICAL THINKING APPLICATION   **23-6**

Michelle, Krysia, and Zac make a list of possible job boards to review frequently for medical assistant postings. They know that sometimes the postings are only available for a short time, so they develop a schedule to review the sites.

- Make a list of five job boards you would like to check for potential jobs.
- What might be other titles that are used for medical assistants in your area?

Traditional Job Search Methods

With the changes in technology, the methods used to find open positions have changed. Networking and checking job boards, as stated in the prior section, are the most effective methods of finding job openings. Mass mailing of résumés to healthcare employers and cold calling to identify opened positions are no longer effective methods. Other methods that remain effective include using the school's placement office resources, newspaper ads (online and print), and employment agencies.

School Career Placement Offices

Students usually have lifetime access to their school placement offices. Take advantage of the opportunities offered, which may include résumé building, job search classes, and interviewing assistance. The school has a vested interest in helping you find employment and the placement office should be the first resource for the student's job search.

Newspaper Ads

Typically, smaller healthcare practices utilize newspaper ads to find potential employees. The ads are run for a set period of time and usually it results in a huge number of applicants for the employer. Many newspaper companies post their ads online, allowing job seekers to look for opened positions.

Applicants need their letter and résumé to stand out from the crowd; people get very creative in how they make this occur. The creative method must stay within the directions given in the ad. For instance, if an employer wants a handwritten cover letter to be included, the applicant needs to follow those directions or the employer may disregard the materials figuring the applicant "can't follow directions." Many employers will provide a mailing address and state no calls or visits will be allowed. If you drop off your materials at the healthcare agency, they may also disregard your documents because the directions were not followed.

Employment Agencies

Employment agencies usually charge a fee for their services. Even when the employer pays the fee, the medical assistant may be offered a lower wage to compensate for the fee. These agencies can be useful, however, especially in salary negotiations. The agency knows the salary range the employer is willing to pay. This means that medical assistants can command a salary within that range and are not short-changed by asking for a salary that is much lower than the employer is willing to pay.

Improving Your Opportunities

Some students and graduates struggle to find jobs. They may not find postings or they may not have success after applying for jobs. This can be stressful, but it is important not to give up.

For those not having success finding job opportunities, it is important to reevaluate your search methods and ask yourself the following questions:

- Am I looking for a very selective opportunity? For instance, are you looking for a dermatology medical assistant position in a specific facility? Those positions may be very limited. Try to broaden your search to other possible opportunities.
- Am I just looking for the correct job title? Remember employers may use a wide range of titles for a medical assistant.
- Am I looking at all agencies that potentially could hire a person with my skill sets? Depending on your area, medical assistants can be in many agencies besides a medical clinic, including a nursing home, hospital, school, or assisted living facility.
- Can I increase the geographical search area for employment opportunities? Can I relocate to an area with greater employment opportunities?

Those finding and applying for job opportunities, yet not having success obtaining a position, may also have to reevaluate their techniques. The lack of success may be related to the content and presentation of the cover letter and résumé or interviewing skills. One of the first places to start is to meet with the school career placement officer. Many times they will review your letter and résumé and provide you with improvement tips. Cover letters and résumés with misspellings and grammar errors may be discarded by employers and are simple items to fix. Sometimes reformatting or revising content is another way to improve one's résumé and cover letter. Having another party review your documents is highly recommended.

Many employers are also checking out social media sites, such as Facebook. Graduates struggling to find positions may want to review their pictures and postings on social media sites. Depending on the site, tightening up security settings and deleting questionable pictures may be helpful. Refraining from inappropriate postings, tweets, and responses may also be useful when looking for employment.

If you are getting interviews, but no job offers, it may be how you dress, your behavior, or how you answer questions during the interview. Again, the school's career placement office may have interview assistance and **mock** interviews that can help you refine your interview skills and behavior.

If you have heard or feel that your résumé lacks skills needed for specific positions you want to obtain, you may want to increase your **skill set**. This can occur through education and experience. Some people increase their job history and skill sets by obtaining temporary employment through temp agencies. Temporary jobs can provide experience and also help you refine your skills. The other way to increase your skill sets through experience is volunteering at a healthcare agency. Depending on the volunteer position, it may help increase your skill sets and also provide you with potential job leads. Volunteer activities should be added to the résumé, because these valuable experiences often can be used in a healthcare setting. It does not matter that the position was not a paid job; experience counts, whether paid or not.

CRITICAL THINKING APPLICATION   **23-7**

Michelle, Krysia, and Zac work together to keep an eye on local newspapers for ads that mention a need for medical assistants.

- What current ads in your local papers are interesting and would prompt sending a résumé?
- What factors might the medical assistant consider in choosing ads to which he or she will respond?
- How can the medical assistant determine which are good potential employers?

Being Organized in Your Job Search

As you identify job openings and submit your résumé and cover letter, it is important that you keep organized. Creating résumés and cover letters will be discussed later in the chapter, but it is important for you to customize both documents for each and every job opening. Keeping organized records is critical.

As you create your word processing documents, keep the documents in an organized system on your computer. For instance, if you are sending out materials for five different postings, keep the customized letter and résumé for each posting in a separate folder on your computer and title it with the name of the organization and the position. If you get notified of an interview for one of the five postings, then you have a record of the materials you sent that agency and you can make a copy of them for your interview.

It is also recommended to make a spreadsheet, word processing document, or handwritten log that indicates the postings you have applied for. The following information will help you remember and stay organized:

- Agency's name
- Position title and job number if available
- Date cover letter and résumé was sent to the agency
- Follow-up information (e.g., status of your application)

As you get notified about the interview, add in the interview information (e.g., date, time, location, interview team members) to your log.

One of the most important things to remember with job searching is that it takes time, stamina, and persistence to find a job. Do not expect to get a job with the first résumé and cover letter you send or with the first interview you have. By keeping good records, you will not apply for the same job twice or overlook job opportunities because you thought you applied for them already.

DEVELOPING A RÉSUMÉ

The purpose of a résumé is to get an employer so interested in you that he or she calls you for an interview. A résumé summarizes an applicant's qualifications, education, and experience. Medical assistants must determine what to include in the résumé, remembering that they are "marketing" themselves to an employer (Procedure 23-1). The résumé should be developed before the cover letter is written or job application is completed so that strengths can be identified and highlighted on all job search documents.

PROCEDURE 23-1 | Prepare a Chronologic Résumé

Goal: To write an effective résumé for use as a tool in obtaining employment.

EQUIPMENT and SUPPLIES

- Computer with word processing software and a printer
- Current job posting
- Résumé paper
- Paper and pen

PROCEDURAL STEPS

1. Apply critical thinking skills as you create a list of the personality traits (wanted by employers), technical skills, and transfer job skills that you possess. Also write down your career goal(s).
   PURPOSE: To determine the strongest aspects of your abilities so that they can be highlighted on the résumé.

2. Using the current job posting, identify the required and recommended qualifications and credentials needed for the position.
   PURPOSE: Identifying what the employer requires and would like will help you tailor your résumé to address these qualifications and credentials.

3. Using the computer with word processing software, create a professional-looking header in the document's header. Include your name, address, telephone number(s), and e-mail address. Select an appropriate font style for your name and a smaller font size for your contact information.
   PURPOSE: To make sure potential employers have a means of contacting you. Using a font style that is bold and a larger size for your name will help your name stand out. Make sure to have your contact information in a smaller nonbold style so it will not detract from your name.

4. In the body of the document, create a section header for "Objective" and type a concise sentence stating your employment objective or goals. These goals should relate to the position being advertised.
   PURPOSE: To give the prospective employer an idea of what you are looking for in a medical assisting position.

5. Create a section header for "Education." For the learning institution(s) you attended, list the school's name, city and state, degree obtained or coursework successfully completed, and the year. Include any additional educational information, like grade point average (GPA), awards, and practicum information.

6. Create a section header for "Work Experience." Provide details about your work experience, including the agency's name, city and state, title of your position, start and end date (month and year), and job duties. The job duties must start with an active verb using the appropriate tense (e.g., a past job would have past tense verbs and a current job would include present tense verbs).
   NOTE: Typically online profiles and applications gather information about past salaries, reasons for leaving, and supervisors' names and contact information. They will also ask for salary expectations for the new position. This information should not be included on the résumé.

PURPOSE: The potential employer will need to know your employment history and all the details.

7. Create a section header for "Special Skills" and list your special language skills, computer proficiencies, and other unique skills you possess that relate to the position.

8. Create a section header for "Certifications and Credentials" and list the active credentials and certifications you have. Include the title of the certification, awarding agency, and the expiration date.
   NOTE: You may want to consider adding in the date you are taking a credential examination. Employers like to know the status of your credential examination.
   PURPOSE: Employers need to know if you have your medical assistant credential (CMA or RMA) and if you have an active cardiopulmonary resuscitation (CPR) and/or first aid card.

9. All information on the résumé needs to appear in reverse chronologic order (i.e., newest information is on top).

10. The résumé needs to look professional and interesting. Utilize font styles (e.g., bold, underline, italic) to highlight important words and phrases. Use professional-looking bullets to list out job duties and other information. Utilize the key words from the posting throughout the résumé.
    PURPOSE: The more professional and interesting a résumé appears, the better chance that it will be reviewed by the potential employer.

11. Proofread the résumé. Correct any spelling, grammar, punctuation, or sentence structure errors you find. If time allows, have another person review the résumé and use the feedback to revise your résumé.
    PURPOSE: Résumés submitted with errors often are discarded without consideration.

12. Print the résumé on résumé paper and proofread one final time. Any errors should be corrected and the document should be reprinted or e-mailed to the instructor.

Résumé Formats

There are three commonly used résumé formats, which include chronologic, combination, and targeted résumés. The résumé format used will depend on the medical assistant's situation.

A chronologic résumé is the most popular format used. It is useful when a person is seeking employment in the same field as his or her education or prior experience. The chronologic résumé focuses on the person's employment history, bulleting out the job duties for each position (Figure 23-6). See Procedure 23-1 for the steps in creating a chronologic résumé.

The combination résumé has been incorrectly described by many as a functional résumé. A true functional résumé showcases a person's skill sets and does not include a work history. Because employers want to see the person's work history, a combination résumé is preferred over a pure functional résumé. A combination résumé lists a person's abilities and skill sets like the functional résumé does, but includes the person's employment history like the chronologic résumé (Figure 23-7). A combination résumé may be used if a person is switching careers and has transferable skills that relate to the new position. It can also be used by applicants that have a gap in their work history to put the focus on the person's skills and ability, rather than the employment history.

The third type of résumé is the targeted résumé, which is customized to a unique job posting (Figure 23-8). Key skills required for the new position are detailed in the résumé, indicating how the applicant has demonstrated those skills and is the best person for the position. This résumé takes longer to create, but can be the most effective format.

Michelle Marison

1234 Cedar Way, Mytown, OH 45458
Home phone: 715.555.1899
Cell phone: 715.555.1355
mmarison@elsevier.net

Objective

To find a full-time medical assistant position in a family practice setting, which will utilize my technical and interpersonal skills.

Education

Community College, Mytown, OH
Medical Assistant Diploma, 20XX
- GPA 3.6

Health Care Experience

Family Practice Associates, Mytown, OH
Medical Assistant Practicum, April to May 20XX (220 hours)
- Performed injections, electrocardiograms, wound care, phlebotomy, throat swabs, and waived tests.
- Obtained vital signs and measurements on children and adults.
- Utilized an electronic health record to document patients' histories, test results, and treatments.
- Answered calls, checked in patients, and updated patients' demographic and insurance information.

Mytown Hospital, Mytown, OH
Volunteer, January to May 20XX
- Provided hospital information to visitors.
- Maintained confidentiality of patients.
- Assisted with deliveries of mail and flowers to patients.
- Assisted nursing staff as needed.

Work Experience

Mytown Family Diner, Mytown, OH
Waitress, June 20XX to present
- Provide efficient, accurate, and timely service to customers.
- Prioritize duties to meet customer needs.
- Provide exceptional customer service.

Special Skills

Fluent in Spanish.
Keyboarding speed: 73 wpm.
Proficient in word processing and spreadsheet software.

Credentials

Certified Medical Assistant, American Association of Medical Assistants (expires May 20XX)
BLS for Healthcare Providers, American Heart Association (expires March 20XX)

FIGURE 23-6 Chronologic résumé.

CRITICAL THINKING APPLICATION   **23-8**

The three friends have very different backgrounds. Michelle has the waitressing experience, Krysia was in the military, and Zac worked in a factory. What type of résumé might each use? Explain your answers.
- What type of résumé would work best for you with your experience and background?

Résumé Content

Between the résumé formats there are similarities and differences in the information presented. The subsequent discussion will describe the content found in the different sections of a résumé. See Procedure 23-1 for the steps in creating a chronologic résumé.

Header

The person's contact information is found in the header of the document. This information or a variation of the information should appear on each sheet if the résumé is more than one page long.

The contact information should include your name, mailing address, professional e-mail address, and phone number. Some applicants will also include their personal websites, such as LinkedIn.

Zacarias Garcia

523 River Way, Mytown OH 45459
Cell phone: 715.555.5472
ZacGarcia@elsevier.net

Objective

To find a full-time medical assistant position in an orthopedic clinic.

Education

Community College, Mytown, OH
Medical Assistant Diploma, 20XX
- Medical Assistant Practicum at Mytown Orthopedic and Massage Center, Mytown, OH
  o Obtained and charted history and vital signs in electronic health record.
  o Assisted providers with tests and treatments.

Credentials

Certified Medical Assistant, American Association of Medical Assistants, expires May 20XX.
BLS for Healthcare Providers, American Heart Association, expires March 20XX.

Skills and Achievement

Strong communication skills
- Supervised 60 employees in a factory setting for over 3 years.
- Initiated procedures to improve communication between employees and management.
- Promoted in union to assist with negotiations with upper management.
- Fluent in Spanish.

Excellent problem-solving skills
- Problem-solved factory issues that delayed shipments to customers.
- Initiated solutions to expedite shipments and increased the profit margin of the company.

Excel in Teamwork
- Assisted team on assembly line, helping fill in when others were absent.
- Promoted to Team Lead within 6 months of hire.
- Received "Outstanding Employee" award in 20XX, 20XX, and 20XX.

Work Experience

Mytown Doors, Mytown, OH
Supervisor (March 20XX – January 20XX)
Team Lead – Door Assembly (January 20XX – March 20XX)
Door Assembler (August 20XX – January 20XX)

FIGURE 23-7 Combination résumé.

Professional e-mail addresses may include your first and last name or first initial and last name. E-mail addresses starting with expressions like: "one_hot_chick" or "party_dude" are not professional and are not used on résumés. If you do not have a professional e-mail, free e-mail sites are available. Like professional e-mails, personal websites should also be professional and contain a professional image of you.

Objective

The objective is a statement indicating to the reader the type of position being sought and the applicant's career goals. The objective should be a concise sentence. "A full-time medical assistant position" is a brief statement, but does not make much of an impression on the reader. A statement like, "To obtain a full-time medical assistant position in a family practice setting, which will utilize my technical and interpersonal skills," is more powerful.

Education

The education section includes information on the schooling the person has received after high school. The information should appear in reverse chronologic order, which means the newest information is on top and the oldest is at the bottom.

If a diploma was obtained, list the school's name, city and state, degree, and the year it was obtained. If a degree was not obtained but coursework was successfully completed, include the earlier mentioned information but summarize the coursework completed in place of the degree information. Additional information that can be included in this section would be academic awards, scholarships, overall GPA if greater than 3.0, and medical assistant practicum information (e.g., location, dates, and duties).

The location of the education section can differ based on the person's situation. If the person is a new graduate, the education section should appear toward the top of the résumé. If the degree is not related to the position or the degree is older, the emphasis would be on the person's achievements or work history; the education section would come toward the end of the résumé.

Work Experience

This section can be titled several different ways, including "Job Experience" and "Related Experience." If people have related

---

Krysia Debski

111 Mall Drive, Mytown, OH 45457
Cell phone: 715.555.6956
KDebski@elsevier.net

Objective
To find a full-time medical assistant position in an internal medicine clinic, which will utilize my technical and interpersonal skills.

Education
Community College, Mytown, OH
A.S. in Medical Assisting, 20XX
- Medical Assistant Practicum at Mytown Associates, Mytown, OH
  - Obtained and charted history and vital signs in electronic health record.
  - Assisted providers with tests and treatments in a busy internal medicine practice.
  - Performed injections, throat swabs, and phlebotomy.

Skills
ORGANIZATION SKILLS
- Organized supplies to expedite restocking procedures and decrease financial loss.
- Exceptional organizational and filing skills utilized to maintain purchase and delivery records for over 300 suppliers.
- Assisted with the installation and training for inventory tracking software for warehouse.

TEAMWORK
- Refined teamwork skills with over ten years in the US Marines.
- Taught teambuilding courses.
- Promoted teamwork among staff by incorporating incentives.

COMMUNICATION SKILLS
- Assertive when working with suppliers to meet deadlines.
- Utilized excellent listening skills to identify needs of various teams that impact the warehouse.
- Composed frequent emails and letters for supervisors.
- Fluent in Spanish and Polish

Credentials
Certified Medical Assistant, American Association of Medical Assistants (expires May 20XX)
BLS for Healthcare Providers, American Heart Association (expires March 20XX)

Work Experience
United States Marines
Supply Administration and Operations Specialist (May 20XX – September 20XX)
Warehouse Clerk (August 20XX – May 20XX)

FIGURE 23-8 Targeted résumé customized for a medical assistant posting. The medical assistant should possess strong organizational skills, experience with teamwork, and exceptional communication skills. The posting indicated it required a person with a Certified Medical Assistant (CMA) credential and a current Basic Life Support (BLS) certification.

healthcare experience that was either volunteer or part of training, using a broader phrase that does not include the words "job" or "work" may be an option. Applicants may want to use "Related Experience" or "Healthcare Experience," which helps draw the attention of the reader. For additional nonrelated experiences, they may use a section called "Other Work Experience." For those with military experience, it is recommended to add a special section to cover the military experience.

The information in this section should be presented in reverse chronologic order. The three most common formats for résumés require the following elements for each position: name of the agency, city and state, title of position, and dates in that position. Employers prefer to see month and year for the dates instead of just a year. This is especially important if the job only lasted a few months or just over a year. If the person has been in the workforce for ten years or

more, employers want to see ten years of employment information. For those working at the same agency for over ten years, it is important to list changes and advancements in the position over the duration of employment. Any gaps in the employment history should be explained to the potential employer during the interview or in the cover letter.

For the chronologic résumé, the most relevant job duties also need to be listed. For instance, if you worked as a housekeeper in a motel, making beds is not related to medical assisting, but providing customer service would be relevant. The statements regarding the duties should be bulleted and begin with an active verb. For present positions, use active verbs in the present tense (e.g., administer, provide); past positions should use active verbs in the past tense (e.g., administered, provided) (Figure 23-9).

Administered	Copied	Performed
Advocated	Developed	Posted
Aided	Distributed	Prepared
Answered	Documented	Processed
Arranged	Established	Provided
Assigned	Filed	Purchased
Assisted	Guided	Reconciled
Balanced	Helped	Restocked
Calculated	Instructed	Reviewed
Cared	Listened	Scanned
Coded	Logged	Scheduled
Collected	Mailed	Sorted
Compiled	Maintained	Supported
Composed	Monitored	Taught
Computed	Operated	Trained
Contacted	Ordered	Wrote
Coordinated	Organized	

FIGURE 23-9 Action verbs in the past tense.

The position of the education section in the résumé is dependent on the résumé format. Chronologic résumés typically have work experience near the top, whereas combination and targeted résumés list the reverse chronologic employment history toward the end of the résumé.

Summary and Skills

A "Summary" section appears just under the "Objective" section in the targeted résumé. This section summarizes why the applicant is the best candidate for the job. By utilizing key words and phrases found in the job description or job posting, the person can create a customized or targeted résumé. The key words are tied with related statements to help show how the applicant demonstrated the skills required in the new position.

A "Skills" or "Skills and Achievement" section is found in combination résumés and showcases specific transferable skills that relate to the new position. These transferable skills may have been obtained in the military, by a stay-at-home parent, or a person switching careers.

Special Skills

A "Special Skills" section typically only appears in a chronologic résumé. The information in this section would appear in the targeted résumé's "Summary" section and in the combination résumé's "Skills and Achievement" section.

Information that would appear in this section might relate to a fluency in another language, including sign language (e.g., fluent in Spanish). It may also contain the person's computer skills and experiences (e.g., "utilized electronic health records during practicum experience"; "keyboarding speed: 85 wpm").

Certifications

Many employers may require specific certifications or credentials for a job position. Regardless of the résumé format used, it is important to include the certifications and credentials that relate to the job position. When listing the information, include the title of the certification or license, awarding agency, and the expiration date (e.g., "Certified Medical Assistant, American Association of Medical Assistants, expires 10/2020" and "BLS for Healthcare Providers, American Heart Association, expires 10/2020").

Appearance of the Résumé

As you create your résumé, keep in mind the eye appeal or interest the résumé will create in the reader. It is recommended to bold only important information; for instance, a job title should be bold, whereas the agency should not be bold. Simple bullets help organize information and provide a neat appearance to the résumé. Changing the font size in certain areas can emphasize more important elements and help keep content on one page.

Spacing is crucial to the appearance of a résumé. Too much spacing creates too much "white space" and can give the reader a negative impression of the résumé. Too little spacing creates a busy, text-heavy résumé that is difficult to read. It is important to keep the same spacing distance between the sections of the résumé and smaller spacing between subsections (e.g., different employment positions).

It is important to have résumé paper available. Even if you submit your résumé online, you should have copies of your résumé on résumé paper available during the interview. Use a light solid-colored résumé paper (e.g., cream, light gray), which will duplicate better than a pattern or dark-colored paper.

Before submitting your résumé, have another person review it. Obtain the person's initial impression of the résumé's appearance. Is there too much white space? Does the résumé look too wordy? Does it look too plain? Does it look too busy? Then have the person read the content in the résumé and provide you with feedback. Use the feedback to revise your résumé. See Figure 23-10 for additional tips on creating a résumé.

CRITICAL THINKING APPLICATION   **23-9**

Zac, Michelle, and Krysia drafted their résumés. They read each other's and provided feedback. Who else might they give their résumés to for proofreading and feedback?

- Think of your circle of family and friends. List three people who might be great candidates to provide feedback on your résumé.

- Don't add clipart or other pictures

- Don't lie or exaggerate the truth

- Don't add unrelated content, like hobbies and interests.

- Don't include "References available upon request" or a similar statement, since it is understood references will be requested and required.

- Don't use personal pronouns, such as "I".

- Don't repeat content.

- Don't include any pay/salary information.

- Always keep the résumé to one page, unless you have been in the workforce for multiple years. Then use an additional page, but your content must fill both pages.

- Be concise and clear.

- Use key terms found in the job posting or job description in your résumé.

- Put important details first.

- Perform a grammar and spelling check on your résumé.

- Limit abbreviations to only the abbreviations used in the job posting (i.e., BLS for basic life support, CPR for cardiopulmonary resuscitation).

FIGURE 23-10 Tips on creating a résumé.

DEVELOPING A COVER LETTER

A cover letter always must accompany the résumé. The cover letter is a critical tool that gains the reader's attention and interest, thus making the reader want to look at the résumé. The advantage of the cover letter over the résumé is that the applicant can include more expression in it; the résumé tends to be more factual. Much attention to detail must occur to create a cover letter that will fulfill its role.

When developing a powerful cover letter to accompany your résumé, follow these strategies:

- Match the appearance of the cover letter and résumé. This means that your header should be identical, along with your font style and margins. Your contact information in the header should match the résumé's contact information. If you are submitting a paper document, use the same paper for both the résumé and cover letter.

- The inside address and the salutation need to be addressed to a specific person. Address the letter to the person who will be hiring the new employee. Use the person's name and job title in the inside address and be formal in the salutation (e.g., Dear Mr. Jones:) (Figure 23-11). You can contact the healthcare facility or utilize online resources like LinkedIn to gather this information. If you are unable to identify the person's name, use "To whom it may concern," "Dear Sir," "Dear Madam," or some variation. Having a specific name will tell the reader you took the time to find out the details and it may distinguish you over other candidates.

- Start the body of your cover letter off with a bang! In the first paragraph show enthusiasm as you summarize why you believe you are the best candidate for the job. *"Having a strong customer service background and a degree in medical assisting, I am confident that I can fulfill your expectations for the family practice medical assistant position (#123)."* Along with your qualities, it is important to include the job title and number so the reader knows what position you are interested in.

- During the second paragraph, sell yourself to the reader by providing a snapshot of your experiences. Weave in the key "requirement" words that the employer included in the job posting. Address the employer's more important requirements first, followed by the lesser requirements or "would like" qualities. You may want to bold these key words to bring more attention to them. If you bullet out your qualifications and abilities, limit the bullets to four or five points. Be concise, yet clear, but do not repeat the résumé; you want the reader to move onto the résumé for the details.

- Start the final paragraph by reaffirming that you are an excellent match for the job by using such phrases as "I believe I have the qualities you require" or "I am confident I will meet your expectations." You can follow this by stating the action you will take in regards to following up (for instance, "I will call the week of …"). Be careful that your tone is not overly aggressive, which might not sit well with the reader. If you chose not to address how you will follow up, finish the paragraph by expressing your interest and enthusiasm in an interview (e.g., "I am very excited about

---

Michelle Marison

1234 Cedar Way, Mytown, OH 45458
Home phone: 715.555.1899
Cell phone: 715.555.1355
mmarison@elsevier.net

May 15, 20XX

Ms. Alex Brown
Medical Assistant Supervisor
Mytown Medical Clinic
555 Clover Drive
Mytown OH 45457

Dear Ms. Brown:

I was excited to see the posting on the Mytown Telegram job board for the medical assistant position (#1243) and would like to be considered for that position. I am graduating from Community College on May 30, 20XX and will be taking my AAMA CMA exam June 2, 20XX.

With two years of customer service experience and five months of being a hospital volunteer, I have learned the importance of prioritizing, teamwork, and communication. During my medical assistant practicum, I have utilized these skills along with my attention to detail and my medical assistant knowledge, as I assist providers with procedures and treatments. The knowledge and skills I am learning in practicum combined with the skills I have developed as a waitress and volunteer will help me provide the best care to my future patients.

I have heard excellent things about Mytown Medical Clinic and would love to be a part of the staff of such a caring agency. I am available for interviews whenever it is convenient for you. I am available either by phone or email.

Thank you so much for considering me for this position.

Sincerely,

Michelle Marison

Enclosure: 1

FIGURE 23-11 Basic cover letter.

---

this opportunity and would enjoy meeting with you to explore how my qualifications could meet your needs."). (See Figure 23-11.)

- Before the closing and signature block, express your thanks to the reader for his or her consideration. Being gracious shows the reader you have good manners.
- When you have completed your letter, review the spelling, punctuation, grammar, and sentence structure. Create a cover letter that is error free and has a professional tone and appearance. Common cover letter weaknesses include:
  - Starting a majority of sentences with "I"
  - Introducing yourself in the first sentence (for instance, "Hi, I am Sally Green.")
  - Spelling, grammar, punctuation, and sentence structure errors
  - Missing parts of the letter (e.g., date, inside address)
  - Missing the position title and posting number

  - Too busy (overuse of font styles), too wordy, or too much "white space"
  - Inappropriate spacing that leads to the body of the letter being too high or too low on the page. Remember the body should be centered vertically on the page.
  - Creating a generic letter that does not contain the key requirement words from the job posting. (Many larger employers utilize software to screen letters and résumés for key words. Those with key words are reviewed closer; those that lack the key words are discarded.)

Use the spell check tool in your word processing software to help identify errors, but do not rely on it solely. **Proofread** your letter and have a few people proofread your letter as well. Use their advice as you make your changes. Refer to the Technology and Written Communication in the Medical Office chapter if you need assistance with composing a business letter. Procedure 23-2 will help guide you in writing a professional cover letter.

PROCEDURE 23-2 | Create a Cover Letter

Goal: *To write an effective cover letter that will accompany the résumé.*

EQUIPMENT and SUPPLIES

- Computer with word processing software and a printer
- Current job posting
- Résumé paper
- Pen

PROCEDURAL STEPS

1. Using the job posting, read through the job description. With a pen, circle the position requirements and the key phrases.
   <u>PURPOSE:</u> Your letter should contain the key phrases and position requirements that are found in the job posting.

2. Using the computer with word processing software, create a professional-looking header in the document's header that matches your résumé header. Include your name, address, telephone number(s), and e-mail address.
   <u>PURPOSE:</u> To ensure potential employers have a means of contacting you. You can increase the professional appearance of your documents by having the same header on each document.

3. Type the date in the correct location using the correct format. Have one blank line between the date line and the last line of the letterhead.
   <u>PURPOSE:</u> All letters require a date for legal purposes.

4. Type the inside address using the correct spelling, punctuation, and location for the information. Leave 1 to 9 blank lines between the date and the inside address, depending on the location of the body of the letter.
   <u>PURPOSE:</u> The body of the letter needs to be centered vertically from top to bottom of the document. More blank lines can be added to move the body to the correct location.

5. Starting on the second line below the inside address, type the salutation using the correct professional format, including the individual's name if known.
   <u>PURPOSE:</u> A proper greeting helps set the tone of the letter.

6. Type the message in the body of the letter using the proper location and format. There should be a blank line after the salutation and between each paragraph. The message should be clear, concise, and professional. Use proper grammar, punctuation, capitalization, and sentence structure.
   <u>PURPOSE:</u> Proper grammar usage helps the message be conveyed more accurately and professionally.

7. The first paragraph should contain the title and number of the job posting. The middle paragraph(s) should summarize your strengths and include key phrases from the posting. The final paragraph should discuss your availability for an interview. The body should end with an expression of gratitude to the reader.
   <u>PURPOSE:</u> It is important to thank the reader for considering you for the position.

8. Type a proper closing, leaving one blank line between the last line of the body and the closing. Use the correct format and location.
   <u>PURPOSE:</u> The closing helps end the message with a proper tone.

9. Type the signature block using the correct format and location. There should be four blank lines between the closing and the signature block.

10. Spell check and proofread the document. Check for proper tone, grammar, punctuation, capitalization, and sentence structure. Check for proper spacing between the parts of the letter.
    <u>PURPOSE:</u> The spell check tool will identify only certain errors; proofreading will help to identify incorrect word usage, improper tone, and errors in formatting. The tone of the letter should be professional, but not aggressive.

11. Make any final corrections. Print the document on résumé paper and sign the letter or e-mail the document to your instructor or employer.

COMPLETING ONLINE PROFILES AND JOB APPLICATIONS

With many healthcare agencies utilizing the Internet during the employment process, the human resource software they use may require applicants to create an online profile before applying for open positions. The online profile collects the information that previously was collected by paper applications.

Online profiles have many advantages over paper applications for both the employer and the applicant. An applicant completes the profile once and updates the information as needed. Typically the agencies keep the profiles active for a long period of time, sometimes for years. Employers can track the activities of applicants, easily read a person's information, and advertise new postings to potential applicants whose profiles meet certain requirements.

If a healthcare agency does not utilize online profiles, then the applicant will need to complete a job application (Figure 23-12). Some organizations require the application to be submitted with the cover letter and résumé but others have applicants arriving for interviews complete the application. If you need to complete an application before an interview, come prepared with your information and arrive at least 20 minutes before the interview. See Procedure 23-3 for the steps in completing a job application.

As you complete the online or paper application, you will be required to read important legal statements and add your signature (or electronic signature). This is a legal document; therefore it should be filled out accurately and completely. Regardless of how you complete the application, you will need to provide the same information. Even if you have the information on your résumé, you still need to

APPLICATION FOR EMPLOYMENT

Date:_____

Name: (First, Middle Initial, Last)_____

Social Security No.:_____   Phone: _____

Address:_____

EDUCATION

	Name, City, State	Graduation Date	Degree Obtained
High School:			
College:			
Other:			

LICENSURE/CERTIFICATION/REGISTRATION

Type of Certification, License or Registration	Agency/State	Registration Name

List any special skills or qualifications which you possess and feel are relevant to health care and the position for which you are applying._____

_____

EMPLOYMENT HISTORY

May we contact and communicate with your present employer? ☐ Yes ☐ No

Employer:	Phone:
Address:	Supervisor:
Employed	Hourly Pay:
Position title and responsibilities:	
Reason for leaving:	

FIGURE 23-12 Application for employment.

add it to the application. Having the information in a word-processed document will save you time. If you are providing the information online, the copy and paste feature will speed up completion time. Information you should include in the word-processed document includes:

- Education information such as: institution's name and address; dates and titles of coursework or diploma.
- Information related to prior and current employers such as: agency name and address; supervisors' names, titles, and contact information; job title, duties, start and end salary, start and end dates; and reason for leaving.
- Information related to certifications and credentials (e.g., certifying agency's name and address; certification/credential; expiration date). A copy of your certification and BLS card may be required by the employer.

- Information related to your references (e.g., names, contact information, type of reference [co-worker, instructor]).

When filling out the application answer the questions carefully. When addressing your availability date, make sure you know how long you have to give notice at your current position if that is pertinent. Usually, most employers have a 2-week notice policy. If you get hired, your new employer will understand that you need to give a 2-week notice.

When completing the reason why you left prior positions, make sure to write the reason using a positive tone. For instance, *"Obtained a position that would advance my skill set"* or *"Resigned to focus more on my education"* sound more professional than *"I hated the job."* If you have a unique situation (e.g., sick parent, new baby), ask the advice of your school's placement counselor if you are unsure what to say in these sections.

PROCEDURE 23-3 | Complete a Job Application

Goal: *To complete an accurate, detailed job application legibly so as to secure a job offer.*

EQUIPMENT and SUPPLIES

- Pen
- Application form
- Information regarding your past education, job experiences, and the skill sets you have obtained (e.g., computer skills, keyboarding speed)
- Contact information for former supervisors and references
- Current résumé

PROCEDURAL STEPS

1. Read the entire job application before completing any part of the document.
   PURPOSE: Reading through the entire application helps prevent errors when filling out the document.
2. Refer to your information on past jobs, education experiences, and skill sets you have obtained as you complete the application. Answers to the questions need to be accurate and honest.
3. Use proper grammar, sentence structure, punctuation, spelling, and capitalization. Handwriting should be legible to the reader.

PURPOSE: Errors on the application or illegible sections may affect whether you are hired.
4. Do not leave any space blank. Answer each question on the document. If the question does not apply, write "not applicable."
   PURPOSE: Leaving a space blank on the application may suggest that the candidate did not want to answer a certain question or accidentally overlooked it. By writing "not applicable" on such questions, the candidate demonstrates competence and attention to detail.
5. Do not write "See résumé" anywhere on the document.
   PURPOSE: Many supervisors view this practice as laziness. Always fill out the job application completely and do not leave blank spaces.
6. Include information on the application that exhibits dependability, punctuality, teamwork, attention to detail, positive work ethics and initiative, the ability to adapt to change, a responsible attitude, and use of technology.
7. Sign the document and date it.
8. Proofread the document and make sure none of the information conflicts with the résumé.
   PURPOSE: Proofreading helps the candidate to catch any errors before submitting the application.

CREATING A CAREER PORTFOLIO

As stated earlier in the chapter, many job seekers claim to have the skill set required by the potential employer, but very few actually show the employer evidence of those qualifications. A career portfolio is a fantastic tool to show a potential employer that you have the skills required for the job. The portfolio should be developed along with the cover letter and résumé. A student may have more than one portfolio if he or she is considering different types of positions (e.g., receptionist, phlebotomist, medical assistant). The portfolio would be customized for each position, highlighting the skills utilized by a person in that position. For a phlebotomist-focused portfolio, evaluations of past venipunctures and related documents would be more useful than content related to coding and billing. The portfolio is utilized during the interview process and shows the interviewer what you have accomplished.

Every career portfolio is unique to the individual. For medical assistants, it is recommended to use a three-ring binder with plastic sheet protectors and divider tabs. (See Procedure 23-4 for the steps in creating a career portfolio.) Typical items found in career portfolios include:

- Cover letter addressed to the interviewer
- Résumé (a copy of what was sent to that facility)
- References document with contact information from three or four people, including one to two instructors, and one to two co-workers or prior supervisors who have given prior consent to be used as references
- Certifications (e.g., copy of BLS card, copy of credentials [e.g., CMA or RMA card])

- Education-related documents:
  - Copy of letters of recommendation
  - Copy of transcripts, awards, and honors
  - A list of the courses successfully completed with a short description of each course (optional, but consider if you are moving to another location where your institution may not be known)
  - Copy of practicum evaluation forms and skill document form
  - Scholarships awarded
  - Copy/details of school-related activities (e.g., officer in student medical assistant group, athlete, volunteer activities)
- Prior employment documents
  - Copy of past employment evaluations
  - Copy of letters of recommendations
  - Documentation showing the student balancing work and education (This can help exhibit a strong work ethic, organizational skills, and prioritizing skills.)
- Examples of work or summary of projects that can provide evidence of abilities and skills
- Criminal background documentation, blood titers, vaccination history, and current tuberculosis (TB) skin test (optional)

The documents placed in the career portfolio binder should be positive and helpful to you in your mission of getting a job. If you have not been very successful in school, you may not want to include your transcript. If you received negative performance evaluations, you should not include those in your portfolio. Be creative as you prepare your portfolio, keeping the appearance professional and neat.

PROCEDURE 23-4   Create a Career Portfolio

Goal: *To create a custom portfolio that provides potential employers evidence of your skills and knowledge as a medical assistant.*

EQUIPMENT and SUPPLIES

- Three-ring binder or folder
- Plastic sleeves for the three-ring binder
- Dividers with tabs for three-ring binder
- Current résumé and cover letter
- Documents providing evidence of your skills and knowledge (e.g., transcripts, job and practicum evaluation forms, practicum skill checklist, projects completed in school, letters of recommendation, copies of certifications [CPR and first aid cards])

PROCEDURAL STEPS

1. Group documents in a logical manner, putting similar documents together. Identify the arrangement for the portfolio. An arrangement could include: cover letter and résumé, education section (e.g., transcript, practicum evaluation form and skills checklist, awards), prior job-related documents (e.g., evaluations), reference letters, and work products (e.g., projects you created in your medical assistant program). Insert a tabbed divider in front of each section. You may want to include a table of contents to identify the tabbed areas.

PURPOSE: Organizing the documents in a logical manner will help the reader identify the important documents. The arrangement will also show the reader your ability to organize content.

2. Neatly write the topic area on the tab of the dividers.
PURPOSE: This will help the reader find the content easier.

3. Insert one document per plastic pocket.
PURPOSE: The plastic pockets will keep the documents clean and neat.

4. Arrange the documents neatly in the binder or folder. Have your cover letter and résumé in the front of all the other documents.
PURPOSE: The reader can review the letter and résumé as needed before looking at the other documents in the portfolio.

5. After the portfolio is assembled, review the entire portfolio to ensure it looks professional and the documents provide positive support of your skill set and knowledge.
PURPOSE: Minimize the negative documents in your portfolio. They will not help you obtain a job as much as the positive, supporting documents.

JOB INTERVIEW

A medical assistant may interview with the office manager, the provider, or both, and other staff members may be brought in for part of the interview. This is especially true in healthcare environments with a cohesive team of employees.

The interview usually is the most stressful of the job search steps. Some individuals dread job interviews and become extremely nervous at the prospect of interviewing. Others are very comfortable and consider the interview to be as much for their own purposes as for the employer's. Either way, the more interviews the medical assistant has, the more comfortable he or she will be with each subsequent interview.

An interview has four phases: preparation for the interview, the interview itself, the follow-up, and the negotiation.

Preparation for the Interview

When preparing for an interview, the medical assistant should learn everything possible about the employer. Look on the Internet for information about the facility. Practice answering possible interview questions. Prepare an outfit to wear to interviews. It is wise to drive to the interview site on a day preceding the interview date if the location is unfamiliar to avoid getting lost on the day of the important event. The better prepared the medical assistant is, the more comfortable he or she will be when interviewing.

The critical part of the interview is the medical assistant's ability to present himself or herself as the best candidate for the job. By preparing to answer interview questions before the interview, the medical assistant will appear much more confident. Although no one can guess exactly what questions will be asked, there are some standard interview questions (Figure 23-13). Review these questions thoroughly, answer them in writing, and then study them before the interview. Then when the medical assistant is asked, "What are your three greatest strengths?" he or she can confidently answer, "I am professional, reliable, and honest." Expanding on these traits will provide additional information to the interviewers on why these are your greatest strengths. Take time to consider your possible answers to some of the standard interview questions. What perception might you be giving to the interviewers by your answer? Is it the perception you want to be giving?

In addition to preparing to answer interview questions, you should prepare two to three questions to ask the interviewer. The organization's website is an excellent source of information. Be familiar with their mission and value statements, the size of the organization, the size of the department that has the open position, and the number of providers. Possible questions might be:

- "I see that there are two providers in this department. Would I be working with both of them?"
- "There are three locations for your clinic on your website; how will I interact with the other locations?"
- "Given the size of your organization is there an opportunity to interact with the other departments?"
- "When will you be making a decision about this position?"

By having questions that relate to the specific organization and department, you are showing that you are truly interested in the position. Asking about their time frame for making a decision on the position will direct your decision about a thank-you card: for example, if they are deciding later that day or the next, you should send a thank-you e-mail; there would not be time for a card to be delivered.

1. Tell me about yourself.	16. What do you know about this facility and our competitors?
2. Why do you want to work for this company?	17. What has been your most rewarding experience at work?
3. Why should I hire you?	18. What was your single most important accomplishment for the company on your last job?
4. How do you work under pressure?	19. What was the toughest problem you have ever solved and how did you do it?
5. How do you handle criticism?	20. How do you see yourself fitting in with our company?
6. What do you think your co-workers think about you?	21. What skills did you learn on your last job that can be used here?
7. Describe your last supervisor.	22. What immediate contribution could you make if you came to work for us today?
8. What would you like to change about yourself?	23. Do you prefer working with others or by yourself?
9. What is your best asset?	24. Can you take instructions or criticism without being upset?
10. What adjectives would you use to describe yourself?	25. What job in this company would you choose if you could?
11. How would you describe the perfect job?	26. What have you done that shows initiative and willingness to work?
12. Why did you leave your last job?	27. What will previous supervisors say about you?
13. Why did you choose this type of profession?	28. Why would you be successful in this job?
14. What are your strongest and weakest personal qualities?	29. Can you explain the gap in your employment history?
15. What personal characteristics are necessary for success in your chosen field?	30. Are you a member of any professional organizations?

FIGURE 23-13 Top 30 interview questions.

When preparing on the day of the interview, be conservative with wardrobe choices. For women a business suit, or skirt or dress pants and blouse, is appropriate. If you choose to wear a skirt or dress it should be of modest length (i.e., at the knee or longer). Your blouse should not be sheer or show cleavage. For men, a business suit, or dress pants and shirt with a tie, is the best choice. Your tie should be professional. Conservative business suits would always be acceptable in an interview. Be sure clothing is fresh, wrinkle-free, and well-fitting and that shoes are clean and shined. For a medical assistant, scrubs would be acceptable for an interview if you do not have

dress clothes. Take care in washing, pressing, and rolling your scrubs for lint before wearing them on an interview.

Pay particular attention to other aspects of appearance (Figure 23-14). Make sure your hair is clean and styled attractively, your teeth are clean, and your breath is fresh. Nails are also important and should be clean and well groomed, because the medical assistant should give the interviewer a firm handshake. Nails should not be excessively long or painted in highly visible colors. Do not wear perfumes or colognes and do not wear excessive jewelry or makeup. Do not chew gum or smoke in your interview attire. Remember the

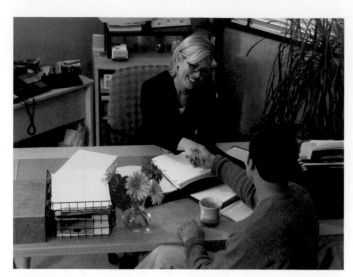

FIGURE 23-14 Present a professional appearance during the job interview and be sure to smile often. (From Yoder-Wise P: *Leading and managing in nursing*, ed 4, 2006, St. Louis, Mosby.)

appearance guidelines that applied to the practicum; some employers will react negatively to tattoos, piercings, extravagant hairstyles, hair colors, or other excessive wardrobe choices. Always dress appropriately and conservatively for an interview. Once hired, the new employee may be allowed to wear more diverse styles that comply with the employee handbook or procedure manual.

Do a test run before the day of the interview to identify the travel time. Always arrive 15 minutes early for the interview. Never take anyone along on a job interview, especially children, even if they are older. Expect to be a little nervous. Any interview can be a stressful situation. The better prepared the medical assistant is, the more of a success the interview will be.

It is a good idea to bring an interview portfolio and a planner or other method of taking notes during the interview; this makes a good impression and indicates interest in the job. The interview portfolio should be reflective of that particular position. It should have a table of contents at the beginning with identified tabbed sections so the interviewer can quickly review materials that he or she finds pertinent. The student should be prepared to leave the portfolio with the interviewer, so no originals should be included. The first items in the portfolio after the table of contents should be a copy of the cover letter and résumé that was sent to the facility; the individual doing the interview may not have received the original documents. A detailed reference list should also be included. Bring a list of questions to ask. If you have not completed an application, bring information regarding former employment (e.g., supervisors' names and contact information, dates of employment, wages, reasons for leaving), education, and any other information that might be needed to accurately complete paperwork; the information could be written down on paper or saved into a document or application in a smart phone. This will help to avoid the embarrassment of asking to look up an address in a phone book or calling to obtain the information while at the interview.

Before the face-to-face interview occurs many organizations will conduct a preliminary phone interview with a human resources representative. This interview is generally done to narrow the applicant pool. It can also give them a very good idea of how you present yourself on the phone. This is an opportunity for you to learn more about the organization. You have provided this potential employer with your phone number, so you should be prepared to receive a phone call. In anticipation of receiving phone calls from a potential employer you should make sure that your voice mail message is appropriate and professional sounding. You should clearly state your name in this message so that they know they have reached the right person. If you receive the call at a time when it is not appropriate to speak, in a noisy location, or in a quiet location where you should not be speaking, let the call go to voice mail. If you are able to answer the call but it is not a good time to speak to them, it is perfectly all right to explain this and offer to call back at a time convenient for the employer.

During the Interview

Whether the interview is conducted over the phone, face-to-face, or via video conference (e.g., Skype, FaceTime), the interviewer should not ask any illegal questions, including those that are related to age, sex, nationality, religion, marital/family status, affiliations/organizations, and disabilities (Figure 23-15).

Employers may ask illegal questions, whether intentionally or accidentally, and the way that the medical assistant answers the questions can influence the employer's hiring decision. If the medical assistant is openly offended, employers may conclude that the applicant will be offended by abrasive comments from patients and will not be able to handle interaction with patients. If the illegal question is answered, the interviewer may use the information in the answer to weed out the medical assistant as a candidate. The best approach is to politely address the question, either by answering it directly or by redirecting the interviewer back to the job requirements. For example, if the interviewer asks if the candidate plans to put children in day care (which might be a way of determining the age of the dependent children and thus the likelihood of absenteeism because of the children's illnesses), the medical assistant could answer, "I will be able to meet the work schedule and the responsibilities that this job requires." Some questions that might normally be considered illegal, such as "What organizations are you a member of?" might be job related. The employer may be interested in knowing that the medical assistant is a member of various professional organizations, such as the AAMA or the AMT.

Phone Interview

A phone interview may be done to screen applicants and narrow the candidate pool or it may replace a face-to-face interview, especially if the candidate is from out of town. If this interview is replacing a face-to-face interview you will be contacted to set up a time for the interview. You should approach this process with the same preparation that you would do for a face-to-face interview. It is important that you are in a quiet, well-lit room that is free from distractions. You should have a copy of your résumé and cover letter in front of you, as well as your list of questions. It would be a good idea to have a glass of water there, as nerves tend to make your throat dry. Be sure to thank the employer for the opportunity to interview with them.

Face-to-Face Interview

During the actual interview, maintain good eye contact. Many supervisors refuse to hire people who seem uncomfortable looking them directly in the eyes. Never take control of the interview. Allow

Topic	Illegal	Legal
RELIABILITY	How many children do you have? Who is going to babysit? What is your marital status? Do you have a car?	What hours and days can you work? Are there specific times that you cannot work? Do you have responsibilities other than work that will interfere with specific job requirements such as traveling?
CITIZENSHIP	What is your national origin? Where are your parents from?	Are you legally eligible for employment in the United States?
REFERENCES	What is your maiden name? What is your father's surname? What are the names of your relatives?	Have you ever worked under a different name?
ARRESTS AND CONVICTIONS	Have you ever been arrested?	Have you ever been convicted of a crime?
DISABILITIES	Do you have any disabilities?	Can you perform the duties of the job you are applying for?
AGE/DATE OF BIRTH	What is your date of birth?	If hired, can you furnish proof that you are over the age of 18?
RELIGION	What church do you attend?	None
EDUCATION	When did you graduate from high school?	Do you have a high school diploma or equivalent?

FIGURE 23-15 Illegal and legal interview questions.

the supervisor to ask questions at his or her own pace. Do not fidget in the chair. Do not volunteer any negative information; be honest and do not exaggerate experience or lengths of employment. Never speak negatively about former employers.

Be careful when answering questions such as, "Tell me about yourself." Most medical assistants might begin to answer this question with a phrase like, "I'm a recent graduate, and I am married and have two children." The answer to this question should not reflect information about personal issues. Focus all answers on professionalism and the strengths that will be an asset to the healthcare setting. Stating "I am a recent graduate and completed a 6-week practicum in a family practice" opens the door to questions that will allow you to highlight your skills.

Remember that the interview is centered on the medical assistant, so freely discuss the skills and attributes that you would bring to the job. The better prepared the medical assistant is, the smoother the interview will go. Be able to prove the skills you claim and explain how they meet the needs of the company or facility. Utilize your interview portfolio during the interview by referencing past job evaluations or your practicum skill checklist/evaluation. Avoid a "know-it-all" attitude, which indicates overconfidence and reluctance to take direction. Always express an interest in the employer and his or her projects, rather than in what the employer can do for the employee. Ask intelligent questions at the end of the interview if given the opportunity. Your first question should never be, "How much will I be paid?" Money, although important, cannot appear to be your primary concern.

Before the interview ends, the medical assistant should ask when a decision will be made and if it would be acceptable to call to follow up (Procedure 23-5).

Video Interview

A third interview possibility is a video interview using technology such as Skype. As with a phone interview, a video interview works well when the candidate is from out of town. There is a certain amount of technology needed for a video interview. Your school's placement office may be able to help you with that, or the organization may have contacts for you to arrange your end of the interview. The benefit of a video interview over a phone interview is that the interviewers can actually see the interviewee. This allows the interviewers to assess the body language and the verbal message being presented. You should dress as you would for a face-to-face interview and have the same materials ready to access during the interview process.

CRITICAL THINKING APPLICATION   **23-10**

Krysia is enjoying a good interview when the interviewer, a male supervisor, asks her if she is married. When Krysia replies that she is not, he asks if she has a steady boyfriend.

- What might the supervisor's motive be with this line of questioning?
- How should Krysia respond?
- Are these questions inappropriate or do they serve a purpose?

PROCEDURE 23-5   Practice Interview Skills During a Mock Interview

Goal: *To project a professional appearance during a job interview and to be able to express the reasons the medical assistant is the best candidate for the position.*

EQUIPMENT and SUPPLIES

- Current job posting
- Résumé
- Cover letter
- Interview portfolio (optional)
- Application (optional)
- Interviewer
- Mock interview questions

PROCEDURAL STEPS

1. Wear interview-appropriate attire and be groomed professionally.
   PURPOSE: Your appearance will influence the first impression made on this potential employer. Most medical facilities prefer conservative dress.
2. Portray a professional image by shaking hands firmly; bringing a copy of the current résumé and cover letter and copies of earned certificates. Do not engage in visible nervous habits such as tapping your foot, bouncing a crossed leg, or drumming fingers.
3. Answer introductory questions by providing only professional information. For example:

Question: "What can you tell us about yourself?"
Response: "I am a recent graduate of an accredited medical assistant program. I have just completed a 6-week practicum experience where I was able to demonstrate proficiency in a variety of clinical and administrative skills."

4. Answer interview questions with open, honest, and positive responses. Completely answer questions, provide information, and do not answer in single sentences or with limited responses.
5. Utilize key words from the job posting when answering the interview questions.
   PURPOSE: Helps to prove the interviewee has exactly what the organization is looking for.
6. Ask the interviewer two to three appropriate questions about the agency or the position.
   PURPOSE: Demonstrates an interest in the organization and the position.
7. Express interest in the job and politely complete the interview by shaking hands and thanking the interviewer for the opportunity for the interview.

Follow-Up After the Interview

Follow-up is critical after an interview. Always send a written thank-you note or letter to the person who conducted the interview (Procedure 23-6). Many employers wait to see who sends a thank-you letter before making the final hiring decision. Limit follow-up calls to one or two a week. Most employers give an indication of when the hiring decision will be made. The company should notify all those who interviewed once a decision has been made, unless specific protocols were set during the interview about follow-up. For instance, if the office manager says a decision will be made on Friday and the final three candidates will be called for a second interview, the medical assistant knows to continue the job search if a call is not received. Although not all companies provide this type of notification, it is considered professional etiquette to tell the candidates who interviewed for the job if they are no longer under consideration. Never place all your hope in one job; continue to search and interview until an offer is made and accepted. In addition, always be on the watch for the next job opportunity.

PROCEDURE 23-6   Create a Thank-You Note for an Interview

Goal: *To create a meaningful thank-you note to be sent after the interview process.*

EQUIPMENT and SUPPLIES

- Computer with word processing software and a printer
- Job description
- Contact name from interview

PROCEDURAL STEPS

1. Using word processing software compose a professional letter using business letter format. Include all of the required elements in the letter. Use correct spacing between the elements.
2. Highlight the particulars of the interview in the body of the letter.
3. Include positive information you wish you had covered in the interview.
   PURPOSE: Allows you to present any missed skills or details in a professional manner.
4. Create a message that is concise and to the point.
5. Sign and send the thank-you note.

Reasons People Do Not Get Hired

The following is a ranked list of reasons interviewers do not hire job candidates, as expressed by surveyed career consultants and reported on www.workoplis.com:

- Not sufficiently differentiating themselves from others
- Failure to successfully transfer past experience to the current job opportunity
- Not showing enough interest and excitement
- Focusing too much on what they want and too little on what the interviewer is saying
- Feeling they can "wing" the interview without preparation
- Not being able to personally connect with the interviewer
- Appearing over- or under-qualified for the job
- Not asking enough or the right questions
- Not researching a potential employer/interviewer
- Lacking humor, warmth, or personality during the interview process

Negotiation

The negotiation stage of job acceptance can be as stressful as the actual interviews. Salary can no longer be the only consideration when determining whether to accept a position or not. Other benefits can play a crucial role in that decision. When a job offer is made there should also be a discussion of the other benefits. If the salary offered is a bit lower than expected, but the employee share of the health insurance premium is less than expected, the salary offer becomes more attractive. A medical assistant should know the lowest salary/benefit combination he or she can afford and should ask for a little more than that figure. Bracket salary requests are often helpful in this: instead of asking for $13 per hour, ask for a salary in the "mid to high twenties." Let the employer mention a figure or a range of salary first. Usually the person who mentions a salary range first has the disadvantage. If the medical assistant requests $13 per hour and the facility was willing to pay $16 per hour, the medical assistant probably will get $13. The organization may have a starting pay level for new employees. To start at higher than that level you will need to show them why you should: for example, proficiency at the required skills for the job or previous work experience in the field. Having a well-designed interview portfolio will allow you to show the interviewer all that you have accomplished.

Never say "no" to a job offer on the spot. Request at least 24 hours to consider the offer. Before accepting or rejecting a job offer, consider whether the position carries any authority, the benefits, the hours, the distance from home, and the potential for advancement. People accept jobs for reasons other than the salary; remember the value of experience.

CRITICAL THINKING APPLICATION   **23-11**

Michelle has been on several interviews and likes the prospect of working for three different physicians. If an offer is made at each office, how can Michelle decide which to accept? What will help Michelle make this decision?

YOU GOT THE JOB!

Once the job offer has been made and accepted, a start date will be determined. Before the first day, use the computer, global positioning system (GPS), or smart phone to map several ways to get to work. If you are unsure of the traffic flow, leave home extra-early the first day so that you are guaranteed to arrive on time.

Most employees are placed on a 30- to 90-day probationary period, during which employment may be terminated for unsatisfactory performance. The probationary period also provides the employer and employee an opportunity to learn about each other. The medical assistant will interact with other co-workers, patients, and providers. A new medical assistant should volunteer to help others and efficiently complete the duties assigned. Use the probationary period as a testing ground, carefully observing ways in which the healthcare facility might run more smoothly. However, do not make numerous suggestions for change during this period. Discover why certain methods are used and make an effort to fit in with the rest of the team before suggesting that the office routine be changed. Remember, the people at the office may have been employed for a substantially longer time and may resent suggestions from a new staff member. Learn the office rhythms, procedures, and culture first and demonstrate a team-oriented attitude. After new employees prove their responsibility and positive attitude, other staff members will be open to suggestions about improvements for the office.

Common Early Mistakes

Some medical assistants make mistakes early on in a new job. Never be disruptive to the office by gossiping or complaining. A medical assistant must realize that procedures may be performed in many different ways and that the way he or she was taught in school probably is not the only correct way. Be open to learning new ideas, concepts, and procedures. Although some mistakes are to be expected, make sure that once a mistake has been pointed out, it is corrected. Do not make the same mistakes over and over.

Supervisors may work closely with the medical assistant, or others may expect the medical assistant to carry out orders independently. Although being diligent about your job is commendable you should never hesitate to ask the more experienced medical assistants if you have any doubt about how to perform a task. Finish all assigned duties in a timely manner and avoid procrastination. When significant problems arise, discuss them openly with the supervisor and attempt to find a quick resolution. Limit absences and tardy days to a minimum and miss work only when absolutely necessary, especially during the probationary period.

Being a Good Employee

A medical assistant can be a good employee in several ways. First and foremost, arrive 15 minutes before the scheduled shift and do not leave early. Even the best medical assistant cannot benefit an office if he or she does not come to work. Be honest and demonstrate trustworthiness and professionalism. Get along with co-workers in the facility. A medical assistant should be able to resolve simple problems with others easily without involving the supervisor. Reflect a friendly attitude toward others, even if they are difficult to get along with. Arrive every single day ready to learn. The medical assistant's education does not end upon graduation from school. The medical field is one of constant change, and those who work in it must learn and change along with it. By choosing to work in the healthcare field you are making a commitment to lifelong learning.

A medical assistant should constantly be performing assigned duties and should not expect frequent breaks in the medical office. Most offices are fast paced, and the supervisor expects the medical assistant to keep up with the activity. Even during slow periods, there is always a counter to clean or documents to scan into the EHR. Be supportive of the leadership in the facility and ask for more responsibility if necessary. Take the initiative to perform duties that are cumbersome or repetitive and get them done quickly.

Always treat patients with compassion and empathy. Remember that they are not always at their best when ill, so be kind and courteous to them and their families. The patients are the reason the facility exists. Treat them with great respect and care.

Remember that medical assistants can be held individually responsible for their actions even though they work as an agent of the physician-employer. Although the provider is usually the person against whom professional liability lawsuits are brought, the medical assistant can still be named in a lawsuit.

CRITICAL THINKING APPLICATION   **23-12**

On Zac's second day at the practicum site, he clearly sees a co-worker taking and using a controlled drug from the storage area.
- What should Zac do?
- What potential problems arise with this situation?
- To whom should Zac report this incident, if anyone?

Dealing With Supervisors

Supervisors appreciate employees who come to them when they have questions, but who are able to handle minor decisions on their own. Never hesitate to approach supervisors when an issue at hand needs their attention. Do not allow a situation to go unaddressed and then say, "I didn't want to bother you with that." The office manager is responsible for dealing with difficult issues, and these should be handled immediately when they arise.

A medical assistant should never attempt to cover up a mistake; admitting the error is a much better approach to solving the problem. When talking with the supervisor, do not hesitate to speak and do not avoid the subject. State the problem clearly and explain what routes are available to **rectify** the situation. Assertive communication skills work best in these situations. Work with the supervisor to resolve issues and accept the advice given with a positive attitude.

Performance Appraisals

Performance appraisals usually are done after the initial probationary period and annually thereafter. The performance appraisal is designed to inform the employee of his or her strengths and weaknesses on the job. An appraisal may be done in a 180-degree style, where you are evaluated by your supervisor. Your supervisor uses his or her observations of your performance over the given time period. An appraisal may also be done using the 360-degree style, where the supervisor asks for input from your co-workers and others that you interact with on a regular basis. Do not expect to receive a perfect appraisal, because employees are seldom perfect in all aspects of their jobs. If the supervisor gives perfect scores to an employee, there is no room for growth or improvement. It is the rare employee who completes all duties and meets every expectation without any errors. Take time to review the job description and honestly evaluate your own performance in all areas.

When asked to sit down with your supervisor for a performance appraisal, expect to address areas where you did not receive a perfect score. These are the areas that need improvement from your supervisor's perspective. If you have had an opportunity to see the performance appraisal before your meeting with your supervisor, pay close attention to those areas where you got less than a perfect rating. Come to the meeting with ways to improve that score. You may be asked about the status of your continuing education units (CEUs) needed to maintain your certification or registration. You should also be prepared to discuss your goals for the coming year. These may be goals for improvement or involvement within the organization. Ask questions and work with the supervisor to improve in the areas that may need more effort or a different approach.

If the employee strongly disagrees with any area of the performance appraisal, he or she should discuss this with the supervisor. There may have been a misunderstanding as to the duties involved. Clarify this calmly and patiently and strive to do better next time.

Pursuing a Raise

Most facilities have some type of schedule for pay increases. Some offer a cost of living increase on an annual basis; others use a merit system, offering raises only when earned and deserved based on performance. The requirements are often outlined in the performance review document.

There may come a time when the medical assistant feels the need to ask for a raise. Before doing so, a little self-reflection is important to determine whether a raise is in order. Has attendance been exemplary? How many times was the medical assistant tardy? Does he or she work well with little supervision? Has he or she performed all the expected duties well and in a timely manner? Has he or she gone above and beyond with patients and/or co-workers? Has he or she met the requirements outlined by the organization?

Make an appointment with the supervisor and ask, in private, how a salary raise might be earned in the near future. Do not expect a raise of more than 3% to 5% at any given time, unless the employee is promoted to another position or given additional duties. If the supervisor is unable to grant a raise, determine whether the reasons are valid. Work with the supervisor to determine what steps you need to take to be able to gain a raise. Is there additional education required, is the supervisor looking for more involvement within the organization, such as participation in a committee, or are there additional responsibilities that can be taken on? If the reasons are not valid, the medical assistant may want to pursue other employment options. The medical assistant will find that finding a job is always easier if one already has a job, so do not quit outright unless the work environment is intolerable. Begin networking again and discover the options available.

Leaving a Job

Always offer at least 2 weeks' notice when resigning from a job. Prepare a written notice of resignation and take it to the supervisor in person. Do not just leave it on a desk or place it in the interoffice mail.

Resigning from a job just as an attempt to get a salary increase is a dangerous practice. Once the employer doubts the employee's loyalty, the future usually is not bright for the employee at that facility. Resign only after a final decision has been made. If the medical assistant is resigning to take another position, the current employer may be expected to make a **counteroffer**. However, be wary about accepting counteroffers. What led you to look for a new job in the first place? Has the situation been resolved? Ask yourself these questions before agreeing to stay with the current employer. Often employees who accept a counteroffer and stay at their original job find that few changes are made, and the employee ends up leaving the position in the long run.

LIFE SKILLS

To be successful in the job search, the medical assistant must have the basic entry-level skills needed to perform in the workplace. Even more important, he or she must develop certain life skills that are essential to excel in any profession. If these skills are not developed and refined, the medical assistant may find fewer opportunities and advancements available, as well as less impressive salaries and benefits. Perhaps even more important, the medical assistant who does not have his or her personal life in order will not be able to offer the employer his or her best performance every day. He or she will be expected to give a full day's work for a full day's pay on every single shift. Although personal issues do affect work performance, the medical assistant must make a good effort to put personal problems aside when working.

The most important life skill one can have is the willingness to change. Many employees insist on doing things the same way they have always been done, and they resist any changes in policy or procedure. However, a medical assistant who does not welcome change and work hard to adjust to change is a failure waiting to happen.

Personal Growth

Personal growth is a comprehensive term that applies to many aspects of a person's mental, physical, and spiritual health. This growth is a result of goals that are set for self-improvement. Without clear goals, people rarely experience personal growth that is initiated from within. Growth may happen as a result of some outside influence, but a conscious effort toward personal growth is an innate decision. One goal may be to get more involved with community by helping out at the local food pantry or free clinic. This opportunity not only will help out the community, but also will expose you to things you might not otherwise see. It can also give you a feeling of accomplishment that you were able to in some way help out those less fortunate. Another goal may be to become more physically active. Starting a lunchtime walking team would be one way to become more active and can also foster teamwork and cooperation within the organization.

Steps for Achieving Goals

- Decide what you want.
- Write down the goal.
- Set the date for accomplishment.
- Read the goal three times a day.
- Think of the goal often.
- See yourself accomplishing the goal.
- Develop a plan of action for reaching the goal.
- Do not discuss the plan with others who might be discouraging.
- Be confident.
- Act successful and you will be!

No matter how great the training or how many opportunities are placed in front of a person, fear and doubt can sabotage efforts to improve the self-image, confidence, and future potential of an individual. Personal growth involves such traits as self-control, self-esteem, problem-solving skills, decision-making skills, and stress management.

Self-Control

Self-control is a vital trait in the medical office. Some patients are not at their best because of their illness, and this may make them less than cordial toward the staff. Remember that this is usually a temporary situation. A medical assistant must exercise self-control and must not respond in kind to patients who are disagreeable.

Self-control in your personal life can influence your professional behaviors in your working life. By choosing to stay home on a work night rather than going out with friends, you will be better prepared for the workday. By choosing to manage your money responsibly you will decrease your stress level and make concentrating on your job easier. Self-control is a key piece in having a successful career as a medical assistant.

Self-Esteem

Everyone has certain strengths and weaknesses. Good self-esteem is the result of knowing what those strengths are and overcoming the weaknesses. It is having a positive outlook about oneself and others. A person with good self-esteem is motivated, able to express love, and capable of handling criticism. A person's self-esteem improves if he or she has developed adaptive skills. Especially in the medical profession, one thing that is guaranteed in the workplace is change. Change can be positive or negative; this depends mostly on the way it is viewed by the individual.

A person is not doomed to live with poor self-esteem forever. Take a good look at what you do each day. How have you contributed to taking care of your patients? How have you made things easier for your co-workers? Are you making a difference? With a degree of effort and openmindedness, an individual can work toward better self-esteem, which can make a tremendous difference in the individual's future potential.

Problem-Solving Skills

For individuals to work together, they must have a degree of trust and be willing to make suggestions for the good of the group. The saying "two heads are better than one" is still true when it comes to problem solving. Employees usually want to play a part in solving

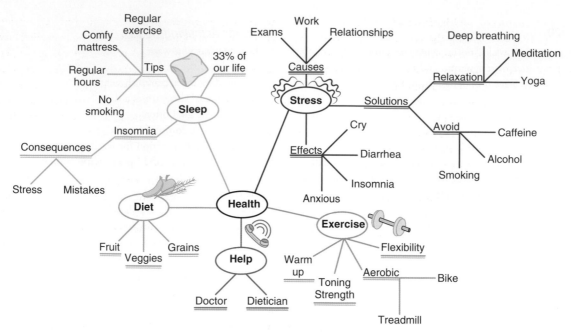

FIGURE 23-16 Mind mapping example.

the problems in the workplace, and they appreciate knowing that their opinions make a difference. Many organizations are looking for the input of their employees. A staff meeting may be called to solicit input when specific issues arise. At this meeting, brainstorming can be a useful problem-solving technique. Everyone should feel free to state his or her ideas, no matter how off-the-wall they are, and participate in the discussion to come up with a solution to the issue. Mind mapping is another problem-solving technique that can help to find a solution to the problem (Figure 23-16). With mind mapping, the problem is shown in the center of a large piece of paper or even on a white board. From this central problem, branches are drawn in all directions with important words or phrases that pertain to the central problem. Additional branches can be added to the important words or phrases until there is a comprehensive diagram of the problem and possible solutions. A medical assistant who can listen to the concerns of others and is willing to give and take will be an excellent problem solver.

Decision-Making Skills

People who know how to make good decisions usually are successful. Thinking through a decision requires logic, and it is best to take some time to think carefully of all the pros and cons. Unfortunately, a medical assistant may not always have time to consider decisions in a leisurely fashion, especially when dealing with emergencies. A good decision maker is honest in identifying the real problems and attempts to keep personal feelings isolated from the process.

There are several steps in making a sound decision. The problem must be specifically defined and evaluated so that the individual understands clearly what needs to happen to resolve the situation. Gather as much information as possible and consider all alternatives. It sometimes is helpful to choose an alternative and consider all the ramifications of making a decision using that alternative. Then, when the best alternative has been determined, the decision should be made and put into action. The last step in this process should be

to evaluate the effectiveness of the decision after a set period of time. Did the decision result in resolution of the problem or should the situation be reevaluated? Care should be taken to avoid making a decision simply because it is easy and comfortable, because more problems could arise later as a result of not addressing the true problem in the beginning.

Professional Development

Many healthcare organizations are looking for credentialed medical assistants. Being credentialed allows you to perform more of the tasks in the organization. If you are a graduate from an accredited program, you are able to take a certification examination. By doing this you are showing a potential or current employer that you are committed to your profession and have been recognized by a national agency for your knowledge about the medical assistant field. The two most common examinations are the CMA credential, given through the AAMA, and the RMA credential, given through the AMT.

Both credentials require that you participate in continuing education to maintain that credential. These CEUs help you to stay current in your field. Both organizations offer many opportunities to earn CEUs in an online format and also through attendance at national, state, or local conventions. Educational opportunities outside of these organizations may also be used for CEU credits if approved by the agency.

Professional development is an ongoing process when working in healthcare. By being committed to continue to learn about your chosen profession you will show your employer that you are a valuable asset to the organization.

Stress Management

The demands of the medical profession make it a stressful environment at times. Stress is not always bad. In fact, some stress is a positive motivator toward a goal. A *stressor* is a stimulus that prompts a reaction from the body. Positive stress, or *eustress,* includes exhilarating activities or success, which often leads to higher expectations from the person experiencing the eustress. The opposite is distress, which includes disappointment, failure, or embarrassment. Stress management is a conscious effort to control the stressors and resulting reactions so that the body and mind operate evenly, even when stress is present in an individual's life.

By learning to recognize the signs of stressful overload, a medical assistant can possibly ward off the negative reactions that are so physically and mentally draining to the body. Many people notice a headache or fatigue when overly stressed. Breathing correctly is one way to reduce stress. Often an accelerated breathing pattern that is quick and shallow is a stress indicator. Breathing from the abdomen at a slower pace, inhaling through the nose, and exhaling through the mouth may help reduce tension. Taking time for relaxing activities and getting plenty of exercise are other methods of stress reduction.

> ## Stress Management Techniques
>
> - Do something you enjoy: gardening, reading, sailing, volunteer work
> - Meditate
> - Exercise
> - Breathe deeply
> - Laugh out loud
> - Keep a gratitude journal

CLOSING COMMENTS

The period surrounding graduation is a celebration but also a busy time that requires much planning. Cooperate with the school in securing a practicum site and make an effort to obtain a site that will be the most beneficial to the career you want. Do not take a practicum site just because it is close to home. Think about the skills that will be offered and learn as much as possible. Then perform well, so that the staff and providers are happy to offer a good reference to potential employers. Strive to attain goals, and once they are reached, set additional goals to continue moving forward in life.

Even though the medical assistant educational experience ends, remember that there is constantly something new to learn in the medical profession. Join professional associations and participate in as many educational seminars and continuing education classes as possible. Remain in a continual state of learning and be determined to be the best medical assistant you can be.

Legal and Ethical Issues

Always be completely honest when completing a job application and offering information on a résumé. Most facilities stipulate that if an individual is not truthful on these documents, his or her employment can be terminated when the deception is discovered. Employers are more interested in honesty and a forthright explanation than in minor problems that affect the job performance.

If a medical assistant has had some brush with the law that requires disclosure on the job application, the best policy is to be honest and to deal with the ramifications of telling the truth. Most businesses can verify whether a potential employee has any type of criminal record. A solid explanation of the facts, admission of a past mistake, and excellent current references often prompt an employer to have faith and make a positive decision about offering employment.

> ## Professional Behaviors
>
> The development of professional behaviors must begin before the start of a new job. Use your time in school to develop those behaviors that employers are looking for: collaboration and interpersonal skills, professionalism, and compassion. By developing these behaviors in school your teachers and practicum mentors will be able to give a recommendation that stresses those skills. By being on time and prepared for class you are showing that you will be on time and prepared for work. By being diligent and self-directed in the classroom you demonstrate that you have a strong work ethic, which is an important characteristic to employers.

SUMMARY OF SCENARIO

Before graduation, Michelle was offered a job at a family practice clinic working with several physicians. She took her instructor's advice and sent a thank-you note to those who interviewed her. When she was offered the job, the supervisor mentioned how thoughtful the note was. During the call, the supervisor summarized the benefits and the starting salary. She mentioned to Michelle that all medical assistants start at the same wage, but after they pass the CMA certification examination, they get a raise. Michelle took 2 days to consider the position and decided to accept the job offer. The wage was lower than what she was hoping for, but the benefits were much better.

Krysia interviewed for several medical assistant positions over the last few weeks, finding that employers respected her service to her country and valued the skills she learned in the military service. She just received her third job offer within the last few days and has decided to accept the position at the local Veterans Affairs (VA) clinic. It is a full-time position with great benefits and the higher wage will help offset the extra mileage that she will be driving to work. She is very excited to be working with other veterans.

Zac struggled identifying what type of clinic he wanted to work for. With his strong leadership skills, he hopes to find a position where he can advance to a supervisory position. He has interviewed for job positions at small and large clinics. He is finding that he is more interested in working with surgeons than with family practitioners. He likes the complexity involved with surgical patients. He is hoping to receive a job offer shortly after graduation. He has decided that if his "dream job" is not offered to him, he will pursue a position in family medicine or internal medicine to get a solid foundation for his new career and then someday move into orthopedics or surgery.

SUMMARY OF LEARNING OBJECTIVES

1. **Define, spell, and pronounce the terms listed in the vocabulary.**
   Spelling and pronouncing terms correctly bolster the medical assistant's credibility. Knowing the definitions of these terms promotes confidence in communication with patients and co-workers.

2. **Describe the four personality traits that are most important to employers.**
   With the cost of training new employees, employers must find the best person to hire. Many employers struggle with assisting new employees to evolve or change personality traits. Thus employers seek people who already have collaboration and interpersonal skills, professionalism, compassion, and a sincere interest in the job. Collaboration and interpersonal skills allow the new employee to blend well with the current staff. Being flexible, dependable, supportive of peers, remaining calm under pressure, listening, and having good manners are just some of the characteristics of a person with great collaboration and interpersonal skills. Being professional includes proper dress and grooming habits, punctuality, honesty, attention to detail, and the abilities to follow directions, prioritize, and manage time efficiently. Providing compassionate and respectful care and supporting the patient's dignity is crucial to good patient care. Lastly, being genuinely interested in the position positively affects the person's attitude and performance in the job.

3. **Explain the three areas that need to be examined to determine one's strengths and skills.**
   A medical assistant must identify the personality traits, technical skills, and transferable job skills that he or she possesses. Using a portfolio will help the interviewee showcase the qualities that he or she has. Technical skills consist of administrative and clinical skills the person has developed during their medical assistant program. Transferable job skills are skills that were utilized in an unrelated position, but relate or transfer to the new position.

4. **Discuss career objectives and describe how personal needs affect the job search.**
   Medical assistants should take some time to think about what they want from their career and develop a career objective. Your personal needs (e.g., wage, benefits, hours, locations) help you determine what job might be right for you so you can focus your job search.

5. **Do the following related to finding a job:**
   - Explain the two best job search methods.
     The two best methods to identify jobs are through networking and using job boards. Networking involves the medical assistant exchanging information with other professionals and family members in hopes of obtaining possible job leads. Job boards are online sites that list positions posted by employers. They can be specific to the healthcare facilities or they can be managed by local media organizations. National job boards can be very helpful for those who want to relocate to another part of the country.
   - Discuss traditional job search methods.
     Traditional job search methods include school career placement offices, newspaper ads, and employment agencies.
   - Describe various ways to improve your opportunities.
     If you are having trouble finding a job, it is important to reevaluate your search methods and ask yourself some questions. Participating in volunteer activities and temporary employment can help.
   - Discuss the importance of being organized in your job search.
     Keeping organized records is critical. Keep the documents in an organized system on your computer, and make a spreadsheet, word processing document, or handwritten log that indicates the postings you have applied for.

6. **Discuss the three types of résumé formats, describe how to prepare a chronologic résumé and cover letter, and discuss the importance and format of both the résumé and cover letter.**
   The three commonly used résumé formats are chronologic, combination, and targeted résumés. Procedures 23-1 and 23-2 describe the steps involved with preparing a résumé and cover letter. As you create your résumé, keep in mind the eye appeal or interest the résumé will create in the reader. A cover letter should always accompany a résumé and much attention to detail is necessary.

7. **Discuss how to complete an online portfolio and job application.**
   Many healthcare agencies utilize the Internet during the employment process, and online portfolios can have many advantages over paper applications. However, not every employer utilizes online portfolios and students may have to fill out job applications as well. Procedure 23-3 describes the steps involved with completing a job application.

8. **Describe how to create a career portfolio.**
   Procedure 23-4 describes the steps involved with creating a career portfolio.

9. **Do the following related to the job interview:**
   - List and describe the four phases of the interview process.
     The four phases of the interview process are the preparation, the actual interview, the follow-up, and the negotiation. The preparation includes all efforts made before the actual interview in obtaining information about the company, deciding on the wardrobe, and making sure nails are groomed and shoes are shined. The interview itself is designed to help the employer and potential employee get to know each other and discover whether they are compatible. The follow-up is perhaps the most critical stage, wherein the medical assistant should send a thank-you letter and continue to stay in touch with the facility until the job is filled. The negotiation includes discussion of the salary and benefits that will be offered to the new employee.
   - List and discuss legal and illegal interview questions.
     Employers may intentionally or accidentally ask illegal interview questions, and the medical assistant has three choices in this situation: (1) refusing to answer the question, which may indicate that he or she will not tolerate difficult patients; (2) answering the question directly, which may cost the medical assistant the position; or (3) relating the question back to the position, which indicates maturity and the ability to be tactful and polite.

- Practice interview skills for a mock interview.
Refer to Procedure 23-5.
- Create a thank-you note for an interview.
Writing a thank-you note for an interview is a way to make you stand out from the other people who have interviewed for the same position. It shows that you are a courteous and conscientious person and also gives you another opportunity to show why you are the right person for the job. Refer to Procedure 23-6.

10. **Do the following related to getting a job:**
- Discuss the importance of the probationary period for a new employee.
The probationary period is a time for the new medical assistant to become oriented to the facility. It also allows the employer to assess whether the medical assistant fits with the team and performs the duties of the job in a satisfactory way. During this time, the medical assistant should demonstrate that he or she is a productive team member with an excellent attitude. There should never be idle time; rather, when all duties are completed, the medical assistant should look for ways to assist others.
- List some common early mistakes of which a new employee should be aware.
A new employee in the medical office should avoid arriving late or being absent, especially during the probationary period. He or she should never participate in office gossip and should make a good attempt to get along with every employee. A medical assistant should not make excessive supervision necessary and should be open to learning new ways of performing procedures. A new employee who fits in with the team finds the job more rewarding.

- Discuss how to be a good employee and how to deal with supervisors.
A medical assistant can be a better employee in several ways: arriving early, being honest, getting along with co-workers, consistently performing assigned duties, treating patients with compassion, and being held responsible for his or her actions. Never hesitate to approach supervisors when an issue at hand needs attention.
- Explain why a performance appraisal rating is usually not perfect.
No employee is perfect, so performance appraisals rarely have perfect ratings. Even an employee who is doing an excellent job has room for improvement in some area. Without comments that suggest improvement, the employee may not feel that the position offers growth potential. Constructive comments help a medical assistant perform better and take on more responsibility.
- Discuss how to pursue a raise and how to leave a job.
Before asking for a raise, self-reflection is necessary. Make an appointment to talk to your supervisor in private and explain why you think you deserve a raise. Do not expect a raise of more than 3% to 5% at any given time. When leaving a job, always offer at least 2 weeks' notice.

11. **Discuss various life skills needed in the workplace.**
To be successful in the job search, the medical assistant must have the basic entry-level skills needed to perform in the workplace. Even more important, he or she must develop certain life skills that are essential to any profession. Personal growth, self-control, self-esteem, problem-solving skills, decision-making skills, professional development, and stress management are all important life skills for a medical assistant to attain and continue to develop over time.

CONNECTIONS

Study Guide Connection: Go to the Chapter 23 Study Guide. Read and complete the activities.

evolve Evolve Connection: Go to the Chapter 23 link at *evolve.elsevier.com/kinn* to complete the Chapter Review Quiz. Check out the other resources listed for this chapter to make the most of what you have learned from Career Development and Life Skills.

GLOSSARY

abandonment   In medical care, the discontinuation of care without proper notice after a patient has been accepted.

ablation (a-bla′-shun)   Amputation or removal of any body part.

abscesses   Localized collections of pus, which may be under the skin or deep in the body, that cause tissue destruction.

abstract   A summary of the diagnostic statement and/or procedures and services performed.

accepting diversity   The practice of accepting every individual, regardless of age, religion, race, disability, and/or gender, in the medical practice.

accommodation   The automatic adjustment of the eye that allows a person to see various sizes of objects at different distances.

accounts payable   Money owed by a company to other companies for services and goods; pertains to paying the bills of the facility.

accreditation (u-kre-duh-ta′-shun)   The process by which an organization is recognized for adherence to a group of standards that meet or exceed the expectations of the accrediting agency.

act   The formal action of a legislative body; a decision or determination of a sovereign state, a legislative council, or a court of justice.

acute   Having a sudden onset, sharp rise, and short course; providing or requiring short-term medical care.

adhesions (ad-he′-zhuns)   Bands of scar tissue that bind together two anatomic surfaces that normally are separate.

adnexal (ad-neks′-uhl)   Pertaining to adjacent or accessory parts.

adrenocorticotropic hormone (ACTH) (uh-dren-o-cor-tih-ko-tro′-pik)   A hormone released by the anterior pituitary gland that stimulates the production and secretion of glucocorticoids.

advocate (ad′-voh-kat)   In medical care, a person who represents the patient when healthcare decisions are made.

affable   Pleasant and at ease in talking to others; characterized by ease and friendliness.

age of majority   The age at which a person is recognized by law to be an adult; it varies by state.

air kerma   Kinetic energy released in matter (Gy$_{-a}$); the SI unit for radiation exposure that represents the amount of radiation in the air that reaches the patient. It is measured in Gray, and a subscript "a" is added to indicate that it is a measurement of the radiation in the air.

albuminuria (al-byoo-muh-nur′-e-uh)   The abnormal presence of albumin protein in the urine.

aliquot (al′-ih-kwaht)   A portion of a well-mixed sample removed for testing.

allegation (al-eh-ga′-shun)   A statement by a party to a legal action of what the party undertakes to prove; an assertion made without proof.

alleviate   To partly remove or correct; to relieve or lessen.

allopathic (al-o-path′-ik)   A system of medical practice that treats disease by the use of remedies, such as medications and surgery, to produce effects different from those caused by the disease under treatment; medical doctors (MDs) and osteopaths (DOs) practice allopathic medicine; also called conventional medicine.

alopecia (al-o-pe′-se-uh)   Partial or complete lack of hair.

alphabetic filing   Any system that arranges names or topics according to the sequence of the letters in the alphabet.

alphanumeric   Of or relating to systems made up of combinations of letters and numbers.

amblyopia (am-ble-o′-pe-uh)   Reduction or dimness of vision with no apparent organic cause; often referred to as *lazy eye syndrome*.

amenity (uh-me′-nuh-te)   Something conducive to comfort, convenience, or enjoyment.

amino acids   The organic compounds that form the chief constituents of protein; they are used by the body to build and repair tissues.

analyte   The substance or chemical being analyzed or detected in a specimen.

anaphylaxis (an-uh-fih-lak′-sis)   An exaggerated hypersensitivity reaction that in severe cases leads to vascular collapse, bronchospasm, and shock.

anaplastic   Relating to an alteration in cells to a more primitive form; a term that describes cancer-producing cells.

anastomosis (uh-nas-tuh-mo′-sis)   The surgical joining of two normally distinct organs.

anemia   A condition marked by a deficiency of red blood cells (RBCs).

angina pectoris (an-ji′-nuh/pek′-tuh-ris)   A spasmlike pain in the chest caused by myocardial anoxia.

angiocardiography (an-je-o-kahr-de-og′-ruh-fe)   Radiography of both the heart and great vessels using an iodine contrast medium.

angiography (an-je-og′-ruh-fe)   The process of producing an image of blood vessels using an iodine contrast medium.

angioplasty (an′-je-o-plas-te)   A technique in which a catheter is used to open or widen a blood vessel narrowed by stenoses or occlusions to improve circulation.

anomaly (uh-nom′-uh-le)   A congenital malformation that occurs during fetal development.

anorexia (ah-nuh-rek′-se-uh)   A lack or loss of appetite for food.

answering service   A business that receives and answers telephone calls for the healthcare facility when it is closed.

anterior (an-tuhr′-e-ohr)   The front part of the body or body part when a person is in anatomic position.

anteroposterior (AP) projection (an-tuhr-o-pos-ter′-e-ohr)   A frontal projection, in which the central ray enters the front of the patient and exits the back to reach the image receptor; the patient is supine or facing the x-ray tube.

anti–kickback statute   A criminal law that prohibits the exchange of anything of value in an effort to reward the referral of a patient sponsored by a government insurance plan

antibodies (an′-tih-bah-dees)   Molecular proteins (immunoglobulins) produced by the blood's plasma cells that specifically destroy a foreign invader or substance that has infected the body.

anticoagulant   Chemicals added to a blood sample after collection to prevent clotting.

antigen (an′-tih-juhn) A foreign invader (e.g., bacterium, virus, toxin, allergen) that generates an immune response, including the production of antibodies.

antimicrobial agents A general term for drugs, chemicals, or other substances that either kill or slow the growth of microbes. Among the antimicrobial agents are antibacterial drugs, antiviral agents, antifungal agents, and antiparasitic drugs.

antiseptic (an-tih-sep′-tik) An agent that inhibits the growth of microorganisms on living tissue (e.g., alcohol and povidone-iodine solution [Betadine]); used to cleanse the skin, wounds, and so on.

anuria The absence of urine production.

aortogram (a-or′-toh-gram) An image of the aorta produced using an iodine contrast medium.

apnea (ap′-ne-uh) Absence or cessation of breathing.

appellate (uh-peh′-lut) A term referring to courts that have the power to review and change the decisions of a lower court.

aqueous (ak′-we-uhs) A waterlike substance; a medication prepared with water.

arbitration (ahr-buh-tra′-shun) A type of alternative dispute resolution that provides parties to a controversy with a choice other than going to court for resolution of a problem. Arbitration is either court-ordered to resolve a conflict, or the two sides select an impartial third party, known as an arbitrator, and agree in advance to comply with the arbitrator's award. The arbitrator's decision is usually final.

arrhythmia An abnormality or irregularity in the heart rhythm.

arteriography (ahr-ter-e-og′-ruh-fe) The technique of producing an image of arteries using an iodine contrast medium.

arteriosclerosis (ahr-ter′-e-o-scler-o-sis) A condition marked by thickening, decreased elasticity, and calcification of arterial walls.

arthritis (ahr-thry′-tis) Inflammation of a joint.

arthrogram (ahr′-thro-gram) Fluoroscopic examination of the soft tissue components of joints, in which a contrast medium is injected directly into the joint capsule.

arthropods (ahr′-throh-pods) A class of invertebrate animals that includes insects, crustaceans, spiders, scorpions, and others.

articular (ahr-tih′-kyuh-luhr) Pertaining to a joint.

artifacts Structures or features not normally present but visible as a result of an external agent or action, such as in a microscopic specimen after fixation or in a radiographic image.

ascites (uh-si′-tez) An abnormal collection of fluid in the peritoneal cavity containing high levels of protein and electrolytes.

assault An intentional attempt to cause bodily harm to another; a threat to cause harm is an assault if it is combined with a physical action (e.g., a raised fist) so that the victim could reasonably assume there would be an assault.

asymptomatic Without symptoms of a disease process.

asystole (a-sis′-toh-le) The absence of a heartbeat.

ataxia (uh-taks′-e-uh) Failure or irregularity of muscle actions and coordination.

atria The two upper chambers of the heart.

atrioventricular (AV) node The part of the cardiac conduction system between the atria and the ventricles.

attenuated (uh-ten′-yoo-wat-ed) Weakened or changed; refers to the virulence of a pathogenic microorganism in reference to vaccine development.

audiologist (aw-de-ah′-loh-jist) Allied healthcare professional who specializes in evaluation of hearing function, detection of hearing impairment, and determination of the anatomic site of impairment.

audit An inspection performed before claims are submitted to examine them for accuracy and completeness.

audit trail A record of computer activity used to monitor users' actions within software, including additions, deletions, and viewing of electronic records.

augment To increase in size or amount; to add to so as to improve or complete.

aura A peculiar sensation that precedes the appearance of a more definite disturbance; commonly seen with migraines or seizure activity.

auscultation The act of listening to body sounds, typically with a stethoscope, to assess various organs throughout the body.

authorized agent A person who has written documentation that he or she can accept a shipment for another individual.

autoimmune (aw-to-im-yoon′) Pertaining to a disturbance in the immune system in which the body reacts against its own tissue. Examples of autoimmune disorders include multiple sclerosis, rheumatoid arthritis, and systemic lupus erythematosus.

automatic call routing A system that distributes incoming calls to a specific group or person based on the caller's need; for example, the individual presses 1 for appointments, 2 for billing questions, and so on.

autonomy (aw-ton′-oh-me) The ability to function independently.

axial projections Radiographs taken with a longitudinal angulation of the x-ray beam; sometimes referred to as *semiaxial projections*.

azotemia (a-zo-te′-me-uh) A condition marked by the retention of excessive quantities of nitrogenous wastes in the blood.

back up The process of copying and archiving computer data so that the duplicate files can be used to restore the original data if a compromise occurs.

backorder An order placed for an item that is temporarily out of stock and will be sent at a later time.

bacteriuria The presence of bacteria in the urine (possible infection).

bailiff An officer of some U.S. courts who usually serves as a messenger or usher and who keeps order at the request of the judge.

Bartholin's cyst A fluid-filled cyst in one of the vestibular glands located on either side of the vaginal orifice.

basement membrane A deep layer of the skin that secures the epithelium to underlying tissue; it separates the epidermis from the dermis.

battery An intentional act of contact with another that causes harm or offends the individual being touched or injured.

benign A tumor or tissue growth that is not cancerous; it may require treatment or removal, depending on its location, and/or for cosmetic reasons.

benign Not cancerous and not recurring.

bevel (bev′-uhl) The angled tip of a needle.

bifurcates Divides from one into two branches.

bilirubin (bih-lih-roo′-bin) An orange pigment in bile; its accumulation leads to jaundice.

bilirubinuria (bi-li-roo-bin-yuhr′-e-uh) The presence of bilirubin in the urine (possible liver damage).

billable service Assistance (i.e., service) that is provided by a healthcare provider that can be billed to the insurance company and/or patient.

biophysical (bi-o-fih′-zih-kuhl) The science of applying physical laws and theories to biologic problems.

blatant Completely obvious, conspicuous, or obtrusive, especially in a crass or offensive manner; brazen.

blood-brain barrier An anatomic-physiologic structure made up of astrocyte glial cells that prevents or slows the transfer of chemicals into the neurons of the central nervous system (CNS).

bonded Referring to a guarantee obtained by an employer from an insurance company (i.e., a fidelity bond) that the company will cover losses from an employee's dishonest acts (e.g., embezzlement, theft).

bounding A term used to describe a pulse that feels full because of increased power of cardiac contraction or as a result of increased blood volume.

bradycardia (brad-ih-kahr′-de-uh) A slow heartbeat; a pulse below 60 beats per minute.

bradypnea (brad-ip′-ne′-uh) Respirations that are regular in rhythm but slower than normal in rate.

broad-spectrum antimicrobial agents Drugs used to treat a wide range of infections.

bronchiectasis (brong-ke-ek′-tuh-sis) Dilation of the bronchi and bronchioles associated with secondary infection or ciliary dysfunction.

bronchoconstriction Narrowing of the bronchiole tubes.

bronchodilator (brahn-ko-di′-la-tuhr) A drug that relaxes contractions of the smooth muscle of the bronchioles to improve lung ventilation.

bruit (broo′-it) An abnormal sound or murmur heard on auscultation of an organ, vessel (e.g., carotid artery), or gland; it is caused by the flow of blood through a narrowed or partially occluded vessel.

Bucky A moving grid device that holds an image receptor and prevents scatter radiation from fogging the image.

buffy coat The layer of white cells or platelets found between the plasma and the packed red blood cells after whole blood has been centrifuged.

bundle of His Specialized muscle fibers that conduct electrical impulses from the AV node to the ventricular myocardium.

bursae (bur′-say) Fluid-filled, saclike membranes that provide cushioning and allow frictionless motion between two tissues.

buying cycle The frequency with which an item is purchased; it depends on how often the item is used and the storage space available for it.

calibration Determining the accuracy of an instrument by comparing its output with that of a known standard or another instrument known to be accurate.

call forwarding A telephone feature that allows calls made to one number to be forwarded to another specified number.

caller ID A feature that identifies and displays the telephone numbers of incoming calls made to a particular line.

candidiasis (kan-dih-di′-uh-sis) An infection caused by a yeast that typically affects the vaginal mucosa and skin.

cannula (kan′-yoo-lah) A rigid tube that surrounds a blunt trocar or a sharp, pointed trocar, which is inserted into the body; when the trocar is withdrawn, fluid may escape from the body through the cannula, depending on the insertion site.

capitation A contract between the health insurance plan and the provider for which the health insurance plan will pay an agreed-upon monthly fee per patient and the provider agrees to provide medical services on a regular basis.

caption A heading, title, or subtitle under which records are filed.

carcinogens (kar-sih′-noh-juhns) Substances or agents that cause the development of cancer or increase its incidence.

cardiac arrest A condition in which cardiac contractions stop completely.

cardioversion The use of electroshock to convert an abnormal cardiac rhythm to a normal one.

cartilage (kahr′-til-ij) A rubbery, smooth, somewhat elastic connective tissue that covers the ends of bones.

cash on hand The amount of money the healthcare practice has in the bank that can be withdrawn as cash.

cassette A special container that holds either film or a phosphorescent screen inside; it is used to transform an x-ray beam into a visible image; also referred to as an *image receptor* when loaded.

cast In kidney disease, a fibrous or protein material molded to the shape of the part in which it has accumulated that is thrown off into the urine. Casts may be identified as hyaline, cellular, granular, or waxy.

cathartics Laxative preparations.

caustic (kos′-tik) A substance that burns or destroys tissue by chemical action.

cell-mediated immunity An immune response that occurs from the action of T lymphocytes rather than from the production of antibodies.

central ray (CR) An imaginary line in the center of the x-ray beam that leaves the tube and reaches the patient.

centrifuge (sen′-trih-fuhj) An apparatus consisting essentially of a compartment that spins about a central axis to separate contained materials of different specific gravities or to separate colloidal particles suspended in a liquid.

Certified Registered Nurse Anesthetist (CRNA) A nursing healthcare professional who is certified to administer anesthesia.

cerumen (seh-room′-en) A waxy secretion in the ear canal; commonly called *ear wax.*

cervical (ser′-vih-kuhl) Pertaining to the neck region containing seven cervical vertebrae.

chain of command A series of executive positions in order of authority.

characteristics Distinguishing traits, qualities, or properties.

Cheyne-Stokes respirations A breathing pattern characterized by rhythmic changes in the depth of respiration. The patient breathes deeply for a short time and then breathes very slightly or stops breathing altogether; the pattern occurs over and over, every 45 seconds to 3 minutes. The Cheyne-Stokes breathing pattern is seen in patients with heart failure or brain damage, but also in healthy individuals who hyperventilate, at high altitudes, and with hypnotic drug or narcotic overdose and sleep apnea.

cholesterol (kuh-les′-tuh-rol) A substance produced by the liver and found in animal fats; it can result in fatty deposits or atherosclerotic plaques in blood vessels.

chordae tendineae (kor′-duh/ten′-din-uh) The tendons that anchor the cusps of the heart valves to the papillary muscles of the myocardium, preventing valvular prolapse.

chromosomes Threadlike molecules that carry hereditary information.

chronic A term describing a disease that manifests over a long period because medical treatment has not been able to resolve it.

chronic bronchitis Recurrent inflammation of the membranes lining the bronchial tubes.

chronic obstructive pulmonary disease (COPD) A progressive, irreversible lung condition that results in diminished lung capacity.

cicatrix Early scar tissue that appears pale, contracted, and firm.

cilia (sil′-e-uh) Hairlike projections capable of movement; in the lungs, cilia waves move unwanted substances (e.g., mucus, dust, and pus) upward; cilia are destroyed by smoking.

cirrhosis (suh-ro′-sis) A chronic, degenerative disease of the liver that interferes with normal liver function.

Clinitest A test tablet commonly used to screen for and confirm glucose and/or to detect other sugars in urine.

clitoris (klih′-tuh-ris) A small, elongated erectile body above the urinary meatus at the superior point of the labia minora.

clubbing Abnormal enlargement of the distal phalanges (fingers and toes); it is associated with cyanotic heart disease or advanced chronic pulmonary disease.

coagulate (ko-ag′-yuh-late) To form into clots.

Coding Clinic A medical coding industry journal that provides insight into the coding of complex medical cases. The journal is sponsored by the American Hospital Association (AHA), which also supports a website (*www.codingclinicadvisor.com*) that can accept questions from coders on specific cases.

cognitive (kog′-nih-tiv) Pertaining to the operation of the mind; referring to the process by which we become aware of perceiving, thinking, and remembering.

cohesive Sticking together tightly; exhibiting or producing cohesion.

coitus Sexual union of a male and a female; also called *intercourse*.

collagen (kah′-luh-jen) The protein that forms the inelastic fibers of tendons, ligaments, and fascia.

colloidal (kah-loid′-uhl) Pertaining to a gluelike substance.

colonoscopy A procedure in which a fiberoptic scope is used to examine the large intestine.

colostrum (koh-lahs′-trum) A thin, yellow, milky fluid secreted by the mammary glands a few days before and after delivery.

coma An unconscious state from which the patient cannot be aroused.

competencies Mastery of the knowledge, skills, and behaviors that are expected of the entry-level medical assistant.

compliance In a medical practice, meeting the standards and regulations of the practice's established policies and procedures.

compression The state of being pressed together.

computed radiography (CR) A modernized x-ray film technique in which a reusable cassette-plate image receptor stores the image, much as a flash drive functions in household computers.

computed tomography (CT) A computerized x-ray imaging modality that provides axial and three-dimensional scans.

computer network A system that links personal computers and peripheral devices to share information and resources.

computer on wheels (COW) Wireless mobile workstation; also called *workstation on wheels* (WOW).

computerized provider/physician order entry (CPOE) The process of entering medication orders or other provider instructions into the electronic health record (EHR).

cones Structures in the retina that make the perception of color possible.

conference call A telephone call in which a caller can speak with several people at the same time.

congenital (kuhn-jen′-ih-tul) An anomaly or defect that is present at birth.

congruence (kon-groo′-ents) Agreement; the state that occurs when the verbal expression of the message matches the sender's nonverbal body language.

contamination (kun-ta-mu-na′-shun) The process by which something becomes harmful or unusable through contact with something unclean; soiled with pathogens or infectious material; nonsterile.

continuing medical education (CME) Activities (e.g., conferences, seminars) that promote further education for physicians and providers.

continuity of care Continuation of care smoothly from one provider to another, so that the patient receives the most benefit and no interruption in care.

contrast media Substances used to enhance the visibility of soft tissues in imaging studies.

contributory negligence Instances in which the individual contributes to the injury or condition; the injury is partly due to the individual's own negligence.

control booth A separated area or room where the radiographer can remain safe from radiation while operating radiography equipment. It is protected by a special wall and/or window lined with lead. This area houses the control console, which contains the settings for the machine.

copulation Sexual intercourse.

corticosteroids (kawr-tih-koh-ster′-oidz) Antiinflammatory hormones, which may be natural or synthetic.

costal Pertaining to the ribs.

counteroffer A return offer made by a person who has rejected an offer or a job.

CPT Assistant An online CPT coding journal, supported by the American Medical Association (AMA), that addresses subjects such as appealing insurance denials, validating coding to auditors, training staff members, and answering day-to-day coding questions.

crash carts Carts stocked with emergency medications and equipment (e.g., oxygen, intravenous [IV], and airway supplies) that are readily available.

creatinine (kre′-a-tuhn-en) Nitrogenous waste from muscle metabolism that is excreted in urine.

credit A bookkeeping entry which increases accounts receivable, or what is owed to the provider

crenate A term describing notched or leaflike, scalloped edges (as seen in shrinking red blood cells).

crepitation (krch-pih-ta′-shun) A dry, crackling sound or sensation.

critical thinking The constant practice of considering all aspects of a situation when deciding what to believe or what to do.

cryosurgery   The technique of exposing tissue to extreme cold to produce a well-defined area of cell destruction.

cryptogenic (krip-tuh-jeh′-nik)   Pertaining to a disease with an unknown cause.

culpability   Meriting condemnation, responsibility, or blame, especially as wrong or harmful.

culture and sensitivity (C&S)   A procedure in which a specimen is cultured on artificial media to detect bacterial or fungal growth; this is followed by appropriate screening for antibiotic sensitivity. C&S is performed in the microbiology referral laboratory.

curettage (kyur-eh-tahjz′)   The act of scraping a body cavity with a surgical instrument, such as a curette.

cuvette   A small tube or specimen container made of plastic or glass designed to hold samples for laboratory tests using light-meter technology (spectrophotometry).

cyanosis (si-an-o′-sis)   A blue coloration of the mucous membranes and body extremities caused by lack of oxygen.

cyst   A small, capsulelike sac that encloses certain organisms in their dormant or larval stage.

cytology (si-tah′-loh-je)   The study of cells using microscopic methods.

damages   Money awarded by a court to an individual who has been injured through the wrongful conduct of another party. Damages attempt to measure in financial terms the extent of harm the victim has suffered. Harm may be an actual physical injury but can also be damage to property or the individual's reputation.

data server   Computer hardware and software that perform data analysis, storage, and archiving; also called a *database server*.

débridement   The surgical removal of dead, damaged, or infected tissue to improve the function of healthy tissue.

decedent (dih-se′-dent)   A legal term for a deceased person.

decryption   The computer process of changing encrypted text to readable or plain text after a user enters a secret key or password.

decubitus ulcer   A sore or ulcer that develops over a bony prominence as the result of ischemia from prolonged pressure; also called a *bed sore*.

defendant   A person required to answer in a legal action or suit; in criminal cases, the person accused of a crime.

defibrillator   A machine that delivers an electroshock to the heart through electrodes placed on the chest wall.

deficiencies (dih-fih′-shun-sees)   Conditions that result from below normal intake of particular substances.

dehiscence   The separation of wound edges or rupture of a wound closure.

demeanor (dih-me′-nur)   Behavior toward others; outward manner.

demographics   Statistical data of a population. In healthcare this includes the patient's name, address, date of birth, employment, and other details.

depreciate   The decline in the value of an item over a certain period; used for tax purposes.

dermatome (dur′-muh-tohm)   An area on the surface of the body that is innervated by nerve fibers from one spinal nerve root.

descendants   Family members that take responsibility over the patient's estate after their death.

detrimental (deh-trih-men′-til)   Obviously harmful or damaging.

diabetes mellitus type 1   A disease in which the beta cells in the pancreas no longer produce insulin. The individual must rely on daily insulin administration to use glucose for energy and prevent complications.

diabetes mellitus type 2   A disease in which the body is unable to use glucose for energy as a result either of inadequate insulin production in the pancreas or resistance to insulin on the cellular level.

diabetic retinopathy   A condition in which microaneurysms and weakness in the capillary wall within the retina result in ischemia and tissue death.

diagnostic statement   Information about a patient's diagnosis or diagnoses that has been extracted from the medical documentation, such as the history and physical findings, operative reports, and encounter form.

diaphoresis (di-uh-fuh-re′-sis)   The profuse excretion of sweat.

diaphysis (di-ah′-fuh-sis)   The midportion of a long bone; it contains the medullary cavity.

diastole   The period of relaxation of the chambers of the heart, during which blood enters the heart from the vascular system and the lungs.

dictation (dik-ta′-shun)   The act or manner of uttering words to be transcribed.

digestion   The process of converting food into chemical substances that can be absorbed and used by the body.

digital radiography (DR)   A radiographic technique that does not use cassettes; instead, the radiographic equipment has built-in image receptors that react to radiation and transmit a digital signal directly to the computer.

dignity   Being worthy of honor and respect from others.

dilation   The opening or widening of the circumference of a body orifice with a dilating instrument; also, the opening of the cervix in the process of labor, measured as 0 to 10 cm.

dilation and curettage (D&C)   The widening of the cervix and scraping of the endometrial wall of the uterus.

diluent   A fluid that makes a solution less concentrated; it is added to vials of powdered medications to create a solution of the drug for injection.

diplopia (dih-plo′-pe-uh)   Double vision.

direct filing system   A filing system in which materials can be located without consulting an intermediary source of reference.

discrepancy   A lack of correspondence between what is stated and what is found; for instance, when what is stated on the packing slip is different from what is found in the box.

discretionary income   Money in a bank account that is not assigned to pay for any office expenses.

disinfectant   A liquid chemical that is capable of eliminating many or all pathogens but is not effective against bacterial spores; it cannot be used on the skin.

disinfected   The state in which pathogenic organisms have been destroyed or rendered inactive (disinfection procedures do not have this effect on spores, tuberculosis bacilli, and certain viruses).

disparaging   Slighting; having a negative or degrading tone.

dispense   To prepare a drug for administration.

disruption   An unexpected event that throws a plan into disorder; an interruption that prevents a system or process from continuing as usual or as expected.

dissect   To cut or separate tissue with a cutting instrument or scissors.

disseminate (dih-se'-muh-na-te) To disburse; to spread around.

diurnal rhythm (di-ur'-nl) A pattern of activity or behavior that follows a day-night cycle.

diverticulosis (di-vuhr-tih-kyuh-lo'-sis) The presence of pouchlike herniations through the muscular layer of the colon.

dosimeter A badge for monitoring the radiation exposure of personnel.

due process A fundamental constitutional guarantee that all legal proceedings will be fair; that one will be given notice of the proceedings and an opportunity to be heard before the government acts to take away life, liberty, or property; a constitutional guarantee that a law will not be unreasonable or arbitrary.

dumb terminal A personal computer that doesn't contain a hard drive and allows the user only limited functions, including access to software, the network, and/or the Internet.

dyspepsia An uncomfortable feeling of fullness, heartburn, bloating, and nausea.

dysphagia Difficulty swallowing.

dysplasia An alteration in cell growth, causing differences in size, shape, and appearance.

dyspnea (disp-ne'-uh) Difficult or painful breathing.

dysuria Painful or difficulty urination.

e-prescribing The use of electronic software to communicate with pharmacies and send prescribing information. It takes the place of writing a prescription by hand and giving it to a patient; most new or refill prescriptions can be submitted electronically, cutting down on fraud and errors.

ecchymosis (eh-kih-moh'-sis) A hemorrhagic skin discoloration, commonly called *bruising*.

ectopic (ek-top'-ik) Originating outside the normal tissue.

edema (ih-de'-muh) An abnormal accumulation of fluid in the interstitial spaces of tissues.

effacement The thinning of the cervix during labor, measured in percentages from 0% to 100%.

elastin An essential part of elastic connective tissue; when moist, it is flexible and elastic.

electrocardiogram (ihlek-tro-kar'-de-uh-gram) A graphic record of electrical conduction through the heart.

electrodesiccation The destruction of cells and tissue by means of short high-frequency electrical sparks.

electronic health record (EHR) An electronic record of health-related information about a patient that conforms to nationally recognized interoperability standards and that can be created, managed, and consulted by authorized clinicians and staff members *from more than one healthcare organization.*

electronic medical record (EMR) An electronic record of health-related information about an individual that can be created, gathered, managed, and consulted by authorized clinicians and staff members *within a single healthcare organization.* An EMR is an electronic version of a paper record.

emancipated minor A person under the age of majority (usually 18) who has been legally separated from his or her parents by the courts. The person is responsible for his or her own care.

embezzlement The misuse of a healthcare facility's funds for personal gain.

embolus A mass of undissolved matter that blocks a blood vessel; frequently a blood clot that has traveled from some other part of the body.

emergency An unexpected, life-threatening situation that requires immediate action.

emetic (eh-met'-ik) A substance that causes vomiting.

empathy (em'-puh-the) Sensitivity to the individual needs and reactions of patients.

emphysema (em-fih-ze'-muh) The pathologic accumulation of air in the alveoli, which results in alveolar destruction and overall oxygen deprivation; the bronchioles become plugged with mucus and lose elasticity.

empower To delegate more responsibilities to employees (a management theory).

encounter Every meeting between a patient and a healthcare provider. The patient's history and chief complaint, in addition to the medical services provided, are documented in the patient's health record.

endemic (en-dem'-ik) A term describing a disease or microorganism that is specific to a particular geographic area.

endocervical curettage The scraping of cells from the wall of the uterus.

endorser The person who signs his or her name on the back of a check for the purpose of transferring all rights in the check to another party.

endoscope (en'-duh-skohp) An illuminated optic instrument for visualization of the inside of the body; it may be inserted through an incision in minimally invasive surgery.

enteric coated A term describing an oral medication that is coated to protect the drug against the stomach juices; this design is used to ensure that the medicine is absorbed in the small intestine.

enunciation The use of articulate, clear sounds when speaking.

enzymatic reaction A specific chemical reaction controlled by an enzyme.

enzymes Complex proteins produced by cells that act as catalysts in specific biochemical reactions.

epiphyseal plate (eh-pih-fiz'-e-uhl) A thin layer of cartilage located at the ends of a long bone where new bone forms.

epiphysis (eh-pih'-fih-sis) The end of a long bone; it contains the growth (epiphyseal) plates.

eponym In medical terms, a name of a medical diagnosis or procedure derived from the name of the person who discovered it.

erythropoietin (ih-rith-ruh-poi'-eh-tuhn) A substance released by the kidneys and liver that promotes red blood cell formation.

eschar Devitalized skin that forms a scab or a dry crust over a burn area.

esophageal varices (ih-sah-fuh-je'-uhl var'-uh-sez) Varicose veins of the esophagus that occur as a result of portal hypertension; these vessels can easily hemorrhage.

essential hypertension Elevated blood pressure of unknown cause that develops for no apparent reason; sometimes called *primary hypertension.*

established patients Patients who are returning to the office who have previously been seen by the provider.

Ethernet A communication system for connecting several computers so information can be shared.

etiology   The cause of a disorder; a claim may be classified according to the etiology.

eukaryote (yoo-kar'-e-oht)   Single-celled or multicellular organism in which each cell contains a distinct membrane-bound nucleus.

evert   To turn the eyelid inside out; this typically is done by the provider to inspect the area for foreign bodies.

exacerbation (ig-zas'-er-ba-shun)   An increase in the seriousness of a disease, marked by greater intensity of the signs.

exclusions   Limitations on an insurance contract for which benefits are not payable.

excoriation (ik-skawr-e-a'-shun)   Inflammation and irritation of the skin; abrasions.

executor   The individual assigned to make financial decisions for a deceased patient.

expediency (ik-spe'-de-en-se)   A means of achieving a particular end, as in a situation requiring haste or caution.

expert witnesses   Individuals who provide testimony to a court as experts in certain fields or subjects to verify facts presented by one or both sides in a lawsuit. They typically are compensated and used to refute or disprove the claims of one party.

Explanation of Benefits (EOB)   A document sent by the insurance company to the provider and the patient explaining the allowed charge amount, the amount reimbursed for services, and the patient's financial responsibilities.

exposure time   The duration of the patient's x-ray exposure, in seconds; the amount of x-rays produced depends on the length of exposure.

extern   A student volunteering in the medical office for experience only; externs do not earn any wages for the work they perform.

exudates (ek'-syu-dats)   Fluids with high concentrations of protein and cellular debris that have escaped from the blood vessels and have been deposited in tissues or on tissue surfaces.

familial   Occurring in or affecting members of a family more than would be expected by chance.

fascia   A sheet or band of fibrous tissue deep in the skin that covers muscles and body organs.

febrile (feb'-ril)   Pertaining to an elevated body temperature.

fecalith (fe'-kuh-lith)   A hard, impacted mass of feces in the colon.

Federal Reserve Bank   The central bank of the United States. The Federal Reserve system consists of a seven-member Board of Governors with headquarters in Washington, D.C., and 12 Federal Reserve banks in major cities throughout the country.

fee-for-service   A reimbursement model in which the health plan pays the provider's fee for every health insurance claim.

fibrillation   Rapid, random, ineffective contractions of the heart.

filtrate   The fluid that remains after a liquid is passed through a filter.

firewall   A program or hardware that acts as a filter between the network and the Internet.

fissures   Narrow slits or clefts in the abdominal wall.

fistula (fis'-chuh-luh)   An abnormal, tubelike passage between internal organs or from an internal organ to the body's surface.

flatus   Gas expelled through the anus.

flora   Microorganisms that live on or within the body; they compete with disease-producing microorganisms and provide a natural immunity against certain infections.

fluoroscopy (floo-ros'-kuh-pe)   Direct observation of an x-ray image in motion.

follicle-stimulating hormone (FSH)   A hormone secreted by the anterior pituitary; it stimulates oogenesis and spermatogenesis.

follow-up appointment   An appointment type used when a patient needs to see the provider after a condition should have been resolved or for monitoring of an ongoing condition, such as hypertension; also known as a *recheck appointment*.

fomites   Contaminated, nonliving objects (e.g., examination room equipment) that can transmit infectious organisms.

fontanelle (fon-tan-el')   A space covered by thick membranes between the sutures of an infant's skull; called the baby's "soft spots"; there are both anterior and posterior fontanelles.

formulary   A list of drugs compiled by a health insurance company that identifies the drugs the insurance company will cover under benefits.

fornix   A recess in the upper part of the vagina caused by protrusion of the cervix into the vaginal wall.

fovea centralis (fo'-ve-uh/sen-trah'-lis)   A small pit in the center of the retina that is considered the center of clearest vision.

free radicals   Compounds with at least one unpaired electron, which makes the compound unstable and highly reactive. Free radicals are believed to damage cell components, ultimately leading to cancer, heart disease, or other diseases.

fundus   The curved, top portion of the uterus; the fundal height can be used as a measurement of fetal growth and estimated gestation.

gait   The manner or style of walking.

gangrene   The death of body tissue as a result of loss of nutritive supply, followed by bacterial invasion and putrefaction.

gantry   A doughnut-shaped portion of a scanner that surrounds the patient and functions, at least partly, to gather imaging data.

gatekeeper   In medical care, the primary care physician, who can approve or deny when the patient seeks additional care via a referral to a specialist or further medical tests.

generic   A medication that is not protected by trademark.

genus   A classification representing a family of microorganisms and all living beings. The genus is the first name assigned to a microorganism and it is italicized and capitalized.

germicides (jur'-mih-sides)   Agents that destroy pathogenic organisms.

girth   The measurement around something; when referring to mail, it is the measurement around the middle of the package that is being shipped.

gleaned   Gathered bit by bit (e.g., information or material); picked over in search of relevant material.

global services   For purposes of CPT coding, medical services and procedures performed for the patient before, during, and after a surgical procedure that is included with the assigned CPT code.

glomerulonephritis (glo-mer'-yoo-lo-neh-fri'-tis)   Inflammation of the glomerulus of the kidney.

gluconeogenesis (glu-kuh-ne-uh-jeh'-nuh-sis)   The formation of glucose in the liver from proteins and fats.

glycogen   The sugar (starch) formed from glucose; it is stored mainly in the liver.

glycosuria   An elevated urinary glucose level (which may be an indicator of diabetes mellitus).

goniometer (goh-ne-om′-ih-ter) An instrument for measuring the degrees of motion in a joint.

gonioscopy (goh-ne-os′-kuh-pe) A procedure in which a mirrored optical instrument is used to visualize the filtration angle of the anterior chamber of the eye; the procedure is used to diagnose glaucoma.

government-sponsored health insurance Health insurance programs that are sponsored by the government and offer coverage for the elderly, disabled, military, and indigent.

gray (Gy) The international unit of radiation dose.

growth hormone (GH) A hormone that stimulates tissue growth and restricts tissue glucose dependence when nutrients are not available; also called *somatotropic hormone*.

guarantor The individual who subscribes to the insurance plan and accepts financial responsibility for the patient.

guardian ad litem An individual who is assigned by the court to be legally responsible for protecting the well-being and interests of a ward, typically a minor or a person who has been declared legally incompetent.

harmonious Marked by accord in sentiment or action; having the parts agreeably related.

healthcare clearinghouses Businesses that receive healthcare transactions from healthcare providers, translate the data from a given format into one acceptable to the intended payer, and forward the processed transaction to designated payers. They include billing services, community health information systems, and private network providers or "value-added" networks that facilitate electronic data interchanges.

hematemesis (hi-mat-uh-me′-sis) Vomiting of bright red blood, indicating rapid upper gastrointestinal (GI) bleeding. Hematemesis is associated with esophageal varices or a peptic ulcer.

hematocrit The percentage by volume of packed red blood cells in a given sample of blood after centrifugation.

hematopoiesis (he-ma-tuh-poi-e′-sis) The formation and development of red blood cells in the bone marrow.

hematuria (he-ma-tuhr′-e-uh) Blood in the urine (may indicate trauma or infection in the urinary tract).

hemoconcentration The condition in which the concentration of blood cells is increased in proportion to the plasma.

hemoglobin (he′-muh-glo-bun) A protein found in erythrocytes that transports molecular oxygen in the blood.

hemoglobinuria Hemoglobin in the urine (from destruction of red blood cells).

hemolysis (he-mah′-luh-sis) The destruction or dissolution of red blood cells, with subsequent release of hemoglobin.

hemolyzed A term used to describe a blood sample in which the red blood cells have ruptured.

hepatomegaly (heh-puh-to-meh′-guh-le) Abnormal enlargement of the liver.

hereditary (heh-re′-duh-ter-e) Pertaining to a characteristic, condition, or disease transmitted from parent to offspring on the DNA chain.

hertz The unit of measurement used in hearing examinations; a wave frequency equal to 1 cycle per second.

holistic (ho-lis′-tik) A form of healing that considers the whole person (i.e., body, mind, spirit, and emotions) in individual treatment plans.

homeostasis Internal adaptation and change in response to environmental factors; multiple functions that attempt to keep the body's functions in balance.

hospice (hos′-pis) A concept of care in which health professionals and volunteers provide medical, psychological, and spiritual support to terminally ill patients and their loved ones.

HR file The human resource file, which contains all documents related to an individual's employment.

human chorionic gonadotropin (HCG) A hormone, secreted by the placenta, found in the urine of pregnant females.

hydrocephaly (hi-dro-seh′-fuh-le) Enlargement of the cranium caused by abnormal accumulation of cerebrospinal fluid in the cerebral system.

hydrogenated (hi-drah′-juh-na-ted) Combined with, treated with, or exposed to hydrogen.

hypercapnia (hi-per-kap′-ne-uh) Excess levels of carbon dioxide in the blood.

hypercholesterolemia (hi-per-kuh-les-tuh-ruh-le′-me-uh) Elevated blood levels of cholesterol.

hyperplasia An increase in the number of normal cells.

hyperpnea (hy-per-ne′-uh) An increase in the depth of breathing.

hypertension High blood pressure.

hyperventilation Abnormally prolonged and deep breathing, usually associated with acute anxiety or emotional tension.

hypotension Blood pressure that is below normal (systolic pressure below 90 mm Hg and diastolic pressure below 50 mm Hg).

iatrogenic A test result or condition caused by medication or treatment.

identity proofing The process by which a credential service provider validates that a person is who he or she claims to be; the provider must complete this verification before being allowed to e-prescribe controlled substances.

idiopathic Pertaining to a condition or a disease that has no known cause.

ileostomy The surgical formation of an opening of the ileum onto the surface of the abdomen, through which fecal material is emptied.

image receptor (IR) A device used to transform an x-ray beam into a visible image; it may include a cassette (with either film or a phosphorescent screen inside) or a special detector that is built into the table or Bucky.

immune globulin A substance made from human plasma that contains antibodies to protect the body from disease.

immunosuppressant A substance that suppresses or prevents an immune system response.

immunotherapy Administration of repeated injections of diluted extracts of a substance that causes an allergy; also called *desensitization*.

impending A term used in the diagnosis of a condition that can be imminently threatening. For example, a patient showing signs of prediabetes may in the near future develop diabetes; therefore, in this case, diabetes is an *impending* condition.

implied contract A contract that lacks a written record or verbal agreement but is assumed to exist. For example, if a patient is being seen in a physician's office for the first time, it is assumed that the patient will provide a comprehensive and accurate health history and that the provider will diagnose and treat the patient in good faith to the best of his or her ability.

in vitro   A term referring to conditions or tests performed outside of a living body.

incentives   Things that incite or spur to action; rewards or reasons for performing a task.

incidental disclosure   A secondary use or disclosure that cannot reasonably be prevented, is limited in nature, and occurs because of another use or disclosure that is permitted.

incompetent   A term describing a person who is not able to manage his or her affairs because of mental deficiency (lack of I.Q., deterioration, illness or psychosis) or sometimes physical disability. The individual cannot comprehend the complexities of a situation and therefore cannot provide informed consent.

indicators   An important point or group of statistical values that, when evaluated, indicates the quality of care provided in a healthcare facility.

indirect filing system   A filing system in which an intermediary source of reference (e.g., a card file) must be consulted to locate specific files.

induration (in-doo-ra'-shuhn)   An abnormally hard, inflamed area.

infarction   An area of tissue that has died from lack of blood supply.

infection   Invasion of body tissues by microorganisms, which then proliferate and damage tissues.

inflammation (in-fluh-ma'-shun)   A tissue reaction to trauma or disease that includes redness, heat, swelling, and pain.

informed consent   Voluntary agreement, usually written, for treatment after being informed of its purpose, methods, procedures, benefits, and risks. The patient must understand the details of the procedure and give his or her consent without duress or undue influence, and the patient must have the right to refuse treatment or voluntarily withdraw from treatment at any time.

intangible   Something of value that cannot be touched physically.

integral (in'-ti-grul)   Essential; being an indispensable part of a whole.

interaction   A two-way communication; mutual or reciprocal action or influence.

intercellular   A term referring to the area between cells.

intercom   A two-way communication system with a microphone and loudspeaker at each station for localized use; often a feature of business telephones.

interferon (in-tuhr-fir'-on)   A protein formed when a cell is exposed to a virus; the protein blocks viral action on the cell and protects against viral invasion

intermittent claudication   Recurring cramping in the calves caused by poor circulation of blood to the muscles of the lower leg.

intermittent pulse   A pulse in which beats occasionally are skipped.

interoperability   The ability to work with other systems.

interpersonal skills   The ability to communicate and interact with others; sometimes referred to as "soft skills."

interval   Space of time between events.

intracellular   A term referring to the area within the cell membrane.

intravenous urogram (IVU)   Radiographic examination of the urinary tract using intravenous injection of an iodine contrast medium; also called an *intravenous pyelogram* (IVP).

inventory   The stored medical and administrative supplies used in the medical office; also, the process of counting the supplies in stock.

invoice   A billing statement that lists the amount owed for goods or services purchased..

ipsilateral (ips-uh-lah'-tehr-uhl)   Pertaining to the same side of the body.

ischemia (is-ke'-me-uh)   Decreased blood flow to a body part or organ, caused by constriction or blockage of the supplying artery.

ischemic (ih-ske'-mik)   Pertaining to a decreased supply of oxygenated blood to a body part.

jargon   The technical terminology or characteristic idioms of a particular group or special activity, as opposed to common, everyday terms.

jaundice   Yellowing of the skin and mucous membranes caused by the deposition of bile pigment, which occurs as a result of excess bilirubin in the blood. Jaundice is not a disease, but rather a sign of a number of diseases, especially liver disorders.

job board   A website that posts jobs submitted by employers and can be used by job seekers to identify open positions.

Kaposi's sarcoma   A malignant tumor of endothelial cells that begins as red, brown, or purple lesions on the ankles or soles.

keloid   A raised, firm scar formation caused by overgrowth of collagen at the site of a skin injury.

keratin   A very hard, tough protein found in the hair, nails, and epidermal tissue.

keratinocytes   The skin cells that synthesize keratin.

ketonuria   Ketones in the urine (possible dehydration or diabetic ketoacidosis).

kilovoltage (kVp)   The electrical control setting that determines the penetrating power of the x-ray beam; the higher the voltage, the shorter the x-ray wavelengths and the greater the energy of the x-ray beam.

kyphotic (ki-fot'-ik)   Relating to the normal convex curvature of the thoracic spine.

lacrimation (lah-krihm-a'-shun)   The secretion or discharge of tears.

laryngoscopy (lar-uhn-gahs'-kuh-pe)   Visual examination of the voice box area through an endoscope equipped with a light and mirrors for illumination.

lateral position   A radiographic position labeled according to which of the patient's sides is facing the image receptor.

law   A binding custom or practice of a community; a rule of conduct or action prescribed or formally recognized as binding or enforceable by a controlling authority.

leads   Electrical connections attached to the body to record the electrical activity of the heart.

learning style   The way an individual perceives and processes information to learn new material.

leukocytosis   An abnormal increase in the number of circulating white blood cells (WBCs); it often occurs with bacterial infections, but not with viral infections.

leukoderma   Lack of skin pigmentation, especially in patches.

liable (li'-uh-buhl)   Obligated according to law or equity; responsible for an act or a circumstance.

liaison   An individual assigned to communicate between multiple parties when settling financial responsibilities of a patient's estate after their death.

libel   A written remark that injures another's reputation or character.

ligaments (lig′-uh-ments) Tough connective tissue bands that hold joints together by attaching to the bones on either side of the joint.

limited radiography A simplified role in radiography, usually in an outpatient setting; also called *practical radiography*. The limited radiographer may be referred to as a *limited operator* or *basic machine operator*.

litigious (lih-tih′-jus) Prone to engage in lawsuits.

loading dose A large dose administered as the first dose of a medication; it usually is used in antibiotic therapy to quickly achieve therapeutic blood levels of the drug.

lordotic (lor-dah′-tik) Relating to the normal concave curvature of the cervical and lumbar spines.

lower gastrointestinal (LGI) series A fluoroscopic examination of the colon; barium sulfate usually is used as a contrast medium and is administered rectally; also called a *barium enema*.

lumbar (lum′-bahr) Relating to the lower back region that contains the five lumbar vertebrae.

lumen An open space, such as within a blood vessel or the intestine, or within a needle or an examining instrument.

luteinizing hormone (LH) (lu-te-uh-niz′-ing) A hormone produced by the anterior pituitary gland that promotes ovulation.

luxation (luhk-sa′-shun) Dislocation of a bone from its normal anatomic location.

lymphedema (limf-uh-de′-muh) Swelling caused by the accumulation of lymph fluid in soft tissues.

lymphadenopathy (lim-fah-deh-nop′-uh-the) Abnormal enlargement of a lymph gland.

lyse To break open cells (e.g., white or red blood cells).

macromolecules The molecules needed for metabolism: carbohydrates, lipids, proteins, and nucleic acids.

macular degeneration A progressive deterioration of the macula of the eye that causes loss of central vision.

magnetic resonance imaging (MRI) An imaging modality that uses a magnetic field and radiofrequency pulses to create computer images of both bones and soft tissues in multiple planes.

magnetism The attraction of materials to magnets; strong magnets can damage magnetic storage devices, such as hard drives.

malaise (muh-layz′) An indefinite feeling of debility or lack of health, often indicating or accompanying the onset of an illness.

malignant A term describing tumor or tissue growth that is cancerous, anaplastic, invasive, and can metastasize.

malpractice A type of negligence in which a licensed professional fails to provide the standard of care, causing harm to a person.

manifestation An indication of the existence, reality, or presence of something, especially an illness; a secondary process.

manipulation Movement or exercise of a body part by means of an externally applied force.

Marfan syndrome An inherited condition characterized by elongation of the bones, joint hypermobility, abnormalities of the eyes, and the development of an aortic aneurysm.

mastication (mas-tih-ka′-shun) Chewing.

matrix Something in which a thing originates, develops, takes shape, or is contained; a base on which to build.

Meaningful Use requirements Requirements established by the Centers for Medicare and Medicaid Services (CMS) as part of the Electronic Health Records (EHRs) Incentives Program. The program provides financial incentives for healthcare organizations that "meaningfully used" their certified EHR technology. The requirements include implementing security measures to ensure the privacy of patients' EHRs.

media A type of communication (e.g., social media sites); with computers, the term refers to data storage devices.

mediastinum (me-de-ast′-uhn-um) The space in the center of the chest under the sternum.

medullary cavity (meh-duhl′-uh-re) The inner portion of the diaphysis; it contains the bone marrow.

Ménière's disease (meyn-yairz′) A chronic disease of the inner ear causing recurrent episodes of vertigo, progressive sensorineural hearing loss, and tinnitus.

meniscus (meh-nis′-kus) The curved surface of liquids in a container.

mentor A steady employee whom a new staff member can approach with questions and concerns.

metabolic alkalosis A condition characterized by significant loss of acid in the body or an increased amount of bicarbonate; severe metabolic alkalosis can lead to coma and death.

metabolite The byproduct of the metabolism of a substance, such as a drug.

metastatic (meh-tas-tah′-tik) Pertaining to the process by which cancerous cells spread from the site of origin to a distant site via lymph and blood circulation.

microcephaly (mi-kroh-seh′-fal-e) Small size of the head in relation to the rest of the body.

microfilm A film with a photographic record of printed or other graphic matter on a reduced scale.

microorganisms Organisms of microscopic or submicroscopic size.

milliamperage (mA) The electrical control setting that determines the amount or concentration of the x-rays by controlling how rapidly the radiation is produced; the higher the mA setting, the more x-rays are produced per second.

miotic (mi-ah′-tik) Any substance or medication that causes constriction of the pupil.

mnemonic A learning device (e.g., an image, a rhyme, or a figure of speech) that a person uses to help him or her remember information.

mock Simulated; intended for imitation or practice.

modem A type of peripheral computer hardware that connects to the router to provide Internet access to the network or computer.

molecule A group of like or different atoms held together by chemical forces.

mononuclear white blood cells Leukocytes with an unsegmented nucleus; monocytes and lymphocytes in particular.

monotone A succession of syllables, words, or sentences spoken in an unvaried key or pitch.

mons pubis The fat pad that covers the symphysis pubis.

multiparous Pertaining to women who have had two or more pregnancies.

multiple-line telephone system A business telephone system that allows for more than one telephone line.

murmur In medical care, an abnormal sound heard during auscultation of the heart that may or may not have a pathologic origin; it is associated with valve disease or a congenital heart defect.

mydriatic (mid-re-at′-ik)   A topical ophthalmic medication that dilates the pupil; it is used in diagnostic procedures of the eye and as treatment for glaucoma.

myelomeningocele   A herniation of a portion of the spinal cord and its meninges that protrudes through a congenital opening in the vertebral column.

myelin sheath   A segmented, fatty tissue that wraps around the axon of the nerve cell and acts as an electrical insulator to speed the conduction of nerve impulses.

myelography (mi-uh-log′-ruh-fe)   Fluoroscopic examination of the spinal canal with spinal injection of an iodine contrast medium.

myocardial (mi-o-kar′-de-uhl)   Pertaining to the heart muscle.

myocardium (mi-o-kar′-de-um)   The muscular lining of the heart.

myoglobinuria   The abnormal presence of a hemoglobin-like chemical of muscle tissue in the urine; it is the result of muscle deterioration.

necrosis (neh-kro′-sis)   The death of cells or tissues.

negligence (neh′-glih-jents)   Failure to show the conduct expected of a reasonably prudent person acting under similar circumstances; it falls below the standards of behavior established by law for the protection of others against unreasonable risk of harm.

neoplasm   A growth of uncontrolled, abnormal tissue; a tumor. The ICD-10-CM assigns diagnostic codes for neoplasms based on six criteria, which can be found in a table that follows the Alphabetic Index.

networking   Exchange of information or services among individuals, groups, or institutions; also, meeting and getting to know individuals in the same or similar career fields and sharing information about available opportunities.

neural tube defects   Congenital malformations of the skull and spinal column caused by failure of the neural tube to close during embryonic development; the neural tube is the origin of the brain, spinal cord, and other central nervous system tissue.

no-show   A patient who fails to keep an appointment without giving advance notice.

nocturia   Frequent urination at night.

nodules (nah′-juhls)   Small lumps, lesions, or swellings that are felt when the skin is palpated.

nonallowed amount   The difference (balance) between the provider's charges and the allowed amount. If the provider is a participating provider, he or she cannot bill the patient for the nonallowed amount. If the provider is not participating in the insurance plan contract, he or she can bill the patient for the nonallowed amount.

nonorganic (nahn-awr-gan′-ik)   A term for a disorder that does not have a cause that can be found in the body.

nonstress tests (NSTs)   Fetal monitoring used in combination with maternal reports of fetal movement to evaluate the fetal heart rate response.

normal flora   Microorganisms normally present on and in our bodies; they perform vital functions and protect the body against infection.

nosocomial infections (nos-uh-ko′-me-uhl)   Infections that are acquired in a healthcare setting.

notations   Instructions or guides for assigning classifications, defining category content, or using subdivision codes. Notations are found in both the Alphabetic Index and the Tabular List.

Notice of Privacy Practices (NPP)   A written document describing the healthcare facilities' privacy practices. The patient must be provided with the NPP and sign an acknowledgment of receipt.

NPO   Nothing by mouth, from the Latin *nil per os.*

nuclear medicine   An imaging modality that uses radioactive materials injected or ingested into the body to provide information about the function of organs and tissues.

numeric filing   The filing of records, correspondence, or cards by number.

obesity   An excessive accumulation of body fat; defined as a body mass index (BMI) of 30 or higher.

objective information   Data obtained through physical examination, laboratory and diagnostic testing, and by measurable information.

oblique position   Radiographic position in which the body or part is rotated at an angle that is neither frontal nor lateral.

obliteration (uh-blih-tuh-ra′-shun)   The act of making undecipherable or imperceptible by obscuring or wearing away.

obturator   A metal rod with a smooth, rounded tip that is placed in hollow instruments to reduce injury to body tissues during insertion of the instrument.

occlude   To close off or block (e.g., a blood vessel).

occlusion   Complete obstruction of an opening.

online provider insurance Web portal   An online service provided by various insurance companies for providers to look up patient insurance benefits, eligibility, claims status, and explanation of benefits.

oophorectomy   Surgical removal of the ovaries.

opaque   Not translucent or transparent; murky.

operating system   Software that acts as the computer's administrator by managing, integrating, and controlling application software and hardware.

opportunistic infections   Infections caused by a normally nonpathogenic organism in a host whose resistance has been decreased.

opportunistic organisms   Microorganisms normally present in low numbers that are capable of causing disease when the conditions are favorable.

optic disc   The region at the back of the eye where the optic nerve meets the retina; it is considered the blind spot of the eye because it contains only nerve fibers and no rods or cones and thus is insensitive to light.

optic nerve   Cranial nerve II, which carries impulses for the sense of sight.

ordinance (or′-di-nens)   An authoritative decree or direction; a law set forth by a governmental authority, specifically municipal regulation.

organelles (or-guh-nels′)   Structures within a cell that perform a specific function.

orthopnea (or-thop′-ne-uh)   A condition in which an individual must sit or stand to breathe comfortably.

orthostatic (postural) hypotension   A temporary fall in blood pressure when a person rapidly changes from a recumbent position to a standing position.

osteoporosis (ah-ste-o-puh-ro′-sis)   Loss of bone density; lack of calcium intake is a major factor in its development.

otitis externa   Inflammation or infection of the external auditory canal; commonly called swimmer's ear.

otosclerosis (o-tuh-skleh-ro'-sis) The formation of spongy bone in the labyrinth of the ear, which often causes the auditory ossicles to become fixed and unable to vibrate when sound enters the ears.

ototoxic (o-tuh-tahk'-sik) A medicine or substance capable of damaging cranial nerve VIII or the organs of hearing and balance.

outguide A sturdy cardboard or plastic file-sized card used to replace a folder temporarily removed from the filing space.

output device Computer hardware that displays the processed data from the computer (e.g., monitors and printers).

over-the-counter (OTC) drugs Medications sold without a prescription.

packing slip A document that accompanies purchased merchandise and shows what is in the box or package.

palliative A substance that relieves or alleviates the symptoms of a disease without curing the disease; also, therapy that relieves or reduces symptoms but does not result in a cure.

palpation The use of touch during the physical examination to assess the size, consistency, and location of certain body parts.

palpitations Pounding or racing of the heart; it may or may not indicate a serious heart disorder.

papilledema Swelling of the optic disc as a result of increased intracranial pressure.

parameters Any set of physical properties, the values of which determine characteristics or behavior.

parenteral (puh-ren'-tuh-ruhl) The injection or introduction of substances into the body by any route other than the digestive tract (e.g., subcutaneous, intravenous, or intramuscular administration).

paresthesia (par-uhs-the'-ze-uh) An abnormal sensation of burning, prickling, or stinging.

paroxysmal (par-ek-siz'-muhl) Pertaining to a sudden recurrence of symptoms; a sudden spasm or convulsion of any kind.

participating provider A physician or other healthcare provider who enters into a contract with a specific insurance company or program and by doing so agrees to abide by certain rules and regulations set forth by that particular third-party payer.

parturition (par-too-rih'-shun) The act or process of giving birth to a child.

patency Open condition of a body cavity or canal.

pathogen An agent that causes disease, especially a living microorganism such as a bacterium or fungus.

pathogenic (path-o-jen'-ik) Pertaining to a disease-causing microorganism.

patient portal A secure online website that gives patients 24-hour access to personal health information using a username and password.

pegboard system A manual bookkeeping system that uses a day sheet to record all financial transactions for the date of service and maintains patient account balances by using physical cards.

perceiving (pur-seev'-ing) How an individual looks at information and sees it as real.

perception A quick, acute, and intuitive cognition; a capacity for comprehension.

perinatal (per-uh-nayt'-l) The period between the 28th week of pregnancy and the 28th day after birth.

periosteum (per-e-os'-te-um) The thin, highly innervated, membranous covering of a bone.

peripheral (puh-rif'-er-uhl) A term that refers to an area outside of or away from an organ or structure.

peripheral neuropathy A problem with the function of the nerves outside the spinal cord; symptoms include weakness, burning pain, and loss of reflexes; a frequent complication of diabetes mellitus.

peristalsis (per-uh-stahl'-sis) The rhythmic, involuntary serial contraction of the smooth muscles lining the gastrointestinal tract.

perjured testimony The voluntary violation of an oath or vow, either by swearing to what is untrue or by omission to do what has been promised under oath; false testimony.

permeable (pur'-me-uh-buhl) Allowing a substance to pass or soak through.

personal health record (PHR) An electronic record of health-related information about an individual that conforms to nationally recognized interoperability standards and that can be drawn from multiple sources but that is managed, shared, and controlled by the individual.

petechiae (peh-te'-ke-uh) Small, purplish hemorrhagic spots on the skin.

phenylalanine (fe-nehl-ah'-luh-neen) An essential amino acid found in milk, eggs, and other foods. Children unable to metabolize this amino acid eliminate it in the urine.

phlebotomy The practice of drawing blood from a vein.

phonetic (fuh-neh'-tik) Constituting an alteration of ordinary spelling that better represents the spoken language, uses only characters of the regular alphabet, and is used in a context of conventional spelling.

photophobia An abnormal sensitivity to light.

pitch The depth of a tone or sound; a distinctive quality of sound.

plaintiff The person or group bringing a case or legal action to court.

plaque In medical care, an abnormal accumulation of a fatty substance.

plasma The liquid portion of a centrifuged whole blood specimen that has not clotted and still contains active clotting agents.

pleurisy Inflammation of the parietal pleura of the lungs; it causes dyspnea and stabbing chest pain, which result in restriction of breathing because of the pain.

point of care Something designed to be used at or near where the patient is seen; point-of-care tools and apps are resources for the provider to use when working directly with the patient.

polycythemia vera (pah-le-si-the'-me-uh/veh'-rah) A condition marked by an abnormally large number of red blood cells (RBCs) in the circulatory system.

polydipsia Excessive thirst.

polymorphonuclear (PMN) white blood cells Leukocytes with a segmented nucleus; also known as segmented neutrophils, which appear in the urine during a bacterial infection.

polyphagia (pah-le-faj'-e-uh) Increased appetite.

polyps (pah'-lips) Outgrowths of tissue found in the mucosal lining of the colon. Polyps are considered precancerous.

polyuria (pah-le-yur'-e-uh) Excretion of abnormally large amounts of urine in 24 hours.

portal circulation The pathway of blood flow through the portal vein from the GI system to the liver.

portal hypertension   Increased venous pressure in the portal circulation caused by cirrhosis or compression of the hepatic vascular system.

portrait orientation   The most common layout for a printed page; the height of the paper is greater than its width.

posterior   The back portion of the body or body part.

posteroanterior (PA) projection   A radiographic view in which the central ray enters the back and exits the front of the patient's body; the patient is prone or facing the image receptor.

postherpetic neuralgia   Pain that lasts longer than a month after a shingles infection and is caused by damage to the nerve; the pain may last for months or years.

power of attorney   A legal statement in which a person authorizes another person to act as his or her attorney or agent. The authority may be limited to the handling of specific procedures. The person authorized to act as the agent is known as the *attorney in fact.*

practice management software   A type of software that allows the user to enter demographic information, schedule appointments, maintain lists of insurance payers, perform billing tasks, and generate reports.

preauthorization   A process required by some insurance carriers in which the provider obtains permission to perform certain procedures or services or refers a patient to a specialist.

precedent (preh′-suh-dent)   A person or thing that serves as a model; something done or said that may serve as an example or rule to authorize or justify a subsequent act of the same kind.

precertification   A process required by some insurance carriers in which the provider must prove medical necessity before performing a procedure.

prerequisite (pre-reh′-kwih-zit)   Something that is necessary to an end or to carry out a function.

present illness   The chief complaint, written in chronologic sequence, with dates of onset.

preservatives   Substances added to a specimen to prevent deterioration of cells or chemicals.

pressboard   A strong, highly glazed composition board resembling vulcanized fiber; heavy card stock.

principal   A capital sum of money due as a debt or used as a fund for which interest is either charged or paid.

privacy filters   Devices attached to the monitor that allow visualization of the screen contents only if the user is directly in front of the screen; also called *monitor filters* or *privacy screens.*

privately sponsored health insurance   Health insurance companies that operate for-profit and use managed care plans to reduce the costs of healthcare.

processing (pro′-ses-ing)   How an individual internalizes new information and makes it his or her own.

procurement (pro-kuhr′-ment)   The act of getting possession of, obtaining, or acquiring; in medicine, this term relates to obtaining organs for transplant.

proficiency (pruh-fi′-shun-se)   Competency as a result of training or practice.

profile testing   A series of laboratory tests associated with a particular organ or disease; also referred to as a "panel" of tests.

progress notes   Notes used in the medical record to track the patient's progress and condition.

prokaryote (pro-kar′-e-oht)   A unicellular organism that lacks a membrane-bound nucleus.

prolactin (PRL)   A hormone secreted by the anterior pituitary gland that stimulates the development of the mammary gland; it also stimulates the production of breast milk.

proofread   To read and mark corrections.

proprioception   The sensation of awareness of body movements and posture; nerve impulses that provide the central nervous system with information about the position of body parts.

prosthesis (prahs-the′-sis)   An artificial replacement for a body part.

proteinuria   Protein in the urine (may indicate kidney destruction, especially if casts are present).

provider   An individual or company that provides medical care and services to a patient or the public.

provider's fee schedule   Fees established by the provider for services rendered.

provisional diagnosis   A temporary diagnosis made before all test results have been received.

prudent   Marked by wisdom or judiciousness; shrewd in the management of practical affairs.

psoriasis (suh-ri′-uh-sis)   A usually chronic, recurrent skin disease marked by bright red patches covered with silvery scales.

psychosocial   Pertaining to a combination of psychological and social factors.

psyllium (sih′-le-um)   A grain found in some cereal products, in certain dietary supplements, and in certain bulk fiber laxatives; a water-soluble fiber.

public domain   A classification of information that indicates the information is open for public review; information or technology that is not protected by a patent or copyright and is available to the public for use without charge.

pulmonary consolidation   In pneumonia, the process by which the lungs become solidified as they fill with exudates.

pulse deficit   A condition in which the radial pulse is less than the apical pulse; it may indicate a peripheral vascular abnormality.

pulse pressure   The difference between the systolic and diastolic blood pressures (30 to 50 mm Hg is considered normal).

purchase order number   Unique number assigned by the ordering facility that allows the facility to track or reference the order. Many vendors will add this number to the order documents (e.g., packing slip and statement).

pure culture   A bacterial or fungal culture that contains a single organism.

purging   The process of moving active files to inactive status.

pyemia (pi-em′-e-uh)   The presence of pus-forming organisms in the blood.

pyloric sphincter   A muscular ring at the distal end of the stomach that separates the stomach from the duodenum of the small intestine.

pyrexia (pi-rek′-se-uh)   A febrile condition or fever.

qualified Medicare beneficiaries (QMB)   Low-income Medicare patients who qualify for Medicaid for their secondary insurance.

qualitative   A laboratory test result expressed as positive or negative.

quality assurance   The process of monitoring all the processes involved before, during, and after a laboratory test is performed so as to ensure reliable patient test results.

quality control An aggregate of activities designed to ensure adequate quality, especially in manufactured products or in the service industries; also, manufactured samples with known values used to determine whether a test method is reliable (i.e., consistently produces accurate and precise results).

quantitative A laboratory test result expressed in numeric units of measure.

quantity to reorder The amount of supplies that need to be ordered.

radiograph An x-ray image taken by a radiographer in the process of radiography.

radiographer One who takes x-rays.

radiography The process of creating an x-ray image to examine internal structures of the body.

radiographic position The placement of a body part as seen by the image receptor.

radiographic projection The path of the central ray from the radiographic tube, through the patient, and to the image receptor. The view as seen by the x-ray tube.

radiologist A physician who specializes in medical imaging or therapeutic applications of radiation.

radiopaque A substance that can easily be visualized on an x-ray film.

rales Abnormal or crackling breath sounds during inspiration.

ramifications (ram-ih-fih-ka'-shuns) Consequences produced by a cause or following from a set of conditions.

range of motion (ROM) The extent of movement possible in a joint; the degree of motion depends on the type of joint and whether a disease process is present; ROM exercises are applied actively (independently) or passively (with assistance) to prevent or treat joint problems.

rapport (rah-por') A relationship of harmony and accord between the patient and the healthcare professional.

reagent (re-a'-gent) A chemical substance used in a test that reacts with the specimen to produce a measurable result.

reagent strips Strips used to test the specific gravity, pH, and chemical analytes in urine.

reasonable cause Circumstances that would make it unreasonable for the covered entity, despite the exercise of ordinary business care and prudence, to comply with the administrative simplification provision (part of Health Information Technology for Economic and Clinical Health Act [HITECH]) that was violated.

reasonable diligence The business care and prudence expected from a person seeking to satisfy a legal requirement under similar circumstances.

recessive Refers to a gene that only produces a particular condition if both the mother and the father carry that particular gene; neither of the parents have the condition.

recheck appointment An appointment type used when a patient needs to see the provider after a condition should have been resolved or to monitor an ongoing condition, such as hypertension. Also known as a *follow-up appointment.*

recourse Turning to something or someone for help or protection.

rectify (rek'-tih-fi) To correct by removing errors.

reduction Return to correct anatomic position, as in reduction of a fracture.

reference range The numeric range of test values for which the general population consistently shows similar results 95% of the time.

referral laboratory A private or hospital-based laboratory that performs a wide variety of tests, many of them specialized; providers often send specimens collected in the office to referral laboratories for testing.

reflection (re-flek'-shun) The process of thinking about new information so as to create new ways of learning. Also, a therapeutic communication technique in which a person responds with a feeling term that indicates how the individual feels about a problem. For example, "You sound angry about being scheduled for this diagnostic test."

registered dietitian (RD) An individual with a minimum of a bachelor's degree in food and nutrition who is concerned with the maintenance and promotion of health and the treatment of diseases through diet; to become an RD, the individual must pass a national examination.

reimbursement The process by which the medical office submits a claim to the insurance company, which then pays the provider for services rendered. All insurance claims must submit diagnoses and procedures as codes, not as descriptions.

relapse The recurrence of the symptoms of a disease after apparent recovery.

release of information A form completed by the patient that authorizes the medical office to release medical records to the insurance company for health insurance reimbursement.

relevant Having significant and demonstrable bearing on the matter at hand.

remission The partial or complete disappearance of the clinical and subjective characteristics of a chronic or malignant disease.

renal threshold The level above which substances cannot be reabsorbed into the blood from the renal tubules and therefore are excreted in the urine (e.g., when glucose reaches its renal threshold, the excess glucose appears in the urine).

renin An enzyme produced and stored in the glomerulus; it is released by a homeostatic response to raise the blood pressure when needed.

reparations (reh-puh-ra'-shuns) Acts of atonement for a wrong or injury.

requisites (reh'-kwih-zitz) Entities considered essential or necessary.

restock Process of replacing the supplies that were used.

retention A term referring to actions taken by management to keep good employees.

retention schedule A method or plan for retaining or keeping health records and for their movement from active to inactive to closed filing.

reverse chronologic order Arranged in order so that the most recent item is on top and older items are filed further back.

rhinitis (rin-i'-tis) Inflammation of the mucous membranes of the nose.

rhinorrhea (ri-no-re'-uh) The discharge of nasal drainage.

rhonchi (ron'-ki) Abnormal sounds heard on auscultation of an airway obstructed by thick secretions; a continuous rumbling sound that is more pronounced on expiration.

rods   Structures in the retina of the eye that form the light-sensitive elements.

Safety Data Sheets (SDSs)   Documents that accompany hazardous chemicals and substances and outline the dangers, composition, safe handling, and disposal of these items. Safety Data Sheets must be formatted to conform to the Globally Harmonized System (GHS), which mandates that SDSs have 16 standardized sections arranged in a strict order.

sanitized   The state of having cleaned equipment and instruments with detergent and water, removing debris, and reducing the number of microorganisms.

sarcoma   A malignant tumor in fibrous, fatty, muscular, synovial, vascular, or neural tissue.

satiety   The state of being satisfied or of feeling full after eating.

sclera   The white part of the eye that forms the orbit.

scleroderma (skleh-rah-der′-muh)   An autoimmune disorder that affects the blood vessels and connective tissue, causing fibrous degeneration of the major organs.

sclerotherapy (skleh-rah-ther′-ah-pe)   The treatment of hemorrhoids, varicose veins, or esophageal varices by means of injection of sclerosing solutions.

scoliosis   An abnormal lateral curvature of the spine.

scored   Referring to a tablet manufactured with an indentation for division through the center.

screening   In medical care, the process of determining the severity of illness that patients experience and prioritizing appointments based on that severity.

seborrhea (seb-uh-re′-uh)   An excessive discharge of sebum from the sebaceous glands, forming greasy scales or cheesy plugs on the body.

secondary hypertension   Elevated blood pressure resulting from another condition, typically kidney disease.

secondary storage devices   Media (e.g., jump drive, hard drive) capable of permanently storing data until it is replaced or deleted by the user.

security risk analysis   Identification of potential threats of computer network breaches, for which action plans are devised.

sediment   Insoluble material that settles to the bottom of a urine specimen and to the bottom of centrifuged urine.

sequentially (sih-kwen′-shuh-le)   Of, relating to, or arranged in a sequence.

serous (seer′-uhs)   A thin, watery, serumlike drainage.

serum   The liquid portion that remains after the blood clot has been removed from a clotted specimen

sievert (Sv) (se′-vuhrt)   The international unit of radiation dose equivalent.

signs   Objective findings determined by a clinician, such as a fever, hypertension, or rash.

sinoatrial (SA) node   The pacemaker of the heart, located in the right atrium.

sinus arrhythmia   An irregular heartbeat that originates in the sinoatrial node (pacemaker).

site map   A list of all Web page links on a website.

skill set   A person's abilities or skills.

slander   An oral defamation or insult; a harmful, false statement made about another person.

small claims court   A last resort option to collect payment from an outstanding patient account in which the healthcare practice can sue the patient for the balance.

social media   Internet-sponsored two-way communication between individuals, individuals and businesses, or businesses to businesses.

sociologic   Oriented or directed toward social needs and problems.

software   A set of electronic instructions to operate and perform different computer tasks.

sonography   A noninvasive procedure used extensively for fetal imaging (often referred to as diagnostic ultrasound); uses high-frequency sound waves to produce echoes in the body, which are used to create images.

source-to-image distance (SID)   The distance between the x-ray tube and the film or other image receptor; the greater the distance, the more widely the x-ray beam is spread and the lower the intensity of the beam.

speakerphone   A telephone with a loudspeaker and a microphone; it can be used without having to pick up and hold the handset.

species   A category of microorganisms below genus in rank; a genetically distinct group. It is the second name given to the microorganism and it is written in all lower case italic letters.

specific gravity   The density of urine compared with an equal volume of water.

specimen   A sample of body fluid, waste product, or tissue collected for analysis.

speed dialing   A telephone function in which a selected stored number can be dialed by pressing only one key.

spermicide (spuhr′-muh-side)   A chemical substance that kills sperm cells.

spirometer   An instrument that measures the volume of air inhaled and exhaled.

spore   A thick-walled, dormant form of bacteria that is very resistant to disinfection measures.

STAT   The medical abbreviation for the Latin term *statum,* meaning immediately; at this moment.

statins   A class of drugs that lowers the level of cholesterol in the blood by reducing the production of cholesterol by the liver; statins block the enzyme in the liver that is responsible for making cholesterol.

stereotactic   Pertaining to an x-ray procedure used to guide the insertion of a needle into a specific area of the breast.

stereotype   Something conforming to a fixed or general pattern; a standardized mental picture that is held in common by many and represents an oversimplified opinion, prejudiced attitude, or uncritical judgment.

sterile (ster′-il)   Free of all microorganisms, pathogenic and nonpathogenic.

sterilization   Complete destruction of all forms of microbial life.

sterilized   The state in which all microorganisms have been removed.

stertorous (stur′-tuh-rus)   A term that describes a strenuous respiratory effort marked by a snoring sound.

stressor   An event, activity, condition, or other stimulus that causes stress.

striated   A muscle that contains fibers divided by bands of cross stripes or striations because of overlapping myofilaments.

stridor (strahy′-dor)   A shrill, harsh respiratory sound heard during inhalation when a laryngeal obstruction is present.

stylus A metal probe that is inserted into or passed through a catheter, needle, or tube used for clearing purposes or to facilitate passage into a body orifice. Also, a pen-shaped device with a variety of tips that is used on touch screens to write, draw, or input commands.

subjective information Data or information elicited from the patient, including the patient's feelings, perceptions, and concerns; obtained through interview or questions.

subluxations (suh-bluk-sa′-shuns) Slight misalignments of the vertebrae or a partial dislocation.

subordinate Submissive to or controlled by authority; placed in or occupying a lower class, rank, or position.

subpoena duces tecum A subpoena for the production of records or documents that pertain to a case as evidence.

supernatant The liquid above the sediment in a centrifuged urine specimen.

suppurative (sup′-yuh-ra-tiv) Characterized by the formation and/ or discharge of pus.

symptoms Subjective complaints reported by the patient, such as pain or visual disturbances.

syncope (sing′-kuh-pe) Fainting; a brief lapse in consciousness.

synovial fluid A clear fluid found in joint cavities that facilitates smooth movements and nourishes joint structures.

systole The period of contraction of the heart.

tachycardia (tak-ih-kahr′-de-uh) A rapid but regular heart rate; one that exceeds 100 beats per minute.

tachypnea (tak-ip-ne′-uh) A condition marked by rapid, shallow respirations.

tactful The quality of having a keen sense of what to do or say to maintain good relations with others or to prevent offense.

telemedicine Healthcare delivered through video conferencing technologies to deliver quality care at a distance.

tendons Tough bands of connective tissue that connect muscle to bone.

teratogen (teh-rah′-tuh-jen) Any substance that interferes with normal prenatal development, resulting in a developmental abnormality.

termination letter A document sent to a patient explaining that the provider is ending the physician-patient relationship and the patient needs to find another provider.

therapeutic range The blood concentration of a drug that produces the desired effect without toxicity.

third-party administrator (TPA) The intermediary and administrator who coordinates patients and providers, as well as processes claims, for self-funded plans.

thixotropic gel A material that appears to be a solid until subjected to a disturbance, such as centrifugation, at which point it becomes a liquid gel that separates blood cells from their serum or plasma.

thready A term describing a pulse that is scarcely perceptible.

thrombolytics Agents that dissolve blood clots.

thrombus A blood clot.

thyroid-stimulating hormone (TSH) A hormone secreted by the anterior pituitary gland that stimulates the secretion of hormones produced by the thyroid gland.

tickler file A chronologic file used as a reminder that something must be dealt with on a certain date.

tinea (tin′-e-uh) Any fungal skin disease that results in scaling, itching, and inflammation.

tinnitus A noise sensation of ringing heard in one or both ears.

tissue culture The technique or process of keeping tissue alive and growing in a culture medium.

tonometer (toh-nom′-ih-ter) An instrument used to measure intraocular pressure.

tracers Special radioactive materials that are swallowed or injected intravenously, to track the activity of cells and determine the location of fractures.

tracheostomy (tra-ke-os′-tuh-me) A surgical opening made through the neck into the trachea to allow breathing.

transcription A written copy of something made either in longhand or by machine.

trans fats Substances that form from hydrogenation of an unsaturated fatty acid; they make a dietary fat more saturated and solid at room temperature.

transection Cross section; a division made by cutting across.

transient ischemic attack (TIA) Temporary neurologic symptoms caused by gradual or partial occlusion of a cerebral blood vessel.

transillumination Inspection of a cavity or organ by passing light through its walls.

transport medium A medium used to keep an organism alive during transport to the laboratory.

transvaginal ultrasound A procedure for examining the vagina, uterus, fallopian tubes, and bladder. An ultrasound transducer (probe) is inserted into the vagina to bounce high-energy sound waves (ultrasound) off internal tissues or organs, resulting in echoes that form a picture (sonogram). The practitioner can identify tumors by looking at the sonogram.

trauma A physical injury or wound caused by external force or violence.

triage The process of sorting patients to determine medical need and the priority of care.

triglyceride (tri-glih′-suh-ride) A fatty acid and glycerol compound that combines with a protein molecule to form high-density or low-density lipoprotein.

trustee The coordinator of financial resources assigned by the court during a bankruptcy case.

tubercle (too′-buhr-kuhl) A nodule produced by the tuberculosis bacillus.

turgor A term referring to normal skin tension; the resistance of the skin to being grasped between the fingers and released. Turgor is decreased with dehydration and increased with edema.

type and cross-match Tests performed to assess the compatibility of blood to be transfused.

unit dose Method used by the pharmacy to prepare individual doses of medication.

unsecured debt Debt that is not guaranteed by something of value; credit card debt is the most common type of unsecured debt.

upcoding A fraudulent practice in which provider services are billed for higher procedural codes than were actually performed, resulting in a higher payment.

upper gastrointestinal (UGI) series Fluoroscopic examination of the esophagus, stomach, and duodenum; barium sulfate is used as a contrast medium and is administered orally.

urea   The major nitrogenous end product of protein metabolism and the chief nitrogenous component of the urine.

urgency   A sudden, compelling desire to urinate and the inability to control the release of urine.

urgent   An acute situation that requires immediate attention but is not life-threatening.

urochrome   The yellow pigment normally found in urine; it is described as straw, yellow, or amber based on its concentration.

urticaria (uhr-tuh-kar′-e-uh)   A skin eruption that creates inflamed wheals; hives.

USB port   The most common type of connector device that allows hardware to be plugged into the computer.

utilization management   A process of managing healthcare costs by influencing patient care decision making through case-by-case assessments of the appropriateness of care.

Valsalva maneuver   The act of attempting to exhale forcibly while keeping the nose and mouth closed, such as occurs when a person strains to defecate or urinate. This causes trapping of blood in the great veins, preventing the blood from entering the chest and right atrium.

vasoconstriction (va-zo-kun-strik′-shun)   Contraction of the muscles lining blood vessels, which narrows the lumen.

vasodilation   An increase in the diameter of a blood vessel.

vectors   Animals or insects (e.g., ticks) that transmit the causative organisms of disease.

vegetations   Abnormal growth of tissue surrounding a valve consisting of fibrin, platelets, and bacteria.

vendor   A company that sells supplies, equipment, or services to another company or individual.

ventricles   The two lower chambers of the heart.

veracity (vuh-rah′-suh-te)   A devotion to or conformity with the truth.

verdict   The finding or decision of a jury on a matter submitted to it in trial.

vertigo   Dizziness; a sensation of spinning or an inability to maintain normal balance.

vested   Granted or endowed with a particular authority, right, or property; to have a special interest in.

viable   Capable of living, developing, or germinating under favorable conditions.

virulent (vir′-yoo-lent)   Exceedingly pathogenic, noxious, or deadly.

viscosity (vis-kos′-ih-te)   The degree of thickness; a substance that is viscous is thick and lacks the capability of easy movement.

vocation   The work in which a person is regularly employed.

voice mail   An electronic system that allows messages from telephone callers to be recorded and stored.

vulva   The external female genitalia, which begins at the mons pubis and terminates at the anus.

waiting period   The amount of time a patient waits for disability insurance to pay cash payments after the date of injury.

wasting syndrome   Physical deterioration resulting in profound weight loss, fatigue, anorexia, and mental confusion.

wet mount   A slide preparation in which a drop of liquid specimen or the like is covered with a coverslip and observed with a microscope.

wheal (weel)   A localized area of edema or a raised lesion.

wheezing   A high-pitched sound heard on expiration; it indicates obstruction or narrowing of respiratory passages.

white noise   The sounds from a television or stereo that muffle or mute the conversation of others, thus helping to protect the confidentiality of patients.

willful neglect   Conscious, intentional failure or reckless indifference to the obligation to comply with the administrative simplification provision violated.

Zip   Software that compresses a file or folder, making it smaller.

zone   A region or geographic area used for shipping.

INDEX

Page numbers followed by "*f*" indicate figures, "*b*" indicate boxes, and "*t*" indicate tables.

505